Veterinary Disaster Response

Veterinary Disaster Response

Wayne E. Wingfield, MS, DVM
Sally B. Palmer, DVM

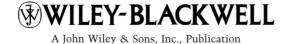

A John Wiley & Sons, Inc., Publication

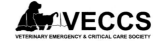

Edition first published 2009
© 2009 Wiley-Blackwell

Blackwell Publishing was acquired by John Wiley & Sons in February 2007. Blackwell's publishing program has been merged with Wiley's global Scientific, Technical, and Medical business to form Wiley-Blackwell.

Editorial Office
2121 State Avenue, Ames, Iowa 50014-8300, USA

For details of our global editorial offices, for customer services, and for information about how to apply for permission to reuse the copyright material in this book, please see our website at www.wiley.com/wiley-blackwell.

Library of Congress Cataloging-in-Publication Data

Veterinary disaster response / [edited by] Wayne E. Wingfield, Sally B. Palmer.
    p. ; cm.
  Includes bibliographical references and index.
  ISBN 978-0-8138-1014-0 (pbk. : alk. paper)
  1. Veterinary emergencies–Management. 2. Veterinary critical care–Management. I. Wingfield, Wayne E. II. Palmer, Sally B., DVM. III. Veterinary Emergency & Critical Care Society.
  [DNLM: 1. Emergencies–veterinary–Outlines. 2. Disaster Planning–organization & administration–Outlines. SF 778 V5867 2009]
  SF778V49 2009
  636.089'6025–dc22

2008040235

A catalog record for this book is available from the U.S. Library of Congress.

Set in 10 on 11.5 pt Sabon by SNP Best-set Typesetter Ltd., Hong Kong
Printed in Singapore by Markono Print Media Pte Ltd

1 2009

DEDICATION

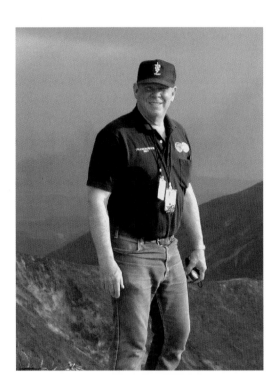

John H. Anderson, DVM, PhD
(1944–2006)

Dr. John H. Anderson will forever be remembered as the "Father of Veterinary Disaster Response" by fellow first responders. John was deployed to respond to our nation's disasters more often than any other veterinarian. He was deployed to North Carolina following Hurricanes Dennis and Floyd, the Houston floods, the World Trade Center after 9/11, the Democratic National Convention in Los Angeles, in support of Secret Service dogs at the United Nations on two occasions, the Alaska Airlines crash off the California coast, two presidential addresses to the nation, and Hurricane Rita, just to mention a few occasions!

John was internationally recognized for his training and support of K-9 police units and search and rescue teams. He taught many first-aid courses for police K-9 handlers all over the country. He was also well known for his overwhelming compassion and willingness to serve those in need, both animal and human, frequently taking long leaves of absence from his practice to volunteer his service and professional skills wherever needed.

As Commander of Veterinary Medical Response Team—4, John led a dedicated group of veterinarians, veterinary technicians, and teammates with a variety of professional occupations. He was adamant that our team be exceptionally well trained. This training covered topics from water and food safety to epidemiology, disaster medicine, wilderness survival, safety in animal handling, communication protocols, and other vitally important topics for responding to disasters. During one of the training weekends, the Simi Valley fires were in progress and suddenly and unexpectedly shifted directions, sending the fires toward John's ranch, where the team was training.

In fewer than 90 minutes, John had the team organized to pack up all the gear and tents for evacuation to Simi Valley. We all vividly recall hearing two visiting officers from the U.S. Army expressing amazement at the way the team worked together with speed and efficiency to accomplish the exodus from the ranch. The morning after we returned to the ranch to find only charred trees and pastures, burned fence posts, and catastrophic losses to the ranch infrastructure where we had been training. Our only losses were a shovel and a livestock chute that had its tires burned off.

John served in the U.S. military. He was wounded twice in Vietnam and received two Purple Hearts, the Bronze Star, and the Silver Star. He also served in the Chemical Corps in the U.S. Army. His association with the army provided him the knowledge and ability to organize numerous trainings of his VMAT with the U.S. Army Veterinary Corps at Camp Pendleton, Fort Lewis, and Simi Valley.

John shared his leadership skills through the Veterinary Emergency and Critical Care Society, serving as recorder, as an at-large executive board member, and as chair of the Veterinary Disaster Preparedness Committee; and he organized several disaster medicine sessions at International Veterinary Emergency and Critical Care Society meetings. John was also president of the American Academy on Veterinary Disaster Medicine.

Dr. John Anderson was a cowboy, owning a ranch near Simi Valley, CA, where he and his son, Logan, bred Texas longhorn cattle and draft horses. John loved to rope and taught his son to rope and ride and start a campfire. John loved to play the harmonica and Jew's harp to entertain his many friends.

John is survived by his wife Karen, daughters Mikaely and Tevyn, and son Logan. The veterinary profession and disaster medicine response were John's other loves. We all miss his leadership, wit, discipline, and teaching skills. Thanks to John, veterinary disaster response is a recognized, necessary, respected, and growing avocation.

To John H. Anderson, DVM, PhD, we the editors of *Veterinary Disaster Response* dedicate this book, our memories, our experiences, and teaching skills. Thank you, John, for lighting the way, blazing the path, and opening the doors.

Wayne E. Wingfield, MS, DVM
Sally B. Palmer, DVM

CONTENTS

CONTRIBUTORS

Eugene A. Adkins, DVM
Small Animal Veterinarian (Retired)
National Veterinary Response Team—4
  Veterinary Medical Officer
  Squad Leader
  National Disaster Medical System
  Department of Health and Human Services

Dennis Michael Baker, MA, LPC
Specialty Certifications: LPC, State of Colorado Full
  Operational Level Evaluator; State of Colorado Full
  Operation Level Sex Offender Evaluator
Staff Clinician, Clinical Coordinator for Sex Offender
  Services, Clinical Supervisor Jail Aftercare Mental
  Health Program
National Medical Response Team—Central USA
  Mental Health Specialist
  National Disaster Medical System
  Department of Health and Human Services
American Red Cross
  Mental Health Team Leader
  Pike Peaks Region Disaster Mental Health Response
  Team

Joan C. Casey
Specialty Certification: Utah Peace Officer
  Certification (expired)
Program Officer, The Animal Assistance Foundation
Colorado State Animal Response Team
  Steering Committee Member

Kevin M. Dennison, DVM
Colorado Veterinary Medical Foundation (CVMF)
  Director of CVMF Animal Emergency Management
  Programs including the Colorado State Animal
  Response Team and the Colorado Veterinary
  Medical Reserve Corps
National Alliance of State Animal and Agricultural
  Emergency Programs, Board of Directors

P. J. (Paula) Havice-Cover, MA, LPC, CAC III
Specialty Certifications: Disaster Mental Health,
  Licensed Professional Counselor, and Certified
  Addictions Counselor—Supervisor

Emergency Management/Disaster Mental Health
  Operations, Planning and Logistics for the State of
  Colorado
  Colorado Department of Human Services, Division
    of Mental Health, Emergency Preparedness and
    Response Department
Mental Health/Public Information Officer
  National Medical Response Team—Central USA
  National Disaster Medical System
  Department of Health and Human Services

Anthony P. Knight, BVSc, MS
Specialty Certification: Diplomate, American College
  of Veterinary Internal Medicine
Professor, Large Animal Medicine
  Animal Population Health Institute, Department of
    Clinical Sciences, College of Veterinary Medicine
    and Biomedical Sciences, Colorado State
    University
Colorado Veterinary Medical Reserve Corps

Lorna L. Lanman, DVM
Owner, Hospital Director, PETSVET Animal Hospital,
  LLC
National Veterinary Response Team—4
  Acting Team Commander
  Veterinary Medical Officer
  National Disaster Medical System
  Department of Health and Human Services

Rebecca S. McConnico, DVM, PhD
Specialty Certification: Diplomate, American College
  of Veterinary Internal Medicine
Associate Professor
  Equine Health Studies Program, School of
    Veterinary Medicine, Louisiana State University,
    Baton Rouge, LA

Paul S. Morley, DVM, PhD
Specialty Certification: Diplomate, American College
  of Veterinary Internal Medicine
Professor
  Animal Population Health Institute, Department of
    Clinical Sciences, College of Veterinary Medicine
    and Biomedical Sciences, Colorado State
    University

Director of Biosecurity, James L. Voss Veterinary Teaching Hospital, College of Veterinary Medicine and Biomedical Sciences, Colorado State University

Lisa A. Murphy, VMD
Specialty Certification: Diplomate, American Board of Toxicology
Assistant Professor of Toxicology
    Department of Pathobiology, University of Pennsylvania School of Veterinary Medicine,
National Veterinary Response Team—2
    Veterinary Medical Officer
    National Disaster Medical System
    Department of Health and Human Services

Ryan Gordon Leon Murphy, MS, PhD Candidate
Center for Meat Safety and Quality, Department of Animal Sciences, College of Agricultural Sciences, Colorado State University

Sherrie L. Nash, MS, DVM
Owner/Veterinarian, Animal Care Clinic, Harlowton, MT
Montana Trichinosis Field Veterinarian
National Veterinary Response Team—4
    Veterinary Medical Officer
    National Disaster Medical System
    Department of Health and Human Services

Terry K. Paik, DVM
Veterinarian, El Cajon, CA
National Veterinary Response Team—4
    Administrative Officer
    Veterinary Medical Officer
    National Disaster Medical System
    Department of Health and Human Services

Sally B. Palmer, DVM
Veterinarian/Owner, Palmer's Animal Wellness Services, PLLC
National Medical Response Team—Central USA
    Veterinary Medical Officer
    National Disaster Medical System
    Department of Health and Human Services

Thomas F. Pedigo, MSc, PA-C
Specialty Certifications: Advanced Radiation Life Support; Wilderness Advanced Life Support; Mass Fatalities Decontamination and Management; National Registry Paramedic
Physician Assistant, OccMed Colorado, LLC
National Medical Response Team—Central USA
    Physician Assistant and Non-Ambulatory Decontamination Unit Leader

National Disaster Medical System
Department of Health and Human Services

Renée A. Poirrier, DVM
Veterinarian, Acadiana Veterinary Clinic
Louisiana State Animal Response Team
    Director

Marc R. Raffe, DVM, MS
Specialty Certifications: Diplomate, American College of Veterinary Anesthesiologists
Diplomate, American College of Veterinary Emergency and Critical Care
Adjunct Professor
    Department of Clinical Sciences, College of Veterinary Medicine and Biomedical Sciences, Colorado State University
    Department of Veterinary Clinical Medicine, College of Veterinary Medicine, University of Illinois
Manager, Veterinary Specialty Team, Pfizer Animal Health

William R. Ray, BS
Regional Epidemiologist Consultant, Colorado Department of Health and Environment, Pueblo, CO
National Medical Response Team—Central USA
    National Disaster Medical System
    Department of Health and Human Services

Gregory A. Rich, DVM
Veterinarian/Owner, West Esplanade Veterinary Clinic, Metairie, LA

Bernard E. Rollin, PhD
University Distinguished Professor of Philosophy, Biomedical Sciences, and Animal Sciences, Colorado State University

Gary L. Stamp, DVM, MS
Specialty Certifications: Diplomate, American College of Veterinary Practitioners
Diplomate, American College of Veterinary Emergency and Critical Care
Executive Director, Veterinary Emergency and Critical Care Society
Small Animal Disaster Response Coordinator, Hurricane Andrew

Lori A. Swenson, BSME, EMT-P
Specialty Certifications: Animal Control Officer
    Aurora Animal Care
Technical Animal Rescuer
    Colorado State Animal Response Team

Jerry J. Upp, DVM
Veterinarian/Owner, Midtown Animal Hospital PC,
  Gering, NE
National Veterinary Response Team—4
  Deputy Commander
  Squad Leader
  National Disaster Medical System
  Department of Health and Human Services

David C. Van Metre, DVM
Specialty Certification: Diplomate, American College
  of Veterinary Internal Medicine
Associate Professor
  Animal Population Health Institute, Department
    of Clinical Sciences, College of Veterinary
    Medicine and Biomedical Sciences, Colorado
    State University
Colorado Veterinary Medical Reserve Corps

Wayne E. Wingfield, MS, DVM
Specialty Certifications: Diplomate, American College
  of Veterinary Surgeons

Diplomate, American College of Veterinary Emergency
  and Critical Care
Emeritus Professor
  Department of Clinical Sciences and Veterinary
    Teaching Hospital, College of Veterinary
    Medicine and Biomedical Sciences, Colorado
    State University
National Medical Response Team—Central USA
  Veterinary Medical Officer
  Squad Leader
  National Disaster Medical System
  Department of Health and Human Services

Dirk B. Yelinek, DVM
Veterinarian/Owner, Redondo Shores Veterinary
  Center
National Veterinary Response Team—4
  Veterinary Medical Officer,
  Deputy Commander
  National Disaster Medical System
  Department of Health and Human Services

INTRODUCTION

Veterinarians and veterinary technicians responding to major disasters have become more organized, better trained, and acquainted with equipment useful in disasters and provide an important service to animal owners and first responders, including working animals and their handlers. These professionals bring a wealth of experience derived not only from service to the profession but also from deployments to a wide variety of local, state, federal, and international disasters affecting animals.

Undoubtedly, animals are injured or killed as frequently as are humans during major disasters. In fact, animals are frequently more at risk because they are not often a priority during preparation or response to a disaster. To add to this dilemma, there will be times when animals may be affected with diseases easily transmitted to humans. Because humans are the priority during any disaster, there may be times when animals must be killed in large numbers to stop the spread of important zoonotic or highly contagious animal diseases that may affect the economy of the country. Thereto, another distressing event during disasters is the knowledge that animals may have to be euthanatized to avoid unnecessary suffering. These points are discussed in the text, and we hope you will find some inner peace after reading about zoonotic and animal diseases, biosecurity concerns, sheltering of large and small animals, and even the psychological and emotional factors affecting veterinary caregivers.

Responding to a disaster is not like everyday practice. There are no radiographic, magnetic resonance, ultrasound, or computed tomography imaging devices available. Laboratory resources are limited to handheld devices (if you are lucky!). Thus, the experienced veterinary team brings common sense, acumen, volunteerism, and a sincere desire to help those unable to help themselves. The challenges are immense! A veterinary practice team may limit themselves to seeing only companion animals (dogs and cats), horses, or food animals (cattle, swine, sheep, etc.), or may be specialists in surgery, critical care, or internal medicine. Undoubtedly, these skills are useful, but during a disaster there is no way to limit oneself to one or two species. All animals are at risk during a disaster, and thus we must train to deal with these animals.

To make the challenge even more real, supplies and medications are extremely limited during most veterinary responses to disasters. We will not have, nor expect to have, unlimited antibiotics, analgesics, parasiticides, etc. Again, we must make do with what we have on hand and be thankful we have some equipment and supplies. Most disaster responses are uncomfortable to the responder. The ground is hard; the environment is unfriendly, cold, hot, humid, or filled with smoke that irritates the senses. As responders, we accept these facts, but in accepting them, we also find them more tolerable if we have been trained and know what to expect and how to minimize these discomforts.

Before responding to a disaster, one needs a very basic understanding of the meaning of "veterinary disaster response." You can't just show up and expect to be a useful addition. If you have never worked under the incident command system; never learned protocols of communication; do not own or have never used a map, compass, or global positioning system (GPS); in talking to the media, have no idea of who, what, or why; and have never been exposed to biosecurity protocols on a large poultry, dairy, or cattle feedlot—then you are not really going to be very useful to the veterinary response team. Unfortunately, training has not been given the highest priority for veterinarians and veterinary technicians prior to a disaster. Too frequently a new veterinary disaster response team member is allowed to deploy and has no concept of expectations, duties, and required skill levels.

With this in mind, the purpose of this basic animal response textbook is to acquaint individuals with the need for training in preparation for assisting animals that become victims of a disaster. With the increased awareness of disaster preparedness, volunteers are being trained to assist. Until now, there has not been a ready resource to assist these individuals.

The book has been divided into five essential elements for disaster response: training, planning, preparation, recovery, and, finally, a contact resource for identifying where to get either more information, supplies, or equipment. The overwhelming majority of this effort is directed to training, as we believe this is the critical element for a successful veterinary disaster response. We have provided a variety of topics based on our experiences and specialties and on your "need to know."

With the able assistance of experienced authors, this response text was written. Too often in the past, we have each been faced with reading through volumes of information in an attempt to extract key information. To help solve this problem, the authors of this text have used their experiences, specialty interests, and expertise to develop a series of key questions and answers often presented in a disaster. In this way, the reader may use the book as a means to learn about the topic or to quickly get an answer to an important question. Did we cover every scenario? You know we didn't! Did we try? Yes, we did!

The exciting parts about disaster responses are the unknowns. We believe each of you will learn from reading this text no matter what your experiences or expertise. If you are a small animal veterinarian, a quick review of some of the large animal topics will serve you well. If you are a large animal veterinarian, farmer, rancher, etc., you undoubtedly will find some relevant information on small animals and even wildlife. If you are an EMS first responder or search-and-rescue individual, you will quickly learn there is not much difference between first aid for humans versus the same for animals.

As I have read and reread this book, there is one word that keeps popping up. The word is "planning." No one plan is going to fit every situation, and thus you will find "planning" as a topic may suffer from perceived overkill. Before you accept that premise, do remember that planning *prior to* a disaster frequently results in a successful outcome. Experience has taught us that failure to plan will result in frustration, complaining, and apathy. If you take nothing else from this text, read about planning, study what the authors are trying to tell you, and then start planning! Our own life experiences surely verify that the failure to plan prior to an activity too often brings unacceptable results.

This book is not intended to be a traditional textbook. Rather, it is designed to provide factual information for the reader and to stimulate further learning and discussion. In preparing this text, we have attempted to take a middle ground between oversimplification and overcomplication. Of necessity, there is jargon in the text material that must be integrated into one's vocabulary to facilitate communication. Additionally, this text provides basic information that will hopefully be used in follow-up field exercises. The old adage of "watch one, do one, and teach one" is the secret to learning. We intend to put that adage to work as we each train to become more prepared for the missions that may be encountered in our future of helping animals.

The authors of this text are truly appreciative of your interest in helping animals in need. We are also indebted to the animals we have learned from during our lifelong experiences. Every animal has taught us something, and it is only proper that we now start to return our debt by training to become better prepared for assisting animals during future disasters.

Wayne E. Wingfield, MS, DVM

Veterinary Disaster Response

SECTION 1
TRAINING

CHAPTER 1.1
AN INTRODUCTION TO THE INCIDENT COMMAND SYSTEM

Lori A. Swenson, BSME, EMT-P

1. Describe the basics of the incident command system (ICS).

The *incident command system*, or ICS, is a standardized, on-scene, all-hazard incident management concept. ICS allows its users to adopt an integrated organizational structure to match the complexities and demands of single or multiple incidents without being hindered by jurisdictional boundaries. ICS has considerable internal flexibility. It can grow or shrink to meet different needs. This flexibility makes it a very cost-effective and efficient management approach for both small and large situations and incidents.

2. What is an "incident"? List some examples.

An *incident* is an occurrence, caused by either humans or a natural phenomenon, that requires response actions to prevent or minimize loss of life or damage to property and/or the environment. Examples of incidents include:

- Fire, both structural and wildland
- Natural disasters, such as tornadoes, floods, ice storms, or earthquakes
- Human and animal disease outbreaks
- Search and rescue missions
- Hazardous materials incidents
- Criminal acts and crime scene investigations
- Terrorist incidents, including the use of weapons of mass destruction
- National special security events, such as presidential visits or the Super Bowl
- Other planned events, such as parades or demonstrations

Given the magnitude of these types of events, it is not always possible for any one agency alone to handle the management and resource needs. Partnerships are often required among local, state, tribal, and federal agencies. These partners must work together in a smooth, coordinated effort under the same management system.

3. Why is it important to understand ICS as a first responder?

A thorough understanding of the ICS structure, principles, and expectations allows emergency personnel to respond to a scene, understand where they fit in the chain of command, and know their operational objectives.

- ICS is a proven management system based on successful business practices.
- ICS is the result of decades of lessons learned in the organization and management of emergency incidents.

- ICS has been tested in more than 30 years of emergency and nonemergency applications, by all levels of government and in the private sector. It represents organizational "best practices," and as a component of the National Incident Management System (NIMS), it has become the standard for emergency management across the country.
- NIMS requires the use of ICS for all domestic responses.
- NIMS also requires that all levels of government, including territories and tribal organizations, adopt ICS as a condition of receiving federal preparedness funding.

The ICS organizational structure develops in a top-down, modular method that is based on the size and complexity of the incident, as well as the specifics of the hazard environment created by the incident. As incident complexity increases, the organization expands from the top down as functional responsibilities are delegated.

The ICS organizational structure is flexible. When needed, separate functional elements can be established and subdivided to enhance internal organizational management and external coordination. As the ICS organizational structure expands, the number of management positions also expands to adequately address the requirements of the incident.

In ICS, only those functions or positions necessary for a particular incident will be filled.

4. What is meant by "management by objectives"?

All levels of a growing ICS organization must have a clear understanding of the functional actions required to manage the incident. Management by objectives is an approach used to communicate functional actions throughout the entire ICS organization. It can be accomplished through the incident action planning process, which includes the following steps:

- Step 1: Understand agency policy and direction.
- Step 2: Assess incident situation.
- Step 3: Establish incident objectives.
- Step 4: Select appropriate strategy or strategies to achieve objectives.
- Step 5: Perform tactical direction (applying tactics appropriate to the strategy, assigning the right resources, and monitoring their performance).
- Step 6: Provide necessary follow-up (changing strategy or tactics, adding or subtracting resources, etc.).

5. List four benefits of using the ICS.

1. It is a flexible system that can be used at an isolated scene involving one response group or a major regional disaster. It has the ability to meet the needs of any incident regardless of kind, size, or complexity.
2. The ICS uses common terminology, including standard titles and names for facilities, to minimize on-scene problems due to communication misunderstandings.
3. ICS allows resources to be managed in support of the incident management activities.
4. ICS relies on an *incident action plan* (IAP) to develop and issue assignments, plans, procedures, and protocols. The IAP provides a means to direct efforts in order to attain specific objectives determined by the ICS command staff.

6. The ICS relies on an IAP. Describe an IAP.

In ICS, considerable emphasis is placed on developing effective IAPs. An IAP is an oral or written plan containing general objectives reflecting the overall strategy for managing an incident. An IAP includes the identification of operational resources and assignments and may include attachments that provide additional direction.

Every incident must have a verbal or written IAP. The purpose of this plan is to provide all incident supervisory personnel with direction for actions to be implemented during the operational period identified in the plan.

IAPs include the measurable strategic operations to be achieved and are prepared around a time frame called an *operational period*. IAPs provide a coherent means of communicating the overall incident objectives in the context of both operational and support activities. The plan may be oral or written, except for hazardous materials incidents, which require a written IAP.

At the simplest level, all IAPs must include four elements:

1. What do we want to do?
2. Who is responsible for doing it?
3. How do we communicate with each other?
4. What is the procedure if someone is injured?

7. What are the five major management components of the ICS?

1. *Incident command* is the first major component of the ICS.

Beneath incident command are four sections:

2. Operations
3. Planning
4. Logistics
5. Administration

Managers of these sections are referred to as *chiefs*. These are set groups that never differ, regardless of the incident. A particular section may not be utilized dependent on the incident; that is, the administration and planning sections may not be staffed for a single medical incident to which the fire department responds (Fig. 1.1.1).

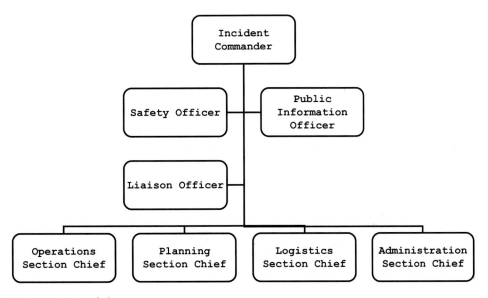

Figure 1.1.1 ICS organizational chart.

8. What are the other "groups or levels" of the ICS called, and how do they differ from each other (Table 1.1.1)?

- Branches fall under the command of the section chiefs. These are used when the span of control needs to be expanded by utilizing divisions or groups. The reason for expanding the span of control may be due to geographical or functional issues. Branch leaders are designated as *directors*.
- Divisions under the branch directors are used to divide an incident geographically. Division managers are called *supervisors*.
- Groups also fall under the branches and are used to divide an incident into functional responsibilities. Group managers are also called *supervisors*.

Table 1.1.1 Organizational Levels, Titles, and Support Positions in an ICS

Organizational Level	Title	Support Position
Incident Command	Incident Commander	Deputy
Command Staff	Officer	Assistant
General Staff (Section)	Chief	Deputy
Branch	Director	Deputy
Division/Group	Supervisor	N/A
Unit	Leader	Manager
Strike Team/Task Force	Leader	Single Resource Boss

9. What is the ICP?

This is the *incident command post*. It is a single location, usually close to, but unaffected by the incident. This is the location from which all incident operations are coordinated and directed.

10. Describe what is meant by the following terms: "staging area," "base," and "camp."

- *Staging areas* are temporary locations at an incident where personnel and equipment are kept while waiting for tactical assignments. The resources in the staging area are always in available status. Staging areas should be located close enough to the incident for a timely response but far enough away to be out of the immediate impact zone. There may be more than one staging area at an incident. Staging areas can be located with the ICP, bases, camps, helibases, or helispots.
- A *base* is the location from which primary logistics and administrative functions are coordinated and administered. The base may be located with the incident command post. There is only one base per incident, and it is designated by the incident name. The base is established and managed by the logistics section. The resources in the base are always out of service.
- A *camp* is the location where resources may be kept to support incident operations if a base is not accessible to all resources. Camps are temporary locations within the general incident area, that are equipped and staffed to provide food, water, sleeping areas, and sanitary services. Camps are designated by geographic location or number. Multiple camps may be used, but not all incidents will have camps.

11. Describe the basic map symbols used to describe the basic ICS facilities (Fig. 1.1.2).

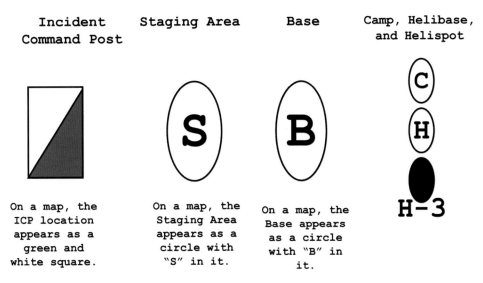

Figure 1.1.2 Map symbols used in identifying ICS components.

12. What is *accountability*, and how is it used during an incident?

Effective accountability during incident operations is essential at all jurisdictional levels and within individual functional areas. Individuals must abide by their agency policies and guidelines and any applicable local, tribal, state, or federal rules and regulations. The following guidelines must be adhered to:

- *Check-in:* All responders, regardless of agency affiliation, must report in to receive an assignment in accordance with the procedures established by the incident commander.
- *IAP:* Response operations must be directed and coordinated as outlined in the IAP.
- *Unity of command:* Each individual involved in incident operations will be assigned to only one supervisor.
- *Span of control:* Supervisors must be able to adequately supervise and control their subordinates, as well as communicate with and manage all resources under their supervision.
- *Resource tracking:* Supervisors must record and report resource status changes as they occur.

13. How would you be expected to participate in accountability during an incident?

Accountability requires that all responders "check in" when they arrive on scene and "check out" when they leave. Each individual "checks in" once through a single supervisor.

14. What is span of control?

Span of control is the number of individuals or resources reporting to any one manager or supervisor that can be effectively controlled.

15. What is the recommended span of control?

The recommended span is between three and seven people, with five being optimal.

16. What do you do when the span of control is exceeded in any one area?

If the number of direct reports is more than seven, the branch, division, or group may be expanded. Likewise, when the number of direct reports is less than three, the branch, division, or group can be contracted.

17. How is communication managed by the ICS?

ICS establishes common terminology and a clear chain of command for communications to flow through. Communications hardware, frequencies, and protocols are also defined by the ICS. Public information dissemination is handled only through the *public information officer* (PIO), who is a member of the command staff.

18. Differentiate between "chain of command" and "unity of command."

- *Chain of command* means that there is an orderly line of authority within the ranks of the organization, with lower levels subordinate to, and connected to, higher levels.
- *Unity of command* means that every individual is accountable to only one designated supervisor to whom they report at the scene of an incident.

19. What is "unified command," and how does it work?

Unified command is a unified team effort comprised of multiple agencies. The agencies work together as an *incident management team* and establish common objectives and strategies, which are used to manage the incident.

20. Describe the "command staff" and their role during an incident.

Depending on the size and complexity of the incident, the incident commander may find it necessary or helpful to assign individuals to provide public information, safety, and liaison services. These individuals report directly to the incident commander and are called "officers": public information officer, safety officer, and liaison officer.

21. What is the purpose of logistics?

Logistics is tasked with all functions necessary to support the Operations. Logistics provides food, transportation, and medical services for the responders. Logistics is also responsible for providing communications planning and resources, and providing facilities used in the support of the incident (i.e., ICP).

22. What is a task force?

A *task force* is any combination of single resources grouped together to accomplish a specific duty.

23. What is the role of the planning section during an incident?

The planning section is responsible for collecting, evaluating, disseminating, and using information about the status of resources and the progress of the incident. The following organizational chart shows an example of planning section units (Fig. 1.1.3).

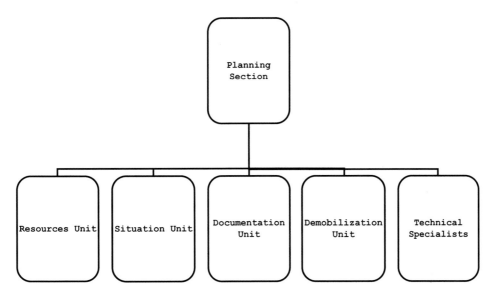

Figure 1.1.3 Planning section organizational chart.

24. What is "resource typing," and why is it beneficial to use it as part of the ICS?

Resource typing describes resource capabilities using common terms. When a resource is requested, "typing" eliminates mistakes based on miscommunication of need.

For instance, air tankers (airplanes) are a "kind" of resource and are "typed" by the Federal Emergency Management Agency (FEMA) as follows:

- *Type 1:* 2000 gallon capacity, 300 gallons per minute (GPM) pump capability
- *Type 2:* 1000 gallon capacity, 120 GPM pump capability
- *Type 3:* 1000 gallon capacity, 50 GPM pump capability

This allows an incident commander at a wildfire to request use of three "type 1 air tankers" from a federal assistance agency and allows both parties to know exactly what is being requested without having to discuss capacity or pump capability.

25. What is a staging area, and what goes on there?

The *staging area* is the physical location where resources that are available wait for assignment.

26. Is demobilization a concern of the ICS? Why?

Yes. Resources need to be released from the scene of an incident in an orderly, safe, and cost-effective manner.

27. What is an EOC, and how does it differ from an ICP?

The EOC is the *emergency operations center*. The EOC is a preestablished location, usually geographically distant from the incident, that is staffed with people who will help ensure that policies are implemented and resources are deployed through the ICP.

28. What is NIMS, and how does it relate to ICS?

NIMS is the National Incident Management System developed as a result of Homeland Security Presidential Directive 5 (HSPD-5). It is intended to provide a cohesive nationwide management system allowing all levels of government and private sector organizations to work together during an incident.

ICS is a component of NIMS along with a Multi-Agency Coordination System (MACS) and the Public Information System.

29. What is the purpose of the National Response Framework?

The purpose of the National Response Framework is to ensure that all response partners across the nation understand domestic incident response roles, responsibilities, and relationships so they can respond more effectively to any type of incident. The Framework is written especially for government executives, private sector and nongovernment organization leaders, and emergency management practitioners.

30. Describe the scope of the National Response Framework.

The Framework provides structure for implementing national-level policy and operational coordination for domestic incident response. The term "response" as used in the Framework includes the following:

• Immediate actions to save lives, protect property and the environment, and meet basic human needs
• The execution of emergency plans and actions to support short-term recovery

31. Describe the response doctrine of the National Response Framework.

Incidents begin and end locally, and most are managed at the local level. Many incidents require unified response from local agencies, the private sector, and nongovernment organizations. Other incidents may require additional support from neighboring jurisdictions or the state. A small number require federal support. National response protocols recognize this and are structured to provide additional, tiered levels of support. A key concept in the National Response Framework is as follows: A basic premise of the Framework is that *incidents are generally handled at the lowest jurisdictional level possible.*

32. How does the National Response Framework work in conjunction with NIMS?

The number, type, and sources of resources must be able to expand rapidly to meet needs associated with a given incident. The Framework builds on NIMS. Together, the Framework and NIMS help to ensure that all response partners use standard command and management structures that allow for scalable, flexible, and adaptable operational capabilities.

33. Provide a bit more information about the National Response Framework and how it relates to disasters.

The National Response Framework is comprised of the core document, the Emergency Support Function (ESF), Support, and Incident Annexes; and the Partner Guides. The core document describes the doctrine that guides our national response, roles and responsibilities, response actions, response organizations, and planning requirements to achieve an effective national response to any incident that occurs.

The following documents provide more detailed information to assist practitioners in implementing the Framework:

- **Emergency Support Function Annexes** group federal resources and capabilities into functional areas that are most frequently needed in a national response (e.g., transportation, firefighting, mass care).
- **Support Annexes** describe essential supporting aspects that are common to all incidents (e.g., financial management, volunteer and donations management, private-sector coordination).
- **Incident Annexes** address the unique aspects of how we respond to seven broad incident categories (e.g., biological, nuclear/radiological, cyber, mass evacuation).
- **Partner Guides** provide ready references describing key roles and actions for local, tribal, state, federal, and private-sector response partners.

These documents are available at the NRF Resource Center, http://www.fema.gov/emergency/nrf/.

34. Is it really important that I know about ICS, NIMS, and the National Response Framework?

Yes, you need to know and understand all of these items. In fact, to be deployed as a temporary federal employee (NVRT, NMRT, etc.), you are required to take the following free, online FEMA courses related to these topics:

- ICS 100
- ICS 200
- ICS 700
- ICS 800

These courses are available to everybody and can be found at the following website: http://training.fema.gov.

35.   How do you prepare for deployment to an incident?

Many incidents last only a short time and may not require travel. Other deployments may require a lengthy assignment away from home. Below are general guidelines for incidents requiring extended stays or travel:

- Assemble a travel kit containing any special technical information (e.g., maps, manuals, contact lists, and reference materials).
- Prepare personal items needed for your estimated length of stay, including medications, cash, credit cards, etc.
- Ensure that family members know your destination and how to contact you.
- Determine appropriate travel authorizations.
- Familiarize yourself with travel and transportation arrangements.
- Determine your return mode of transportation (if possible).
- Determine payroll procedures (at incident or through home agency).
- If you are going on a foreign assignment, be sure to take your passport.

36.   How do you determine your role and authority during deployment?

In addition to preparing for your travel arrangements, it is important to understand your role and authorities.

- Review your emergency assignment. Know who you will report to and what your position will be.
- Establish a clear understanding of your decision making authority.
- Determine communications procedures for contacting your headquarters or home office (if necessary).
- Identify purchasing authority and procedures.
- Identify procedures for obtaining food and lodging.

37.   What should be discussed with you prior to a deployment?

Upon receiving an incident assignment, your deployment briefing should include, but may not be limited to, the following information:

- Incident type and name or designation
- Descriptive location and response area
- Incident check-in location
- Specific assignment
- Reporting date and time
- Travel instructions
- Communications instructions (e.g., incident frequencies)
- Special support requirements (facilities, equipment transportation and off-loading, etc.)
- Travel authorization for air, rental car, lodging, meals, and incidental expenses

Suggested Reading
FEMA Emergency Management Institute. IS-100. **An Introduction to Incident Command System,**
    I-100. Available at http://training.fema.gov/emiweb/is/is100.asp. Accessed September 5, 2008.
FEMA Emergency Management Institute. **IS-700. National Incident Management System (NIMS),**
    An Introduction. Available at http://training.fema.gov/emiweb/is/is700.asp. http://training.fema.gov/emiweb/is/
    is100.asp. Accessed September 5, 2008.

CHAPTER 1.2
LEADERSHIP DURING A DISASTER

Eugene A. Adkins, DVM

1. What are the principals of leadership?

Leaders are required to show themselves as good examples of virtue, honor, patriotism, and subordination; to be vigilant in inspecting the conduct of all persons who are placed under their command; and to promote and safeguard the morale, physical well-being, and general welfare of all those persons under their command.

2. What are the attributes of a leader?

- The contagion of example (lead by example): It is not enough to know a leader's qualities, and not enough to proclaim them. You must exhibit them.
- To exact discipline, you must first possess self-discipline.
- Command presence is the product of dignity, carriage, neat and well-fitting uniform, firm and unhurried speech, and self-confidence.
- Your personal resolution and tenacity characterize an unfaltering determination to achieve the mission assigned.
- Leaders are able to teach and communicate effectively.
- Loyalty downward means protecting your team members and assuming responsibility for their actions and mistakes, and ensuring that they receive all credit due them.
- Encourage subordinates by giving them all the initiative and latitude they can handle.
- Professional competence will elicit the team's respect.
- Physical readiness is essential for every leader.
- The spirit of "can do" and "make do" marks you as a leader.
- Adaptability means staying loose and rolling with the punches.

3. What about delegating authority?

You can delegate authority but not responsibility. Tell subordinates what results you want and leave the "how" to them. Never oversupervise. Assign missions clearly and then get out of the way and observe how the mission is carried out. Request progress reports daily (weekly?) and tell your delegates to come to you if they have problems. One vital component of leadership that is often overlooked is the backup/deputy leader. This person should be kept continually apprised of the situation.

4. How close should you get to your people?

Develop a genuine interest in everyone and study each person's personality. Remember that familiarity breeds contempt.

5. When should you praise and reprimand?

Praise in public and reprimand in private. An acronym to remember is P.N.P. When offering a critique, say something positive, then negative, and end with something positive. This softens the criticism.

6. What does being responsible mean?

Being responsible means sometimes upsetting people.

7. What are other characteristics of a good leader?

A leader must be a person of decision and action, be calm in crisis and decisive in action, be a good judge of people and a good picker of subordinates, be tough and ruthless in dealing with inefficiency, and be prepared to take charge when the situation requires boldness. Everyone will be in a potentially dangerous situation, and you must remember two key points:

1. You and your colleagues will be afraid. This is a normal response, but the leader must keep his or her fears within, because good, clear decisions have to be made quickly. These decisions cannot be made logically or correctly if the leader panics.
2. If at all possible, remove yourself and your team from the situation if you believe it to be too dangerous.

8. Describe the relationships among leadership, power, and responsibility.

There is absolutely nothing as intoxicating as leadership power. With that power comes an equal, if not greater, responsibility—for the people you lead and your mission. You as an individual are not important. The people you are honored to lead are the important ones. Being a true leader is a humbling and tremendously self-satisfying experience.

9. How important is the mission?

The safety of your people is primary, and this is followed in importance by accomplishment of the mission.

10. What are the seven Ps used in leadership?

Prior proper planning and preparation prevent poor performance.

11. How important is a clear objective?

Take no action until you have a clear objective.

12. How do you judge people?

Look for intelligence and judgment and a capacity to anticipate changes ("seeing around the corners"). You should value loyalty, integrity, a high energy level, a balanced ego, and a drive to get things done.

13. How does a leader make decisions?

Develop all the information you can; then go with your instincts. Does it sound, smell, feel, and fit right? Don't make quick decisions, but make timely ones.

14. Who should get the credit for a successful mission?

There is no end to what you can accomplish if you don't care who gets the credit.

15. How important are details?

Never neglect details.

16. What about getting opinions from subordinates?

A wise leader gets opinions and suggestions from their subordinates *before* he or she offers his or her own and, more important, makes any decisions. That way your people say what they think, not what you want to hear.

17. How important are issuing and enforcing orders?

Promulgation of an order represents 10% of your responsibility. The remaining 90% consists of ensuring, through personal supervision by you and staff, proper and vigorous execution.

18. How important is looking out for your people?

In the final analysis, the essence of leadership is looking out for your people.

19. Just how important is response to stress?

You never know how people will react under stress until they are in a stressful situation, regardless of the training they have undergone.

20. How can a leader make certain an assignment is understood?

Have the person to whom you have given the order tell you what he or she is supposed to do.

21. How can a leader know if the assignment is being carried out?

A timely proven axiom is, "If it is not inspected, it will be neglected." A leader continually checks to see if his or her assignments are being fulfilled.

22. What is one way of ensuring an assignment is a good one?

Running the projected assignment by a trusted subordinate and eliciting their opinion.

23. What are Colin Powell's 13 rules of leadership?

1. It ain't as bad as you think. It will look better in the morning.
2. Get mad, and then get over it.
3. Avoid having your ego so close to your position that when your position falls, your ego goes with it.
4. It can be done!
5. Be careful what you choose. You may get it.
6. Don't let adverse facts stand in the way of a good decision.
7. You can't make someone else's choices. You shouldn't let someone else make yours.
8. Check small things.
9. Share credit.
10. Remain calm. Be kind.
11. Have a vision. Be demanding.
12. Don't take counsel of your fears or naysayers.
13. Perpetual optimism is a force multiplier.

24. Why is it important to provide an orientation to your team prior to deployment each day?

An orientation will help team members relate to their location, mission objective, routes of travel, and environmental concerns in the area.

25. When briefing your team, list the five major items that must be included each time.

1. Situation overview
2. Mission
3. Execution or concept of operation summary
4. Administration and logistics
5. Command and signals

26. What information is included when providing the "situation overview" to your team?

• Provide a general overview of events past, present, and future.
• Define new problems you will face.

- List the assets available to your team.
- List the team assignments and when their duties commence and end for the day.
- Provide the team with your assessment of the events likely to occur.

27. In providing the team with an overview of the situation, list the factors you should include in your assessment of the problems you will face, and provide the acronym for recalling this list of problems.

- Size of the disaster/objective
- Activity at the objective
- Location of the objective
- Unit (farm, kennel, herd)
- Time
- Equipment

The acronym is **SALUTE.**

28. What should be included when defining "mission" to your team?

The mission statement must be a clear concise definition of your mission and should include these five Ws:

1. Who?
2. What?
3. Where?
4. When?
5. Why?

29. What is included in the "execution *or concept of operation summary*" item?

First, you give a concept of the operation, a summary statement of how the operation will be conducted. A list of target objectives and descriptions are given.

30. What is the next item to be elucidated?

- Each unit is assigned a specific task.
- Missions are assigned to units, teams, elements, and individuals both in and out of the objective area.
- Reserve or backup if required
- Coordinating instructions: contains instructions common to two or more units/teams, coordinating details and control measures applicable to the unit/team as a whole (starting time, area to be covered, rallying points, actions in the objective area, debriefing, emergency procedures, other actions)

31. What is included in the "administration and logistics" item?

Food, water, medical supplies, animals to be picked up or that need attention, and conditions that need to be corrected.

32. Last, what is included in "command and signals" item?

- *Command relationships:* used in large operations or when relationships are unusual
- *Signal:* radio procedures, call signs, hand and arm signals, whistle procedures
- *Command posts:* location of leaders and next higher unit commander's location

33. Briefly summarize the five items you need to include in each day's orientation to your team.

1. Situation
   a. General overview
   b. Problems you will face (SALUTE)
      S = size
      A = activity
      L = location
      U = unit
      T = time
      E = equipment
   c. Assets (HAS)
      H = higher unit's mission
      A = adjacent unit's mission
      S = supporting unit's mission
2. Mission
   (5 Ws = who, what, where, when, why)
3. Execution
   Concept of operation
   a. Each unit assigned specific task
   b. Missions assigned to teams, units, elements, and individuals
   c. Reserve if required
   d. Coordinating instructions
4. Administration and logistics
   a. Food, water, medical, animals
5. Command and signals
   a. Command relationships
   b. Signal: radio, call signs, hand and arm, whistle and location of leaders, and next higher unit commander's location
   c. Command posts: location of leaders and location of next higher unit's commander's location.

Suggested Reading

Grant US, Kaltman A. *Cigars, Whiskey & Winning Leadership Lessons from General Ulysses S. Grant.* New York, Prentice-Hall, 1998.
Pitino R, Reynolds B. *Success Is a Choice.* New York, Broadway Books, 1997.
Powell CL. *My American Journey.* New York, Random House, 1995.
Thomas GC, Heinl RD, Ageton AA. *The Marine Officers Guide,* 3rd ed. Annapolis, MD, US Naval Institute Press, 1967.
Wooden J. *Wooden on Leadership.* New York, McGraw-Hill, 2005.

CHAPTER 1.3
COMMUNICATIONS

Lori A. Swenson, BSME, EMT-P

1. List methods of communication that you could use at an incident.

- Two-way radio (public safety, GMRS, FRS, HAM, CB)
- Written instructions
- Face-to-face verbal
- Hand signals
- Whistles
- Cell and satellite phones

2. Describe what you need to know with regard to radio frequencies used in the event of an emergency.

- Most two-way radio frequencies are licensed and managed by the Federal Communications Commission (FCC); therefore, you cannot just pick a frequency and begin transmitting. Public safety radios and GMRS (General Mobile Radio Service) radios require FCC licensure.
- Family Radio Service (FRS) radios do not require the user to license the frequencies used. When on a federal deployment, use of these radios is not allowed.

3. Who determines which channel or frequency a responder will use on the scene of an incident?

The incident commander and command staff will know which frequencies are accessible and which are restricted. Your team leader will assign you a frequency.

4. What are GMRS and FRS radios?

These are both examples of consumer walkie-talkies (e.g., Motorola's "Walkabout" radios). Generally, the GMRS radios are used for commercial purposes like road or construction crew communications and require an FCC license. FRS radios, on the other hand, are designed for family recreation use such as camping, keeping in touch with your kids at large public events, and so on, and do not require FCC licensure.

5. Describe the difference between a mobile radio and a handheld radio (packset).

A mobile radio is one that is installed in a car or communications vehicle and uses power from the vehicle to operate. These radios can have up to 100 W of transmission power.

Handheld radios (packsets) are battery powered and have a limited range of transmission. Packsets are limited to 5 W of power by the FCC.

6. What is meant by "clear text" or "clear speech"?

"Clear text" or "clear speech" is a method of communication that does not involve codes or proprietary phrases. It is simply speaking on the radio as you would in person.

7. What is a "repeater"?

This is an antenna site set up to "repeat" messages. Repeaters serve as bridges in areas where transmission is difficult due to obstacles, such as mountains, canyons, buildings, etc. They are also used when there is a long distance between transmitters and receivers.

8. What is a "call sign"?

A call sign is the identifier assigned to each radio user. For example, your call sign may be "Ops 3" and your supervisor may be "Ops 1."

9. You have never used the radio before and are a little nervous about using it now. What steps can you take to ensure your message sounds calm and professional?

First, take a minute to think about what you want to say. Rehearse it if needed, to minimize mistakes when actually transmitting. Jotting down notes to cue you may also be helpful. Keep messages short, direct, and relevant. If you are in a high-stress situation, take a deep breath and calm yourself before speaking.

When you are ready, make sure there is no other radio traffic, key the microphone, and wait 2 seconds before speaking. This will ensure you do not cut yourself off by speaking before the radio actually starts to transmit. Relay your message, release the microphone, and wait for acknowledgment of your transmission.

10. Every time you key the microphone, you hear a high-pitched screech. What is wrong?

What you are hearing is "squelch." This occurs when another radio or pager is in close proximity to the radio you are using and is tuned to the same frequency. When you hear this, check to make sure there are no mobile radios, pagers, other packsets, etc. near you while you are transmitting. If there are other devices in close proximity, turn them off before you transmit.

While most radios in use these days have an "automatic squelch" that cannot be adjusted, some older radios have a squelch that can be adjusted. To adjust these properly, turn the squelch knob all the way down (counterclockwise) and then slowly rotate the knob clockwise until the static stops. Turn the knob just slightly more clockwise from the point that the static stopped. If you continue to hear a lot of static on the radio, readjust the squelch until it goes away again.

11. What is the proper way to initiate radio communications?

Wait until the channel is free of traffic, depress (key) your microphone, and wait for 2 seconds. State the name, number, or title of the person you are trying to reach followed by your name, number, or title. An easy way to remember this is to remember, "Hey you! It's me!"

Example: "South Command, 3189." The other person will come back and say something to the effect of "3189, South Command, go ahead." This response is frequently shortened to "Go ahead, 3189" or even just "3189." You should be prepared for a variety of responses but know that all of them are acknowledgments that you have a message to transmit.

12. Describe why one does not use personal names, telephone numbers, or specific locations when calling on the radio.

Radio frequencies are easily monitored and it is important that sensitive information not be broadcast. This is especially important in response to an animal welfare incident with owners present or during a terrorist attack, where the terrorist could gain information about responders and perhaps initiate a secondary attack on these persons.

13. What if you attempt to contact someone and get no acknowledgment?

If radio traffic is heavy, it may take awhile for the other party to get back to you. If you do not hear an acknowledgment after a few minutes, try again and repeat your transmission.

14. What is the proper way to acknowledge a transmission has been received and understood?

If the message is long or complex or you would like clarification, it is a good idea to repeat the message to ensure you understand exactly what was said. This will give the other person an opportunity to correct any misunderstanding or rephrase it in a way that is more understandable. Once you are comfortable that you understand the information, respond with the phrase "Unit X copies" or "Affirmative." If you have no more information to relay, you can say "Unit X clear"; this will let everyone else know you are finished transmitting.

15. You have an urgent message that you need to relay to your incident commander, but radio traffic is heavy and you have not been able to make contact. What should you do?

The proper way to "get a word in" is to key the microphone and state "BREAK." You do not need to wait for radio traffic to cease to issue this command. Once others on the radio hear the "BREAK" command, they should cease all traffic and wait for your transmission.

16. You are in a mountainous area and can only transmit and receive intermittently. What kinds of things might you do to fix this problem?

If you are using a packset you might try to switch to a mobile radio with more power. You can try to find a clearing or open area where mountains or other obstacles will not interfere with transmissions. You can also try to raise your radio antennae as high as possible (e.g., stand on a rock and raise your radio, etc.). If you are using a traditional cell phone, chances are you will not be able to fix this issue until your phone can acquire a signal from a cell site. This will require you to physically move to another location.

17. You need to relay a long message to your group supervisor. What is the best way to accomplish this?

Single transmissions should not exceed 45 seconds, with less than 30 seconds being the optimal length. When your transmission is longer than this, you will break your transmission into multiple, smaller transmissions separated by the "break" command. You resume your transmission when acknowledged by the person to whom you are talking.

The following is an example of a responder who has arrived on scene of a motor vehicle accident and is giving dispatch an update on the scene survey.

> **Responder:** "Communications, 3189 is arrival at a 3 vehicle rollover accident, break."
> **Dispatch:** "Go ahead 3189."
> **Responder:** "We have a pickup on its top, confirmed parties pinned, break."
> **Dispatch:** "Go ahead."
> **Responder:** Second vehicle is an SUV on its side, unable to visualize occupants at the moment, break."
> **Dispatch:** "Go ahead."
> **Responder:** "Third vehicle is a sedan on its wheels in the creek, occupied by two, airbags deployed, 3189 will be investigating further."

Note: The use of the word "*break*" in this instance is different from when you have an emergency transmission and state "BREAK" in order to interrupt radio traffic.

18. You are talking to another member of your team using a packset. You can clearly hear your teammate, but he keeps asking you to repeat your transmission. What is the most likely problem?

Since packsets are battery operated, loss of the ability to transmit is your first indication that the battery in your packset is dying. It takes less energy to receive than to transmit, so you may still be able to hear others, even when you cannot transmit. Thus, one of the most important items to carry will be an extra, fully charged battery set.

19. After almost an hour on scene of a geographically diverse animal welfare incident, your supervisor radios you and asks for "your status." How do you respond?

Your supervisor wants to know how you and your team are proceeding. This includes number of team members and physical and mental conditions. If you were a team of six and you are all okay, you would respond by saying

"Status 6, everyone's fine." If you have team members working in an area away from you and are not certain of their status, let the supervisor know that you need to get back to them by stating "Status 6, stand by for more." Once you determine the remainder of your team is okay, you can then get back to your supervisor and update him or her.

20. What are the different frequency bands, and how do they work together?

Currently, there are four main frequency bands in use for public safety communications. They are VHF (very high frequency), UHF (ultra high frequency), 700 MHz, and 800 MHz. VHF radios operate between 136 and 174 MHz, UHF radios operate between 470 and 512 MHz, and 700- and 800-MHz radios operate within the 700 and 800 MHz bands, respectively.

None of these bands are interoperable. A VHF radio cannot transmit to a UHF radio or an 800-MHz radio. This is why it is important for responders to all have the same type of radio.

21. You have been given a command to perform a particular task that you believe is unsafe. How do you handle this?

Understanding that no commanding officer should knowingly issue such a command, sometimes the commanding officers do not have all the information available to the personnel on the scene and this may lead to orders being given that are not in the best interest of the organization or responder. After clarifying and providing the commander with any pertinent information, if the person is still asked to carry out an order that is unsafe, unlawful, or unethical, he or she is obligated to refuse to carry out such task or order. After refusal of such order, a report should be made to the incident commander.

Remember: REPEAT – REFUSE – REPORT.

22. What are two whistle sounds you need to know during an incident?

- Two sounds = gather around (usually at a predetermined location)
- Three sounds = emergency

23. How would you use the radio to indicate you are not safe or need help without letting someone who is with you know that you are alerting others?

It is important for your group to have a prearranged code that will signal danger for anyone using it. There should be a code for command officers to alert field personnel that they need to drop what they are doing and leave the area NOW! There should also be a code to alert team members or command officers that someone in the field is in danger. The code should be distinctive and known only to the rescuers and not the general public. For example, if you believe you need to leave the immediate area, stating that you "Forgot to set the brake on the truck" should trigger an egress.

Also, if fire trucks are on scene and you hear all the air horns going off at one time, this is a signal to evacuate the area.

24. What is the "phonetic alphabet"?

The phonetic alphabet is a group of words representing individual letters that is used when an individual needs to spell something over the radio or phone. Sometimes it is difficult to understand the person on the other end of the line due to accents, background noise, poor enunciation, etc. Using the phonetic alphabet ensures that the correct letter is used and eliminates the problem of a "d" sounding like a "p", a "c" sounding like an "e", and so on (Table 1.3.1).

Table 1.3.1 Phonetic Alphabets

Phonetic alphabets: There are two main sets of phonetic alphabets. One is used primarily by law enforcement personnel and the other by military or governmental personnel. Although you will only use one set in your organization, you should be familiar with both sets. This will assist you with communicating with someone who uses the other set.

Military/international Version

Alpha	Juliet	Sierra
Bravo	Kilo	Tango
Charlie	Lima	Uniform
Delta	Mike	Victor
Echo	November	Whiskey
Foxtrot	Oscar	X-ray
Golf	Papa	Yankee
Hotel	Quebec	Zulu
India	Romeo	

Law Enforcement Version

Adam	John	Sam
Boy	King	Tom
Charles	Lincoln	Union
David	Mary	Victor
Edward	Nora	William
Frank	Ocean	X-ray
George	Paul	Young
Henry	Queen	Zebra
Ida	Robert	

25. You need to spell the last name of an animal owner to your supervisor. The owner's last name is Dixon. How do you relay this information?

Say the name first and then spell it phonetically.

"Dixon; Delta India X–ray Oscar November"

26. You are on the scene of a geographically diverse incident with a major roadway cutting through the middle of the scene. Traffic needs to be controlled and only one lane is available for travel. Because of the terrain, you cannot communicate with radios. How do you manage this traffic control task?

First, stop all traffic in all directions until a safe plan can be put into action. Brief all team members prior to putting a plan into action. Make sure everyone understands the procedures, objectives, and strategies for safety.

One way to manage this specific task would be to agree that eastbound traffic will be released first. Westbound traffic will be held until the road is clear. Give the driver of the last eastbound vehicle a baton and instruct them to give the baton to the traffic control person at the other end. When the westbound responder receives the baton they know that there is no more eastbound traffic and they can release westbound travelers. Repeat passing the baton until a better method of communication becomes available. This same method of communication can be accomplished with a flag, a note, etc., on a variety of scenes.

27. Describe what is meant by communications "pro words."

These are words used by the public safety community to relay standard information. When you hear these "pro words" (procedural words), or use these words, it is generally understood that other parties will understand your meaning. These words are a type of shorthand to relay pertinent information in the least possible number of words (Table 1.3.2).

Table 1.3.2 Procedural Words (Pro Words) Used in Communications

Pro Word	Meaning
Affirmative, Affirm	Yes or I understand
Break	Important, urgent information to relay
Clear	Transmission completed
Copy	Message heard and understood
Correction	Erroneous info relayed, correct info forthcoming
Decimal	Use instead of "point"
FREEZE	Everybody stop immediately, danger identified
Go Ahead	I am ready for the next communication
Monitoring	Actively listening to radio
Negative	No or refusal of request
Off the air	You will not be available to speak on radio
Out	End of transmission, no response necessary
Over	End of transmission, a response is necessary
Please repeat last	I did not get all the information, say again
Relay	Please repeat my information to specified party
Roger	Message heard and understood
Stand by	Wait
Wilco	I understand and will comply

28. What are considered essential features of a good communications system?

It should be reliable, interoperable, scaleable, readily available, resilient, durable, and redundant. Ease of use is also a consideration, as well as cost to implement.

29. A message has just been transmitted from incident command stating, "All responders should report to the staging area at nineteen hundred hours." What does this mean?

All radio time designations are given in military time, so this message is telling you that all responders should be back to the staging area by 7:00 p.m. (Table 1.3.3).

Table 1.3.3 Time Conversions

When communicating time during a response, it is convention to use military time. This is not as confusing as some believe it to be. For the first 12 hours of the day, military time is the same numerical value as regular time. For example 1:00 A.M. is 0100 (stated "zero one hundred). 1:52 A.M. is 0152 and stated as "zero one fifty two." After noon, military time is determined by adding 12 to the current time. So, 1:00 P.M. in regular time is 1300 (12 + 1 P.M.) in military time. Stating convention is the same; this would be thirteen hundred hours. Midnight can either be stated as 2400 or 0000; stated "twenty four hundred hours or zero hundred hours."

Midnight = 0000 or 2400	Noon or 12 p.m. = 1200
1 A.M. = 0100	1:00 P.M. = 1300
2 A.M. = 0200	2:00 P.M. = 1400
3 A.M. = 0300	3:00 P.M. = 1500
4 A.M. = 0400	4:00 P.M. = 1600
5 A.M. = 0500	5:00 P.M. = 1700
6 A.M. = 0600	6:00 P.M. = 1800
7 A.M. = 0700	7:00 P.M. = 1900
8 A.M. = 0800	8:00 P.M. = 2000
9 A.M. = 0900	9:00 P.M. = 2100
10 A.M. = 1000	10:00 P.M. = 2200
11 A.M. = 1100	11:00 P.M. = 2300

CONTROVERSIES

30. Discuss some pros and cons of using "10 codes" on the radio versus clear speech.

PROS
• General public does not know codes; helps keep sensitive communications private
• Replaces lengthier sentences to keep transmissions short

CONS
• Regionally variable. Same code may have a different meaning in a different area.
• May not save time in some instances, e.g., "Can I give you a Code 2?" versus "Can I call you?"
• Must be memorized

31. List some of the pros and cons of using hand signals in the field.

PROS
• Good when on a noisy scene that prohibits clear verbal communication by radio or face-to-face contact
• Generally simple to interpret when preestablished

CONS
• The same signal may mean different things on different scenes or in different regions.
    Example: You are doing a swift-water rescue and you are the "swimmer." As you travel downstream, one of your downstream safeties has identified a hazard and needs to communicate this to you so that you can avoid it. Because you are in loud and fast water and cannot see the hazard, you are relying on hand signals from the safety.
    In some areas of the country, the safety will *point at* the hazard and you will attempt to avoid that area. In other areas of the country, the downstream safety will *point away* from the hazard in an attempt to tell you where to go and thereby miss the hazard. This is a single hand signal (the pointing), but not knowing the actual meaning of this signal can literally kill you.

- Must be within visual range to be seen easily and not misinterpreted
- Require consistent practice and utilization to be effective. You must also be diligent about rehearsing hand signals and their meanings prior to putting any rescue into action in order to refresh people's memories and make sure everyone is on the same page.

32. Give the pros and cons of using a whistle for communication.

PROS
- Good for relatively close areas when hands are tied up, such as holding a rope, hanging on rocks, trying to maintain balance in a boat, etc.
- Good for close areas that are visually obscured, e.g. around the bend of a river, in heavy forest, etc.
- Loud enough to be heard on moderately noisy scenes

CONS
- Not commonly used; easy to forget signal combinations
- If speaking on a radio to someone in a remote location, you cannot keep the whistle in your mouth and talk on the radio. Frequently, people forget to replace the whistle when they are done talking.
- Depending on the noise level, whistle sounds can be difficult to distinguish from other noise and become part of the background.

Selected Reading

Federal Communications Commission. Home page. Available at http://www.fcc.gov/.
FEMA. NIMS guide. Available at http://www.fema.gov/emergency/nims/rm/guide_standards.shtm.
FEMA Library. NIMS Guide for Communication and Information Management Standards. Available at http://www.fema.gov/library/viewRecord.do?id=3138.
GMRS. General Mobile Radio Service. Home page. Available at http://www.gmrs.org/, 2007.

CHAPTER 1.4
BASIC MAP, COMPASS, AND GLOBAL POSITIONING SYSTEM SKILLS

Sally B. Palmer, DVM

For this section, I recommend having a topographic map at hand to refer to as various topics are discussed. Topographic (or topo) maps are inexpensive and can be found at mountaineering stores or via the Internet by going to www.usgs.gov and following the links to purchase topo maps. National Geographic Trails Illustrated Maps™ also produce some outdoor recreation topographic maps. These can be found at www.natgeomaps.com. Having a compass and Global Positioning System (GPS) receiver available would also be helpful when reading this chapter, but they are fairly expensive and are not critical. With so many options available, it is best to thoroughly investigate the different brands and models to find the compass and/or GPS receiver that is right for your use.

MAPS

1. Why is it important for (animal) disaster responders to be familiar with maps, compasses, and the Global Positioning Systems and receivers?

A responder may be in unfamiliar territory or communicating with others who are unfamiliar with the area. They may be operating in the backcountry or in an urban, suburban, or rural area where street signs and other directional infrastructure is lacking or has been destroyed. Navigating in a disaster and communicating specific location information to others rely upon everyone having at least a basic understanding of maps, compasses, and the Global Positioning Systems and receivers.

2. What is a map?

For our purposes, a *map* is a two-dimensional representation of the Earth's surface. Different types of maps convey different information.

3. What are some different types of maps that can be helpful to disaster responders and emergency managers?

- Road maps: city, county, state, and country
- Topographic maps (USGS maps, topo maps, 7.5′ or 15′ quadrangles)
  - Topographic maps use contour lines to show the relief of the terrain and convey a three-dimensional representation. They also show certain vegetative features and other items of interest including roads, trails, buildings, landing strips, etc. For locations in the United States, topographic maps are made by the U.S. Geological Survey (USGS) and therefore are also referred to as USGS maps. Because USGS maps cover an area of 7.5′ or 15′ (7½ minutes or 15 minutes) of longitude and latitude, they may also be referred to as 7.5′quadrangles, 15′ quadrangles, or simply "quadrangles."
- U.S. Forest Service (USFS) National Forest System maps
  - These maps cover the various National Forests and surrounding land, and aside from marking roads (including Forest Service roads) and trails, these maps indicate ownership of land: National Forest, private, Bureau of Land

Management (BLM), State Park, National Park, etc. Identifying private property areas in relation to public property can be very helpful in emergency planning and response. Generally, National Forest System maps are drawn to a smaller scale than topo maps, providing a broader perspective of an area, albeit at the expense of detail.
- USGS–U.S. Department of Agriculture (USDA) Forest Service Joint Mapping Program
  - In 1993, the USGS and the U.S. Forest Service signed an interagency agreement to produce and maintain single-edition primary series topographic maps for quadrangles containing National Forest System lands. These maps contain features of the USGS maps and features of the USFS maps.
- Charts:
  - Charts are essentially the nautical version of a topographic map.

4. What is the map legend?

The *map legend* contains pertinent information about that map. Usually the map legend is in the margin(s) of the map. Common elements found in the *map legend* include:

- A *title* of the area represented (Fig. 1.4.1)
- The *year* the map was made (Fig. 1.4.1)
- The *scale* of the map (Fig. 1.4.2)
- The *map datum* (Fig. 1.4.2)
- A *direction marker* indicating True north (Fig. 1.4.3)
- Interpretation of at least some of the symbols used on the map (Figs. 1.4.1 and 1.4.2). A booklet detailing all of the symbols used on USGS maps can be obtained by following the links on their website (http://www.usgs. gov. [www.usgs.gov → MAPS IMAGERY PUBLICATIONS → Publications → Booklets → Mapping and Geography tools → Topographic Map symbols]). A listing of nautical chart symbols, abbreviations, and terms (officially termed *Chart No. 1*) can be accessed via the National Oceanic and Atmospheric Administration (NOAA) website (http://www.nauticalcharts.noaa.gov/mcd/chartno1.htm).

HIGHWAYS AND ROADS

Interstate 5

U. S. 101

State 79

County 6

National Forest, suitable for passenger cars .... 105 | 61

National Forest, suitable for high clearance vehicles 105

National Forest Trail 384

Primary highway ....

Secondary highway..................

Light-duty road

    Composition: Unspecified...

                Paved...........

                Gravel ....

                Dirt ....

Unimproved; 4 wheel drive 4WD

Trail ....

Gate; Barrier............................

JOHNNY MOORE MOUNTAIN, CO
2000

40106-F1-TF-024
NIMA 4765 II NE-SERIES V877

Figure 1.4.1 In this part of the margin on a U.S. Geological Survey (USGS) map, those common elements found in the map legend include the title of the area represented, the year it was made, and symbols used on the map.

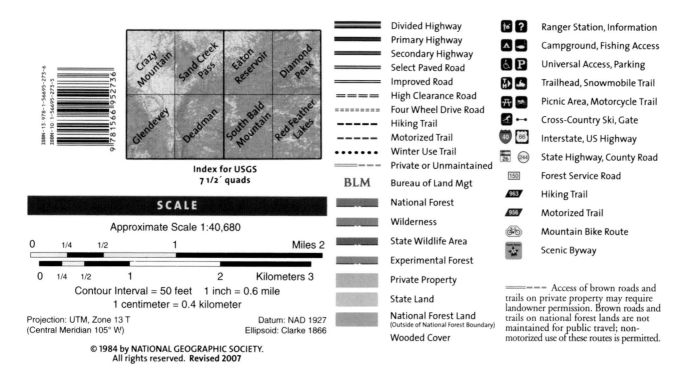

Figure 1.4.2   In this part of the margin of a National Geographic Trails Illustrated™ map, common elements found in the map legend include the year it was made, the scale, the map datum, and symbols used on the map. Additional information is included in this legend: the corresponding USGS 7.5′ quadrangles, the contour interval, the UTM Grid Zone, and the Central Meridian. (Map: Courtesy of National Geographic Trails Illustrated Map™.)

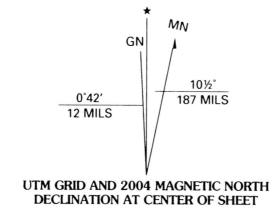

**UTM GRID AND 2004 MAGNETIC NORTH
DECLINATION AT CENTER OF SHEET**

Figure 1.4.3   True north is a common element found on all maps. A variety of symbols may be used to indicate True north including a compass graphic, or an arrow indicating north. This graphic from a USGS map represents True north with a "*" and details Grid north and Magnetic north as well. On USGS topographic maps, True north is always toward the top of the map. The right- and left-hand edges of the map are longitudes, and as such, are indicators of True north direction.

5.   What additional information is displayed in the legend on topographic maps?

- The m*agnetic declination* or *magnetic variation* for the area represented by that map is displayed (Fig. 1.4.3).
- The *grid declination* for the area represented by that map is displayed (Fig. 1.4.3).
- The *contour interval* for that map is given (Fig. 1.4.2).
- The latitude and longitude are noted (Fig. 1.4.4).

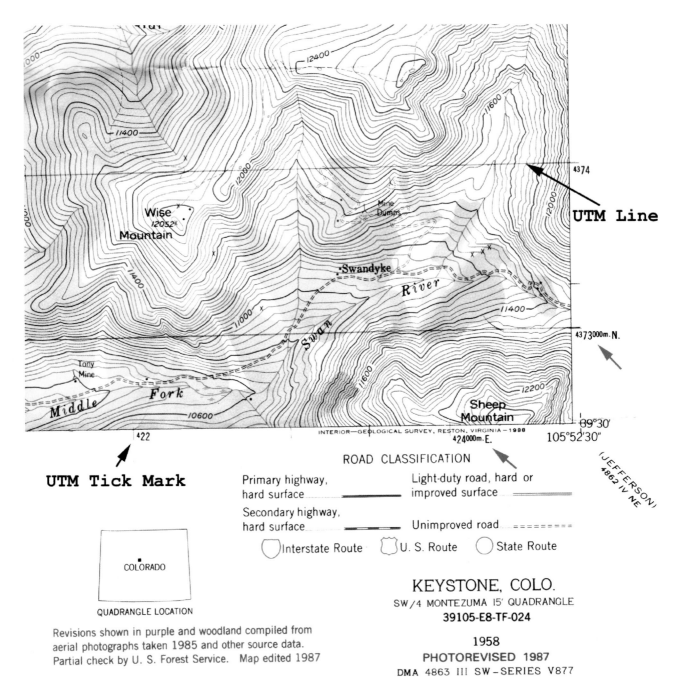

UTM Line

UTM Tick Mark

ROAD CLASSIFICATION

Primary highway, hard surface _____

Secondary highway, hard surface _____

Light-duty road, hard or improved surface ======

Unimproved road =========

Interstate Route   U. S. Route   State Route

COLORADO

QUADRANGLE LOCATION

Revisions shown in purple and woodland compiled from aerial photographs taken 1985 and other source data. Partial check by U. S. Forest Service. Map edited 1987

KEYSTONE, COLO.

SW/4 MONTEZUMA 15' QUADRANGLE

39105-E8-TF-024

1958

PHOTOREVISED 1987

DMA 4863 III SW — SERIES V877

Figure 1.4.4 Additional information that can be found in the margins and legends of USGS topographic maps includes the latitude and longitude (at the corners of the map), UTM grid blue tick marks (*short black arrow*), and UTM Easting and Northing Coordinates (*red arrows*). Adjacent topographic maps are noted in parentheses; in this case, the map adjacent to the southeast corner of this map is "(JEFFERSON)." If using the UTM grid system, *prior* to taking the map into the field, it is advisable to connect the UTM tick marks and lightly draw in the UTM lines (*long black arrow*), thereby completing the grid.

- Universal Transverse Meridian (UTM) grid marks, or ticks, and their corresponding meter values are displayed (Fig. 1.4.4).
- The *Grid Zone* is stated (Fig. 1.4.2).
- For maps utilizing the Military Grid Reference System (MGRS) or the U.S. National Grid (USNG) system, the 100,000 m Square Identification(s) is(are) also noted.
- Other surrounding maps are noted. This may be represented in a graphic or by adjacent map titles printed in the top, bottom, and corner margins (Figs. 1.4.4 and 1.4.5).

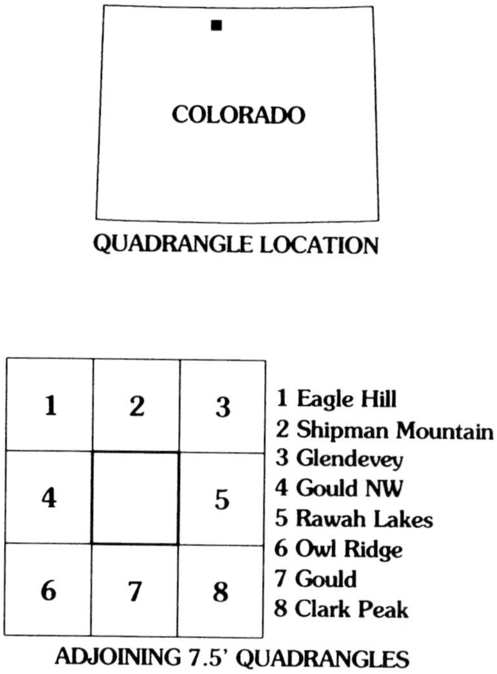

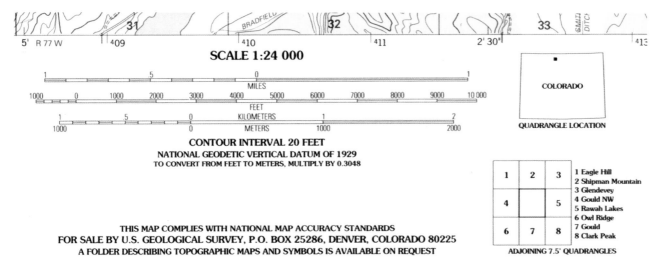

Figure 1.4.5 To readily obtain the titles of adjacent maps, USGS maps, nautical charts, and National Geographic Trails Illustrated™ maps, among others, will state this information either in parentheses in the respective margins, as seen in Figure 1.4.4, or as a graphic. This graphic is from a USGS topographic map. Having this information readily available allows responders to plan ahead and secure their mapping needs.

Figure 1.4.6 The scale on this USGS map is displayed as a bar scale and as a ratio (1:24,000). The bar scale favors easy visualization of distances, while the ratio scale allows one to readily compare and communicate scale size if looking for additional maps of the area in a smaller or larger scale. If working in UTM/MGRS/USNG grid systems, the ratio scale quickly identifies the proper scale of grid reader to use, or the kilometer bar scale (complete with 100 m divisions) can be used to make your own grid reader.

6. What is the scale on a map?

A scale is the relationship between a distance on the map and the actual distance in the field. Scales may be represented by a bar scale or they may be indicated as fractions (e.g., 1/250,000) or as ratios (e.g., 1:250,000). This fraction or ratio means that 1 unit on the map is equivalent to 250,000 of those same units in the field; 1 inch on the map is equivalent to 250,000 inches in the field, or 1 cm on the map is equivalent to 250,000 cm in the field. Some commonly used map scales are:

- 1:250,000 equates to approximately 1 inch on the map = 4 miles in the field.
- 1:62,000 equates to approximately 1 inch on the map = 1 mile in the field.
- 1:24,000 equates to 1 inch on the map = 2,000 feet in the field (Fig. 1.4.6).

Maps may be described as "small-scale" or "large-scale" maps. Small-scale maps cover a larger area in less detail, and large-scale maps tend to cover a smaller area in greater detail. An easy way to understand and remember this is to think about the scale size in terms of the size of the fraction of the scale: 1/250,000 is a much *smaller* number than 1/24,000; therefore, 1/250,000 is a small-scale map compared to a map scaled 1/24,000. By understanding that the length of 1 unit on the map represents a distance of 250,000 units in the field versus just 24,000 units, it is readily apparent that the smaller scale covers a larger area.

An example of small- and large-scale maps can be seen in a road atlas of the United States. The first one or two pages show a *small-scale* map of the whole country with minimal detail—only the interstates and major highways are displayed—but it provides a good overview of the whole country. The bar scale indicates that 1 inch (″) on the map equates to approximately 140 miles in the field. Translated into a fraction scale, this would be 1/8,870,400. The maps of the individual states are of a larger scale and can show more detail (more cities, towns, roads, etc.). The bar scale indicates 1″ on the map is the equivalent of approximately 22 miles in the field. Translated into a fraction scale, this is approximately 1/1,400,000. The side boxes or pages dedicated to maps of a single city are even larger-scale maps. For example, the bar scale may indicate that 1 inch is equivalent to 2 miles in the field. Translated into a fraction scale, this would be approximately 1/125,000.

It is helpful to have both small- and large-scale maps of an area impacted by disaster, as they both have important information to offer.

7. How is the relief of the terrain displayed on a topographic map?

Elevation features are shown with thin brown lines called *contour lines*. Every point on a given contour line is the same elevation. Every fifth line is an *index contour line* that is slightly thicker and contains a number, which is the elevation of that line. The contour lines in between the index contour lines are called *intermediate contour lines*, and their elevation is derived from knowing the *contour interval* for the map. The contour interval will be stated on the map or can be calculated by taking the difference in elevation between two index contour lines and dividing by 5.

One can determine how relatively steep or flat the terrain by how close together or far apart the contour lines are to one another and how large or small the contour interval. Where a contour line crosses a stream or river, it takes on a V-shape with the point of the "V" pointing uphill and upstream. One can recognize these "V"s at a glance and quickly determine the uphill direction (Fig. 1.4.7).

8. What is "map datum," and why is it so important to us?

Map datum indicates the mathematical model used to describe the shape of the Earth and the resulting surveys upon which a map is based, and this in turn impacts the latitude/longitude framework on that map. While this one sentence explanation is a bit overwhelming, a little historical information may help illuminate the concept.

For thousands of years humans have been making maps representing the world around them. A bit of understanding as to how maps were (are) created, leads one to appreciate the amazing genius of surveyors. In the early days, surveyors started from a single point (whose location was determined by fairly accurate astronomical observations) and then painstakingly measured horizontal distances—sometimes over many miles—and even correcting for changes in elevations. Because the Earth was thought to be a perfect sphere, angular measurements were then taken from each end of this baseline to a third position, and spherical trigonometry established the distances to this third point. This process was then repeated until a triangular "patchwork" charted the surveyed area. By making additional astronomical sightings from different points, it was possible to establish a latitude and longitude framework (coordinate system) and then apply this framework to that survey.

By the seventeenth century, instrumentation for obtaining accurate astronomical observations and distance measurements had improved such that it was discovered that a degree of latitude in one part of the world did not cover the same distance as a degree of latitude in another part of the world—this discovery illuminated the fact that the Earth is not a perfect sphere.

The challenge, then, was to find a model for the Earth that was mathematically predictable and could demonstrate the changing relationship between distance on the ground and the mapped latitude and longitude framework, with actual observed latitudes and longitudes. The accepted model became an *ellipsoid* or spheroid, where the Earth's poles are flattened and the radius at the equator is lengthened—similar to pressing down on a tennis ball

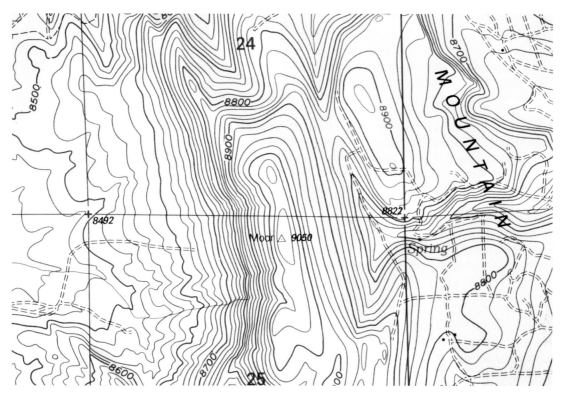

Figure 1.4.7 Topography of an area is conveyed with the use of contour lines. Index contour lines are thicker and note the elevation of that line. The elevation of the intermediate contour lines is derived from the contour interval. How steep or flat the terrain is readily apparent from how close together or far apart the contour lines are. Note that where a contour line crosses a stream (*thin blue line*), it takes on a "V" shape with the point of the "V" pointing upstream and therefore uphill.

and shortening that axis while the middle of the ball bulges out increasing its radius. The next questions asked were, How much are the poles flattened? And how much bulging occurs at the equator? In other words, how squished is the tennis ball?

During the nineteenth century, years were spent determining the answers to those questions as ellipsoid models of the Earth were used to map the continents. Preliminary astronomical observations and baseline distances were measured and used to calculate the key dimensions of the shape of an ellipsoid that best fit that area and would underlie the survey of that area.

As an example, Sir George Airy developed an ellipsoid model of the Earth that allowed him to create a detailed survey of the British Isles in 1830. The ellipsoid dimensions that he calculated fit the shape of this part of the world extremely well and his survey was exceedingly accurate—in other words, distances on the map and the latitude/longitude framework on the map matched the real world and could be confirmed with astronomical observations. Maps of the British Isles that use this datum now reference it as "*Map Datum: Airy 1830*", and it is still in use today.

Other people were doing similar work in other parts of the world. Preliminary work established an underlying ellipsoid model that supported accurate surveys in the field for the area in which they were working. In 1866, a man named Alexander Clarke developed an ellipsoid model fitting the shape of the Earth in the area of the United States. In the twentieth century, other people used Clarke's ellipsoid model, and starting from a single astronomically determined point in the middle of the country in Kansas, fanned out from there, mapping the whole country (measuring distances, taking astronomical sights, making mathematical calculations, etc.). Again, the accuracy of their data (distances and the latitude/longitude framework on the map correlating with distances and latitude/longitude coordinates as determined by astronomical observations) was superb. This *map datum* became known as *North American Datum of 1927 (NAD 27)*.

What is clear from these two examples is that different people determined different ellipsoid models (i.e., different map datums) that fit the part of the world in which they were working, and the ellipsoid that fit their part of the world could not be extrapolated to fit other parts of the world. Once again, a single mathematically predictable model did not fit the whole Earth. The bottom line is that there is no single mathematically predictable model that can perfectly describe the whole Earth because the Earth does not have a uniform shape! The term used to describe this irregular, mathematically unpredictable shape is *geoid*.

While there is no single perfect ellipsoid that can be applied the world over, these (different) ellipsoids can be used to accurately model large areas of the world, resulting in very accurate maps. When operating in an area that "has" a specific best-fit ellipsoid, using maps of that datum in that area will be most accurate. Since these "local" ellipsoids do not correlate with one another, these datums cannot be extrapolated to "fit" other parts of the world. Essentially, this extrapolation would result in an inaccurate coordinate framework of that area. Most ellipsoids that fit a particular area of the world include that area in their descriptive title—for example, *North American Datum 1983, South American 69, Mahe 1971,* and *European 1979.*

So the question remained, How to solve the problem of coming up with an accurate datum that could describe the *whole* geoid with reasonable and acceptable accuracy?

Enter the space age. Difficulties in accurately measuring great distances, such as across oceans, were overcome with satellites and other advancements in technology. These satellite-derived data are termed *World Geodetic Systems (WGS).* As more data were collected, improvements were made to the model over the years, hence *WGS 66* (i.e., *WGS 1966*), *WGS 72* (i.e., *WGS 1972*), and the latest *WGS 84* (i.e., *WGS 1984*). WGS 84 is still an ellipsoid model, in this case having a "best fit" for the Earth as a *whole*, rather than just a part of the Earth. Distances and coordinate locations on maps from around the world based on this datum correlate well with the real world.

Of note, however, for some areas of the world, other (local) ellipsoids (and surveys) (i.e., another map datum) may be a more accurate representation of that particular *part* of the earth. As an example, for the British Isles, maps and charts created using *Map Datum: Ord Srvy GB* may be more accurate for that area of the world than maps and charts using *Map Datum: WGS 84.* In North America, the *WGS 84* ellipsoid and the *NAD 83* ellipsoid match very well and many consider them "the same" for this area of the Earth.

To summarize, the *Map Datum* tells us what ellipsoid model of the Earth the mapmakers used to create the survey of an area and its latitude/longitude framework. The goal is to have the latitude/longitude framework and distances on a map synchronized with the latitude/longitude coordinates and distances in the real world, which are verified by astronomical observation (Fig. 1.4.8).

Whew! So, that answers the first part of the question—what is map datum? Now, why is it important to us? Map datum becomes important to us because we, the common man, woman, and child, now have ready access to a device called a GPS receiver, which pinpoints location with astounding accuracy. **GPS receivers identify a location's coordinates based on the particular map datum in which the GPS receiver is operating.** Location coordinates become helpful when you place them on a map and can then "see" that location and how it relates to its surroundings. Coordinates from a GPS receiver can be transferred onto a map or, conversely, coordinates from a map can be entered into the GPS receiver and stored as a location *"waypoint"* (more about that later when we discuss GPS receivers in detail). Either way, location coordinates are flowing from GPS to map and map to GPS. Now it becomes obvious that for the GPS coordinates to correlate with those same coordinates on a map (i.e., where the GPS derived location coordinates appear on a particular map), **BOTH** that map and the GPS receiver **have to be** using the same map datum.

GPS receivers have the capability to use a variety of map datums. The map datum is selected from a list of options accessed on a menu screen in the GPS receiver.

This is why ALL maps should have the map datum stated, and why ALL GPS coordinates should state which map datum is being referenced. One should *always* check to ensure their GPS receiver is set to read the same map datum as stated on their map. When using more than one map, be aware that they may be of different datums.

It has been said that if a map datum is not referenced (either on the map or a stated waypoint), one should *assume* it is WGS 84. Having to make this "assumption" is a little unsettling, as there are many maps in use today that use a map datum other than WGS 84, and too, sometime in the future it is possible that a new model of the Earth will become an even more accurate representation of this geoid. Anyone creating maps, working with coordinate systems, relaying or referencing waypoints, etc. should follow protocol and state the map datum. In the words of one of my professors, *"Assumption is the mother of all screwups."*

9. What are coordinates?

Coordinates form the link between a position in the real world and that location on a map. There are various coordinate systems including latitude/longitude, UTM/MGRS/USNG grids, or even simple road map systems that

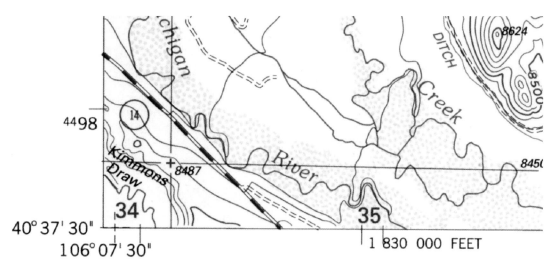

Produced by the United States Geological Survey 1956 Revision within and adjacent to National Forest System lands by USDA Forest Service 2000

Topography compiled 1952. Planimetry derived from imagery taken 1999 and other sources. Public Land Survey System and survey control current as of 2001. Boundaries current as of 2001

North American Datum of 1927 (NAD 27). Projection and 10,000-foot ticks: Colorado coordinate system, north zone (Lambert conformal conic) Blue 1000-meter Universal Transverse Mercator ticks, zone 13

North American Datum of 1983 (NAD 83) is shown by dashed corner ticks The values of the shift between NAD 27 and NAD 83 for 7.5-minute intersections are obtainable from National Geodetic Survey NADCON software

Non-National Forest System lands within the National Forest Inholdings may exist in other National or State reservations

This map is not a legal land line or ownership document. Public lands are subject to change and leasing, and may have access restrictions; check with local offices. Obtain permission before entering private lands

Figure 1.4.8 The map datum is displayed in the map legend. This USGS topographic map, initially produced in 1956, states the map datum is North American Datum of 1927 (NAD 27), and this map is still based on the ellipsoid, survey, and latitude/longitude framework of NAD 27. The map was revised in 2000, noting a shift in the coordinate framework when using a different map datum of this area, North American Datum of 1983 (NAD 83). The difference in the two data and the corresponding shift in the latitude/longitude framework is "... shown by dashed corner ticks," with a reference to obtain software for the shift in values. When using this map and transferring location coordinates between map and a GPS receiver, one would set the GPS map datum to NAD 27.

label columns with letters and rows with numbers. All these coordinate systems describe an east-west component and a north-south component. Sometimes multiple coordinate systems will be displayed on a map; for example, latitude/longitude and UTM grid coordinates (Fig. 1.4.9).

In a disaster response, it is helpful for everyone to be using the same coordinate system, but this is dependent on all the maps having that system in place, everyone being familiar with using that system, and having GPS receivers capable of working in that system.

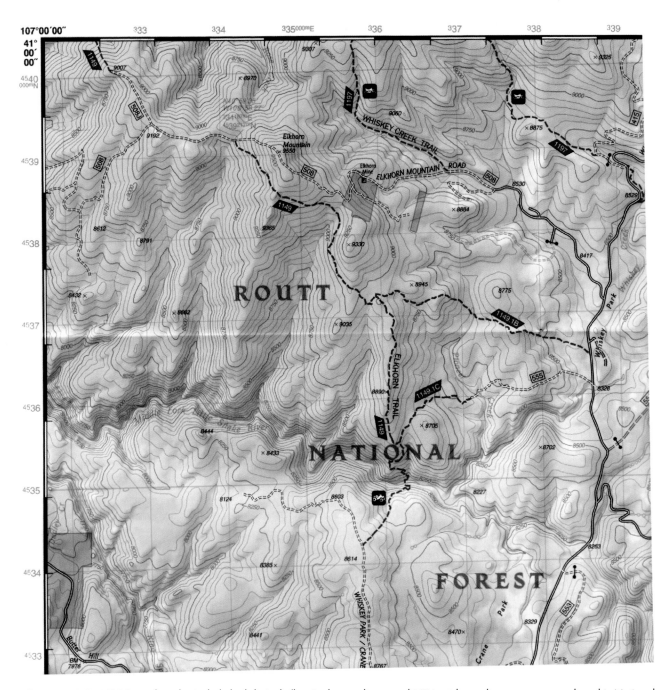

Figure 1.4.9 USGS quadrangles include both latitude/longitude coordinate and UTM grid coordinate systems, as does this National Geographic Trails Illustrated™ map. The latitude/longitude coordinates are in black in the upper left-hand corner of this map section. The left edge of the map graphic is longitude 107°00′00″. The top edge of the map graphic is latitude 41°00′00″. The light blue UTM grid lines establish 1,000 m × 1,000 m squares. The UTM coordinates that correspond with these grid lines are in light blue in the outer margins. (Map: Courtesy of National Geographic Trails Illustrated Map™ Hahns Peak Steamboat Lake Colorado, USA.)

10. Describe the latitude/longitude coordinate system.

Latitude refers to the angle measured from the center of the Earth above (north) or below (south) the *Equator*, with the Equator being 0° and the North and South Pole being 90° north and 90° south, respectively (Fig. 1.4.10). Lines of latitude circle the Earth and never intersect one another, so they are also referred to as *parallels*. Latitude is the north-south coordinate (Fig. 1.4.11).

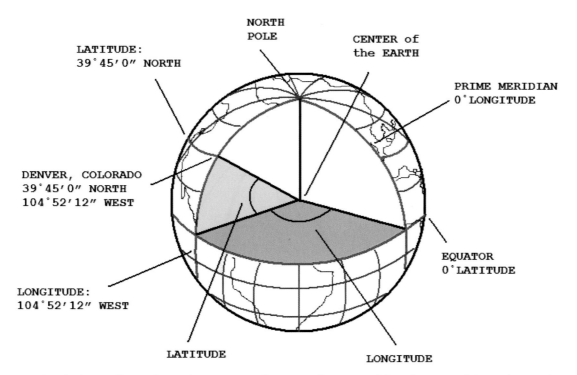

Figure 1.4.10 The latitude/longitude coordinate system relates to angles measured from the center of the Earth. Latitude measures the angle north or south of the Equator and longitude measures the angle east or west of 0°, also known as the Prime Meridian.

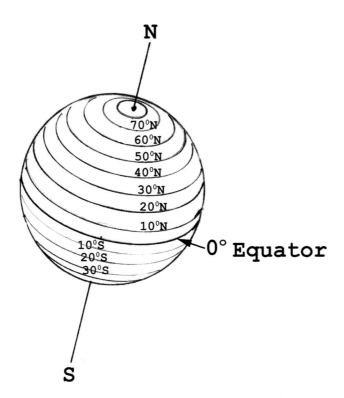

Figure 1.4.11 The latitude coordinate measures the angle, from the center of the Earth, north or south of the Equator. Lines of latitude circle the globe and never intersect one another; because of this, they are also called "parallels."

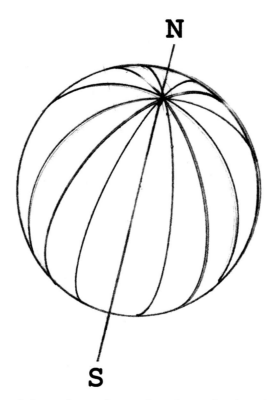

Figure 1.4.12 Longitudes are also called "meridians." They run from the North Pole to the South Pole. The longitude coordinate measures the angle, from the center of the Earth, east or west of 0° longitude, which is known as the Prime Meridian.

Longitude, also referred to as a *meridian,* is the angle measured from the center of the Earth west (up to 180° west) or east (up to 180° east) of 0° longitude—180° east and 180° west longitude are the same meridian. The term *meridian* comes from the Latin word *meri*—a variation of *medius* which denotes "middle", and *diem* which means "day". At noon, the Sun was said to be "passing meridian", and since all points on the same line of longitude experience noon at the same time they were said to be on the same meridian line, which became shortened to meridian. 0° Longitude is also called the *Prime Meridian,* and it runs through the Royal Astronomical Observatory in Greenwich, England (Fig. 1.4.10). The lines of longitude run north and south from the North Pole to the South Pole, and they measure the east-west coordinate (Fig. 1.4.12).

Some countries use a different prime meridian, which would be important to recognize if you are part of an IMSURT unit deployed to one of these countries. For our purposes, we will consider Greenwich, England, as the Prime Meridian, 0°.

11. How are the angular measurements of latitude and longitude expressed?

The angular measurements are expressed in *degrees, minutes,* and *seconds of arc.* A circle (i.e., the circumference of a sphere) is divided into 360°, so 1° represents 1/360th of the way around the circumference of the Earth. (Even though the Earth is not a perfect sphere, for our purposes we will consider it to be.) Minutes of arc and seconds of arc describe the fractions of a degree of arc. Each degree of arc contains 60 minutes of arc and each minute of arc contains 60 seconds of arc. The terms *degree of arc* (°), *minutes of arc* ('), and *seconds of arc* (") are shortened to *degrees, minutes,* and *seconds* (DMS). These minutes and seconds of *arc* are not to be confused with minutes and seconds of *time,* and their symbols are not to be confused with those for feet (') and inches (").

When describing a location, the descriptive "North" or "South" must be added to the latitude coordinate, and "East" or "West" must be added to the longitude coordinate. As an example, the coordinates for a location in Denver, Colorado, are as follows: 39° 45' 0" North and 104° 52' 12" West.

12. What is the relationship of distance to degrees, minutes, and seconds of arc?

A *great circle* is a circle drawn, in *any* direction, around the circumference of a sphere such that the plane of that circle passes through the center of the sphere. The Equator is a *great circle* as are all meridians part of a *great circle*, but lines of latitude (other than the Equator) circling the globe are not GREAT circles.

The circumference of the earth is about 24,880 statute miles. By dividing this circumference by 360, each *degree* around this circle (which is a *great circle*) equates to approximately 69 statute miles (5,280 feet/mile), or 60 nautical miles (6,080.27 feet/mile). As previously mentioned, 1° contains 60' of arc; as 1° equates to 60 nautical miles (on a *great circle*), then 1' equates to 1 nautical mile. The length for the nautical mile was chosen because it is practically the length of 1 minute of arc on a *great circle* of the Earth.

Because meridians run from pole to pole, the distance *between* meridians changes depending upon latitude (Fig. 1.4.13). At the poles where all meridians meet the distance has been reduced to a point, whereas at the equator (which is a *great circle*), the distance between two meridians 1° apart is 60 nautical miles.

At a given latitude, the distance between two meridians 1° apart can be determined by taking the cosine of that latitude and multiplying it by 1 nautical mile [Cos (latitude °) × 1 nautical mile = distance between 2 meridians 1° apart at that given latitude]. For example, at the Equator, the latitude is 0°, Cos 0 = 1; therefore, 1 × 1 nautical mile = 1 nautical mile between each degree of longitude. At the Poles, the latitude is 90°, Cos 90 = 0; therefore, 0 × 1 nautical mile = 0 nautical miles between each degree of longitude, which is readily apparent since the lines of longitude converge at the poles to a single point. At 60° latitude, Cos 60 = 0.5, therefore, the distance between two meridians 1° apart at latitude 60 is 0.5 × 1 nautical mile = 0.5 nautical mile. In other words, when traveling along latitude 60°, you will travel 0.5 nautical mile for every 1° change in longitude. Memorizing cosines is not practical, but understanding that distance **between** *longitudes* changes with latitude is important.

When traveling north or south **along** a *longitude*, one is on a *great circle*; therefore, each 1° of latitude change equates to 60 nautical miles. The distances **between** *latitudes* remain constant at 60 nautical miles per degree. This

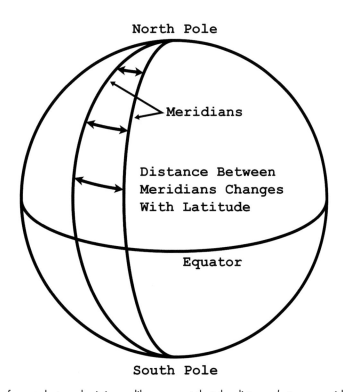

Figure 1.4.13 As longitudes run from pole to pole, it is readily apparent that the distance *between* meridians changes with latitude. At the Equator, a Great Circle, the distance between two longitudes 1° apart is 60 nautical miles. At the Poles, the meridians meet and the distance between them is reduced to a single point.

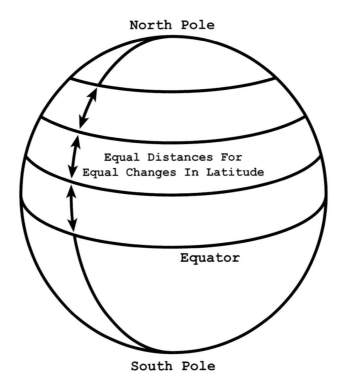

Figure 1.4.14 When traveling *along* a longitude (part of a Great Circle) the distance *between* latitudes remains constant at 60 nautical miles per degree of change. Because of this, latitude is used for all measurements of distances.

is the reason that latitude is used for taking off *all* measurements for distance, and dividers make quick work of this (Fig. 1.4.14).

The latitude/longitude system is really quite straightforward and easy to use. As with anything, the more you use a system, the more familiar and intuitive it becomes. It is important to understand the basics of latitude/longitude, because other coordinate systems have their basis in this system, and limitations and challenges of other systems can be appreciated in light of an understanding of the latitude/longitude system.

13. What is a grid coordinate system, and how does it work?

To avoid dealing with angular measurements of latitude and longitude (degrees, minutes, and seconds of arc), grid coordinate systems were developed that superimpose rectangles and squares (grids) onto a flat map projection of the Earth. Rectangular measurements describing distance in meters, relative to a designated origin, are used for the coordinates. This is known as a *Cartesian coordinate system.*

We will use the *Universal Transverse Mercator* (UTM) grid to explain how grid systems work and then discuss the *Military Grid Reference System* (MGRS) and the *United States National Grid* (USNG).

The *Universal Transverse Mercator Grid* (UTM Grid) system can be found on USGS maps. The UTM system places a grid onto a Transverse Mercator projection of the Earth. Trying to represent a spheroid object in a flat two-dimensional representation (i.e., transverse Mercator projection) still incurs some distortion and poses limitations on the ability to lay a single predictable grid system over the whole spheroid. Therefore, the UTM grid covers from 80° South latitude to 84° North latitude. A separate grid system, the Universal Polar Stereographic (UPS) grid, covers the North and South polar regions.

The UTM grid is created by making 60 *Zones* (6° of longitude wide), and 20 *Bands* (8° of latitude tall, with the most northerly band being 12° of latitude). The *Zones* are numbered from 1 through 60, starting at 180° West longitude and moving *easterly* around the globe. The *Bands* are lettered starting with the letter "C" at 80° South latitude and moving in a *northerly* direction through the letter "X." The letters "I" and "O" are not used, to avoid any misinterpretation as a "1" (one) or "0" (zero) (Fig. 1.4.15).

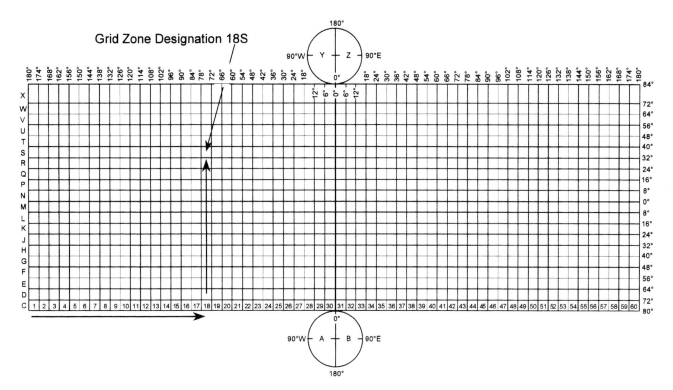

Figure 1.4.15 The UTM Grid, MGRS, and USNG systems use this underlying grid layout. The grid covers from 80° South latitude to 84° North latitude. There are 60 Zones, 6° of longitude wide, numbered 1 through 60 starting at 180° West longitude; moving in an easterly direction around the world. There are 20 Bands, 8° of latitude tall (Band "X" is 12°), lettered from "C" to "X" ("I" and "O" are not used). Each Zone number and Band letter provides a unique alphanumeric Grid Zone designation.

Coincidentally, *Band* "N" is from 0° latitude to 8° North latitude; therefore, it is easy to remember that "N" and any letter past "N" is in the Northern Hemisphere. Each, *Zone* number and *Band* letter provide a unique alphanumeric designation, from 1C to 60X, for each *Grid Zone*. (Note that the term *Grid Zone* refers to the rectangle formed by the 6° wide *Zone* **and** the 8° tall *Band* and is NOT to be confused with the term *Zone*, which refers to the whole 6° wide zone from 84° North latitude to 80° South latitude.) The 48 contiguous states of the U.S. fall within *Zones* 10 through 19 and *Bands* R, S, T, and U.

Each *Zone* is centered on a longitude, which is called its *Central Meridian*. Because each *Zone* spans 6° of longitude, the Central Meridian is 3° of longitude from either edge (Fig. 1.4.16). For example, *Zone* 13 is from 108° West longitude to 102° West longitude. The Central Meridian for *Zone* 13 is 105° West longitude.

EACH *Zone* is an independent Cartesian coordinate system that has its own *Origin*. The Origin for each *Zone* is where that *Zone's* Central Meridian crosses the Equator. In the UTM grid system, the Cartesian coordinates relate the number of meters west or east relative to the Central Meridian, and the number of meters north or south relative to the Equator.

The Central Meridian has been given the arbitrary value of 500,000 meters (m). Numbers less than 500,000 m indicate the coordinate is west of the Central Meridian, and numbers greater than 500,000 m indicate the coordinate is east of the Central Meridian. For the Northern Hemisphere, the Equator has been given the arbitrary value of 0 m, and heading toward the North Pole from the Equator, the values increase toward 10,000,000 m. For the Southern Hemisphere, the Equator is given the arbitrary value of 10,000,000 m, and as you head toward the South Pole, the numbers decrease toward 0 m (Fig. 1.4.17).

Why were these numbers chosen? The widest distance spanned by a *Zone* 6° of longitude wide (i.e., at the Equator) is less than 1,000,000 m, so by assigning the Central Meridian (the middle of the zone) a value of 500,000 m, this ensures that coordinates west of the Central Meridian will always be a positive number. By the same token, when working in the Southern Hemisphere, the distance between the Equator and 80° South latitude does not exceed 10,000,000 m. By assigning the Equator a value of 10,000,000 m, this ensures that coordinates in the Southern Hemisphere will always be a positive number. In addition to not having negative numbers, the coordinate numbers are *always* increasing as you move east within a zone and as you move north; this becomes important when determining grid coordinates.

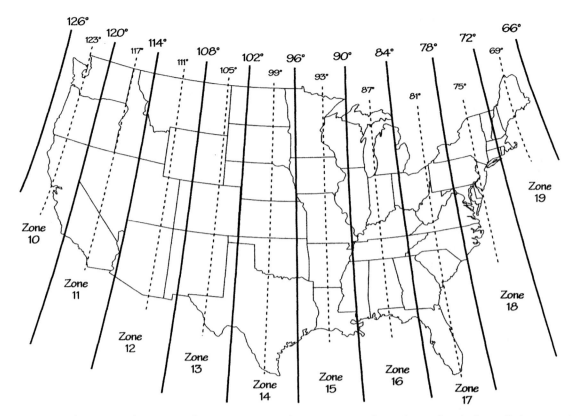

Figure 1.4.16 In the UTM Grid, MGRS, and USNG systems, each Zone is centered on a longitude, which is called its Central Meridian (*dashed lines*). The intersection of the Central Meridian and the Equator is termed the Origin of that Zone. (Illustration: Courtesy of *GPS Land Navigation*, 1997. Ferguson, Michael. Boise, ID: Glassford Publishing.)

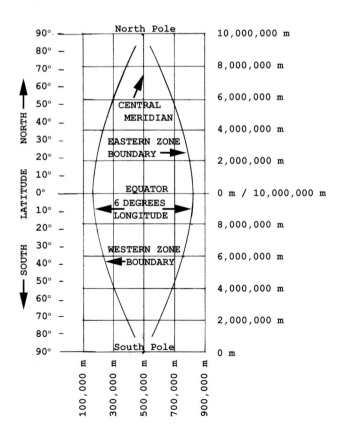

Figure 1.4.17 Each Zone, 6° of longitude wide, is an independent Cartesian coordinate system that has its own Origin where the Central Meridian crosses the Equator. The Central Meridian is given the arbitrary value of 500,000 m, and the Equator is given the arbitrary value of 0 m or 10,000,000 m depending on whether one is working in the Northern or Southern Hemisphere, respectively. Grid coordinates relate the number of meters east or west of the Central Meridian and the number of meters north or south of the Equator.

On a map, grid lines will either be drawn in completely or their position noted by blue tick marks in the margins. On most maps, these "working" grid lines form 1,000 m × 1,000 m squares (Fig. 1.4.9).

To use the UTM grid system and determine the grid coordinates of a location on the map, the grid lines must be present on the map. If you have a map that has just the blue tick marks in the margins, you should find a large flat area and, using a straight edge, lightly draw in the lines connecting the tick marks, thus creating a complete grid. (It is best to do this before you have to use the map in the field.)

The numbers along the top and bottom margins of the map next to each blue line or tick mark running "vertically" relate, in meters, the position of that line relative to the Central Meridian. Coordinates relating to the Central Meridian are termed *Easting Coordinates*. As previously mentioned, any number less than 500,000 m is west of the Central Meridian, and any number greater than 500,000 m is east of the Central Meridian. Regardless of whether a coordinate lies east or west of the Central Meridian, it is still referred to as the Easting Coordinate. For example, 355,000 mE means that grid line is at 355,000 m, which also means it is 145,000 m west of the Central Meridian (500,000 m − 355,000 m = 145,000 m), and the "E" stands for Easting Coordinate.

The numbers in the left- and right-hand margins of the map next to each blue line or tick mark running "horizontally" relate, in meters, the position of that line relative to the Equator. Coordinates relating to the Equator are termed *Northing Coordinates* regardless of whether the coordinate lies north or south of the Equator (Fig. 1.4.18).

To determine if a coordinate is in the Northern or Southern Hemisphere, one must look at the *Band* letter of the *Grid Zone*. C-M are Southern Hemisphere *Bands* and N-X are Northern Hemisphere *Bands*. For example, 13T 4535000mN means that grid line is 4,535,000 m north of the Equator, and the "N" stands for Northing Coordinate. 13F 4535000mN means that grid line is in the Southern Hemisphere and is 5,465,000 m south of the Equator (10,000,000 m − 4,535,000 m = 5,465,000 m), and the "N" still refers to Northing Coordinate.

Because *each Zone* is a separate coordinate system, and the Central Meridian and Equator were arbitrarily given their values of 500,000 m and 0 m/10,000,000 m, respectively, the Origin is also referred to as *False Origin*; and because the meter distances are related to this False Origin, the terms *False Easting and False Northing* are sometimes used as well.

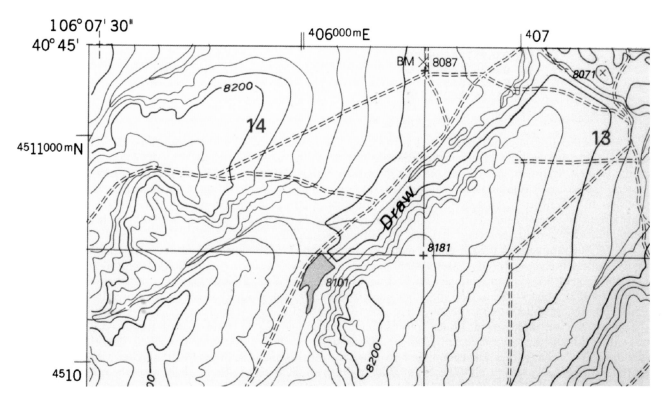

Figure 1.4.18 The numbers associated with the UTM grid lines (or tick marks, as on this USGS topographic map) are the UTM coordinates for that grid line. In this figure, the Easting Coordinates are 406000 mE and 407, and the Northing Coordinates are 4511000 mN and 4510. Note the latitude and longitude (40°45' and 106°07'30" respectively) in the upper left corner margin.

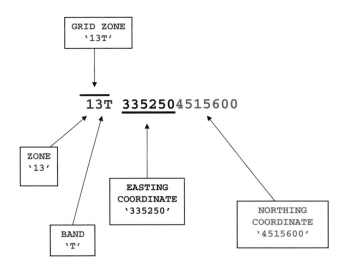

Figure 1.4.19 UTM grid coordinate dissected. The Grid Zone is written first and establishes the Zone and Band of the coordinates. The Grid Zone makes it a unique location. The Easting and Northing Coordinates are written in a continuous stream with the Easting Coordinate always written first. Note that the Easting Coordinate contains one less number than the Northing Coordinate. This set of coordinates is carried out to the "ones place column" so this coordinate denotes a square 1 m × 1 m.

Table 1.4.1 For the Easting and Northing Coordinates, the "place column" described is highlighted in red. The "millions" place column for the Easting Coordinate will always have a value of "0" and therefore it is not written when recording UTM coordinates, but one should appreciate that technically it is present. Each successive place column represents a 10-fold change in the size or resolution of the square that the coordinates describe. Grid coordinates printed in the map margins associated with the grid lines are carried out to the "ones" place column.

UTM Coordinate	Place Column
13T 03625184535270	Ones
13T 03625184535270	Tens
13T 03625184535270	Hundreds
13T 03625184535270	Thousands
13T 03625184535270	Ten Thousands
13T 03625184535270	Hundred Thousands
13T 03625184535270	Millions

When recording grid coordinates, the Easting Coordinate is given first, and the Northing Coordinate is given second. These numbers are written in a continuous stream, so by convention, the first "half" of the numbers relates to the Central Meridian, and the second "half" of the numbers relates to the Equator (Fig. 1.4.19). In the UTM system, the Easting Coordinate is *recorded* with one less digit than the Northing Coordinate; because an Easting Coordinate will never reach 1,000,000 m, the "millions" place column will always have a value of "0" and, therefore, it is generally not written. Rather than record an Easting Coordinate as 0500000 m, it is recorded as 500000 m. One should appreciate that the "0" is there technically.

The UTM coordinates in the margins of maps are often abbreviated and printed in such a way that the "principle digits" representing the 1,000 m and 10,000 m place columns are accentuated—**bolded** and/or made slightly larger (Table 1.4.1). As an example, an Easting Coordinate of 335,000 mE may be printed in the margin as 335000 mE, or abbreviated to 335 m. A Northing Coordinate of 4,516,000 mN may be printed in the margin as 4516000 mN, or abbreviated to 4516 m (Fig. 1.4.18). These abbreviated coordinates still represent a coordinate that has been "measured" to the "ones" place column and should not be confused with truncated coordinates.

Grid coordinates specify the *lower left* corner of a square, but they are actually *describing* that **square** and not just the point of that corner. Depending on how exact the measurement is, the size of that square may be as small as 1 m × 1 m or as large as 100,000 m × 100,000 m. One can tell the size of the square from the number of digits reported in each coordinate (Table 1.4.2). If 14 digits are used (i.e., 7 digits in the Easting Coordinate—remember the "0" in the millions column is technically there—and 7 digits in the Northing Coordinate), the measurement has been carried out 7 places to the "ones column," so that coordinate is describing a square 1 m × 1 m.

Table 1.4.2 The number of digits or "place columns" recorded in the coordinate corresponds to the size of the square described. Grid coordinates **specify** the lower left corner of a square, but they are actually describing the square as a whole. In other words, if a point of interest is noted by a set of coordinates carried out to the "hundreds" place column, this establishes a square 100 m × 100 m, and the point of interest is somewhere within that square.

UTM Coordinate	Zone	Band	Easting Coordinate	Northing Coordinate	Size of the Square
13T 3345484514297	13	T	334548	4514297	1 m × 1 m
13T 33454451429	13	T	33454	451429	10 m × 10 m
13T 334545142	13	T	3345	45142	100 m × 100 m
13T 3344514	13	T	334	4514	1,000 m × 1,000 m
13T 33451	13	T	33	451	10,000 m × 10,000 m
13T 345	13	T	3	45	100,000 m × 100,000 m

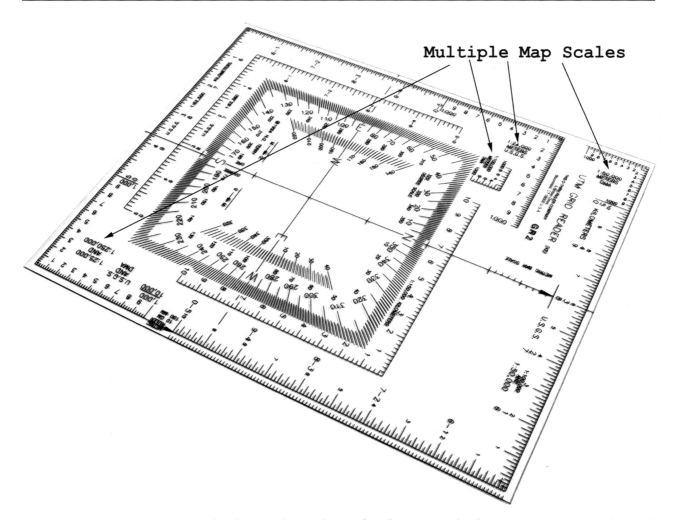

Figure 1.4.20 Grid readers are used to determine the coordinates of smaller squares within the 1,000 m × 1,000 m "working" grid squares printed on USGS topographic maps and other maps such as National Geographic Trails Illustrated™ maps. This commercial grid reader has multiple scales present, making it useful for a variety of maps of differing scales.

As previously mentioned, a common size for working grid squares on maps is 1,000 m × 1,000 m. *Grid readers* are used to determine the coordinates of a smaller square within these 1,000 m × 1,000 m squares (Fig. 1.4.20). How small a square the grid reader can determine is based on the scale of the map. For most maps, the scale is such that a grid reader can discern a point that describes a 10 m × 10 m square; for this reason, the "ones" place will frequently be recorded as "0." When using a grid reader, the scale of the grid reader must match the scale of the map (Fig. 1.4.21).

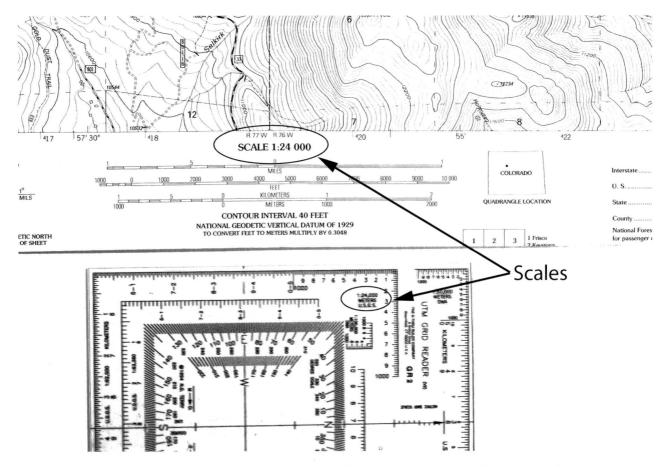

Figure 1.4.21 The scale of the grid reader must match the scale of the map. Here, the scale of this USGS quadrangle is 1:24,000 and a corresponding scale is present on the grid reader.

If a commercially made grid reader is not available or it does not match the scale on your map, it is very simple to make your own grid reader (Fig. 1.4.22).

1. Take a blank white card or piece of paper.
2. Align the upper right corner of your paper to the upper right corner of a grid square on your map.
3. Mark the upper left edge of the grid's square on your paper. This will become the horizontal axis.
4. Mark the lower right edge of the grid's square on your paper. This will become the vertical axis.
5. Place marks dividing these axes into tenths, which represent 100 meter increments.

To obtain grid coordinates, place the corner of the grid reader on the *lower left corner* of the square that contains the location in which you are interested (Fig. 1.4.23). The grid coordinates for this corner (i.e., intersection of grid lines) are found in the margins of the map. Next, move the corner of the grid reader to the *right* along the (bottom) horizontal line of the square in an *easterly* direction until aligned with your location. Next, move the grid reader *upward* in a *northerly* direction to intersect your location of interest. The horizontal axis of the grid reader tells you the number of meters to add to the lower left corner's Easting grid line value. This is termed *easting*, and this will be the location's Easting Coordinate. The vertical axis of the grid reader tells you the number of meters to add to the lower left corner's Northing grid line. This is termed *northing*, and this will be the location's Northing Coordinate. This process is often referred to as "read right—then up" (Fig. 1.4.24).

While a grid reader (commercial or homemade) offers a certain level of accuracy, one of the advantages of the UTM grid system is that coordinates can be estimated within a 1,000 m × 1,000 m grid square without the need for *any* special equipment. One can simply "eyeball" along the horizontal axis and up the vertical axis to a location and obtain a quick and reasonably accurate measure (to within approximately 50–100 m) of the coordinates for that location.

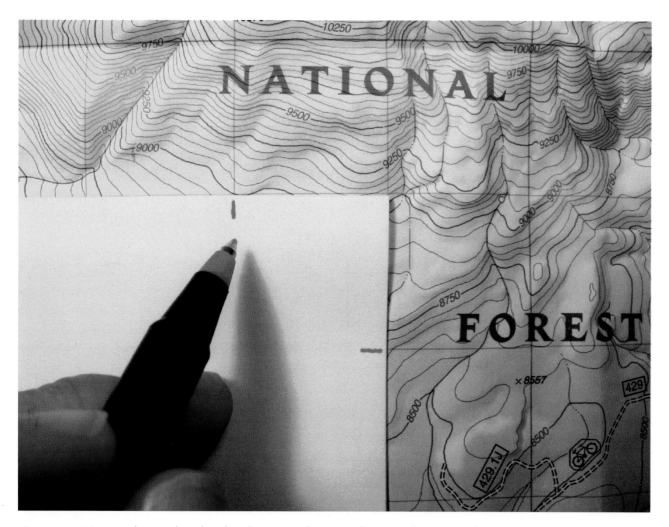

Figure 1.4.22 To make a grid reader, align the upper right corner of a piece of paper with the upper right corner of a 1,000 m × 1,000 m grid square on your map. Mark the upper left edge of the square on your paper, which will become the horizontal axis, and the lower right edge of the square, which will become the vertical axis. Divide these axes into tenths, which represent 100 m increments. If a kilometer bar scale is present on the map, it may display 100 m increments, which facilitates the division of your grid reader axes. (Map: Courtesy of National Geographic Trails Illustrated Map™ Hahns Peak Steamboat Lake Colorado, USA.)

14. Provide a summary of how the UTM grid system works.

- A grid is superimposed over a flat Transverse Mercator map projection of the Earth.
- The grid consists of *Zones:* 6° of longitude wide, which are numbered from 1 to 60 starting at 180° West longitude and proceeding in an easterly direction, and *Bands:* 8° of latitude tall (12° for band "X"), which are lettered from C to X starting at 80° South latitude and moving north to 84° North latitude. (Letters "I" and "O" are not used.)
- The *Grid Zones* are identified by their *Zone* number and *Band* letter, for example 13T.
- Each *Zone* is an independent Cartesian coordinate system with its own Origin.
- Each *Zone* is centered on a line of longitude that is called the Central Meridian.
- The Origin for each *Zone* is where the Central Meridian crosses the Equator.
- Coordinates in the UTM grid system describe, in meters, a position east or west of the Central Meridian, and a position north or south of the Equator.
- The Central Meridian is given the arbitrary value of 500,000 m. The Equator is given the arbitrary value of 0 m when working in the Northern Hemisphere, and 10,000,000 m when working in the Southern Hemisphere.
- The coordinate that describes the position east or west of the Central Meridian is called the Easting Coordinate, and it is recorded first.

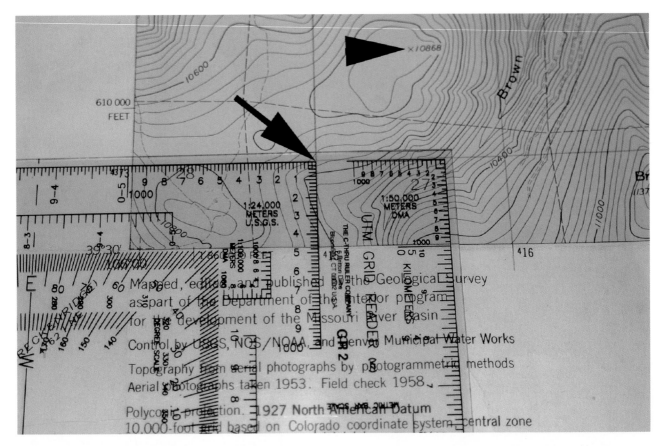

Figure 1.4.23 Figures 1.4.23 and 1.4.24 demonstrate how to obtain grid coordinates. This is a USGS quadrangle; lightly drawn pencil lines connect the UTM blue tick marks to complete the 1,000 m × 1,000 m grid squares. The grid reader scaled "1:24,000 METERS U.S.G.S." has been selected as it corresponds to this map's scale. In this example, the point of interest is the peak of a mountain, "× 10868" (*arrowhead*). The lower left corner of the square containing the point of interest is identified (*arrow*) and the coordinates of these grid lines noted. Although difficult to see through the writing on the grid reader, the Easting Coordinate is 415 (i.e., 415,000 mE), and the Northing Coordinate is 4373 (i.e., 4,373,000 mN). The corner of the grid reader is placed on this lower left corner and will be moved easterly and northerly to intersect the point of interest.

- The coordinate that describes the position north or south of the Equator is called the Northing Coordinate, and it is recorded second.
- Coordinates identify the lower left corner of a square. The size of this square is determined by the number of digits used to describe the coordinate. The more digits, the more exact is the measurement and therefore, the smaller the square.
- To determine a position on a map, grid lines forming squares (typically 1,000 m × 1,000 m) need to be drawn on the map.
- The meter values for these established grid lines are recorded in the margins of the map.
- A grid reader (either commercially available or home made) is used to determine a position within a particular 1,000 m × 1,000 m square.
- The grid reader must be in the same scale as the map.
- The corner of the grid reader is placed on the lower left corner of the square that contains the location of interest, and these coordinates are noted.
- "READ RIGHT THEN UP": The grid reader is moved to the right (in an easterly direction) until aligned with the point of interest, and the grid reader is then moved upward (in a northerly direction) to intersect the point of interest. The meters on the horizontal scale are added to the Easting Coordinate of the 1,000 m × 1,000 m square, and the meters on the vertical scale are added to the Northing Coordinate of the 1,000 m × 1,000 m square.
- The complete coordinate is recorded as *Grid Zone* Easting Coordinate Northing Coordinate (*Map Datum*, to be complete).

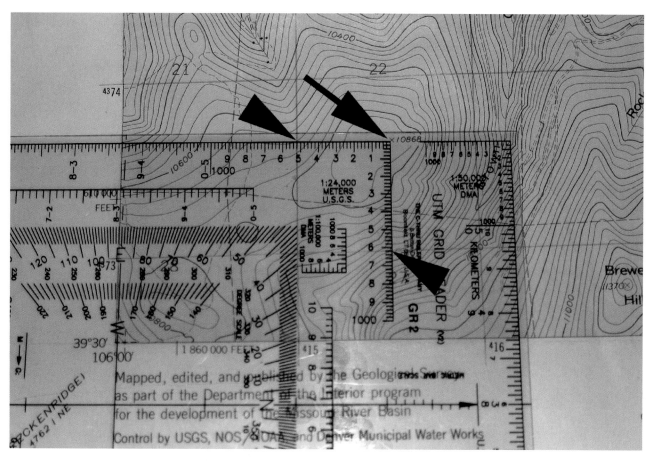

Figure 1.4.24 As noted in Figure 1.4.23, the grid reader is moved easterly and northerly ("read right—then up") until the corner of the grid reader intersects " × 10868" (*arrow*). The horizontal axis of the grid reader intersects the grid line of the 1,000 m × 1,000 m square (*upper arrowhead*) and indicates 520 m are to be added to the Easting grid coordinate, 415,520mE. The vertical axis of the grid reader intersects the grid line of the 1,000 m × 1,000 m square (*lower arrowhead*) and indicates 620 m are to be added to the Northing grid coordinate, 4,373,620mN. The complete UTM coordinate for peak " × 10868" is 13S 4155204373620.

15. How does the Military Grid Reference System (MGRS) differ from the UTM grid system?

The MGRS is similar to the UTM grid system. It uses the same *Zone* designations (1–60) and the same *Band* designations (C through X, no "I" or "O"), and therefore the same *Grid Zone* designations (Fig. 1.4.15). The difference is that, in each *Grid Zone*, there is an additional grid of 100,000 m × 100,000 m squares. Each of these squares is given a two-letter designation. The first letter refers to the Easting Coordinate, and the second letter refers to the Northing Coordinate. This is called the *100,000 m Square Identification* (Fig. 1.4.25).

These squares are labeled starting with the letter "A" in the lower left corner of a *Grid Zone* and proceeding through the alphabet as you move east and north; again, "I" and "O" are not used. The *Grid Zone* designation is required to make these 100,000 m × 100,000 m squares unique, as the two-letter 100,000 m Square Identifications repeat themselves about every 18° (approximately 1,000 nautical miles). The 100,000 m Square Identification (or Identifications if the map extends into another 100,000 m × 100,000 m square) will be printed in the map legend (Fig. 1.4.26).

The 100,000 m Square Identification *replaces* the digits in the "hundred thousands" place columns of a UTM coordinate. (To demonstrate this more clearly, a "/" has been placed between the Easting Coordinate and the Northing Coordinate.)

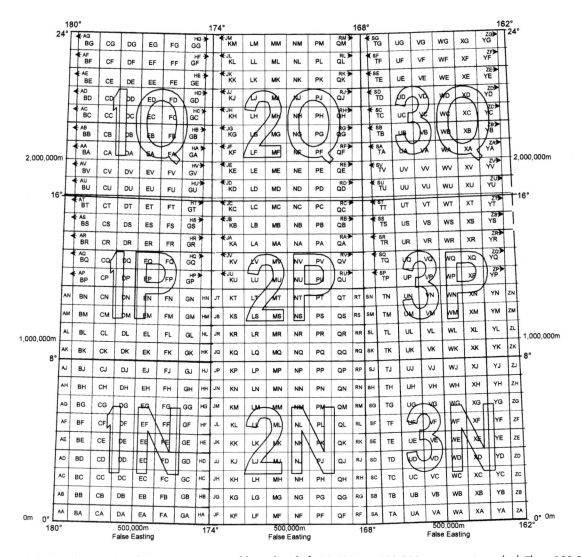

Figure 1.4.25 In the MGRS and USNG systems, an additional grid of 100,000 m × 100,000 m squares is applied. These 100,000 m × 100,000 m squares are given a two-letter designation (AA, BA, CA, AB, AC, etc.), called the 100,000 m Square Identification. The larger alphanumeric labels, 1 N, 2 N, 1P, etc., are the Grid Zone designations.

- UTM coordinate   15S 362518/2135270

The 300,000 and 2,100,000 are replaced with L and G, respectively, resulting in:

- MGRS coordinate   15S LG62518/35270

Note that the remaining digits are still the same, and in the MGRS system the Easting value and the Northing value have the same number of digits, in this case 5 × 5. In the UTM grid system, 14 digits describes a square 1 m × 1 m; in the MGRS grid system, 10 digits describes a square 1 m × 1 m, as the ones, tens, hundreds, thousands, and ten thousands place columns are the same as in the UTM system (Table 1.4.3).

Finding a location using the MGRS system is similar to using the UTM grid system. To pinpoint the above coordinates on a map: First, identify *Grid Zone* 15S → Find the 100,000 m × 100,000 m Square Identification labeled LG → on the 1,000 m × 1,000 m grid lines on the map → I identify the Easting grid line **62** and the Northing grid line **35** → Place the grid reader where these lines intersect → Move right (east) 518 m and up (north) 270 m.

Just as other coordinate systems relate to the map datum on which they are based, so, too, does the MGRS coordinate system. As the MGRS has developed over the years, changes have been made to it as map datums have

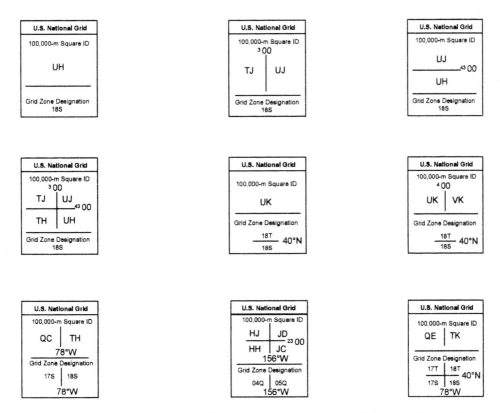

Figure 1.4.26 Maps may cover single or multiple 100,000 m × 100,000 m squares, Grid Zones, and Zones. Here are some examples detailing how this information may be displayed in the map legend.

Table 1.4.3 This table demonstrates the relationship between UTM grid coordinates and MGRS/USNG coordinates. Not including the Grid Zone designation (15S), the letters and numbers in black correspond to the Easting Coordinate, and the letters and numbers in red correspond to the Northing Coordinate. Note that the "hundred thousands" place columns of the UTM coordinate are replaced with the two letters of the 100,000 m Square Identification. This table also relates the size of the square described by these coordinate systems to the number of place columns recorded

Square Size	UTM Coordinate	MGRS/USNG Coordinate
1 m × 1 m	15S 3625182135270	15S LG6251835270
10 m × 10 m	15S 36251213527	15S LG62513527
100 m × 100 m	15S 362521352	15S LG625352
1,000 m × 1,000 m	15S 3622135	15S LG6235
10,000 m × 10,000 m	15S 36213	15S LG63
100,000 m × 100,000 m	15S 321	15S LG

changed. Here in the United States, in an effort to make the coordinate differences more obvious between the "old MGRS" using map datum NAD 27 and the "new MGRS" using WGS 84, the Northing letters in the 100,000 m Square Identifications were "shifted" 10 letters. A square identified as UT when using NAD 27 is now identified as UH with map datum WGS 84. Once again, this highlights the importance of (1) stating the map datum on every map, (2) noting the map datum of a recorded or reported coordinate, and (3) checking that map and GPS receiver are operating in the same map datum.

16. What is the United States National Grid (USNG)?

In 1997, a group of citizens formed the Public XY Mapping Project, as a nonprofit science and education corporation dedicated to the development and implementation of spatial addressing (i.e., another grid system) in the United

States. This private group approached the federal government with a proposal to develop and establish standards for a national system. The Federal Geographic Data Committee (FGDC) and National Spatial Data Infrastructure (NSDI) Standards Working Group published the standards for the USNG in December 2001.

The USNG uses the same *Zones*, *Bands*, two letter 100,000 m Square Identification, and UTM metric system as the MGRS. The FGDC established the standard datum for USNG coordinates to be North American Datum 83 (NAD 83), which correlates well in the United States with the MGRS using World Geodetic System 84 (WGS 84). One of the proposed benefits of the USNG system is that during a disaster, civilian and military responders would be operating in essentially compatible systems, which would facilitate communication of location coordinates between these two entities. An attempt is under way to encourage everyone to "add" the USNG coordinates to their home, business, etc. address information; in a disaster, these coordinates would be used to guide responders to a location. Older GPS units may not have "USNG" as a coordinates (position format) menu option, but they may have "MGRS" listed. Selecting "MGRS" and Map Datum WGS 84 would allow a responder to report GPS coordinates compatible with USNG coordinates.

17. What is the difference between "truncating" and "rounding" of digits?

When decreasing the resolution of the square that your coordinates are describing, the affected column(s) is(are) eliminated. For example, going from a 1 m × 1 m square to a 10 m × 10 m square, the "ones" column is eliminated. If "rounding," the "tens" column stays the same when the "ones" column is less than 5, but it would increase if the "ones" column was 5 to 9. In "truncating," the "ones" column is dropped and the "tens" column does not change regardless of the value in the "ones" column (Table 1.4.4). **In UTM, MRGS, and USNG grid systems, the proper method is to** *truncate*.

Table 1.4.4   This table uses an MGRS/USNG coordinate to demonstrate the difference between Rounding (incorrect) and Truncating (correct) coordinates. The same principle applies to UTM grid coordinates as well. In this example, the "ones" column is underlined and the "tens" column is in red. When the resolution of a square is decreased, in this example from 1 m × 1 m to 10 m × 10 m, note that the "tens" column of the Easting Coordinate changes to "8" if Rounding, but remains the same, "7", when Truncating. Because coordinates identify the lower left corner of the square, but are actually describing that square as a whole, rounding results in a shift of the entire square. Therefore, the correct method for decreasing resolution is to truncate; the square is getting bigger, but it does not move.

Coordinate 1 m × 1 m square	Rounding 10 m × 10 m square	Truncating 10 m × 10 m square
11T NJ6457629733	11T NJ64582973	11T NJ64572973

18. What are "legal descriptions"?

Legal descriptions are primarily used for real estate purposes. They describe a piece of property in relation to previously established range and section markers. These legal descriptions should NOT be used by emergency or disaster personnel to communicate location.

19. What is the difference between True north, Magnetic north, and Grid north?

True north refers to the geographic North Pole, where the axis, upon which the Earth rotates, "exits" the Earth. All lines of longitude meet at this point, and therefore, all lines of longitude run in a True north direction (Fig. 1.4.12).

Basically, *Magnetic north* is what a compass points to as "north" and this has to do with the Earth acting as a magnet. A magnetic field is produced by electrical currents that originate in the outer core of the Earth, which results in one end of a magnet being in the north and the other end in the south. The north end of this magnet attracts a magnetized needle (i.e., compass needle) to point to it, and so it is called Magnetic north. Changes in natural conditions affect the electrical currents and therefore the magnetic field. Because of this, Magnetic north moves around approximately 10 kilometers (km) per year.

The angle between True north and Magnetic north is called the *magnetic declination*. This is also referred to as *magnetic variation*. (Declination/variation should not be confused with *deviation*, which has to do with a compass needle deviating away from Magnetic north because of local magnetic disturbance.) Depending on where you are, the declination will be either east or west of True north (i.e., Magnetic north will be either east or west of True north) (Fig. 1.4.27).

Grid north describes the relationship between a vertical grid line and True north. When a rectangular grid is applied to a *Zone* 6° of longitude wide, the vertical lines of the grid will not align with the outlying lines of longitude in the *Zone*, as the longitude lines *appear* to "curve" to meet at the North Pole. Only on the Central Meridian will the direction of a vertical grid line and the longitude match. As **all** lines of longitude run in a True north direction, the angle of the vertical grid line (Grid north) relative to True north is called *grid declination* (Fig. 1.4.28). West of the Central Meridian, Grid north will be west of True north and grid declination will be west. East of the Central Meridian, Grid north will be east of True north and the grid declination will be east.

True north, Magnetic north, and Grid north will be detailed on USGS maps (Fig. 1.4.3). Because Magnetic north moves, the magnetic declination may be out of date on older maps. Current declination information is available at http://www.ngs.noah.gov.

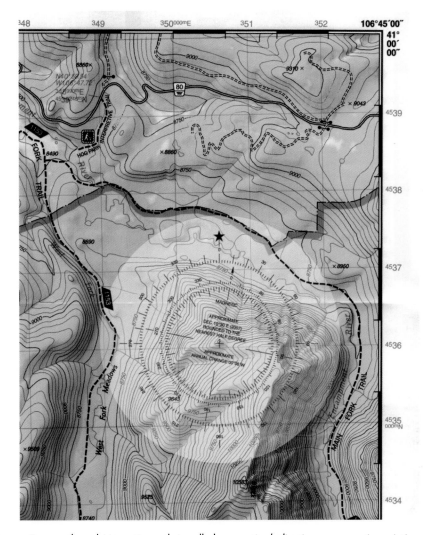

Figure 1.4.27 The angle between True north and Magnetic north is called *magnetic declination* or *magnetic variation*. This may be noted on a map with a "Compass Rose" (named for their "rose" color on nautical charts) highlighted here. The True north azimuth compass is on the outer ring, and the Magnetic north azimuth compass is on the inner ring. (Map: Courtesy of National Geographic Trails Illustrated Map™ Hahns Peak Steamboat Lake Colorado, USA.)

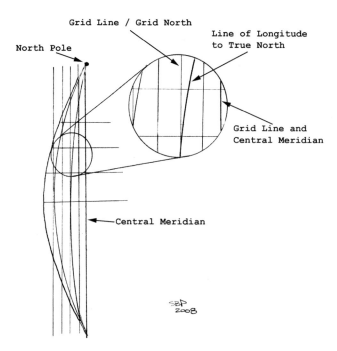

Figure 1.4.28 This illustration of one-half of a Zone demonstrates the relationship of a flat grid to the spheroid Earth. Lines of longitude run from pole to pole and therefore indicate True north. The vertical lines of the grid will not align with the outlying lines of longitude. This angle between a grid line indicating Grid north and True north is called *grid declination*. Grid north and True north are the same on the Central Meridian.

COMPASS

20. What is a compass?

In its simplest form, a *compass* is an instrument that allows a free swinging magnetized needle to point toward Magnetic north. The function of a compass is to determine direction which can be used to plan a direction of travel or to determine a location.

Horizontal direction from one point to another point is called the *azimuth*. An azimuth compass circle is divided into 360°. By convention, north is 0°; moving *clockwise*, east is 90°, south is 180°, west is 270°, and back around to north is 360°. 0° and 360° are the same direction, north (Fig. 1.4.29). The azimuth describes direction as an angle relative to north, always in a clockwise direction (Fig. 1.4.30). It is important to note that latitude/longitude is also a system based on a 360° circle, but it is separate from the "compass system" using a 360° circle to describe direction.

Other types of compasses may divide the circle differently, such as 6,400 Mils used by the military. (Note the "Mils" information on the declination legend in a topo map margin; Fig.1.4.3.)

21. To which "north" (True, Magnetic, or Grid) does the azimuth relate?

Since azimuth describes direction as an angle relative to "north," it is important to indicate which "north" is being used. "True," "Magnetic," or "Grid" must be stated with the azimuth (e.g., 90° True, 20° Magnetic, 0° Grid, etc.). This is very important because *maps* are based on True north, and *compasses* are based on Magnetic north, so a responder must be comfortable translating azimuths back and forth between True, Magnetic, and/or Grid.

For example, the area you are working in has a magnetic declination of 13° East. When your *compass* points to "north," 0° on the compass housing, it is pointing to Magnetic north. This direction is 0° Magnetic. The declination tells us that Magnetic north is 13° East of True north, so as an azimuth related to True north it is 13° True.

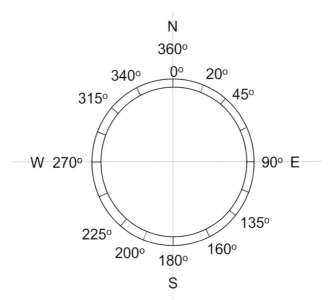

Figure 1.4.29 Horizontal direction from one point to another is called the *azimuth*. An azimuth compass circle is divided into 360°. By convention, north is 0°; turning clockwise, east is 90°, south is 180°, and west is 270°, circling back around to north at 360°/0°.

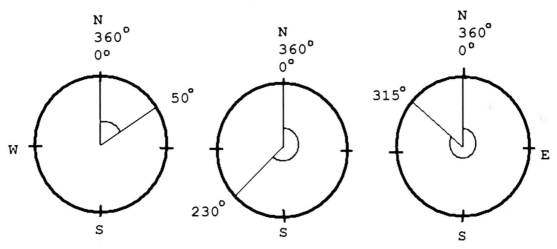

Figure 1.4.30 North is both 0° and 360°. Azimuths describe direction as an angle relative to north. On an azimuth compass this angle is always in a clockwise direction.

If your compass shows a heading of 110°, this is 110° Magnetic, which translates to 123° True. Conversely, your map indicates the direction to your base camp from your current location is 270° True. The direction on the compass that you would follow to arrive at base would be 257° Magnetic.

As another example, the area you are working in has a magnetic declination of 10° West. When your *compass* points to "north," 0° on the compass housing, it is pointing to Magnetic north. This direction is 0° Magnetic. The declination tells us that Magnetic north is 10° West of True north, so as an azimuth related to True north, it is 350° True. If your compass shows a heading of 40°, this is 40° Magnetic, which corresponds to 30° True. On your map, if the direction to the Command Post (CP) from your current location is 60° True, the compass direction that you would follow to arrive at the CP would be 70° Magnetic.

"Compass to True, add East" is a phrase to help you remember when to add or subtract. When the magnetic declination is "East," add the declination to the compass azimuth to obtain the corresponding true azimuth. Accounting for grid declination is handled in the same way.

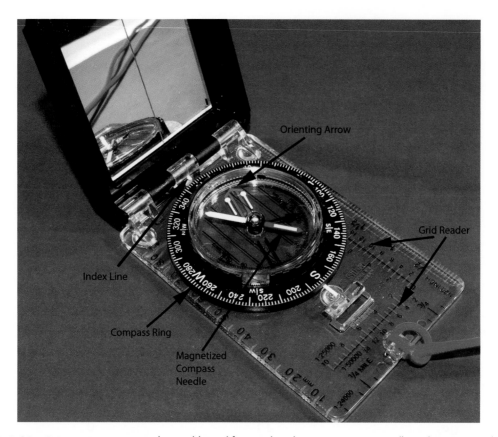

Figure 1.4.31 Orienteering compasses have additional features besides just a compass needle and 360° azimuth circle. The *orienting arrow* and *index line* are used for determining bearings. Using the mirror increases accuracy when taking a sighting on an object. Some orienteering compasses will have a large arrow on the base plate indicating "Direction of Travel." On this particular compass, the compass is oriented so that the hinge of the cover is toward the "Direction of Travel."

When working with map and compass, azimuths will have to be translated back and forth, so it is paramount to indicate whether an azimuth is True, Magnetic, or Grid. In addition to stating True, Magnetic, or Grid, it may be helpful in a disaster to establish a standard operating procedure (SOP) that azimuths be reported in "True" format. Even if an SOP is in place, the word "True" should be added to avoid any confusion.

Some orienteering compasses can be adjusted to account for declination. This eliminates having to make any calculations when working between map (True) and compass (Magnetic), and all azimuths will be "True." This "heading reference" option is also available on GPS receivers. If you are using another compass in addition to the compass in a GPS receiver, confirm that both are "operating" in the same "heading reference."

22. What are some other features available on an "orienteering compass"?

An orienteering compass will have features besides a compass needle and 360° azimuth circle (Fig. 1.4.31). These may include:

- Compass Ring or Housing
- Base plate
- Index line
- Orienting arrow
- Direction of travel arrow
- Grid reader
- Mirror (to assist in taking accurate sightings)

There are a variety of brands and styles of compasses that are of excellent quality and a good value.

23. How does one use a compass to determine direction?

For this discussion, we will simplify the steps by having 0° magnetic declination; in other words, True north and Magnetic north are the same. (If they are not the same, then the additional steps converting magnetic azimuths [compass readings] to true azimuths [map readings], and vice versa, must be done.)

To determine an azimuth, (also called a *"bearing,"*) on a map:

- Draw a line on the map between two points, A and B. Point A is where you are starting from, and point B is where you want to finish.
- Place the edge of the *base plate* of the compass along this line, with the *direction of travel arrow* directed toward point B.
- Turn the compass housing until the *orienting arrow* points True north on the map. The degree mark lined up with the *index line* will be the bearing **from** point A **to** point B.

To determine a bearing in the field:

- Pick a point or object (tree, mountain top, building, etc.) to which you want to determine the bearing.
- Orient the compass so that the *direction of travel arrow* is pointing away from you and toward that point.
- Carefully sight in your point or object.
- Turn the compass housing so that the north end of the compass needle lines up inside the *orienting arrow*.
- The degree marking lined up with the *index line* will be the bearing to that object.

To orient yourself on a bearing:

- Orient the compass so that the *direction of travel arrow* is pointing away from you.
- Turn the compass housing so that your desired bearing is lined up with the *index line*.
- Turn your body until the north end of the compass needle lines up inside the *orienting arrow*. You will now be facing your desired bearing.

If you are trying to follow a specific bearing, generally it is easier to identify an object (a tree, building, etc.) on that bearing; walk to it; sight the bearing again and identify another object on that bearing and walk to it, etc.

24. What is a reciprocal bearing?

Sighting in one direction determines the azimuth or bearing. The exact opposite direction is 180° from that bearing and is called the *reciprocal bearing*. Reciprocal bearings are used to determine one's position. If the azimuth from point A to point B is 90° True, then the reciprocal bearing from point B to point A is 270° True. If the bearing from point A to point B is 324° True, then the reciprocal bearing from point B to point A is 144° True.

25. How can one find their location on a map using a compass?

Triangulate position or *triangulation* refers to finding one's location on a map. Bearings and reciprocal bearings are used to triangulate position. Triangulation is done by determining the azimuth from you to two separate and distinct points that are identifiable on your map—for example, two separate mountain peaks. These three points, your position plus the two bearing points, form a triangle, hence the term *triangulation*.

The bearings to the separate points are converted to reciprocal bearings so that these lines of direction can be drawn on the map FROM these points TO you. These two lines will intersect, and that intersection is your location. Sighting on more than two points will improve the accuracy of determining your position.

GLOBAL POSITIONING SYSTEM (GPS)

26. What is GPS?

GPS stands for *global positioning system*. A GPS receiver provides the coordinates of your location.

GPS is a navigation system that utilizes satellites to send radio signals from space that are received by a GPS receiver and converted into position, velocity, and time. The radio waves sent by the satellites are electromagnetic energy traveling at the speed of light, approximately 186,000 miles per second. The term "acquired" is used when a GPS receiver picks up a satellite's radio signal. The GPS receiver calculates how far the radio signal traveled by timing how long it took the signal to arrive from a given satellite, thus determining the distance between the satellite and the GPS receiver. Satellites are placed in six orbital planes with at least four satellites in each plane, and each satellite orbits the Earth in 12 hours. This satellite arrangement allows a GPS receiver to acquire four to eight satellites from any point on Earth at any given time, thereby determining its position by calculating the distance to each satellite.

27. How accurate is a GPS position?

Our GPS navigational satellite system was developed by the U.S. Department of Defense (DOD) and then made available to civilians. The system has two levels of accuracy: a standard level of accuracy for civilian use and a more precise level for use by the military. The standard level has an accuracy of about 100 m horizontally, 150 m vertically, and 340 nanoseconds. Since it was first made available to civilians, the DOD has allowed for greater accuracy in the civilian system by implementing WAAS.

28. What is WAAS?

WAAS stands for *wide area augmentation system*. These are special satellites that the GPS receiver uses to produce a more accurate position fix. WAAS satellites transmit data for correction differentials in the GPS satellite signals. Using WAAS increases accuracy to approximately 3 m. A GPS receiver must be *enabled* to receive data from the WAAS satellites. On the Satellite Page of a GPS receiver, WAAS satellites are displayed with numbers of 33 or greater.

29. Describe the different features available on GPS Receivers.

Technically, the GPS system provides a position and reports this position as coordinates. Manufacturers of GPS receivers have added multiple features to these units to make them complete navigational systems. We will use the Garmin eTrex Vista GPS receiver to describe basic features that are applicable to many different brands and models of GPS receivers. This is not an endorsement of Garmin eTrex Vista over other brands and/or models; there are many excellent GPS units available.

The Garmin eTrex Vista has six main display screens, which are called *Main Pages* (Fig. 1.4.32).

Whenever a Main Page is in the display screen, an *options menu* can be opened that pertains to that page. On the Garmin eTrex Vista, the "single page" icon button in the upper right-hand corner of the Main Pages opens these option menus (Fig. 1.4.32). The options menu opens a secondary page that allows you to select options, preferences for data information, or reset data screens that relate to that page.

The six Main Pages are as follows.

SATELLITE PAGE (FIG. 1.4.33)
When the GPS unit is turned "on," the Satellite Page appears. The GPS receiver has to acquire satellites in order to determine position, and this page shows which satellites are acquired and their radio signal strength. Satellites with a number 33 or greater are WAAS satellites. When enough satellites (three or more) have been acquired, this page displays your location coordinates, and states "Ready to Navigate," plus the accuracy of your location coordinates.

MAP PAGE (FIG. 1.4.34)
The Map Page places your location on a map with a "position icon." The position icon notes your direction of movement, and as you travel the display leaves a "trail," or *track log*, of your movements. The Garmin eTrex Vista comes with a basic map program installed, but a number of maps can be downloaded into this unit using a CD-ROM mapping program. You can change the scale of the map in the display by using the "zoom in" and "zoom out" buttons on the side of the GPS Receiver.

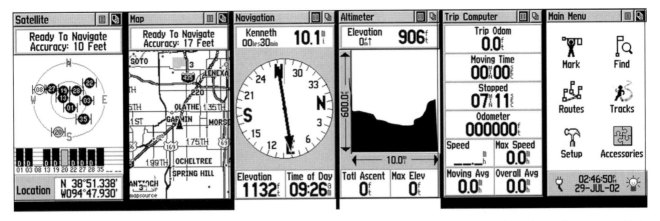

Figure 1.4.32 Many handheld GPS receivers have a similar page layout to the Garmin eTrex Vista shown here. There are six Main Page displays, with each page titled at the top. On each Main Page to the right of the title, is an icon that appears as a single sheet. This icon opens the Options Menu for each page. Selecting it, takes you to additional pages that pertain to that Main Page. To the right of this is an icon that appears as multiple sheets of paper. Selecting this icon brings up a menu displaying the six Main Pages to facilitate moving between these screens. (Graphic: Courtesy of Garmin International, Inc.)

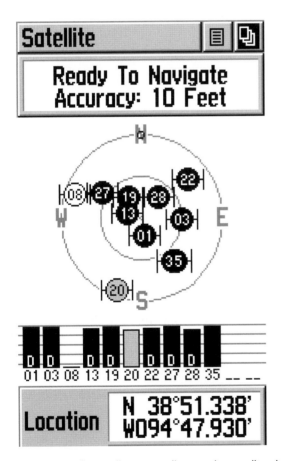

Figure 1.4.33 The Satellite Page tells you what satellites have been acquired and what your location is. When enough satellites have been acquired to establish your position, the GPS receiver indicates that it is "Ready To Navigate" and the accuracy of the coordinates. In this graphic of a Satellite Page, a WAAS Satellite (#35) has been acquired, and the location coordinate display is in the hddd.mm.mmm' latitude/longitude position format. (Graphic: Courtesy of Garmin International, Inc.)

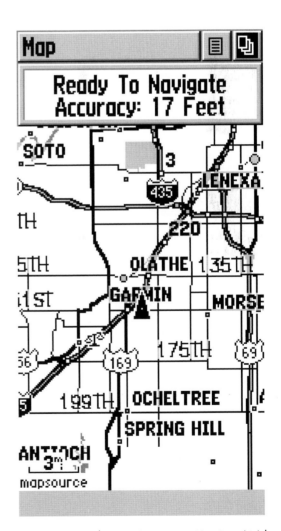

Figure 1.4.34 On the Map Page, a position icon (▲) locates your position and notes your direction of movement. You can change the scale of the map by using the Zoom In or Zoom Out buttons on the receiver. Aside from the factory installed map program, additional maps may be downloaded into many GPS receivers. (Graphic: Courtesy of Garmin International, Inc.)

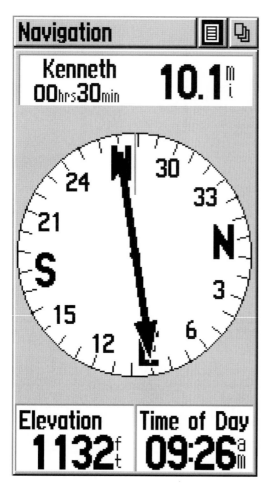

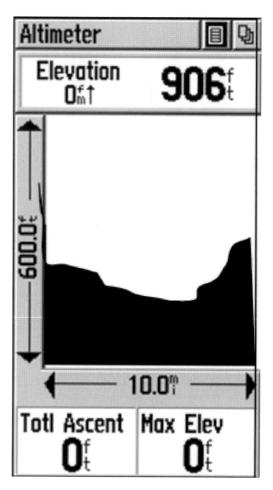

Figure 1.4.35 The Navigation Page displays information to guide you to another location. This page is where the *compass* and *bearing pointer* are to be found. Note the two data fields at the bottom of this page; in the Garmin eTrex Vista, there are over 20 different data options from which to select for these fields. (Graphic: Courtesy of Garmin International, Inc.)

Figure 1.4.36 The Altimeter Page. (Graphic: Courtesy of Garmin International, Inc.)

NAVIGATION PAGE (FIG. 1.4.35)
The Navigation Page displays information to help guide you to another location. The compass ring is displayed on this page, as is the bearing pointer, to help stay on a particular bearing to a destination. There are a variety of menu options for this page, and the bottom of the page has two data fields with over 20 different data options.

ALTIMETER PAGE (FIG. 1.4.36)
The Altimeter Page provides a variety of altitude information, including current elevation, current rate of ascent/descent, changes in elevation over time, and other selectable data fields from its menu options.

TRIP COMPUTER PAGE (FIG. 1.4.37)
The Trip Computer Page provides a variety of data field options that are selected from its menu options. The default settings include a trip odometer, moving time, stopped time, odometer, speed, max speed, moving average, and overall average. This page also allows access to deleting all waypoints, tracks, and routes.

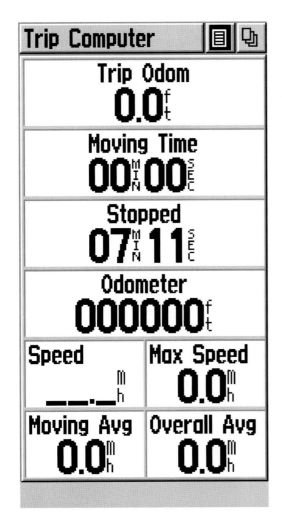

Figure 1.4.37 The Trip Computer Page. (Graphic: Courtesy of Garmin International, Inc.)

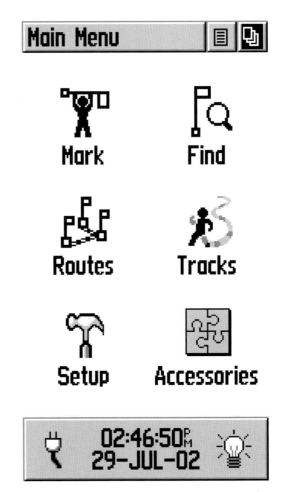

Figure 1.4.38 The Main Menu Page displays six different Feature Icons that mark waypoints, navigate to waypoints, establish routes, and set up the receiver to correlate with your maps/charts and personal preferences. These Feature Icons are used frequently. When operating on battery, this page also keeps track of the battery capacity—an important function when out in the field. (Graphic: Courtesy of Garmin International, Inc.)

MAIN MENU PAGE (FIG. 1.4.38)
The Main Menu Page displays six different icons, called *Feature Icons*. In addition, this page displays battery capacity, time/date, and backlighting status.

The Feature Icons on the Main Menu Page are as follows:

Mark (Fig. 1.4.39)
"Mark" stands for *mark waypoint*. When this icon is selected, the screen displayed allows you to mark, name, and record your current location, or enter and name a set of coordinates to record a waypoint at another location for later use.

Find
The "Find" icon allows you to *find* and *GoTo* a location or waypoint.

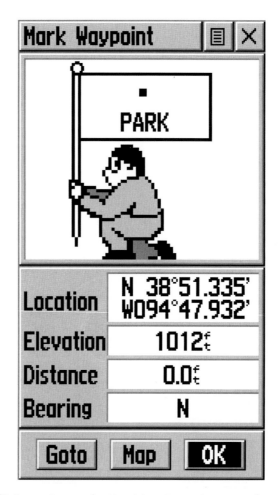

Figure 1.4.39 Selecting the "Mark" Feature Icon on the Main Menu Page takes you to the "Mark Waypoint" page. Waypoints are a set of coordinates for a location or "Point Along the Way." The default setting in the GPS receiver assigns sequential numbers to the waypoints entered, but you can rename any waypoint. In this case, the waypoint has been renamed "Park." In this example, note that the "Location" coordinates are displayed in the hddd.mm.mmm' latitude/longitude format. This format was selected from the Main Menu Page → (Feature Icon) Setup → Units → Position Format menu. This Waypoint marks the user's current location as the Distance to it is 0.0 ft. Coordinates of a distant location can also be entered and named on this screen. In this scenario, the "Distance" data field will display how far it is to that Waypoint, and the "Bearing" data field will indicate the azimuth to that Waypoint from your current location. (Graphic: Courtesy of Garmin International, Inc.)

Routes (Fig. 1.4.40)
When this icon is selected, it allows you to *create* a route to a destination by entering successive waypoints, effectively dividing a route into "legs" that will lead you to the end point.

Tracks
Selecting the "Tracks" icon allows you to save a *track log* and navigate a previous path of travel. This track log is saved from information the GPS receiver collects as an electronic "bread crumb trail."

Accessories (Fig. 1.4.41)
Selecting the Accessories icon from the Main Menu Page, takes you to a page where additional icon options are available including Sun and Moon positions and a calendar, among other things.

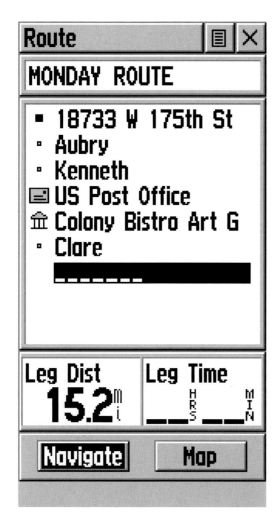

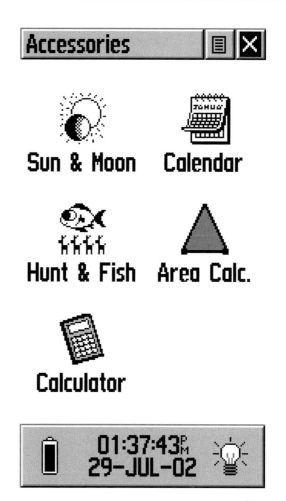

Figure 1.4.40 The Route Feature Icon allows you to populate a series of waypoints ahead of time to sequentially guide you along a route to your destination. You can also reverse this route and use it to retrace a journey back along the same route. This feature can be extremely useful. (Graphic: Courtesy of Garmin International, Inc.)

Figure 1.4.41 The Accessories Page on the Garmin eTrex Vista has a very fun Sun and Moon Page. This feature provides a graphic display of both Sun and Moon positioning for a certain date, time, and location. It can also display the different phases of the Moon. (Graphic: Courtesy of Garmin International, Inc.)

Setup
The Setup icon is very important. When selected, it takes you to a menu page displaying six other icon options (Fig. 1.4.42):

• Time
• Units
• Display
• Heading
• Interface
• System

Selecting the Units icon takes you to a page where preferences are selected for the *position format* (latitude/longitude, UTM grid, MGRS grid, etc.), the *map datum* (WGS 84, NAD 83, NAD 27, etc.), *distance/speed* (statute miles, nautical miles, kilometers), and *elevation units* (feet, meters).

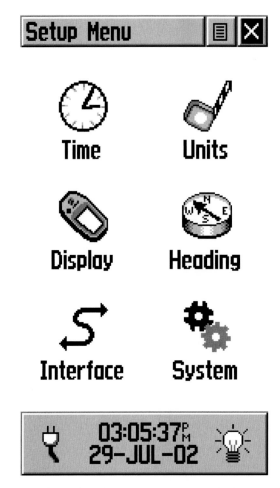

Figure 1.4.42 When the Setup Feature Icon is selected from the Main Menu Page, it displays six other icon options. The "Units" page is very important, as Position Format, Map Datum, Distance/Speed units, and Elevation units are all set from this screen. Menu options for the compass are found on the Heading page. The System page is where WAAS is enabled. (Graphic: Courtesy of Garmin International, Inc.)

The Heading page relates to the compass. The compass can display degrees, mils, or cardinal letters. There are four north reference options: True, Magnetic, Grid, or user. If "user" is selected, you must correct for the magnetic variation using data entry techniques.

The System page allows you to choose from four modes of operation: normal, battery saver, use with GPS off, and demo mode. This page is also where WAAS is enabled.

A page button on the side of the GPS receiver allows you to cycle through the six Main Pages. The Garmin eTrex Vista also has a "click stick" that facilitates moving between the Pages, accessing their menu options pages, and selecting Feature Icons and their menu options. The click stick directs a highlight cursor around the screen by pushing the stick left, right, up, or down, and then selects the highlighted option by pressing down and releasing it. The "click stick" can also be used to mark your current location as a "waypoint" by pressing down and holding this button. This is extremely handy, because you can set a waypoint regardless of which Page is on the screen. In an emergency, such as a man overboard, you can press and hold to mark that location instantly.

30. What is a "waypoint"?

A *waypoint* is a set of coordinates marking a location. Waypoints are stored in the GPS receiver as a GPS default assigned number, or they can be renamed by you (Fig. 1.4.39). A waypoint may be your current location, which can be entered by depressing and holding the "click stick," or by displaying the Main Menu Page and selecting the "Mark" Feature Icon. They can also be entered and named ahead of time to facilitate reference to them at a later time. As previously mentioned, using the "Route" Feature Icon on the Main Menu Page allows you to enter multiple waypoints ahead of time to guide you along a particular route to a destination.

31. What are bearing, heading, and course over ground?

"Bearing," "heading," and "course over ground" all indicate a compass direction between two points. GPS uses the term "bearing" to indicate the direction to a waypoint and the term "heading" to indicate the direction you are traveling; they may or may not be the same. When you have selected a waypoint to "GoTo" ("Find" Feature Icon on the Main Menu Page), the GPS gives you a bearing, which is a straight line direction from your location to that waypoint. This bearing does not see any obstacles (cliffs, rapids, buildings, etc.) that you may have to navigate around in order to reach your waypoint. As you change your heading (i.e., the direction you are traveling), to maneuver around an obstacle, the bearing will adjust to continuously show the direction and distance to the waypoint. Another term that describes the direction you are traveling is "course over ground" (COG). The GPS has other features available to assist in navigating to a waypoint, such as Cross Track Error (XTE) or Course Deviation Indicator. When you get a GPS receiver, reading through the manual will help you select the different data fields for display.

32. Describe the latitude/longitude coordinate options in the GPS receiver's Setup-Units–Position Format.

It is not uncommon for rescue operations to involve different groups and specialties such as air operations and ground search and rescue. While ground operations may prefer to work in UTM/MGRS/USNG coordinates, air operations prefer latitude/longitude coordinates. When GPS receivers are used, it is easy for people to convert back and forth between coordinate systems by changing the Position Format in the Setup. Enter a set of coordinates in one format → change the Position Format in the Units Setup screen → and the GPS converts the coordinates to the new format.

It is important to recognize that latitude/longitude coordinates have *three* different format options. Latitude/longitude can be entered as:

- Degrees, minutes, thousandths of a minute (hddd.mm.mmm')
- Degrees, minutes, seconds, tenths of a second (hddd.mm'.ss.s")
- Degrees, decimal degrees (hddd.ddddd)

40°20.500' North is an example of the hddd.mm.mmm' format. Verbally, this is read as "forty degrees, twenty decimal five hundred minutes North." An equivalent coordinate is 40°20'30.0" North; this is an example of the hddd.mm.ss.s" option. It is read as "forty degrees, twenty minutes, thirty decimal zero seconds North." Both of the coordinates above are equivalent to 40.34167° North, which is an example of the hddd.ddddd option for recording latitude/longitude coordinates. This is read as "forty decimal three four one six seven degrees North."

Key points that can be helpful as a means to understanding the different formats are:

- There are 60" (of arc) per 1' (of arc).
- There are 60' (of arc) per 1° (of arc).
- Both seconds tenths of a second (ss.s") *and* thousandths of a minute (.mmm') are fractions of 1' (of arc).
- Both minutes seconds tenths of a second (mm'ss.s") *and* minutes thousandths of a minute (mm.mmm') are fractions of 1° (of arc).

- A nautical mile is 6,080.27 feet.
- On a *great circle*, the distance of 1′ (of arc) is essentially 1 nautical mile, and therefore, the distance of 1° (of arc) is essentially 60 nautical miles. By the same token, the distance of 60″ (of arc) is essentially 1 nautical mile.
- On a great circle, by *approximating* a nautical mile to 6,000 feet, each thousandths of a minute (of arc) is equivalent to 6 feet, and each tenth of a second (of arc) is equivalent to 10 feet.

Understanding how the conversion is made between the three format options may help you to recognize *what* the different display options are so you can select the correct format when requested.

To convert from thousandths of a minute (.mmm′) to seconds (ss.s″), divide the thousandths of a minute by 1,000 and multiply that number by 60.

40°20.500′ (hddd.mm.mmm′)
40°20 (500′/1,000′) × 60″ = 30.0″
40°20′30.0″ (hddd.mm′.ss.s ″)

To convert from seconds (ss.s″) to thousandths of a minute (.mmm′), divide the seconds by 60 and multiply that number by 1,000.

40°20′30.0″ (hddd.mm.′ss.s″)
40°20′ (30.0″/60″) × 1,000 = 500
40°20.500′ (hddd.mm.mmm′)

To convert a degrees minutes seconds (DMS) format to a decimal degrees (DD) format, divide the seconds by 60 to convert to decimal minutes, then divide the decimal minutes by 60 to convert them to a decimal degrees.

40°20′30.0″ (hddd.mm′.ss.s ″)
40°20 (30.0/60) = 40° 20.50′
40° (20.50/60) = 40.34167° (hddd.ddddd)

The key point here is not to manually perform these conversions but to understand the different formats so that the correct menu option can be selected for the GPS unit to make the conversion.

33. Are there times when a GPS receiver will not work?

There are times when GPS receivers will not work. GPS receivers need to "see" the satellites in order to acquire them, so anything that interferes with this line of sight, such as a canopy of trees, high close canyon walls or buildings, or being inside a building, may prevent a GPS receiver from acquiring the satellites. Too, handheld units can be at risk of running out of battery power.

34. If you have a GPS receiver, do you need to have a paper map and a separate compass?

ABSOLUTELY! Even though a GPS receiver may seem to be all inclusive, it has limitations. The screen on a GPS receiver (especially the handheld receivers) is very small, so using it as your only map reference can be a mistake. The compass feature on a GPS requires a fair amount of battery power, so using a separate compass and turning "off" the GPS compass can extend the battery life. A map and compass are mandatory backups to a GPS in case of battery failure or inability to acquire satellite signals. Using a map, compass, and GPS receiver together is best.

CONTROVERSIES

35. What are the drawbacks to mandating the USNG system be the standard coordinate system for emergency and disaster response at this time?

Many different types of disasters (hurricanes, wildfires, blizzards, oil spills, etc.) necessitate land, air, and/or water operations, which may involve both civilian and military entities (i.e., Civil Air Patrol, Air National Guard, Army National Guard, U.S. Coast Guard, etc.). Air and water operations are better suited to using the latitude/longitude coordinate system because of their speed of travel and ability to cover very large areas. The latitude/longitude system is the best system for them. Grid systems work well for ground operations. A disaster may involve a very large ground area, but individual responders generally operate within a limited area, move more slowly (walking/driving), and can easily stop and obtain location coordinates. Standardizing to the USNG system for all disaster response, including air and water, would not work well. As previously mentioned, air operations (utilizing latitude/longitude) and ground search and rescue (utilizing UTM grids) are able to work together and this arrangement is likely to continue.

In terms of all ground operations standardizing to the USNG system, there is another hurdle as well. While USGS 7.5 minute and 15 minute quadrangles (which cover the entire United States) and other recreational maps include UTM grids on their maps, the MGRS/USNG 100,000 m Square Identifications have not been implemented on very many maps readily available to civilians and civilian emergency and disaster responders to date. In a disaster/emergency, if the area of operations is limited to a single 100,000 m square, there is little risk of miscommunicating location coordinates as the 10,000 m–1 m place columns of UTM coordinates are identical to the 10,000 m–1 m place columns of the MGRS/USNG coordinates, (obviously, the 100,000 m place columns remain constant). The risk for error increases when an area of operations involves multiple 100,000 m squares or spans across more than one *Zone*. When certain groups are using maps with MGRS/USNG information and others are relying on more readily available maps with only the UTM grid system, coordinates must be translated between the two systems. GPS receivers make this translation quite easily; however, errors may occur because of the steps involved in the flow of coordinate information between maps and the GPS and selecting the correct options for translation. These steps may include:

- Determining coordinates from a map and entering them into the GPS.
- From the Setup/Units page, selecting the proper menu options for Position Format *and* map datum.
- Communicating the translated coordinates to others.
- Receiving coordinate information that may need to be translated to a grid system that is applicable to your map.

Each step has the potential for error, which tends to increase with stress, exhaustion, and chaos—all of which are possible during a significant disaster. The addition of 100,000 m Square Identifications to the already established latitude/longitude and UTM grid coordinate systems is one hurdle that must be overcome if the USNG is to become the mandatory coordinate system used for disaster response in the United States, as has been proposed.

If a system is mandated, it will be decided upon by the powers that be, but *most important to the disaster responder* is having *knowledge* and *understanding* of ALL three systems (latitude/longitude, UTM grid, MGRS/USNG) so as to be able to operate in any or all systems depending on the situation.

Suggested Reading
Burns B, Burns M. *Wilderness Navigation*, 2nd ed. Seattle, The Mountaineers Books, 2004.
Calder N. *How to Read a Nautical Chart*. Camden, ME, International Marine/McGraw-Hill, 2003.
Ferguson M. *GPS Land Navigation*. Boise, ID: Glassford Publishing, 1997.
Kjellstrom B. *Be Expert With Map and Compass*. New York: Charles Scribner's Sons, 1976.
National Geographic Trails Illustrated Maps™. Available at www.natgeomaps.com.
National Oceanic and Atmospheric Administration (NOAA). Available at http://www.nauticalcharts.noaa.gov/mcd/chartno1.htm.
Sweet RJ. *GPS for Mariners*, Camden, ME, International Marine/McGraw-Hill, 2003.
United States Geological Survey. Available at http://www.usgs.gov.

CHAPTER 1.5
RECORDS AND ANIMAL IDENTIFICATION

Lori A. Swenson, BSME, EMT-P

1. Why is complete and accurate information important to document?

All documentation and forms are considered legal documents. Incidents that go to court may not get there until 12 to 24 months later, long after you have forgotten the particulars of a scene. Complete documentation will help jog your memory years later, and if you practice good documentation skills, you can be confident that what you wrote was what you did, even if you do not remember the specific event.

Also, legally speaking, "If it isn't written, it wasn't done." Remember to write it down.

2. Explain why you would want to document and record your actions at the scene of an animal welfare incident.

Any animal welfare incident scene should be considered a crime scene. It is critical that you document with video, photographs, and written records the observations and events during the entire time you are on scene. Often, your records of the scene will be the only proof that an incident occurred once time has passed and animal owners have corrected the original problem.

In the event that an incident goes to trial, this will most likely occur months after the initial response. If you have not clearly documented your activities and observations, you will be less likely to recall them after the fact. You should also document who was on scene and where they went. Remember that one of the rules of crime scene investigation is that everyone brings something into the scene and everyone takes something from the scene when they leave.

3. Describe some components of documentation or record keeping you would want to maintain during any incident involving animals.

- Document where the animal came from: addresses, building descriptions, locations of animals found at large, using cross streets, global positioning system (GPS), landmarks, etc.
- Physical descriptions of the animal
- Photographs or sketches that remain with the written document
- Numerical tags, leg bands, nylon tie tags, or other means of correlating an animal with a document
- Brands or tattoos on herd animals can be photographed or sketched and kept with written documentation.
- Any preexisting tag or microchip numbers
- Any medical information or treatments administered to the animal
- Documentation of euthanasia or death of animal while in your custody

Editor's Note: The Humane Society of the United States (HSUS) has some excellent forms that may be copied and used in preparing for an emergency. These forms are located at the following website: http://www.animalsheltering.org/resource_library/policies_and_guidelines/disaster_forms_insert.pdf.

It is important to have the forms available for filling out prior to a disaster!

4. Describe some simple ways to mark or affix identification to animals.

- Leg banding for birds or reptiles
- Grease pens for writing on hard exoskeletons
- Snap-on plastic or adhesive Mylar collars that can be written on
- Clip-on wing bands
- Paint sticks on livestock
- Ankle bands on livestock
- Cable ties and write-on tags
- Spray paint
- Veterinary emergency tag (VET) (see Chapter 1.9)

5. List some resources that would be helpful during documentation at an incident.

- Camera and/or video recorder with extra tapes, batteries, and film/digital cards
- Digital cards (smart cards, flash memory, etc.) and method of downloading to a computer
- Laptop computer
- Log books, preestablished forms
- Audio recorder
- Nylon ties and rubber bands
- Bags and containers for evidence collection
- Waterproof markers, grease pens
- Numbered tags or write-on tags
- Extra batteries

6. List some ways an animal owner might provide positive identification or proof of ownership.

- Microchip documentation
- Photograph of animal
- Brand registration
- Address corresponding to a tag found on animal with positive description
- Tattoo registration
- Registration papers (i.e., AKC, UKC)
- Rabies tag or county/parish license certificates

7. What are some methods used by owners to mark or identify livestock or large animals?

- Heat brands
- Freeze brands
- Freeze markings
- Visual tags (ear and neck)
- Barcode tags
- Radiofrequency identification technology (RFID) tags

- Microchips
- Tattoos
- Retinal scans
- Ankle bands

8. Describe ways to ensure that documentation and information relevant to specific animals do not become separated from the animal during operations.

- Attach photographs to documents, and record tag or ID numbers of animals on documents and photographs.
- Attach traveling documents to the cage or carrier when possible, preferably in a plastic bag or container.
- Follow all procedures for processing paperwork in the standard manner.
- Back up all information when possible so that data may be restored in the event something happens to the hard copy.

9. What should be documented when you take an animal from a home/residence?

- Address and description of home/residence
- Description of animal, identifying features, tag numbers, etc.
- Date and time taken
- Reason for taking animal
- Any requests or permissions from owners
- Condition of home or environment at time of collection
- Any equipment taken with animal, such as leash, halter, cage, etc.

10. Describe some of the ways you might describe a domestic animal.

- Species (canine, feline, caprine, ovine, bovine, equine, etc.)
- Breed
- Color, length, and texture of hair or fur
- Gender (neutered or intact)
- Eye, nose, and/or tongue color
- Body shape
- Claws intact or declawed
- Identification, collars, or halters, etc.
- Approximate age, weight, and height

11. You are collecting animals from a herpitarium; how do you provide identification for snakes or amphibians?

Keep them in their enclosure and place a tag or label on the cage with pertinent information.

12. You have recovered three birds from a home. What types of identification would you look for to determine ownership?

- Leg bands
- Tattoos
- Microchips

13. Besides verification of ownership, list some other reasons for individual identification of livestock.

- Can make breed registration and ancestry lines easier to trace
- In the event of a biosecurity event, facilitates tracking of infected or suspect animals
- Quarantine procedures will also be easier to establish when you can monitor individuals.
- Helps with evaluation of response to treatment in commingled populations
- Can assist with determining scope of recalls for contaminated product

14. Explain what the NAIS is and when the data would be used.

The National Animal Identification System (NAIS) is an information system that helps producers and animal health officials respond quickly and effectively to animal disease events in the United States. The NAIS is designed to accomplish the following:

- Increase the disease response capabilities of the United States.
- Limit the spread of animal diseases.
- Minimize animal losses and economic impact.
- Protect producers' livelihoods.
- Maintain market access.

   Participation in this program is voluntary to producers and animal owners of livestock or poultry. Livestock includes horses.

15. How does a producer participate in the NAIS?

There are several ways for producers to participate in NAIS.

- Premises registration—Identification of the geographic location where animals are raised, housed, or boarded through a premises identification number (PIN)
- Animal identification—Individual or group identification that remains with the animal for its lifetime
- Animal tracing—Access to timely, accurate animal movement records to quickly locate at-risk animals in the event of a disease outbreak

16. How are animals identified in the NAIS?

If you choose to identify your animals, there are two potential options:

- Individual identification—Individual identification is a good option for many situations. Any animal can be identified individually if you prefer. The method of identification varies by species. The U.S. Department of Agriculture recommends using new 840 animal ID devices whenever official animal identification is needed. Available in RFID ear tags and injectable transponders, 840 devices use a standardized 15-digit numbering system. The resulting number is known as an animal identification number (AIN). The AIN stays with the animal throughout its life.
- Group/lot identification—Group/lot identification is best suited for animals that are raised and move through the production chain as one group. These animals can be identified by a group/lot identification number (GIN), rather than individual numbers. The GIN is a 15-character number consisting of the 7-character PIN; the date that the group or lot of animals was assembled; and a 2-digit number to reflect the count of groups assembled at the same premises on the same day.

17. What are the basic requirements/characteristics of AIN ear tags?

- All AIN tags are one-time use (tamper proof).
- AIN tags are imprinted with the following:
  - AIN (15-digit number beginning with "840")
  - US shield (US)
  - Unlawful to remove
  - Manufacturer's logo or trademark (printed or impression of)
- The de facto standard for some species is a visual ear tag. For these species, ear tags with radiofrequency identification technology (RFID) may be encased in the visual tag when the above printing criteria are met. Such technology is considered supplemental identification (the visual tag remains the animal's official identifier). Tags with RFID must have all 15 digits of the AIN printed on the tag pieces that contain the transponder.
- RFID button tags (button front and button back pieces) must have the AIN imprinted on the tag piece with the transponder. The US Shield and text "Unlawful to Remove" must be printed on the other piece (most commonly, the male tag). Imprinting the AIN on the male tag is optional. In such cases, the tag set is packaged in containers or trays to keep the front and back tag piece together as a pair before being applied. Figures 1.5.1 through 1.5.7 show the AIN devices approved by the USDA as of June 19, 2008 (http://animalid.aphis.usda.gov/nais/naislibrary/documents/guidelines/NAIS_ID_Tag_Web_Listing.pdf).

18. Using the key below, determine the meaning of this freeze mark (Figs. 1.5.8 and 1.5.9).

This mark indicates that this horse was registered to the U.S. government, born in (19)95, and has a registration number of 560994.

19. What is a microchip?

A microchip is about the size of a grain of rice. It consists of a tiny computer chip housed in a type of glass made to be compatible with living tissue. The microchip is implanted between the pet's shoulder blades under the skin with use of a needle and special syringe. Little to no pain is experienced. Once in place, the microchip can be detected immediately with a handheld device (scanner) that uses radio waves to read the chip. This device scans

AIN Devices				
Manufacturer	Allflex USA, Inc. P. O. Box 612266 2805 East 14th Street Dallas Ft. Worth Airport, Texas 75261-2266		(800) 989-TAGS [8247] (972) 456-3686 (972) 456-3882/FAX www.allflexusa.com	
Images of Devices	Front (inside of ear) 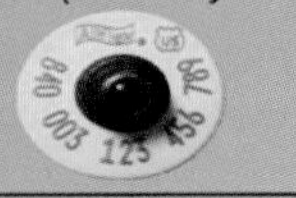	Back (outside of ear) 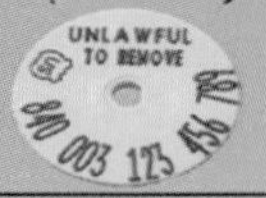	Front (inside of ear) 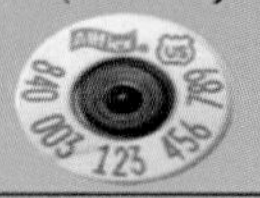	Back (outside of ear) 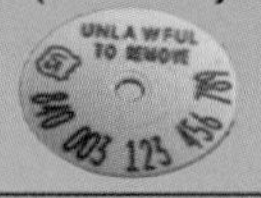
Mfr. Product Name	FDX Ultra EID Tag		HDX High Performance Ultra ED Tag	
NAIS Product Code	NAIS 0003		NAIS 0004	
Recommended Species	Bison, Cattle, Deer/Elk, Pigs		Bison, Cattle, Deer/Elk, Pigs	
Description	RFID Button ear tag ISO 11784/11785 Compliant; Full Duplex Front Tag: Diameter = 30.8 mm Weight = 5.8 grams		RFID Button ear tag ISO 11784/85 Compliant; Half Duplex Front Tag: Diameter = 29.9 mm Weight = 8.9 grams	

Figure 1.5.1 Animal identification number devices and manufacturer. (From http://animalid.aphis.usda.gov/nais/naislibrary/documents/guidelines/NAIS_ID_Tag_Web_Listing.pdf).

Manufacturer	Allflex USA, Inc. P. O. Box 612266 2805 East 14th Street Dallas Ft. Worth Airport, Texas 75261-2266	(800) 989-TAGS [8247] (972) 456-3686 (972) 456-3882/FAX www.allflexusa.com
Images of Devices	Front (inside of ear) 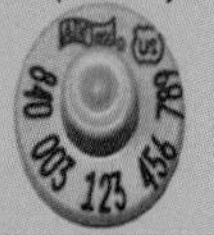	Back (outside of ear) 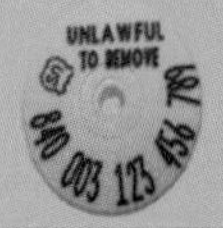
Mfr. Product Name	Allflex Lightweight EID Tag	
NAIS Product Code	NAIS 0010	
Recommended Species	Deer, Elk, Sheep/Goat, Pigs	
Description	RFID Button ISO 11784/85 Compliant; Full Duplex Front Tag: Diameter = 26.5 mm Weight = 3.3 grams	

Figure 1.5.2 Animal identification number devices and manufacturer. (From http://animalid.aphis.usda.gov/nais/naislibrary/documents/guidelines/NAIS_ID_Tag_Web_Listing.pdf).

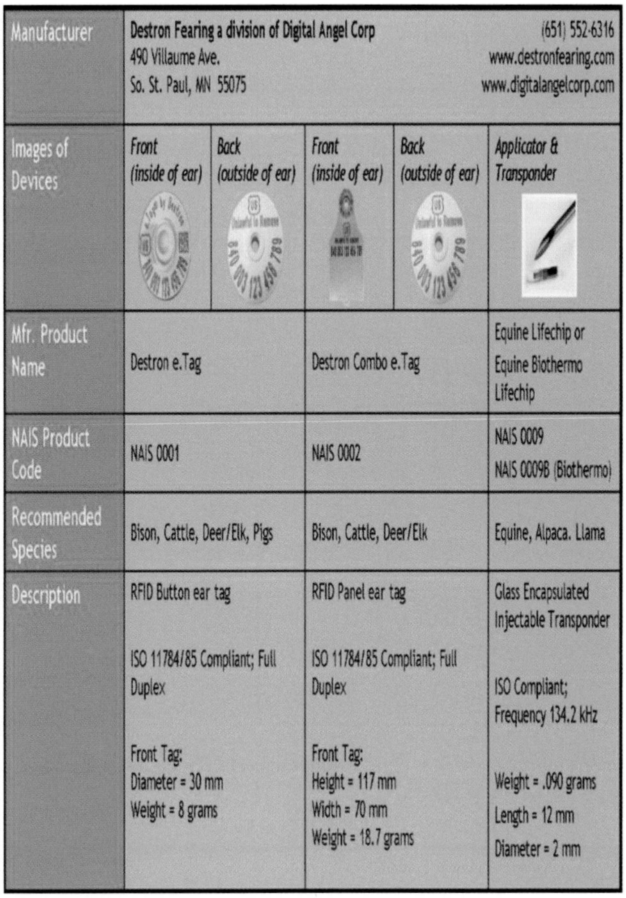

Manufacturer	Destron Fearing a division of Digital Angel Corp 490 Villaume Ave. So. St. Paul, MN 55075				(651) 552-6316 www.destronfearing.com www.digitalangelcorp.com
Images of Devices	Front (inside of ear)	Back (outside of ear)	Front (inside of ear)	Back (outside of ear)	Applicator & Transponder
Mfr. Product Name	Destron e.Tag		Destron Combo e.Tag		Equine Lifechip or Equine Biothermo Lifechip
NAIS Product Code	NAIS 0001		NAIS 0002		NAIS 0009 NAIS 0009B (Biothermo)
Recommended Species	Bison, Cattle, Deer/Elk, Pigs		Bison, Cattle, Deer/Elk		Equine, Alpaca. Llama
Description	RFID Button ear tag ISO 11784/85 Compliant; Full Duplex Front Tag: Diameter = 30 mm Weight = 8 grams		RFID Panel ear tag ISO 11784/85 Compliant; Full Duplex Front Tag: Height = 117 mm Width = 70 mm Weight = 18.7 grams		Glass Encapsulated Injectable Transponder ISO Compliant; Frequency 134.2 kHz Weight = .090 grams Length = 12 mm Diameter = 2 mm

Figure 1.5.3 Animal identification number devices and manufacturer. (From http://animalid.aphis.usda.gov/nais/naislibrary/documents/guidelines/NAIS_ID_Tag_Web_Listing.pdf).

the microchip and then displays a unique alphanumeric code. The pet must then be registered with the microchip company, usually for a one-time fee, so that if can be traced back to the owner if found. Microchips are designed to last for the life of the pet. They do not need to be charged or replaced. Some microchips have been known to migrate from the area between the shoulder blades, but the instructions for scanning emphasize the need to scan the pet's entire body.

20. Should every pet be microchipped?

No method of identification is perfect. The best thing anyone can do to protect their dog is to be a responsible owner. Keep current identification tags on the pet at all times, consider microchipping as reinforcement, and never allow the dog to roam free. If the pet does become lost, especially during a major disaster, more identification can increase the odds of finding the dog's home and owner.

21. What is all the controversy regarding microchips in animals?

There are two microchip "standards." The "ISO chip" calls for a microchip that transmits data at a frequency of 134.2 kHz. This frequency is endorsed by the International Standards Organization and is the chip most often

Manufacturer	Global Animal Management/Geissler Technologies 556 Morris Avenue Summit, NJ 07901 (800) 235-9824 http://www.mygamonline.com/gamweb/index.html		Y-Tex Corporation 1825 Big Horn Avenue Cody, WY 82414 307-527-6433 www.ytex.com	
Images of Devices	Front (inside of ear) 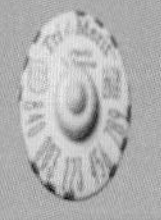 	Back (outside of ear) 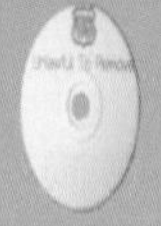 	Front (inside of ear) 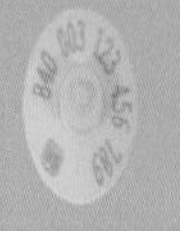 	Back (outside of ear) 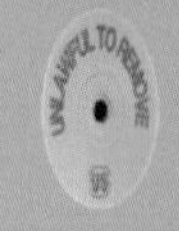
Mfr. Product Name	g.TAG/TriMerit		Y-Tex Round RFID Tag	
NAIS Product Code	NAIS 0006		NAIS 0007	
Recommended Species	Bison, Cattle, Deer/Elk, Sheep/Goats, Pigs		Bison, Cattle, Deer/Elk, Pigs	
Description	RFID Button ear tag ISO 11784/11785 Compliant; Full Duplex Front Tag: Diameter = 30.5 mm Weight = 8.8 grams		RFID Button ear tag ISO 11784/85 Compliant; Full Duplex Front Tag: Diameter = 32.05 mm Weight = 6.17 grams	

Figure 1.5.4 Animal identification number devices and manufacturer. (From http://animalid.aphis.usda.gov/nais/naislibrary/ documents/guidelines/NAIS_ID_Tag_Web_Listing.pdf).

Manufacturer	Leader Products 465 Humo Highway Craigieburn, VIC 3064 Australia www.leaderproducts.com.auLeader	**U.S. Distributer** **EZid Livestock Identification** Greeley, CO (877) 330-3943, (970) 351-7701 (970) 351-7711/FAX www.EZIDavid/let.html
Images of Devices	Front (inside of ear) 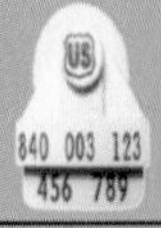 	Back (outside of ear) 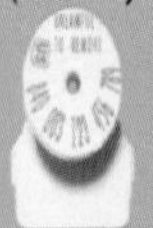
Mfr. Product Name	Leadertronic HDX	
NAIS Product Code	NAIS 0008	
Recommended Species	Bison, Cattle, Deer/Elk, Pigs	
Description	RFID Ear tag ISO 11784/85 Compliant; Half Duplex Front Tag: Width = 36mm Weight = 7 grams	Length = 35 mm Height = 12mm

Figure 1.5.5 Animal identification number devices and manufacturer. (From http://animalid.aphis.usda.gov/nais/naislibrary/ documents/guidelines/NAIS_ID_Tag_Web_Listing.pdf).

Manufacturer	ITW Fastex 195 Algonquin Road Des Plaines, IL 60016-6197 (847) 375-6711 www.itw-fastex.com	
Images of Devices	*Front (inside of ear)* 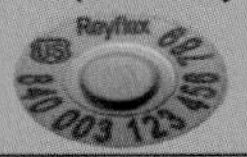	*Back (outside of ear)* 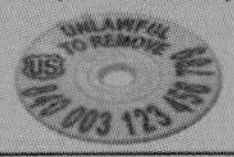
Mfr. Product Name	ReyFID Tag	
NAIS Product Code	NAIS 0011	
Recommended Species	Bison, Cattle, Deer/Elk, Pigs	
Description	RFID Button ear tag ISO 11784/11785 Compliant; Full Duplex Front Tag: Diameter = 30.5 mm Weight = 4.85 grams	

Figure 1.5.6 Animal identification number devices and manufacturer. (From http://animalid.aphis.usda.gov/nais/naislibrary/documents/guidelines/NAIS_ID_Tag_Web_Listing.pdf).

Other		
Manufacturer	**Destron Fearing a division of Digital Angel Corp** 490 Villaume Ave. So. St. Paul, MN 55075 (651) 552-6316 www.destronfearing.com www.digitalangelcorp.com	
Images of Devices	*Front (inside of ear)* 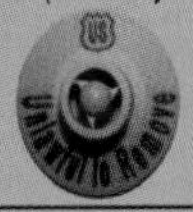	*Back (outside of ear)* 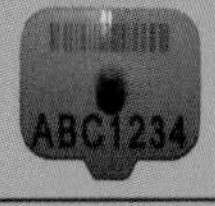
Mfr. Product Name	Hog Max TE	
NAIS Product Code	NAIS 0012	
Recommended Species	Slaughter Swine	
Description	Button ear tag Front Tag: Diameter = 28.5 mm Weight = 1.8 grams	

Figure 1.5.7 Animal identification number devices and manufacturer. (From http://animalid.aphis.usda.gov/nais/naislibrary/documents/guidelines/NAIS_ID_Tag_Web_Listing.pdf).

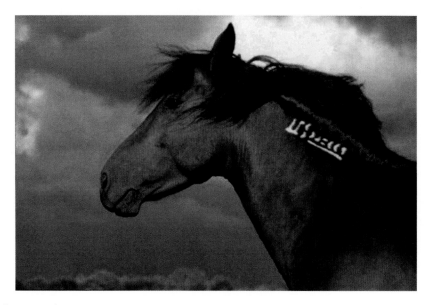

Figure 1.5.8 BLM freeze mark.

Key to the Alpha Angle Symbol

Read each angle to determine the freeze mark number

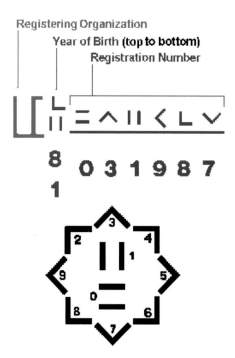

Figure 1.5.9 BLM freeze mark key.

used in other countries. In the United States, the majority of microchips transmit data at a frequency of 125 kHz. Most shelters, rescues, and veterinary offices in the United States are equipped to read chips at this frequency. Two companies, Avid and Digital Angel, manufacture these chips.

Avid has been blamed for not making readers that will read the ISO chip. However, Avid does make them—in fact, they make "multifrequency" readers that detect either frequency, but they do not distribute them in the United

States. Avid is also accused of trying to prevent competition by encoding the data using a proprietary encryption method. This makes it impractical for other companies to sell multifrequency readers in the United States. Because of all this, the ISO chips have not gained a foothold. Moreover, Avid has also been blamed for seeding the marketplace, by distributing their specialized readers to animal shelters, rescues, and veterinary clinics for free.

The controversy really started when Banfield (a chain of veterinary clinics found in PetSmart stores across the United States) began selling ISO chips. Pet owners who bought the ISO chips from Banfield complained that when their animals got loose and ended up in shelters, the microchips were not detected. Some of these owners failed to check the nearby shelters in a timely manner, resulting in the deaths of their pets. This all came about because shelters either were not equipped with ISO readers or simply did not want to scan each animal twice. In effect, Banfield was selling chips not readily scannable in the United States.

22. Do all microchip readers work with the various microchips on the market?

The recent introduction of chips operating at various different radio frequencies has created quite a bit of confusion. Although it seems impossible to sort out, it is really quite simple. Veterinarians in the United States have used the 125-kHz system for nearly 20 years. All scanners being used to scan pets today are designed to read the 125-kHz microchip. Additionally, the USDA Pet Microchip Report states that 80% of these scanners read **only** the 125-kHz chip and **not those of other frequencies**. Table 1.5.1 lists the microchip and frequency.

Table 1.5.1 Microchip Manufacturers and Chip Frequencies

125 kHz	128 kHz	134.2 kHz
Allflex	Bayer ResQ Chip	AKC Trovan
Avid Euro	Datamars (Swiss)	
Avid Secure Encrypted		
Destron Fearing		
HomeAgain		
Microchip ID Products		
TravelChip		

23. Do microchips cause cancer in pets?

Studies conducted in the 1990s suggesting that microchips may cause cancer have recently resurfaced. This time published by the Associated Press, the story gained some momentum and was picked up by *The New York Times*, ABC and Fox News, and other major media sources. The fact remains that in the past 10 years, no evidence has been found that in any way demonstrates the existence of a correlation between microchip implantation and occurrence of cancer in cats and dogs. It has long been known that anything that gains entrance to the body and incites inflammation may be a trigger for cancer. This is extremely rare, although there appears to be a higher incidence in certain families or lines of animals, indicating a genetic predisposition. This predisposition does not simply apply to microchips but to ALL products or items that end up in a subcutaneous location, including vaccines, surgical implants, foreign bodies, etc., and even trauma. Additionally, the aforementioned studies were flawed from an epidemiological perspective because the mice used (e.g., 4279 CBA/J mice) are genetically selected to be prone to cancer; therefore, they are not representative of the general population of animals kept as pets. Additionally, it is well recognized that one cannot extrapolate from studies in one species (e.g., mice) to another (e.g., cats and dogs). A literature search shows only two case reports of a suspected inflammation-induced fibrosarcoma at the microchip implantation site; however, there was no definitive cause-effect conclusion as other injections had been given in the same area. The British Small Animal Veterinary Association (BSAVA) has had a microchip adverse reaction surveillance system in place for over 10 years with only two reports of cancer associated with a microchip implant. Again, there was no causality assessment assigned and this may simply be a coincidental occurrence. Even so, based on all adverse reports received by the BSAVA, this equates to only a 0.6% incidence, which is extremely low, especially when one factors in the high rate of microchip use in the United Kingdom, where the majority of dogs and cats are implanted with a microchip.

Suggested Reading

Ball DJ, Argentieri G, Krause R, Lipinski M, Robison RL, Stoll RE, Visscher GE. Evaluation of a microchip implant system used for animal identification in rats. *Lab Anim Sci* 1999;41:185–186.

Murasugi E, Koie H, Okano M, Watanabe T, Asano R. Histological reactions to microchip implants in dogs. *Vet Rec* 2003;153:328–330.

National Animal Identification System. Identification devices with the animal identification numbers (AIN) and other official identification. Available at http://animalid.aphis.usda.gov/nais/naislibrary/documents/guidelines/ NAIS_ID_Tag_Web_Listing.pdf.

Rao GN, Edmondson J. Tissue reaction to an implantable identification device in mice. *Toxicol Pathol* 1990;18:412–416.

U.S. Bureau of Land Management. Sale and adoption of wild horses and burros. Available at http://www.blm. gov/wo/st/en/prog/wild_horse_and_burro.html.

U.S. Department of Agriculture, Animal and Plant Health Inspection Service. Animal identification. Available at http://animalid.aphis.usda.gov/nais/animal_id/why_840.shtml.

U.S. Department of Agriculture, Animal and Plant Health Inspection Service. National animal identification system (NAIS). Available at http://animalid.aphis.usda.gov/nais.

U.S. Department of Agriculture, Animal and Plant Health Inspection Service (APHIS). USDA approves three additional animal identification devices for use in the national animal identification system. Available at http://www.aphis.usda.gov/publications/animal_health/content/printable_version/sa_nais3tag_vs.pdf.

CHAPTER 1.6
VETERINARY RISK ASSESSMENT OF THE DISASTER SITE

Wayne E. Wingfield, MS, DVM

1. What is the purpose of risk assessment in a disaster?

The overall purpose of an initial risk assessment is to provide emergency services agencies and incident command with information and recommendations to make timely decisions regarding disaster response.

2. List important tasks to be performed in veterinary risk assessment.

- Identify the impact a disaster has had on animals in the community and the ability of that community to cope.
- Identify the most vulnerable populations, especially pets and food animals that need to be targeted for assistance.
- Identify the most urgent food and nonfood requirements and potential methods of providing assistance in the most effective manner.
- Identify the level of response by the affected community, county, or state and its internal capacities to cope with the situation, including those of the affected population.
- Identify the priorities of the affected population and their preferred strategies for meeting those priorities.
- Identify the level of response from other donor groups, private voluntary organizations (PVOs), and nongovernment organizations (NGOs).
- Make recommendations to incident command that define and prioritize the actions and resources needed for immediate response. Recommendations should include possibilities for facilitating and expediting recovery and development.
- Identify which types of in-depth assessments should be undertaken.
- Highlight special concerns that would not immediately be evident to nonveterinarian persons.

3. Why are initial assessments of the disaster scene so important?

Initial assessments provide baseline data as a reference for further monitoring. Monitoring systems should be identified so that relief officials will be able to determine whether a situation is improving or deteriorating. The systems must also provide a means of measuring the effectiveness of relief activities. Each assessment or survey should be designed to build on previous surveys and expand the assessment or survey database.

4. Describe why the initial assessment team must be professional in their actions.

The assessment team must be sensitive to the situation of the affected community and needs to structure its assessment questions so that unreasonable expectations are not created. The assessment team must also be aware of the pressures it will feel from the affected parties and others to "identify needs." A recommendation of "no additional assistance is required" may be a valid response, given that the on-the-ground site visit yields a disaster that is not as severe as indicated in third-hand reports and media coverage. The assessment team is supporting the response management team and will have a strong desire to help. However, the assessment team must also consider the local/state/regional animal response team's desire to help, and thus it must be prepared to advise on the limitations of this response team and realize they cannot solve all of the disaster problems alone.

5.   What are the types of assessment?

Assessment teams collect two types of information: (1) what has happened as a result of the disaster and (2) what is needed. The type of information that is usually available first to an assessment team concerns the effects of the disaster. Collecting this information is referred to as a "situation or disaster assessment." It identifies the magnitude and extent of the disaster and its effects on the community. The other information gathered is a "needs assessment." It defines the level and type of assistance required for the affected population. The gathering of information for the situation assessment and needs assessment can be done concurrently. The information collected in the initial assessment is the basis for determining the type and amount of relief needed during the immediate response phase of the disaster. It may also identify the need for continued monitoring and reassessing of the unfolding disaster.

6.   What type of information is collected in a "situation or disaster assessment"?

This assessment gathers information regarding the magnitude of the disaster and the extent of its impact on both the animal and human populations and the infrastructure of the community. Areas assessed and reported on include, but are not limited to, the following:

- Area affected by the disaster (location and size)
- Number of animals affected by the disaster
- Mortality and morbidity rates
- Types of injuries and illness
- Characteristics and condition of the affected population
- Emergency veterinary, health, nutritional, water, and sanitation situations
- Level of continuing or emerging threats (natural and human causes)
- Damage to infrastructure and critical facilities
- Damage to animal husbandry buildings
- Damage to agriculture and food supply system
- Damage to economic resources and social organization
- Vulnerability of the population to continuing or expanding impacts of the disaster over the coming weeks and months
- Level of response by the affected community and internal capacities to cope with the situation
- Level of response from other PVOs and NGOs

7.   What type of information is included in a "needs assessment"?

The initial needs assessment identifies resources and services for immediate emergency measures to save and sustain the lives of the affected animal population. It is conducted at the site of a disaster or at the location of a displaced animal population. A quick response based on this information should help reduce excessive death rates and stabilize the nutritional, health, and living conditions among the population at risk. A quick response to urgent needs must never be delayed because a comprehensive assessment has not yet been completed.

8. What individuals should be included in a risk assessment team?

An ideal assessment team is composed of three or four people. The assessment team is lead by a team leader (TL), who is usually selected from within the local/county/state team. Team leaders should be experienced and familiar with the local/county/state mandate, mission, and response capabilities. The scope of work for the assessment team is defined by disaster management and the local, county, or state authorities.

9. What are the six basic elements of any assessment?

- Preparedness planning
- Survey and data collection
- Interpretation
- Forecasting
- Reporting
- Monitoring

10. What is preparedness planning?

An accurate assessment depends on thorough planning, design, and preparation. Most information needs can be identified well in advance. The means of collecting the necessary data, and the selection of formats for collection and presentation of the information, should be established as part of an organization's predisaster planning. Seek advice from survey specialists, statisticians, and epidemiologists. Be prepared to undertake assessments well in advance of an emergency: Both the data required and the process most appropriate for its accurate and speedy collection can be identified and refined prior to the emergency. Proper design of sampling and survey methods can substantially increase the accuracy and usefulness of assessment data. Standard survey techniques, questionnaires, checklists, and procedures should be prepared to ensure that all areas are examined and that the information is reported using standard terminology and classifications. Also, consideration of local factors, social organization, and hierarchies of power at this stage can help greatly in formulating interview methods and identifying useful sources of information.

11. Describe what might be included in survey and data collection.

The gathering of the information must proceed rapidly and thoroughly. In an initial reconnaissance, surveyors should look for patterns and indicators of potential problems. Using the procedures developed earlier, key problem areas are thoroughly checked. Sources of all information should be identified. Examples include whether it was observed, reported by an informant in a discussion, collected through a survey of a randomly sampled population, heard by rumor, etc. The information will be more meaningful to those interpreting it, especially when there are conflicting reports, if a source is recorded.

12. Describe why interpretation is important during an assessment.

Thorough analysis of information gathered is critical. Those performing the analysis must be trained to detect and recognize trends and indicators of problems, to interpret the information, and to link the information to action programs.

13.   Describe the relevance of forecasting in risk assessment.

Using the collected data, the assessment team must construct estimates about how the situation might develop in the future so that contingency plans can be developed to prepare for and mitigate negative impacts. Forecasting requires input from many specialists, especially persons who have extensive experience in previous emergencies and who might detect trends and provide insights as to what course an emergency might follow.

14.   Discuss the importance of reporting in an assessment.

When data analysis and forecasting are complete, it is necessary to report and disseminate the results in a format that enables managers to make decisions and formulate plans and projects. Essential information should be presented and structured so that the main patterns and trends are clear.

15.   Why is monitoring such an important part of assessment?

An assessment should not be seen as an end result in itself, but rather as one part of a continuing process of reevaluating the needs and the appropriateness of responses to the disaster. This is particularly true in long-term, complex disasters.

16.   Distinguish the terms "data" and "information."

Data simply mean a structured collection of words, numbers, and other characters. *Information* means "useful data." Data become information when they are useful, meaningful, relevant, and understandable to particular people at particular times and places and for particular purposes. What is information to one person may simply be useless data to another.

17.   List three important considerations in assessment data collection.

- The need for accuracy—The information must agree with the reality it represents. The data on which it is based must be accurate.
- The need for timeliness and adequate frequency—Information must be produced as and when it is wanted. The frequency of data collection and reporting must match the rate of change in the situation being assessed.
- The question of availability of and access to information—Who should get what information? The way in which data are collected or the access to the data can affect the way they are routed, who they reach, and where their flow may be blocked.

18.   List the means by which data are collected.

- Automatic initial self-assessment and local assessment are key elements in the system—For example, staff of "lifeline" systems can involve preplanned damage reporting by civil authorities and military units.
- Visual inspection and interviews by specialists—Methods can include overflight, actions by special point assessment teams (including preplanned visits), and sample surveys to achieve rapid appraisal of area damage.

- Sample surveying of specific characteristics of affected populations by specialist teams—Well-conducted surveys have a number of advantages, not the least of which is the relative confidence that may be attached to data collected using formal statistical sampling methods. There are several different types of sample surveys:
  - *Simple random sampling:* Every member of the target population is equally likely to be selected, and the selection of a particular member of the target population has no effect on the other selections.
  - *Systematic random sampling:* Every fifth or tenth member on a numbered list is chosen (may be wildly inaccurate if the lists are structured in certain ways).
  - *Stratified random sampling:* The population is divided into categories (or strata); members from each category are then selected by simple or systematic random sampling and then combined to give an overall sample.
  - *Cluster sampling:* The sample is restricted to a limited number of geographical areas, known as "clusters", for each of the geographical areas chosen; a sample is selected by simple or random sampling. Sub-samples are then combined to get an overall sample.
  - *"Sentinel" surveillance:* This is a method used widely in emergency health monitoring, where professional staff establish a reporting system that detects early signs of particular problems at specific sites such as veterinary hospitals or sales yards. The method can be applied to a variety of other problems where early warning is particularly important.
  - *Detailed critical sector assessments by specialist:* This involves technical inspections and assessments by experts. It is required in sectors such as health and nutrition, food, water supply, electrical power, and other infrastructure systems in particular. Critical sector assessments may be compiled from reports by specialist of these systems or by visits by specialist teams from outside.
  - *Continuing surveillance by regular "polling" visits:* This again is a technique that is well developed in epidemiological surveillance of casualty care requirements and emergency health problems.
  - *Continuing surveillance by routing reporting:* As the situation develops, it will be especially useful if routine reporting systems can be adapted and used to develop a comprehensive picture of the events.
  - *Interviews with key informants:* Interviews with government and PVO/NGO/information officers and within particular groups of affected people, local veterinarians, livestock producers, local officials, local community leaders, and (especially in food and displacement emergencies) leaders of groups of displaced people.

19. Describe factors that will lead to a successful veterinary assessment.

- Identify the users—Every element of an assessment should be designed to collect information for a specific user. The potential users should specify their data needs during the design phase. For example, health workers need certain types of information that will only be useful in certain formats, usually tables, while a procurement officer may need more quantitative or statistical data.
- Identify the information needed to plan specific programs—Too often, assessment teams collect incomplete information or information of little value for planning relief programs or specific interventions. In many cases, information is anecdotal rather than substantive; in others, valuable time is wasted collecting detailed information when representative data would be just as useful. Determine what information is vital, what method is best to obtain this information, and how much detail is necessary for the information to be useful. The type of assistance usually provided by an agency should be considered when listing the data to be collected. For example, an agency that provides livestock or pet animal food will need to know about the availability of transport and fuel, road conditions, etc.
- Consider the format—It is important to collect, organize, and present the data in a form useful to analysts and program planners. The results must be presented in a format that makes the implications very clear so that priorities can be set quickly. By applying baselines and standards to the presentation, key relationships can be quickly noted.
- Consider the timing of the assessment—Timing may affect the accuracy of an assessment because situations and needs can change dramatically from day to day. Various types of assessments need to be timed to collect the necessary information when it is available and most useful. Relief needs are always relative but, as a general rule, initial surveys should be broad in scope and should determine overall patterns and trends. More detailed information can wait until emergency operations are well established.

- Determine the best places to obtain accurate information—If the information must be obtained from sample surveys, it is important that the areas to be surveyed provide an accurate picture of needs and priorities. For example, carrying out a health survey in a veterinary hospital would yield a distorted view of the overall health situation, because only sick or severely malnourished animals would be in the veterinary medical center.
- Distinguish between emergency and chronic needs—Virtually all geographical areas, especially those prone to natural disasters, have longstanding chronic needs. It is important to design an assessment that will distinguish between chronic and emergency needs. Attempt to acquire baseline data, reference data, and/or recognized and accepted standards in each area. The surveyors must differentiate between what is normal for the location and what is occurring as a result of the disaster, so that emergency first aid and health care can be provided to those most in need. It should be remembered that assessments may bring to light previously unrecognized or unacknowledged problems in a society. Thus, the data collection system should be careful to structure the information so that critical data such as health status, etc., can be used for long-term planning.
- Assess needs and vulnerabilities in relation to capacities—Needs are immediate requirements for survival. Vulnerabilities are potential areas for harm and include factors that increase the risks to the affected population. Vulnerabilities create unequal levels of risk between groups. Needs are assessed after an emergency has occurred, whereas vulnerabilities can be assessed both before and during the emergency. Needs are expressed in terms of requirements (food, water, shelter, etc.); vulnerabilities are expressed in terms of their origins (physical/material, social/organization, or motivational/attitudinal). The antidote to needs and vulnerabilities are capacities. Capacities are means and resources that can be mobilized by the affected population to meet their own needs and reduce vulnerability. Assessing vulnerabilities and capacities as well as needs provides a way of:
  ○ Preventing a widening of the emergency in which today's vulnerabilities become tomorrow's needs.
  ○ Targeting assistance to the most vulnerable groups.
  ○ Affecting a sustainable recovery, based on local resources and institutions.
  ○ Requiring direct engagement of members of the affected population in order to ensure that the required information is being shared. This last point is a particularly important contribution of capacity assessment, since externally provided assistance can actually slow recovery and impede a return to development if it is not given in a way that supports the efforts of the local populations to secure their own means of long-term survival.
- Use recognized terminology, standards, and procedures—Assessments will invariably be carried out by a variety of people operating independently. To provide a basis for evaluating the information, generally accepted terminology, ratings, and classifications should be used in classifying and reporting. The use of standard survey forms with clear guidelines for descriptive terms is usually the best way to ensure that all information is reported on a uniform basis.

20. Describe how assessment recommendations might impact recovery.

- It is important that the recommendations made by the assessment team do not have a detrimental effect on the long-term recovery efforts of an affected region. Relief programs can set the stage for rapid recovery or prolong the length of the recovery period. Every action in an emergency response will have a direct effect on the manner and cost of reconstruction.
- Many common relief programs can create dependencies and severely reduce the survivors' ability to cope with the next disaster. For example, food commodities (i.e., hay and grain) brought into a disaster area without consideration for the local agricultural system can destroy the local market system and cause future food shortages where self-sufficiency had been the norm. Another example is when relief supplies, equipment, or technology are sent in that are not sustainable in the socioeconomic environment of the survivors. When this assistance wears out or is used up, the survivors may be left in the same condition as immediately following the disaster.
- Sustainable recovery depends on restoring the affected populations' own capacity to meet their basic food, shelter, water, and sanitation needs. The victims have the most immediate and direct interest in recovering from a disaster, and most disaster survivors do so using their own resources. Consequently, they may place a high priority on restoring their means of livelihood. Understanding their priorities and providing assistance that supports the affected population's efforts to restore viable socioeconomic systems is critical to achieving a long-lasting, sustainable recovery.

- Recommendations should be simple, support the use of local materials and systems, and be sustainable by the affected area. Do not discount alternative interventions that may be against "conventional wisdom," collide with bureaucratic obstacles, or need increased relief agency capacity. In the long run, they may be more cost effective and sustainable.

21. In summary of risk assessment, list the main points to consider.

- An assessment is only a "snapshot in time."
- Information changes over time.
- The significance of information changes over time.
- If a disaster manager can identify the unfolding scenarios, monitoring will ultimately be more important than assessment.
- What you cannot see is often more important than what you can see.
- It is vital to use the first assessment to establish an ongoing data collection and analysis system.
- Most reports should be iterative, not detailed.
- The initial assessment should provide information that feeds directly into the program planning process.
- Timing of the report is vital. Without a point of reference, most assessment data is of little value.
- Communication of information is vitally important.

CHAPTER 1.7
RISK COMMUNICATION AND DEALING WITH THE MEDIA

Wayne E. Wingfield, MS, DVM

1. Describe what is meant by "risk communication".

Risk communication is the art of responding effectively to public outrage. Risk communication IS NOT a means to obscure facts, manipulate public opinion, or avoid responsible action. Risk communication is how to communicate while operating in a low trust and/or high concern environment. This is the type of environment that you will find yourself in during most deployments. The local veterinary infrastructure, humane organizations, and even local and state agencies may have little trust or knowledge of federal/state/county animal response teams.

2. What is the overriding goal of effective risk communication?

The goal of risk communication should be to produce an informed public that is involved, solution oriented, and collaborative. It should not be a goal to diffuse public concerns or become a substitute for action. Risk communication is a two-way activity based on mutual respect, trust, and the open exchange of information.

3. During a disaster, who is considered the "public"?

Following deployment, the public may be, but is not limited to, members of the affected veterinary infrastructure; agricultural members of the community; various local, state, or federal agency employees; humane organizations; and the general population of an area.

4. It is sometimes useful to subdivide the public in accordance with their awareness during a disaster. List the three subdivisions of the public.

- Passive public (largely unaware)
- Attentive public (relatively aware)
- Active public (seeking to affect decisions and make its views known)

Important point: different messages and channels may be needed for these different groups and those in different stages of awareness and activity.

5. Describe how risk communication is likely to be handled during large disasters.

Under ICS, the Public Information Officer is a key member of the command staff. The PIO advises the incident command on all public information matters related to the management of the incident, including media and public inquiries, emergency public information and warnings, rumor monitoring and control, media monitoring, and other functions required to coordinate, clear with proper authorities, and disseminate accurate and timely information related to the incident. The PIO establishes and operates within the parameters established for the joint Information System (JIS). The JIS provides an organized, integrated, and coordinated mechanism for providing information to the public during an emergency. The JIS includes plans, protocols, and structures used to provide information to the public. It encompasses all public information related to the incident.

Key elements of a JIS include interagency coordination and integration, developing and delivering coordinated messages, and support for decision makers. The PIO, using the JIS, ensures that decision makers—and the public—are fully informed throughout a domestic incident response.

During emergencies, the public may receive information from a variety of sources. Part of the PIO's job is ensuring that the information the public receives is accurate, coordinated, timely, and easy to understand. One way to ensure the coordination of public information is by establishing a joint information center (JIC). Using the JIC as a central location, information can be coordinated and integrated across jurisdictions and agencies, and among all government partners, the private sector, and nongovernment agencies.

6. List the seven cardinal rules of risk communication.

1. Accept and involve the public as a legitimate partner.
2. Plan carefully and evaluate your efforts.
3. Listen to the public's specific concerns. (Communication is a two-way activity: sender—receiver).
4. Be honest, frank, and open.
5. Coordinate and collaborate with other credible sources. Allies can be effective in helping communicate risk.
6. Meet the needs of the media (WHEN DEPLOYED, THIS HAS TO BE APPROVED BY THE PUBLIC INFORMATION OFFICER [PIO] OR THE COMMANDER ON THE SCENE.)
7. Speak clearly and with compassion.

7. Describe what is involved with accepting and involving the public as a legitimate partner during risk communication.

• People and communities have a right to participate in decisions that affect their lives, property, and the things they value (veterinarians in a disaster area may be particularly sensitive to this).
• Involve the community early (attempt to contact representatives from all stakeholders in the area).
• Remember that as a volunteer animal response person, you are there to assist the public.

Point to consider: The goal of risk communication should be to produce an informed public that is involved, interested, reasonable, thoughtful, and collaborative. It should not be to diffuse public concerns or replace action.

8. Describe how to carefully explain and evaluate your efforts in risk communication.

• Begin with clear, explicit objectives (if you do not know what your mission is, then it is difficult to communicate objectives that are needed to complete the mission).
• Evaluate all the information you have about risks and know the strengths and weaknesses.
• Identify the various groups in your audience and aim your communications toward the specific groups (local veterinarians versus humane organizations).

- Train all team members in communication skills (out in the field, how you are perceived and communicate makes a difference).
- Pretest your messages (run your messages by someone).
- Evaluate your efforts and learn from mistakes. You cannot manage what you cannot measure (determine if the message you deliver is being understood).

9. Describe how to listen to the public's concerns during a disaster.

- Do not make assumptions about what people know, think, or want done (various groups or organizations may have their own agendas).
- Let all parties with an interest be heard (do not shut out anyone).
- Identify with your audience. Try to put yourself in their place.
- Recognize emotion, symbolic meanings, and broader economic and political considerations that underlie and complicate risk communication (be aware of the short-term and LONG-TERM problems or consequences of the disaster).

Point to consider: People in a community are often more concerned about such issues as trust, credibility, competence, control, fairness, caring, and compassion than about mortality or morbidity statistics and the details of quantitative risk assessment.

10. Why is it important to be open, frank, and honest in risk communication activities?

- Trust and credibility are difficult to obtain. Once lost, they are almost impossible to regain completely.
- If you are not trusted, this will lead to lack of cooperation, anger, obstructive acts, and impediments to action.

Point to consider: When a lower-credibility source attacks the credibility of a higher-credibility source, the lower-credibility source loses further credibility.

11. Offer some guidelines on how to effectively communicate your assessment of the disaster.

- State your credentials, but do not ask or expect to be trusted.
- If you do not know the answer or are uncertain, say so. Get back to people with answers. Admit mistakes.
- Disclose risk information as soon as possible.
- Do not minimize or exaggerate the level of risk.
- Discuss data uncertainties, strengths, and weaknesses, including those identified by other credible sources.

12. Describe how to collaborate and communicate with other credible sources.

- Take time to coordinate all communication (whether it is from teams you have placed out in the field or from other agencies or organizations).
- Devote effort and resources to the slow, hard work of building bridges with other organizations (this will vary depending on the disaster deployment but it is an absolute necessity).
- Try to issue communications jointly with other trustworthy sources (if possible, join with the state public health service when communicating about public health and the local or state veterinary medical association regarding animal issues).

Point to consider: Few things make risk communication more difficult than conflicts or public disagreements with other credible sources.

13. Why is the media viewed as a problem during a disaster?

It is the nature of the beast. The news business is aggressive, highly competitive, and getting more so everyday. Media pursue the stories that attract viewers/listeners/readers . . . and advertising dollars. They want what sells: the gore, the suffering, the drama, the conflict, the tragedy; the unique and emotional images; the colorful and compelling quotes; the poignant human-interest angles. A story with a cute dog, cat, horse, or sheep that has survived a disaster often meets the needs of the media and these animals and their owners are thus exploited.

14. Describe how to integrate risk communication into a disaster response plan.

View the media as an ally, not an adversary. Use the news media to your advantage, as a tool to inform, educate, and enlist support and assistance. Media can help quickly convey your message to a very large audience; they might be useful in local activation of a disaster response and mobilization of volunteers; they can also stimulate disaster relief from individuals and the private sector.

Media relations should be an integral part of your emergency response plan. You and your PIO need to know your local reporters and assignment editors and their needs and deadlines (and personal styles). Find out how they plan to respond during natural disasters and how they would handle something like an animal rescue or mass death/euthanasia. Tell them about your organization. Invite them to your drills. Develop a fact book or background material to familiarize the media reporters with animal issues and terminology.

In most situations making a media representative a part of your disaster response planning team will work wonders when you call on them for help. If you use prepositioned news releases, ask the media for input when updating them. This will make them feel needed, while actually helping you to come up with something easier for the public to understand. Make sure the media has a thorough understanding of the time frame under which you hope to operate in advance of any emergencies.

Use every media opportunity presented. The more exposure you get, the greater your name recognition among those in the public sector. If the general public does not know you, they will not be inclined to place much credibility in what you say during an emergency, when getting the public to take quick action might mean the difference between living and dying.

Take advantage of all forms of media, no matter what the situation. Do not take a defensive posture with the media. Make periodic telephone calls to your media outlets, checking on staff changes and simply letting them know you are aware of their existence. If you play your cards right, you will always get what you want out of the media to advance your program, while still satisfying their need for information.

Always return telephone calls from the media promptly. This is not to say that you must leap on the telephone immediately; however, you should never disregard a media call or dismiss it as unimportant. It may be something that will promote your program. Painful as it might seem, never make the mistake of telling the media not to call you at home.

15. How does one meet the needs of the media during a disaster?

- *Communication with the media will come from the public information officer of the management support team (MST) commander.*
- Be open and accessible (This does not mean you have to answer all media questions.)
- Provide risk information tailored to the needs of each type of media.
- Prepare in advance and provide background material on complex risk issues (know of what you speak).

- Do not hesitate to follow up on stories with praise or to temper public criticism. It is very important for the public to see their agencies as a cohesive group.
- Try to establish long-term relationships of trust with specific editors and reporters (individual PIOs of a team may do this so they can provide approved postdeployment and/or predeployment information).

Point to consider: The media are frequently more interested in politics than in risk; more interested in simplicity than in complexity; and more interested in danger than in safety.

16. Undoubtedly, we have all experienced the arrogant media crew that insists on being in the middle of a disaster. How should one deal with these people during a disaster?

Always designate one person as your media liaison (PIO) and make certain all personnel know that contact person. A well-informed spokesperson can greatly reduce demands on other key personnel and explain activities or actions that otherwise might be misinterpreted by reporters (and other observers). Also, remember that detaining or excluding the news media is always counterproductive. If reporters or camera operators are in your way, find a better place for them as close to the action as possible. If danger exists, tell them about it and suggest a safer location, but never use danger as an excuse for keeping reporters away from the disaster scene. You are not responsible for their safety!

17. Provide some guidance in conducting an interview during a disaster.

You must be the one to set the ground rules when agreeing to be the subject of any interview. The topic(s) to be discussed should be mutually agreed on at the outset. If you are not prepared to discuss a certain subject, do not attempt it just for the sake of the interview. If you know nothing about the topic, do not lose your credibility by trying to bluff your way through the interview. There is nothing wrong with using the phrase, "I don't know, but I will do my best to get you an answer to that important question!" Do not be afraid to ask questions of your interviewer. Find out where the reporter stands in terms of subject knowledge. This may allow you to determine what direction the interview will take. Never make a habit of doing "off-the-cuff" interviews.

Document your contacts with the media: date, time, reporter's name, place, and subject. Mistakes will be made in media coverage; do not make a big deal out of minor glitches. Remember that while there are big egos in every profession, most reporters you encounter will be (1) regular human beings, (2) eager to do their job in a professional manner, and (3) perhaps a bit anxious because they are on unfamiliar turf—your turf. Be empathetic to these people.

18. Describe the most common reasons for interview (communication) failures.

- *Failure to take charge.* A spokesperson must be a leader. His or her role is not just to answer questions but also to disseminate information.
- *Failure to anticipate questions.* Prepare for obvious questions. Remember, the public wants to know, "Is it safe?"
- *Failure to develop key message.* This is your opportunity to communicate with the public.
- *Failure to stick to the facts.* Speculating can get you into trouble.
- *Failure to keep calm.* Do not let questions get under your skin. Keep cool.
- *Failure to keep the interview brief!*

19. List some important tips in speaking clearly and communicating effectively during a disaster.

- Use simple, nontechnical language, and avoid professional jargon. Be prepared to provide an expert opinion to a non-expert. Make your information concise and understandable.
- Say the "important stuff" first.
- Be sensitive to local norms, such as speech and dress.
- Be open and friendly, but be careful with humor.
- Use vivid concrete images that communicate on a personal level.
- Acknowledge and respond to the emotions that people express—anxiety, fear, anger, outrage, and helplessness.
- Acknowledge and respond to the distinction that public views are important in evaluating risk (do not just brush off information because it comes from a local or public source).
- Use risk comparisons to help put risks in perspective, but avoid comparisons that ignore distinctions that people consider important.
- Tell people what you cannot do. Promise only what you can do. Do what you promise.
- Know who you are talking to and establish how the information is going to be used.
- Know your subject and be clear on the message you are trying to convey. Stick to the facts and avoid speculation.
- Anticipate questions. In addition to the usual who, what, when, where, why, and what, anticipate the toughest questions the reporter is likely to ask. Think about your answers. Is there possible controversy?
- Fill in the background if you think there are gaps in the audience's or reporter's knowledge and/or understanding of the situation.
- Don't be afraid to say, "I don't know," but always get back to them with the answer.
- Never say, "No comment." (Do you have something to hide?).
- Never ask to speak "off the record"; always assume that you are speaking on the record.

Point to consider: Never let your efforts to inform people about risks prevent you from acknowledging that any illness, injury, or loss of life is a tragedy.

20. List some tips that might be useful during a television interview.

- If you are standing for your interview, put one foot slightly in front of the other so that you do not sway. If you are seated, lean forward slightly so you do not look like you are slouching.
- Maintain eye contact with the reporter, not the camera lens. The slightest movement (up/down, sideways) will be exaggerated on camera and could make you look nervous or unreliable; limit head and arm movement.
- Try to breathe normally; keep your voice slow and steady.
- If you make a mistake, say so right away and try again. This will hopefully be edited out before being broadcast.
- Fight the urge to fill "dead air"; that is the reporter's problem, not yours.
- Avoid giving "yes/no" answers.
- Act as if you are on camera until you are absolutely certain that you are not!

21. What's different about an interview for print media?

- Print media can address complex subjects better than electronic media. Reporters generally want detailed information and lots of it.
- Respond to questions in simple concise sentences.
- Repeat yourself if necessary to make certain the reporter is getting all the information.
- Newspaper photographers must have excellent photos in order to compete with television, so try to be accommodating.

22. Provide more detail regarding a JIC during a major disaster.

A JIC is the physical location where public information staff involved in incident management activities can co-locate to perform critical emergency information, crisis communications, and public affairs functions. JICs provide the organizational structure for coordinating and disseminating official information. Incident commanders and multiagency coordination entities are responsible for establishing and overseeing JICs, including processes for coordinating and clearing public communications. In the case of a unified command, those contributing to joint public information management do not lose their individual identities or responsibilities. Rather, each entity contributes to the overall unified message. JICs may be established at various levels of government. All JICs must communicate and coordinate with each other on an ongoing basis using established JIS protocols. When multiple JICs are established, information must be coordinated among them to ensure that a consistent message is disseminated to the public.

23. Summarize some of the dos and don'ts to remember during risk communication.

- Do remember, no matter what you believe, what you say IS ALWAYS ON THE RECORD!
- Do be careful around microphones and tape recorders.
- Do correct any mistakes you may have made in question and answer sessions.
- Do be honest and accurate. Your credibility depends on it.
- Do stick to key points.
- Do state your conclusions, first to get your main points across, and then back them up with facts.
- Don't assume that a microphone is ever off.
- Don't assume the interview/conference is over. Remember that directional microphones can hear you even when you are at a distance and cameras can certainly still be taking photographs!
- Don't get your message lost in a morass of detail.
- Don't hesitate to refuse to give proprietary information.
- Don't believe you know it all.
- Don't improvise.
- Don't lie.
- Don't try to fool the public or a reporter.

Acknowledgment

The author is appreciative of guidance and assistance provided while preparing this chapter by Dr. John H. Anderson, Commander, National Veterinary Response Team—4, American Veterinary Hospital, Simi Valley, CA.

CHAPTER 1.8
BIOSECURITY FUNDAMENTALS FOR ANIMAL RESPONSE PERSONNEL IN A FARM/LIVESTOCK DISASTER

Wayne E. Wingfield, MS, DVM, and Anthony P. Knight, BVSc, MS

1. What is biosecurity?

Biosecurity (biological risk management), in the context of animal responders during a disaster, refers to measures taken to keep disease agents out of populations, herds, flocks, or groups of animals where they do not already exist and to measures taken to prevent animal responders from spreading a disease when leaving the site of an emergency.

2. Which U.S. government agency is most often associated with biosecurity measures involving farm animals?

The U.S. Department of Agriculture (USDA)—A comprehensive international biosecurity resource available through the United Nations Food and Agriculture Organization (FAO), is the FAO Biosecurity Toolkit that provides practical guidance to developing and implementing a national integrated biosecurity program.

3. Who might implement biosecurity measures?

Biosecurity measures can be implemented on a national, state, and even a herd, flock, farm, etc. level; by responsible persons at the national and state level; and locally by animal owners, feedlot managers, veterinarians, etc.

4. Give some examples of diseases that are of particular concern to the United States.

- Foreign animal diseases such as foot-and-mouth disease, Rift Valley fever, Rinderpest, African swine fever, classical swine fever, etc.
- Brucellosis
- Tuberculosis
- Pseudorabies
- Exotic Newcastle disease, avian influenza

5. List some diseases a farm owner or management team would like to exclude.

- Mastitis
- Bovine virus diarrhea, salmonellosis
- Ovine progressive pneumonia
- Swine dysentery
- Porcine respiratory and reproductive syndrome (PRRS)
- Exotic Newcastle disease, avian influenza

6. Describe the basics of a valid farm biosecurity plan.

- First identify the most likely risks and "control points" on the farm where biosecurity measures can be readily implemented to prevent the introduction of diseases. A useful biosecurity assessment questionnaire is available on the University of Vermont website (http://www.uvm.edu/~ascibios/?Page=assessment.html).
- Introduction of new animals to the farm or animals returning from a livestock show is the greatest risk for introducing disease. Having a plan to isolate "new" animals well away from other animals for at least 2 weeks is very important.
- Determine how members of the public, tradesman, veterinarians, and vehicle traffic will be regulated to minimize the risks of introducing disease.
- Decide on effective cleaning and disinfection procedures to reduce pathogen levels.

7. Why should a herd or flock manager adopt a biosecurity plan?

"An ounce of prevention is worth a pound of cure." Every flock or herd manager hopes to raise livestock profitably and it is well documented that diseased animals are not as profitable; thus, it is in the producer's best interest to adopt a biosecurity plan (Fig. 1.8.1).

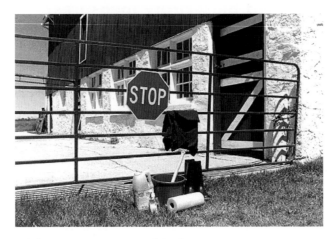

Figure 1.8.1 Biosecurity starts with limiting access to areas of the farm.

8. What does farm biosecurity have to do with animal disaster response personnel?

Comprehensive biosecurity programs have already been adopted by many poultry and pork producers. With the relatively large number of birds or pigs housed in a modern production unit, disease prevention, rather than disease treatment, is already in practice. In the event of a disaster, animal response personnel may be asked to assist *and* do not want to be responsible for further breakdowns in biosecurity. Biological risk management procedures must be followed before and after entering animal facilities. Efforts must be prioritized to address those factors posing the greatest risk of disease introduction.

9. What is the most common way contagious diseases are introduced to a herd/flock?

Adding new animals to a farm is the most common way contagious diseases are introduced. Merely excluding obviously sick animals is not sufficient to prevent disease introduction; new stock may be incubating diseases to which they were recently exposed, or they may be carriers and shedders of disease organisms. In these cases, it is likely that they will have no apparent signs of disease upon arrival at their new home. There is also a risk of disease introduction by people traveling between groups of animals.

10. Describe the risk variables for animal response personnel traveling between groups of animals during a disaster.

- The specific disease agent—Some agents persist on fomites better than others.
- The extent of animal contact—Increases the chances of contamination
- The time elapsed since the last animal contact—Extended periods between animal contacts decrease the potential for disease spread
- The preventive measures used—Ineffective personal protection equipment and disinfection increase the risk of spreading disease

11. Describe general guidelines that should be adopted to reduce the risk of introducing diseases with new additions to the herd/flock.

- The health status of the herd-of-origin should be reviewed. The number of source herds should be minimized; single-source animals are preferred over commingled animals. If there are diseases present in the herd-of-origin that are not in the recipient farm, the acceptability of the animals should be questioned. Obtaining animals where commingling is common (fairs, shows, livestock sales/auctions) generally increases the risk of introducing disease.
- All new or returning animals should be isolated from the herd for at least 2 weeks and preferably 4 weeks. Many swine herds now require a strict 30-day isolation period followed by a 30-day acclimation period before new animals are introduced.

12. How should one isolate new or returning animals in a biosecurity plan?

- The isolation facility should be at least several hundred yards from the rest of the herd when possible and positioned so that surface water drainage and prevailing winds do not carry contamination to the herd/flock.

As a rule of thumb, the isolation facility should be far enough away so that it is not readily and easily accessible to personnel as they perform other regular farm duties.

- The isolation facility should be managed as "all-in/all-out." In other words, no animal should be moved from the isolation facility to the recipient herd until the most recent addition has completed the testing protocol or isolation period.
- Animals must be carefully observed on a daily basis in the isolation facility. Those showing signs of illness must be penned separately and examined by a veterinarian.
- Tests for diseases of specific interest can be accomplished before the isolation period ends. Acceptable test results should be received before animals are released from isolation.
- Preventive treatments such as deworming and vaccination can be started in preparation for moving to the herd.
- Outerwear (boots, coveralls, coats, gloves, hats) worn while tending these isolation animals should be restricted to the isolation facility.
- Duties should be sequenced so the person caring for the isolation animals does not come into contact with other animals later that day. If possible, the person(s) taking care of isolation animals would have no other animal contact duties.
- Equipment such as feed containers, snares, halters, blankets, shovels, pitchforks, scrapers, etc., used in the isolation facility should not be used in other farm animal units. Particular attention needs to be paid to the use of mechanized equipment (front-end loaders) used for cleaning corals, pens, moving hay, etc., to be sure they are not used in both the isolation facility and the regular animals' pens without appropriate disinfection (Fig. 1.8.2).

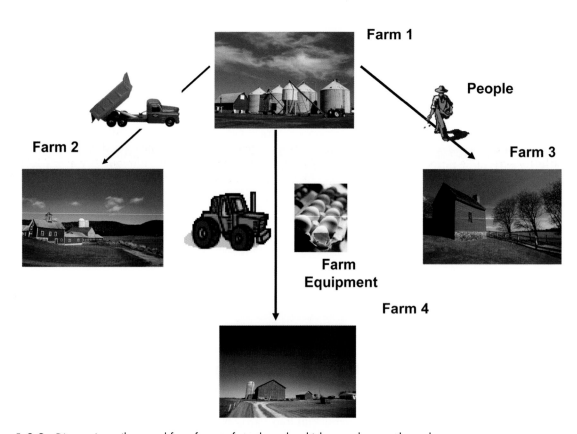

Figure 1.8.2 Disease is easily spread from farm to farm through vehicles, produce, and people.

13. Describe who might be considered a low-risk responder/visitor to a farm.

Responders from urban areas who have had little or no livestock contact are likely low-risk visitors (Table 1.8.1).

Table 1.8.1 Guidelines for Responder/Visitor Risk Assessment

	Low Risk	Moderate Risk	High Risk
Number of farm visits per day	No other farm contact	One or occasionally more than one farm per day	Routinely visits many farms or auctions
Protective Clothing	Wears sanitized shoes or boots. One pair of clean coveralls per site	Wears sanitized shoes or boots— If clean, may not change coveralls	Does not wear clean or protective clothing
Animal Ownership	Does not own and/or care for livestock	Owns and/or cares for a different species	Owns and/or cares for a similar species and production type
Contact with animals	No animal contact	Minimal or no direct contact— exposure to housing facilities	Regular direct contact with animals
Biosecurity knowledge	Understands and promotes biosecurity for industry	Aware of basic biosecurity principles but is not an advocate	Little appreciation or understanding of biosecurity principles
Foreign travel	Does not travel out of USA	Limited travel outside of USA without animal contact	Travel to foreign countries with animal contact in those countries

Source: http://www.omafra.gov.on.ca/english/livestock/vet/facts/04-003.htm.

14. Describe some precautions that should be followed by the low-risk responder to a farm.

- Wear freshly laundered outerwear and clean footwear. Disposable gloves, plastic boots, and coveralls (Tyvek) are an added precaution. This not only reduces the disease risk for animals on the farm but also prevents responders from contaminating their clothing with disease agents on the farm being visited.
- Foot baths for scrubbing one's boots are commonplace but their effectiveness is quite questionable. Unless boots are scrubbed before immersion and adequate contact time in the disinfectant is permitted—usually at least 5 minutes—disinfection is unreliable. Use boots that have no or minimal cleats to facilitate easy cleaning (Fig. 1.8.3).

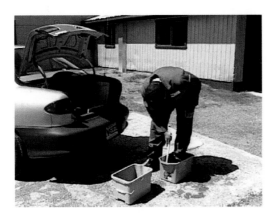

Figure 1.8.3 Foot baths, disinfectant, and scrubbing boots are all part of biosecurity procedures.

- Responders should minimize entry into animal pens, walking through feed alleys, and should only touch animals if absolutely necessary.
- Responders should never bring food articles with them onto the farm.
- All disposable clothing and boots should be collected in a plastic bag for disposal. Boots should be scrubbed before leaving the premises. All responders must wash and disinfect their hands before leaving the farm.

15. Describe a responder who might be considered a moderate-risk visitor to a farm.

Moderate-risk responders are those people who routinely visit farms but have little or no actual contact with animals. Salespersons, feed and fuel delivery drivers, and maintenance workers are examples of this group.

16. List the precautions that should be followed by the moderate-risk responder to a farm.

- The moderate-risk responder must at least follow all the guidelines of the low-risk responder (see No. 13).
- Moderate-risk responders should wear clean coveralls and boots if there is any contact with animal feed, animals, soil, or manure.
- Any sampling equipment should be properly cleaned and disinfected between uses.
- Dirty boots should be cleaned and disinfected, and coveralls should be removed and placed in a clean plastic bag or container before reentering the vehicle.

17. Who would be considered a high-risk responder to a farm's biosecurity?

High-risk visitors are those people who come into direct contact with livestock in their work and would include veterinarians, veterinary technicians, inseminators, livestock haulers, and even livestock-owning responders. These people generally have direct contact with animals and their bodily discharges. In a disaster, animal responders will have multiple animal/farm contacts and therefore *all* will be considered "high risk" to the farm.

18. What precautions should be followed as a high-risk responder to a farm?

- All items noted for the low- and moderate-risk responders should be followed.
- Vehicles should be clean and free of visible manure on the tires and wheel wells and should be kept away from animal areas and driveways used by the farm's own vehicles. If possible park off the premises and walk in after donning appropriate personal protection equipment. Vehicle interiors should be clean and easily cleanable. Livestock trucks and trailers should be clean and dry, and preferably disinfected, before arrival at the farm.
- All responders should arrive with clean clothing, boots, and equipment. Equipment and instruments that have direct animal contact should be cleaned and disinfected (or sterilized) after use and maintained in such a way that they do not become contaminated.
- Disposable clothing and gloves should be worn whenever there is the possibility of direct contact with bodily discharges or animal tissues.
- Before leaving the farm, dirty equipment and footwear must be cleaned and disinfected with an appropriate chemical agent. Soiled coveralls should be removed before reentering the vehicle. Hands and forearms should be washed and disinfected.
- Vehicles that have been at the site of a disaster involving an infectious disease (especially a potential foreign animal disease) should have the tires and wheel wells disinfected with a suitable disinfectant (see Chapter 1.22). Ideally, the vehicle should be put through a car wash before going to the next animal premise (Fig. 1.8.4).

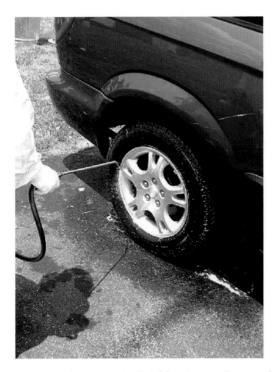

Figure 1.8.4 Spraying the vehicle tires with disinfectant can be helpful in limiting the spread of infectious agents between farms.

- Responders with livestock at their own home are required to report with clean clothes that have not been exposed to their livestock. Prior to returning home, it is in the responder's best interest to again don clean clothes to prevent a breach of one's own animal biosecurity.

19. When planning to respond to a farm disaster, what procedures should be followed prior to entry?

- If possible, contact the farm to discuss the farm's requirements for biosecurity in terms of clothing, animal contact, showing, etc. If no specific requirements are defined, the responder will, at a minimum, set the example by using measures that would seem prudent for a well-managed farm.
- Expect to be asked, or at the very least, inform the farm manager of your recent contact with animals in other herds or visits to foreign countries.
- Avoid unnecessary animal contact when responding to livestock facilities. For observing outside buildings or fences, new disposable plastic boots or footwear should be used.
- All outerwear of the responder must be clean (not worn on any other farm since being cleaned and disinfected) if it is necessary to be in buildings, alleyways, lots, pens, or pastures normally accessible to the herd. Disposable coveralls and disposable plastic boots and gloves are recommended. Clean laundered coveralls and clean disinfected boots may be acceptable. Protective face masks and head covers may be necessary in situations where responders may be exposed to dusty animal housing or if there is potential for aerosol transmission of zoonotic diseases (e.g., Q fever, avian influenza). If an emergency responder is entering a premise in which there is known zoonotic disease such as avian influenza, a higher level of eye and respiratory protection will be necessary such as a full face mask with air filters (Figs. 1.8.5 and 1.8.6).
- Plastic storage containers with sealing lids can be used for storing and transporting the new and/or clean coveralls and disposable boots, head covers and dust masks, etc.
- When leaving the farm, protective outer clothing worn on the farm should be removed before entering the vehicle and left on that farm if at all possible for appropriate disposal. Reusable clothing should be placed in a plastic bag and sealed until they can be laundered. Reusable boots should be scrubbed free of debris with water, soaked in disinfectant solution, and then placed in a plastic bag or other container for transport allowing the disinfectant to dry upon them (Fig. 1.8.7).

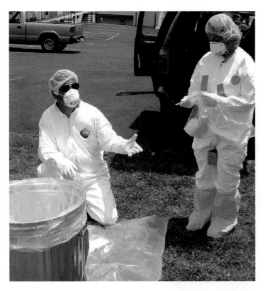

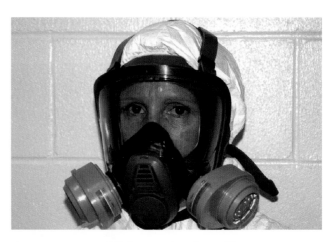

Figure 1.8.6 A full face mask with air filters is appropriate where a known zoonotic disease is present in an animal facility.

Figure 1.8.5 Appropriate personal protective equipment not only provides protection to the responder, but since this equipment does not leave the farm, it also is part of the biosecurity prevention of further spread of disease.

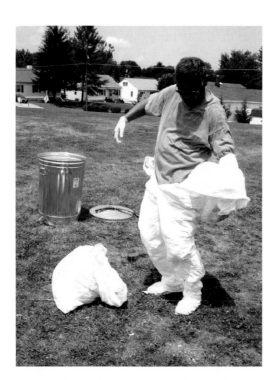

Figure 1.8.7 Disposable personal protective equipment is removed and left at the farm.

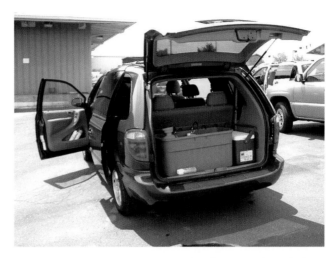

Figure 1.8.8 All clean and contaminated items are to be transported in the responder' vehicle. Separate containers for each should be used to prevent cross-contamination.

20. What other guidelines are suggested when the responder must visit multiple farms?

- Visit as few farms as possible having the same species on any given day.
- Farms with a full-time livestock production unit should be visited first.
- Keep the number of responders to the minimum required to do the job. For biosecurity, it would be better to have multiple small response teams visiting multiple farms rather than one large response team that visits all the farms.
- Use disposable plastic boots if the visit requires entering animal facilities. If animal contact is necessary, disposable gloves, boots, and coveralls should be worn and disposed of appropriately before going to another animal facility.
- Request that each farm supply as much equipment as possible for use on their own animals (nose-leads, snares, buckets, brushes, etc.). Clean and sanitize all transported equipment before and after use at each location.
- Leave used disposable items (boots, coveralls, gloves, etc.) at the farm where they were used. All items can be sealed in a small trash bag for convenient disposal by the owner. If clean and contaminated items are to be transported in the responder's vehicle, separate containers for each should be used to prevent cross-contamination (Fig. 1.8.8).

21. What are the key elements of a biological risk management/ biosecurity plan for a farm?

- Recognize the means by which diseases can be transmitted on a farm—aerosols, direct contact, fomites, orally, and vectors.
- Take control of how diseases enter and spread in a herd/flock by managing animals, manure, pests, pets, wildlife, people, water, and feed sources.
- Obtain replacement animals from a single source that provides a herd health history.
- Develop a comprehensive vaccination program for purchased and home-raised animals.
- Isolate new animals on arrival at the farm.
- Transport purchased animals in clean trucks, while minimizing the stress of transportation.
- Control other species (i.e., cats, dogs, birds, rodents, and wildlife) to reduce contact with the herd/flock.
- Manage manure to prevent contamination of young stock and feed.

22.   Any final thoughts on biosecurity and the animal responder in a disaster?

Any disaster is going to have catastrophic impacts on the farm. Not only will there be significant financial consequences, but there are numerous psychological impacts on the farmer who has spent his or her lifetime developing profitable livestock. A disaster will be devastating. Animal responders are there to help. Do not add to the devastation through carelessness or a lack of knowledge. Show compassion for the animals and for the animal owners!

Suggested Reading

Center for Food Safety and Public Health, Iowa State University. Available at: http://www.cfsph.iastate.edu/ and http://www.cfsph.iastate.edu/BRMForProducers/default.htm.

Compendium of measures to prevent disease associated with animals in public settings, 2005. Available at: www.cdc.gov/nasd/docs/d001801-d001900/d001804/d001804.html.

FAO Biosecurity Toolkit 2007. Available at: http://www.fao.org/docrep/010/a1140e/a1140e00.html.

The University of Vermont. Farm biosecurity risk assessment and biosecurity. Available at: http://www.uvm.edu/~ascibios/Assessment/Farm_Biosecurity_Risk_Assessment.html.

CHAPTER 1.9
VETERINARY TRIAGE

Wayne E. Wingfield, MS, DVM

In disasters, triage is conducted with the purpose of doing the greatest good for the largest number of animals.

1. What is triage?

Triage is a medical decision-making process used to identify the most seriously injured. *Triage* comes from the French word *trier* which means "to sort." It originally meant "to sort wool." Without doubt, conventional triage is only the first step in a dynamic decision-making process.

2. Describe the principal objective of triage.

Triage functions as an analytical sorting process with one objective, doing the greatest good for the greatest number of animals. The focus is on efficiency!

3. How important is triage in a disaster?

Triage is one of the most important missions of any medical response. In triage, one must balance two important factors:

- Medical needs of the patient(s)
- Available medical resources

With any disaster, the number of casualties can easily overwhelm the medical resources. Conversely, severe damage to the medical resources will result in the facility being overwhelmed with only a few casualties.

4. How does veterinary triage differ from the classic description of triage?

In veterinary disasters, there will usually be large numbers of casualties and there is often a large geographic/demographic area.

5. List some of the factors that result in triage and treatment decisions being different in human and veterinary medicine.

- The option of euthanasia
- Little tolerance for fair to poor outcomes of animal patients including long-term/permanent disabilities or intensive nursing care requirements

- Transport difficulties for large numbers of animals or certain species
- Limited veterinary medical resources (facilities, equipment, supplies, personnel, and varying 24-hour emergency care capabilities)
- Additional considerations that impact triage decisions within veterinary medicine include the following:
  - Companion animals (dogs, cats, horses, pocket pets, birds, etc.) versus livestock animals (cattle, sheep, pigs, poultry, etc.)
  - Small animals versus large animals
  - Presently, in veterinary medicine, there is no such designation of a level I, II, III, or IV trauma clinic or hospital.
    - Most veterinary practices fall into two broad categories: general practice (of one or more species) or specialty practice (surgery, medicine, critical care, emergency, etc.).
    - Specialty practices tend to be limited to the larger metropolitan areas and academic institutions. Many areas of the country are limited in their access to general practice care. Therefore, destination options may be limited, and triage will focus on identifying medical needs of the patient in light of available transport and medical resources, as well as the professional competency of the veterinarian.
- Recognizing that the treatment of animals is still dependent on the animal owner's disposable income, "medical resources" includes not only facilities, supplies, equipment, personnel, and time but also money. In a disaster, **all animals** will receive first-aid care regardless of the owner's ability to pay.

6. List several factors delaying animal rescue in veterinary disasters.

- Veterinary disasters often result in catastrophic casualty management (poultry, swine, and fish) where there are large numbers of victims.
- Severely limited medical resources
- Poorly trained local rescue personnel
- Animals caught in a disaster often remain at the disaster scene for a protracted period of time.

7. What are the three triage techniques used in veterinary medicine?

1. Field
2. Medical
3. Mobile veterinary unit

8. Describe veterinary field triage.

- Requires *experienced* veterinarians or rescuers
- Usually does not involve the individual examination of animals. More commonly, the animals are observed and decisions are made.
- Designed to identify animals most likely to benefit from the available care under austere conditions
- Usually does not involve the individual examination of the animal. It is more likely that the animals are observed from a distance and triage decisions are made.

9. Who conducts field triage at the disaster site?

First responders are usually local citizens when the disaster is sudden and are often tasked with field triage of affected animals. These responders usually have limited resources and training in veterinary issues.

10. How are veterinary patients categorized during field triage (Table 1.9.1)?

- Those that will likely die regardless of how much care they receive. Coded color = black
- Those that will survive whether or not they receive care. Coded color = green
- Those that will benefit significantly from austere interventions. Coded color = red.

Table 1.9.1 Triage Color Codes Used in Veterinary Field Triage

Triage Color	Triage Category	Explanation
	Immediate	Might benefit from austere interventions
	Minor	Walking wounded but likely to survive
	Dead, dying, or euthanatize	Dead, dying, or euthanatize

11. Exercise:

Using the field triage technique, assign a color (red, green, or black) beside each of the following disaster victims. **Red tag** = those that will benefit significantly from emergency interventions conducted with minimal equipment, facilities, and veterinary personnel. **Green tag** = those that will survive regardless of whether they receive care. **Black tag** = those that will die regardless of how much care they receive.
Using the field technique of triage, assign a number beside each of the following disaster victims.

_____ Fractured femur from yesterday
_____ Anemic with symptoms
_____ Dilated cardiomyopathy with ventricular tachycardia
_____ Laryngeal paralysis with respiratory distress
_____ Acute intervertebral disc prolapse with rear limb paralysis
_____ Acute pancreatitis with vomiting and diarrhea

Answers:
Green—Fractured femur from yesterday
Green—Anemic animal with symptoms
Black—Dilated cardiomyopathy with ventricular tachycardia
Red—Laryngeal paralysis with respiratory distress
Red—Acute intervertebral disc prolapse with rear limb paralysis
Red—Acute pancreatitis with vomiting and diarrhea

We are teaching principles in this exercise and fully realize you will have either examined and/or collected laboratory data to make such a diagnosis. Unfortunately, this is the only way I could envision giving you an opportunity to see how the system works!

12. List some of the advantages of field triage.

- Focuses resources appropriately
- Requires an experienced triage team
- Tough decisions are made and adhered to.
- After the disaster is over, the team retrospectively examines decisions and improves performance.

13. What is involved in medical triage?

Medical triage is done rapidly and involves examining individual animals.

14. What technique is recommended during medical triage?

One approach is to use the following four physiological criteria (RPPN):

1. Respirations/minute
2. Pulse rate/minute
3. Pulse pressure
   ○ Although subjective, pulse pressure has a linear relationship to stroke volume. Therefore, if the pulse pressure is decreased (as you might see in shock) the stroke volume is also likely decreased.

$$Cardiac\ Output = Heart\ Rate \times Stroke\ Volume$$

4. Neurological status

15. How are animals coded during medical triage (Table 1.9.2)?

Table 1.9.2 Veterinary Medical Triage Technique

Category	Color	RPPN
Immediate		Abnormal RPP
Urgent		Abnormal PPN
Minor		"Normal RPPN"
Dead, Dying, or Euthanatize		Mortal Wounds or *Severely* Abnormal Neurological

RPPN: respiration, pulse rate, pulse pressure, and neurologic status.

16. Describe some points to recall as you perform medical triage to animals.

- In veterinary medical triage, it is important to recognize that limitations of treatment and injuries for certain species will affect the triage assessment.
  ○ For example, a fractured femur in a dog may be tagged yellow, but a fractured femur in a horse will be tagged black.
- A relatively small number of animals can overwhelm the veterinary medical system, necessitating the implementation of the field triage system discussed earlier.
- Medical triage always begins with a reassessment of patients.
- Immediate and urgent patients go to the treatment area, where they are treated based on severity and resources. Those patients who need limited resources with a high probability of surviving will probably be treated first.
- Minor casualties go to an observation area where they are periodically reassessed.
- Patients who do not respond to treatment are retagged and sent to the observation area or euthanatized.
- One critical difference in veterinary, versus human triage, is that patients that will die regardless of how much care they receive and those that will suffer for the lack of care will be euthanatized.
- Therefore, it is very important to properly identify those animals who will survive regardless of whether they receive care and those who will benefit significantly from available interventions.
- Of note, while euthanatizing an injured animal is done for humane reasons, these decisions need to be well documented and supported.
  ○ Most commonly, there is a written protocol for euthanasia and it often requires two veterinarians agreeing this is the best option considering the patient and the patient's condition.
  ○ It is not uncommon for some animals (horses especially) to be insured, and the insurance company must authorize the euthanasia when possible. When contacting the insurance company is not feasible, documentation and witnesses are very important.

17. Study the following flow chart to learn the techniques of using RPPN in veterinary medical triage (Fig. 1.9.1).

Medical Triage Using RPPN

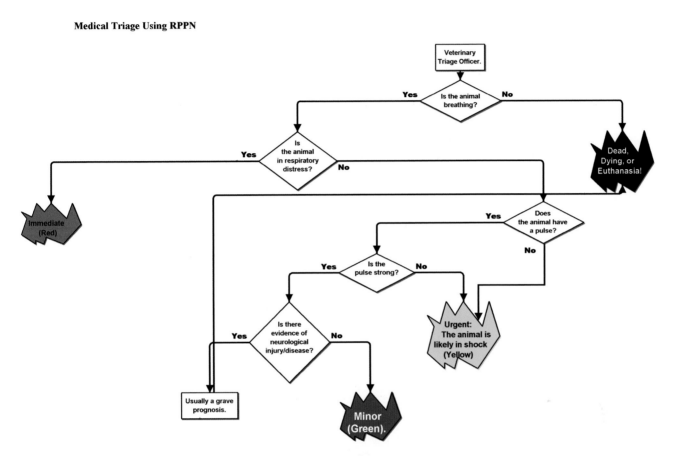

Figure 1.9.1   Decision tree demonstrating the use of RPPN in medical triage.

18. How are animals to be identified during triage?

- Ribbons of the appropriate triage color may be attached to the animal. These will have no information regarding the patient.
- Appropriately colored chalks or spray paint might be used.
- An alternative would be to attach a triage tag to the animal (Fig. 1.9.2). This tag uses an image of a dog, but this should not deter its use on other veterinary species. The idea is to identify wounds, fractures, burns, etc. by marking an approximate location on the triage tag image. It is also important that the behavioral disposition of the animal be identified to make other responders aware of potential aggressiveness.

19. What technique is used in mobile veterinary unit triage?

V-START.

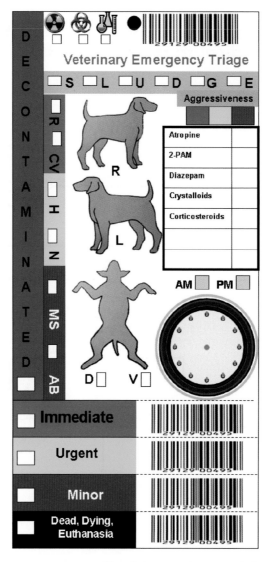

Figure 1.9.2 Proposed triage tag for veterinary patients. Although there is a dog pictured, the image can represent any animal species. Notice "aggressiveness" is listed and should be identified before the animal moves to the next treatment (shelter) area.

20. What does the acronym V-START stand for?

- Veterinary
- Systems
- Triage
- And
- Rapid
- Treatment

21. In animals, V-START uses physiologic systems to categorize animals during mobile veterinary unit triage. List the system's priorities.

1. Respiratory
2. Cardiovascular
3. Hemorrhage
4. Neurological
5. Musculoskeletal
6. Abdominal or other injuries

22. Using the V-START technique, a series of colors will define the priorities in triage (Table 1.9.3). Identify the colors, the triage priority, and the physiological system of each (Table 1.9.4).

Table 1.9.3 Types of Injury May Influence the Triage Category. Also, the species may be an influence. Notice that animals decontaminated will be tagged with a blue color indicating the animal is less of a risk to the rescuer.

Group	Color	Types of Injuries
Immediate	Red	Critical: May survive if life-saving measures are administered.
Urgent	Yellow	Likely to survive if care is given within hours.
Minor	Green	Minor injuries: Care may be delayed while other patients receive treatment.
All Groups	Blue	Animal has been decontaminated.
Dead, Dying, or Euthanasia	Black	Dead or severely injured and not expected to survive

Table 1.9.4 Guidelines for Using Physiologic Systems in Mobile Veterinary Unit Triage

Triage Color	Triage Category	Physiologic System Involvement
Red	Immediate	Respiratory, Cardiovascular, (Hypothermia, Hyperthermia)
Yellow	Urgent	Cardiovascular, Musculoskeletal, Neurologic, Abdominal Injuries
Green	Minor	Musculoskeletal, Neurologic, Abdominal Injuries
Black	Dead, Dying, or Euthanasia	Dead or dying when initially assessed. Mortal wounds not compatible with "Quality of Life" issues. Euthanasia.

23. Examine the following three flow charts to learn guidelines on how to use the V-START technique used in veterinary mobile unit triage (Figs. 1.9.3 through 1.9.5).

24. If an animal is exposed to a hazardous material, would you decontaminate first or address your concerns to the physiologic system affected?

- Tough question! Life-saving measures may be necessary but you must remember that your life is even more important.
- **Decontamination always precedes triage!**
- If the animal was not first decontaminated, it would likely expose other animals (and rescuers) to the hazardous material.

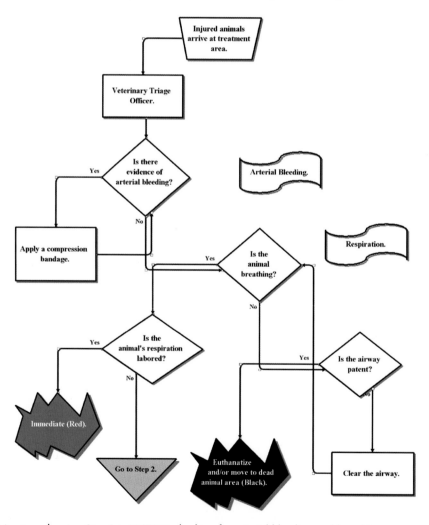

Veterinary Systems Triage and Rapid Treatment (V-START)
Step 1: Check for Arterial Bleeding and Breathing

Figure 1.9.3 Decision tree showing Step 1 in V-START, checking for arterial bleeding and breathing.

Step 2: Check Circulation and Control Hemorrhage

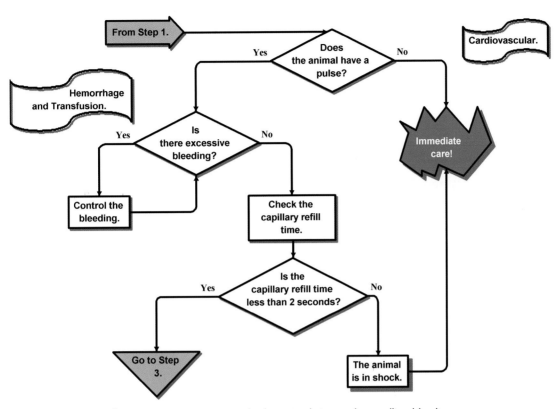

Figure 1.9.4 Decision tree showing Step 2 in V-START, checking circulation and controlling bleeding.

Step 3: Check for Neurological, Musculoskeletal, and Abdominal Injuries

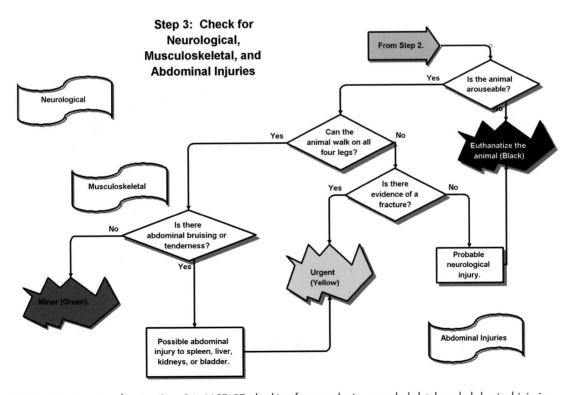

Figure 1.9.5 Decision tree showing Step 3 in V-START, checking for neurologic, musculoskeletal, and abdominal injuries.

25. List individuals who are important resources for triage during a disaster.

- Animal owners
- Livestock and poultry producers
- Owner/manager of a kennel or cattery
- Animal attendants from the zoo

26. How do preexisting illnesses or multiple injuries affect triage?

- When a disaster hits a veterinary hospital, an injury to a hospitalized animal will compound the seriousness of the previous illness/injury.
- These things must be considered when making triage decisions.

27. How do newly acquired illnesses affect triage decisions?

- Newly acquired illnesses or exacerbation of chronic illnesses require diagnosis and treatment.
- These animals should be treated by their regular veterinarian if possible, or a veterinary colleague temporarily.
- These animals should not be included in triage techniques!

28. List three important facts regarding the application of triage in a disaster.

- Participants must be trained in triage.
- Hard rules are developed and followed.
- Reassessment following the disaster is mandatory.

Suggested Reading
Bozeman WP. Mass casualty incident triage. *Ann Emerg Med* 2003;41:582–583.
Buono CJ, Lyon J, Huang J, et al. Comparison of mass casualty incident triage acuity status accuracy by traditional paper method, electronic tag, and provider PDA algorithm. *Ann Emerg Med* 2007;50:S12–S13.
Ducharme J, Tanabe P, Todd K, et al. A comparison of triage systems and their impact on initial pain management: A multicenter study. *Ann Emerg Med* 2006;48:61.
Fox PR, Puschner B, Ebel JG. 2008. Assessment of acute injuries, exposure to environmental toxins, and five-year health surveillance of New York Police Department working dogs following the September 11, 2001, World Trade Center terrorist attack. *J Am Vet Med Assoc* 2008;233:48–59.
Garner A, Lee A, Harrison K, Schultz CH. Comparative analysis of multiple-casualty incident triage algorithms. *Ann Emerg Med* 2001;38:541–548.
Hirshberg A, Holcomb JB, Mattox KL. Hospital trauma care in multiple-casualty incidents: A critical view. *Ann Emerg Med* 2001;37:647–652.
Iserson KV, Moskop JC. Triage in medicine, Part I: Concept, history, and types. *Ann Emerg Med* 2007;49:275–281.
Meredith W, Rutledge R, Hansen AR, et al. Field triage of trauma patients based upon the ability to follow commands: A study in 29,573 injured patients. *J Trauma* 1995;38:129–135.
Moskop JC, Iserson KV. Triage in medicine, Part II: Underlying values and principles. *Ann Emerg Med* 2007;49:282–287.
Pesik N, Keim ME, Iserson KV. Terrorism and the ethics of emergency medical care. *Ann Emerg Med* 2001;37:642–646.

Richards ME, Nufer KE. Simple triage and rapid treatment: Does it predict transportation and referral needs in patients evaluated by disaster medical assistance teams? *Ann Emerg Med* 2004;44:S33–S34.

Ross SE, Leipold C, Terregino C, O'Malley KF. Efficacy of the motor component of the Glasgow Coma Scale in trauma triage. *J Trauma* 1998;45:42–44.

Torres HC, Moreno-Walton L, Radeos M. The reliability of triage classification as a predictor of severity in major trauma. *Ann Emerg Med* 2007;50:S106–S107.

APPENDIX 1.9.1

1. Cite important factors learned from the Oakland firestorms regarding small animals caught in a disaster.

- Cats are less likely to be evacuated than are dogs.
- Pets are abandoned in disasters.
- Pets are not motivational priorities during a disaster.
- People who take their animals regularly to a veterinarian usually evacuate their pets.
- The longer an animal was lost, the less likely it was to be found.
- Animals wearing collars with the owner's name and address had a 10-fold increased likelihood of being reunited.
- Few animals were reunited after 4 weeks.

From Heath SE, et al: JAMA 212:504, 1998.

2. Describe some of the large-animal issues following Hurricane Floyd in North Carolina.

- 30,000 hogs, 2.9 million chickens and turkeys, 680 cattle, and 12 horses drowned.
- Few evacuation resources were available.
- Livestock producers are often the rescuers.
- There was a tremendous economic and emotional impact on the farmers.

CHAPTER 1.10
INTRODUCTION TO WEAPONS OF MASS DESTRUCTION

Jerry J. Upp, DVM

1. What are weapons of mass destruction?

Weapons of mass destruction (WMDs) include chemicals, biologics, nuclear and radiologics, incendiaries, and explosives. Any of these separately or in conjunction with each other has the ability of causing large numbers of injuries, illnesses, and death. Probably more important to the perpetrators, WMDs cause *terror* (Fig. 1.10.1).

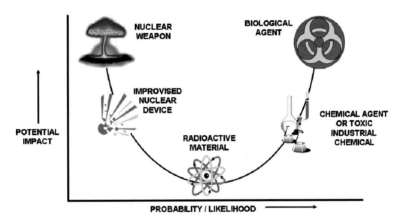

Figure 1.10.1. Weapons of mass destruction showing the potential impact versus the probability or likelihood of occurrence.

2. Why are animals important when discussing WMDs?

Many of the chemicals used as a weapon can affect animals in similar ways as they affect humans. This is important when dealing with our service animals such as search and rescue dogs, law enforcement animals, and our pets.

A large percentage of the biologics used as WMDs are zoonotic agents. This means that humans and animals can be affected by the same organism. Some of these agents can cause disease in animals or the animals can be carriers of the disease.

Radiation will cause similar signs and symptoms in animals as in people. This is important in the field. If large numbers of animals are suddenly found to show signs of radiation poisoning, this could be a red flag for first responders when entering a disaster.

3. List some of the chemical agents that may pose a WMD threat.

Chemical agents can fall into different categories depending on their composition and their effects. The major groups that can be seen are as follows:

• Blood agents
• Pulmonary or choking agents

- Nerve agents
- Vesicants or blister agents
- Riot control agents

The most likely agent to be seen in a chemical attack is one of these agents. The FBI has listed the top 10 most likely chemicals: ammonia, arsine, chlorine, cyanide, hydrogen sulfide, methyl isocyanate, phosgene, phosphine, sulfur dioxide, and fluorine. There are no nerve agents on this list, but they need to be included. These agents have been used in the past in acts of chemical terrorism and can cause a great deal of harm and deaths.

4.   What are blood agents?

The most likely blood agents to be encountered in a chemical attack are cyanide, or its derivatives, and arsine. Inhalation would be the most likely route of exposure for these agents.

Cyanide works at the cellular level by binding with cytochrome oxidase and disrupting cellular oxygen use. This leads to cellular asphyxiation and cell death. Cyanide may have a slight almond odor but not in every case. Cyanide may also be used as a food or water contaminate.

Arsine is a gas formed from arsenic. It binds in the red blood cell and causes an intravascular hemolysis. Inhalation is the primary route of exposure, but absorption through mucous membranes can occur.

5.   Describe the signs and symptoms of blood agents.

The signs and symptoms of the blood agents are related to damage at the cellular level. Cyanide exposure causes hypoxia, and the patient will have some form of cyanosis depending on exposure. Headache and dizziness are usually the initial complaints in humans, and these are followed by nausea and vomiting. Severe cases will involve respiratory and cardiac signs, comas, seizures, and death. Cyanide signs in a terrorist event are usually seen immediately after exposure.

Signs and symptoms of arsine exposure are not as immediate as those of cyanide. This can make it more desirable as a weapon since detection will be more difficult. It is not very irritating and exposure may not be known for as long as 1 day later. Intravascular hemolysis and renal failure occur. Similar early signs of headache can occur with possible vomiting. Death may occur within 1 day if a large exposure has occurred.

6.   What are pulmonary agents?

Pulmonary, or choking, agents are chemicals that affect the pulmonary system including both the upper and lower respiratory tracts. Inhalation is the most likely route of exposure, but ocular and dermal problems may also occur. There are many pulmonary agents, but the most likely in a terrorist event are ammonia, chlorine, phosgene, and phosphine.

Ammonia is most commonly found as anhydrous ammonia and is used especially in agriculture and as a coolant in large buildings, breweries, and sports arenas. It is colorless but has a strong odor and when combined with water forms a strong alkali called *ammonium hydroxide*.

Chlorine is a gas that is commonly used in industry. It also has a strong odor and when combined with water produces hydrochloric acid.

Phosgene is also used commonly in industry. When combined with water, it also forms carbon dioxide and hydrochloric acid.

Phosphine is another industrial chemical. It not only affects the respiratory system but can also lead to renal and cardiac failure. These chemicals are all fairly easy to obtain and should be considered likely choices in a terrorist chemical attack.

7.   Describe the signs and symptoms of pulmonary agents.

Ammonia will cause upper airway irritation including the eyes, laryngeal edema, coughing, wheezing, respiratory distress (dyspnea), and pulmonary edema. Death may occur with larger exposures. If contacted with the skin, it will cause burns and frostbite-type lesions.

Chlorine gas shows signs similar to ammonia. Ocular and upper airway irritation will occur and may progress to coughing, respiratory distress, and pulmonary edema. Death may also result following exposure.

Phosgene tends to have a more delayed action. It is not as water soluble and thus produces hydrochloric acid somewhat slower. It irritates the eyes and upper airways early following exposure but is slower to produce the pulmonary edema. It has a latent period after the initial upper airway signs but can progress to respiratory distress and hypoxia.

Phosphine will also cause the upper respiratory signs but can also cause vomiting, coughing, and chest and abdominal pain and can lead to renal and cardiac failure. On contact, it can cause frostbite-type lesions.

8. What are nerve agents?

Nerve agents may be the most well known of the chemical agents but are harder for the terrorists to obtain or produce. This puts their likelihood in a terrorist attack lower than the previously listed agents. These chemicals include *tabun* (GA), *sarin* (GB), *soman* (GD), and VX. The "G" in the nomenclature comes from their original production by the Germans before and during World War II. Sarin was used in the 1995 attack on the Tokyo subway by the Aum Shinrikyo terrorist sect. All of the nerve agents are organophosphate compounds and cause organophosphate poisoning. Of the four listed, VX is the only one that dissipates slowly. It is a very persistent, nonvolatile liquid and evaporates very slowly.

9. Describe the signs and symptoms of nerve agents.

Nerve agent exposure follows signs seen in organophosphate poisoning. The acronym **SLUDGEM** describes salivation, lacrimation, urination, defecation, gastrointestinal upset, emesis, and miosis. You may also see muscle weakness, increased heart rates, and eventual mydriasis. Central nervous system signs may include seizures and coma. Death can occur without expedient treatments. Tabun, sarin, and soman are very volatile and can be used in aerosol form, so inhalation of vapors is a primary concern during a terrorist release. Absorption of droplets is another slower route of entry. VX is nonvolatile, so dermal absorption is the more likely route of entry.

10. What are blister agents?

Blister agents, also known as *vesicants*, are agents that cause an injury like their name. They produce lesions on the skin, eyes, and any part of the body they contact. Burns and blisters are their primary mode of injury. Some of these agents were used as early as World War I and include sulfur mustard, Lewisite, and phosgene oxime. Of these, sulfur mustard has been used most in battle to incapacitate enemy troops.

11. Describe the signs and symptoms of blister agents.

Sulfur mustard causes burns and blisters and will be absorbed systemically or accidentally ingested. The signs are slightly delayed until the blisters form. This can happen within hours to 1 to 2 days later. The initial contact is not painful. Other signs that may become apparent are corneal burns, conjunctivitis, upper respiratory irritation, and gastrointestinal signs such as vomiting and diarrhea. If large enough doses are absorbed, bone marrow signs may be present. Anemias, leukopenias, and thrombocytopenias have been known to occur.

Lewisite differs from sulfur mustard in that it causes immediate pain and more immediate blisters. It also causes ocular signs much more quickly. Corneal ulcers and conjunctival edema may develop within minutes. Respiratory signs may include pulmonary edema in addition to respiratory irritation. High doses can cause death within minutes due to hypovolemic shock. Kidney and liver necrosis may also be systemic effects.

12. Describe what is meant by riot control agents, and provide expected clinical signs from exposure.

The riot control agents (RCAs) are chemicals that rapidly produce sensory irritation or disabling physical effects that disappear within a short time following termination of exposure. The standard tear-producing agents are *o*-chlorobenzylidene (CS), other agents in the same family (CS1, CS2, CSX), and dibenz(**b,f**)1:4-oxazepine (CR). Generally, they produce a rapid onset of effects (seconds to several minutes) and they have a relatively brief duration of effects (15 to 30 minutes) once the victim has escaped the contaminated atmosphere and the contamination has been removed from clothing or hair coat. Because tear compounds produce only transient casualties, they are widely used for training, riot control, and situations where long-term incapacitation is unacceptable. When released indoors, they may cause serious illness or death. It is not uncommon for working animals (WAs) to become exposed to RCAs. Many of these agents will cause temporary discomfort but seldom have long-term or fatal effects. Tests have been conducted by various credible organizations and it has been determined that working dogs can often continue with their operations even after being exposed to these chemicals. If the environment requires the handler to a wear protective mask, one should avoid taking a WA into that environment.

Clinical signs include an initial burning feeling or irritation to the eyes that progresses to pain accompanied by blepharospasm and lacrimation. The mucous membranes of the mouth have a sensation of discomfort or burning, with excess salivation. Rhinorrhea is accompanied by pain inside the nose. When inhaled, these compounds cause a burning sensation or a feeling of tightness in the chest, with coughing, sneezing, and increased secretions. On unprotected skin, especially if the air is warm and moist, these agents cause tingling or burning.

Specific treatment is generally not required since the signs and symptoms subside on their own once animals have been moved to fresh air. The eyes should be rinsed with either sterile water or saline. A topical ophthalmic ointment can then be applied to soothe and reduce inflammation caused by the contamination.

During decontamination, no form of hypochlorite (bleach) should be used in an attempt to decontaminate RCAs. Bleach reacts with riot control agents to form a strong irritant.

Move the animal to fresh air, and brush or vacuum powders from the hair coat. Flush the skin with plain water, soap and water, or a weak solution of sodium bicarbonate (baking soda). Water and soap may cause a temporary worsening of the burning sensation, but it will not cause additional damage.

13. List the most likely biologic agents to be used as WMDs.

The Centers for Disease Control and Prevention in Atlanta, Georgia, has put the biologic agents into categories based on their dissemination and transmissibility, high morbidity and mortality, public perception, and difficulty of public health response. These categories include Class A, Class B, and Class C agents.

- **Class A** agents include the organisms for anthrax, botulism, plague, smallpox, tularemia, and the viral hemorrhagic fevers (arenaviruses, bunyaviruses, filoviruses, and flaviviruses). Class A agents cause the most severe health effects if encountered in a terrorist event.
- **Class B** agents include agents for brucellosis, *Clostridium perfringens*, glanders, meliodosis, psittacosis, Q-fever, ricin toxin, staphylococcal enterotoxin B, typhus, viral encephalitis agents, and food and water threats such as *Salmonella* spp., *Escherichia coli (E. coli)*, *Shigella* spp., *Vibrio* spp., and *Cryptosporidium* spp.
- **Class C** agents are emerging agents such as Hantavirus and Nipah virus.

14. Describe the cause, routes of exposure, and clinical signs of anthrax exposure.

Anthrax is caused by the bacterium *Bacillus anthracis*. It is a zoonotic disease but does not have person-to-person transmission. This bacteria forms spores that are very resistant in the environment (Fig. 1.10.2).

The spores can cause signs depending on contact, inhalation, or ingestion. Three forms of the disease can occur and each gives different signs and symptoms of disease. The three forms of anthrax are cutaneous anthrax, gastrointestinal anthrax, and inhalational anthrax. Of these, *inhalational anthrax* is the most deadly and most likely

Bacteriology of *Bacillus anthracis*

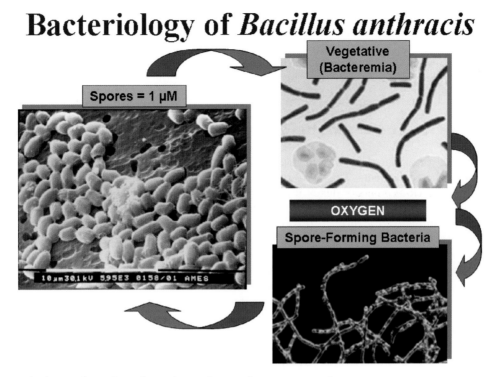

Figure 1.10.2. The bacteriology of *Bacillus anthracis* showing the vegetative and spores.

in a terrorist event. The biologic event after 9/11 involved anthrax and resultant deaths were due to inhalation. The spores can be weaponized by adding an electrical charge to cause greater dispersal and therefore greater transmission. Interestingly, dogs seem to be extremely resistant to the inhalation route of exposure to anthrax organisms. It is conjectured that the longer nasal passages of the dog "filter out" the organism.

Cutaneous anthrax occurs from contact and is the most common natural form of the disease in humans. It starts as a cutaneous skin lesion that becomes ulcerated and becomes a blackened lesion within 2 to 3 days. These lesions are usually not painful. Regional lymph node enlargement may occur. If left untreated, cutaneous anthrax can have a mortality rate of 20% in humans.

Gastrointestinal anthrax comes from ingestion of the spores. This is the least likely presentation in a terrorist event for people but may be likely in dogs if they ingest contaminated meat. Signs include vomiting, diarrhea, sepsis, and possible death if not treated. The most likely route of infection is consuming contaminated meat.

Inhalational anthrax is the most severe form for humans and is the most likely exposure route in a terrorist event. It is the rarest form in nature. Inhalation of the spores sets up the disease process. The spores release a toxin, which decreases the chance of successful treatment. Initial diagnosis is difficult due to the commonality of signs compared with flulike symptoms. Expedient diagnosis is imperative due to the severity of the disease and lack of response to treatment in the later stages. The respiratory disease progresses quickly and includes flulike symptoms, shortness of breath, coughing, and tightening of the chest. The second stage of the disease is caused by the bacteremia and includes respiratory distress, cyanosis, shock, and death. Thoracic radiographs reveal mediastinal widening, which is indicative of the disease. A high mortality rate will occur without early treatment.

15. Describe the cause, routes of infection, and clinical signs of botulism.

Botulism is caused by the bacteria *Clostridium botulinum*, which produces a potent toxin. Like anthrax, *C. botulinum* produces spores, which in turn release the toxin. These toxins are the most lethal known toxins and can easily be produced for dissemination. The most likely natural route of infection is ingestion. This route could be used in a terrorist event, but aerosol dispersal is a bigger concern due to the ability of affecting more people. Once again, there is no person-to-person transmission. The disease may occur by ingestion, wound penetration, or inhalation. Inhalation is *least* likely in nature. If inhalation botulism is suspected, terrorism should be considered likely. The signs are the same no matter how it occurs. Botulism tends to be a neurologic disease that shows descending weakness or flaccid paralysis without fever or altered mental status. Signs in people may begin as difficulty speaking, swallowing, abnormal vision, facial nerve paralysis, dry mouth, constipation or diarrhea, weakness, and dyspnea. Phrenic nerve involvement can occur, necessitating the use of a ventilator.

16.   Describe the cause, routes of infection, and clinical signs of plague.

Plague is a bacterial disease caused by the bacteria *Yersinia pestis*. It is a naturally occurring disease spread by fleas that have fed on infected rodents. The initial host will eventually die and the fleas will have a greater tendency to seek out other hosts such as humans (Fig. 1.10.3).

Plague is a favorable choice for terrorists since the organism can be aerosolized, is highly contagious, can have a high mortality rate, and is well identified to cause terror when released. There are three forms of plague and signs differ between the three. The three forms are bubonic plague, pneumonic plague, and septicemic plague.

Bubonic plague is the most common form of plague seen in natural infections. It is characterized by enlarged lymph nodes in the area of a flea bite called *buboes*. Fever occurs with malaise, dizziness, and possible recumbency. Septicemia can occur with a disseminated intravascular coagulopathy (DIC), shock, and death. Unless large numbers of plague-infected fleas are released in a populated setting, bubonic plague may not be the most likely form to be seen in a terror event. Bubonic plague is not transmitted person-to-person unless a secondary pneumonia has occurred. This is not very common. Without treatment, approximately one-half of the cases of bubonic plague will die.

Pneumonic plague is the *least* likely form of plague to be seen in natural infections but may be the most likely form in a terrorist event. If the bacteria are aerosolized and dispersed, inhalation of the bacteria may occur and large numbers of people will become infected. Pneumonic plague has an almost 100% mortality rate if left untreated and can be spread person-to-person. If pneumonic plague is diagnosed, terrorism should be considered. Symptoms can occur very quickly. The incubation period is from a few hours to 3 days. Sudden onset of dyspnea, bloody sputum, chest pain, fever, and cough with severe pneumonia occurs. Signs can rapidly lead to septicemia, DIC, multiorgan failure, and death.

Septicemic plague is plague without primary pneumonia or buboe formation and has a very rapid onset and course. Fever with severe gastrointestinal symptoms leading to DIC, shock, and multiorgan failure will occur. The mortality rate without treatment approaches 100%, and even with treatment the rate approaches 50%. Primary septicemic plague is not transmitted person-to-person but can spread if a secondary pneumonia is present.

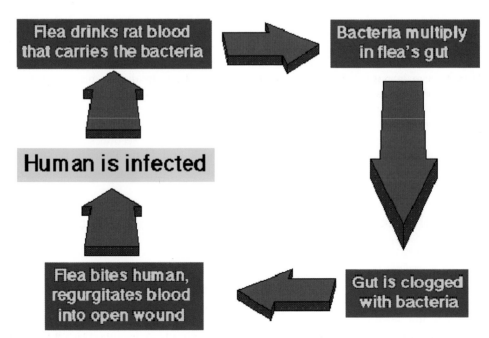

Figure 1.10.3 Plague cycle in animals.

17. Describe the cause, routes of infection, and clinical signs of smallpox.

Smallpox (variola) is a viral disease caused by an orthopox virus. It has been eradicated worldwide, and the World Health Organization declared it eradicated on May 8, 1980. A vaccine is available but until recently it had not been used since 1972 in the United States. The terrorist concern with smallpox results from possible unknown storehouses of the virus since eradication. The CDC has one storehouse and the former Soviet Union has the other. There is a possibility that some of the latter could have made its way into rogue states that sponsor terrorism. For of this reason, the CDC has put it on their Class A list. It is the only Class A organism that does not have an animal source or vector. It is highly contagious and has a mortality rate of approximately 30%. There are no proven treatments for the virus, and little is known on how current antiviral agents will work against this virus. Widespread panic would ensue with a release, which makes it desirable for a terrorist.

Smallpox is transmitted as an aerosol and replicates in the respiratory mucosa. The incubation period from exposure to clinical manifestation of disease is generally 12 to 14 days but can range from 7 to 14 days. The initial signs are fever, headache, and malaise with characteristic skin lesions starting in the mouth and face and spreading to the trunk and extremities. Smallpox lesions progress from a rash to macules, papules, vesicles, pustules, and then to scabs. The person-to-person spread occurs once the rash moves to the scab stage, which is usually around 14 to 20 days. It can be easy to confuse chickenpox lesions with smallpox lesions, but some differences do exist. Smallpox lesions tend to occur in larger numbers on the face and extremities, whereas chickenpox lesions accumulate more on the trunk. Smallpox lesions evolve together, whereas chickenpox lesions occur at different stages.

18. Describe the cause, routes of infection, and clinical signs of tularemia.

Tularemia is a disease caused by the bacterium *Francisella tularensis*. It is a naturally occurring disease that most commonly occurs following handling rodents or lagomorphs (especially rabbits). The other route involves the bite of infected ticks or the deer fly. Person-to-person transmission does not occur with tularemia. There are various forms of the disease. The most common forms seen in the natural setting are the ulceroglandular and glandular forms. The ulceroglandular form gives a cutaneous ulcer with enlarged lymph nodes. The glandular form causes enlarged lymph nodes without the cutaneous lesion. The signs of these include fever, malaise, muscle pain, weakness, headache, joint pain, and cough. Although debilitating, the mortality rate of these forms is low. Less common forms are the oropharyngel, oculoglandular, and pneumonic forms. These forms would be more likely in a terrorist event since they are spread more through aerosol dispersal. A higher mortality rate is expected with the pneumonic form. Aerosol dispersal of the agent would infect a larger number of people, and according to the World Health Organization (WHO), a dispersal of 50 kg of agent in a metropolitan area of 5 million people would result in 250,000 cases and 19,000 deaths.

The incubation period of *F. tularensis* in the pneumonic form is usually 3 to 5 days after inhalation. Signs include coughing, fever, and dyspnea. Cases rapidly deteriorate and mental capacity can be lost. Flulike signs will also be present. If the oropharyngeal form is present, cervical lymphadenitis along with pharyngitis will be present. The oculoglandular form results from ocular exposure in the aerosol release and can exhibit corneal ulcers, conjunctivitis, and periorbital edema.

19. Describe the cause, routes of infection, and clinical signs of the viral hemorrhagic fevers.

The viral hemorrhagic fevers (VHF) are large classes of viral diseases causing varying degrees of fever and hemorrhage from any site in the body. The course and severity of disease vary depending on the agent. The four families of viruses that cause VHF are the Arenaviruses, Bunyaviruses, Filoviruses, and Flaviviruses. Included in these families are the following diseases: Ebola, Marburg, Lassa, Hantaan, Rift Valley fever, Argentine hemorrhagic fever, Bolivian hemorrhagic fever, Crimean-Congo hemorrhagic fever, and others. The incubation periods vary between the diseases, as do the mortality rates. None of these diseases are seen in the United States, so any diagnosis without foreign travel is very suggestive of a terrorist release. These agents are thought to be attractive to terrorists due to their disease severities, high transmissibility, and, in some cases, high morbidity and mortality rates. For example, Ebola Zaire has a mortality of 90%.

The VHFs cause multisystem failure resulting in bleeding. Most of the bleeding problems relate to low thrombocyte counts and bleeding can be present in any organ system. They are all febrile diseases and can transmit person-to-person. The VHF all tend to have an animal or arthropod reservoir, but in the cases of Ebola and Marburg, the animal or arthropod has yet to be identified. Because of the transmissibility of these diseases, a small release of organism could snowball into a large-scale medical emergency if not recognized early. This is what makes them attractive agents to terrorists. Most of the diseases begin with a few days of flulike symptoms, which then lead to bleeding manifestations. Additional signs may include multiorgan failure, bleeding from any orifice, bleeding under the skin, hypovolemia, shock, and death.

20. Are there any other biologic agents that may be used as a weapon?

Question Nos. 13 through 18 covered the CDC Class A agents—There are other agents and diseases in the Class B and Class C levels; these include brucellosis, C. perfringens, glanders, meliodosis, psittacosis, Q-fever, ricin toxin, staphylococcal enterotoxin B, typhus, viral encephalitis agents, and food and water threats such as Salmonella, E. coli, Shigella, Vibrio, and Cryptosporidium. Class C agents are emerging agents such as Hantavirus and Nipah virus. The CDC does not downplay these agents, but they are not as likely to be seen in a terrorist release. High mortality rates still occur with some of these agents, such as ricin toxin, but the chance of large-scale release is not as high. Some of these diseases such as Q-fever, brucellosis, glanders, and meliodosis tend to have lower mortality rates but are very debilitating. They can be used especially against the military to incapacitate the troops and their animals. Food and water threats can severely affect people, but the chance of affecting large-scale numbers of people is not good.

21. How can radiation be used as a WMD?

Radiation could be used by terrorists in many different ways. These releases may range from highly sophisticated releases from a nuclear bomb or a suitcase bomb to less-sophisticated releases from a dirty bomb or by merely planting a radioactive substance in a public place. The more highly technical the device, the less likely it is that a terrorist could get his or her hands on the technology or the radiation needed. Public perception of radiation has the Hiroshima or Nagasaki connotations, whereas an actual terrorist attack would almost certainly be much less severe. Just mentioning a radiation attack will cause panic until public education and awareness can come into play.

22. What is a nuclear blast?

A nuclear blast is the actual detonation of a nuclear bomb. This is what the public fears most, but it is much less likely in the hands of terror groups. The reaction actually involves fission or fusion and requires radioactive materials that are much harder to obtain. Enriched uranium or plutonium is needed, and it is not likely for terrorists to use unless they have terror-sponsoring countries behind them. The mushroom cloud occurs from these sorts of blasts, and tremendous destruction will occur. The detonations involving Hiroshima and Nagasaki in World War II involved nuclear blasts.

23. What is a "suitcase" bomb?

A "suitcase" bomb is an actual nuclear device that can form a nuclear blast like the larger nuclear bombs. These bombs are generally equivalent to a 1 kiloton explosion of dynamite. Compared to the bomb at Hiroshima, which was 12½ kilotons, they are much smaller but can still produce a very destructive explosion. Once again, fission or fusion is required but the bombs are much smaller and can fit into a suitcase. The old Soviet Union (Russia) and the United States supposedly produced these smaller bombs during the Cold War, and when the Soviet Union collapsed, there has been some uncertainty as to whether some of the suitcase bombs may be missing. According to a CBS television *60 Minutes* interview of former Russian National Security Adviser Alexandr Labed, in 1997, as many as 100 of 250 suitcase bombs are missing after the dissolution of the Soviet Union in 1991. An article produced by Fox News on January 29, 2003, also speaks of a possibility that Osama Bin Laden may have purchased suitcase bombs from Chechen-organized crime groups.

24. What is a "dirty" bomb?

A "dirty" bomb differs from a nuclear or suitcase bomb because it does not require fission or fusion reactions. Another name for a dirty bomb is a radiological dispersion device (RDD). This name explains how it works. It disperses the radiation from a conventional type blast such as dynamite. The radiation is dispersed from the blast and leads to contamination of the immediate area. The dirty bomb has also been called a weapon of mass *disruption*. It is thought in a lot of scenarios that the *initial blast* will likely produce more harm than the radiation. Here is where the public perception of a radiation emergency will have to be altered soon after an attack to help alleviate widespread panic. The radiation from a dirty bomb is not equal to the radiation from a nuclear bomb or suitcase bomb. Time, distance, and shielding are the most important things to remember in any radiological event. In other words, minimize your exposure time, maximize your distance from the event, and shield yourself from ionizing radiation.

25. What are some of the radioactive materials that may be used in a dirty bomb?

There are many possible radioactive substances that may be encountered. The following are some of the more common, and one should be familiar with some of their basic characteristics:

*   *Americium* is *not* a naturally occurring substance. Instead, it is a manmade metal produced from plutonium. The isotope has uses in industry and medicine and is called Americium-241, or Am-241. The most common place that Am-241 is found is in household smoke detectors.
*   *Cesium* is a naturally occurring element found in rock and granite. The radioactive form of cesium is cesium 137, or Cs-137. It is formed by the fission of uranium and is used commercially to calibrate radiation detection equipment, used medically as a cancer treatment, and used in industry to detect flow rates of some liquids. Cs-137 was one of the major isotopes found in the 1986 Chernobyl nuclear plant accident.
*   *Cobalt* occurs naturally in many metals and has been used as a blue coloring in glass and pottery. Radioactive cobalt, or Co-60, is used medically as a cancer therapy and is used commercially in plastic manufacturing and food sterilization.
*   The radioactive form of *iodine* is I-131. Its greatest use is in the medical field. Iodine is taken up in the thyroid gland of humans and animals. I-131 is used in the treatment of thyroid disorders and tumors.
*   *Plutonium* is listed here due to its familiarity in the public, but is probably farther down the list as a possibility in a dirty bomb. Plutonium is used almost exclusively in nuclear facilities and would be fairly hard to obtain by a terrorist. It is produced by a fission reaction and is a byproduct in weapon production and in nuclear power plants.
*   Strontium-90 is the most radioactive isotope of *strontium*. It is actually a waste product from fission reactions. A medical isotope of strontium is Sr-89, which is used for pain relief in certain bone cancers. Sr-90 gives off heat when decaying and is also used as a power source in space vehicles.
*   *Uranium* has three major isotopes of concern. They are U-234, U-235, and U-238. U-235 is the enriched or concentrated form. U-235 is the most talked about isotope, when dealing with nuclear reactors and power sources. Uranium is also used in armor-piercing shells due to its extremely hard structure. It is 65% more dense than lead. Once again, emergency responders will probably not be confronted with a uranium release due to the difficulty in obtaining enriched uranium.

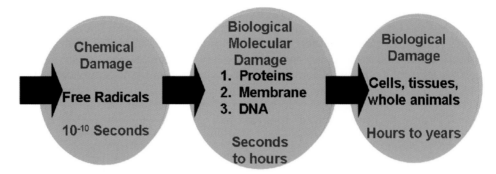

Figure 1.10.4. The basics of radiation injury to an animal.

26.   What are signs and symptoms of radiation exposure?

Acute and chronic medical problems due to radiation can result. The problems seen in animals will correlate closely with human signs and symptoms (Fig. 1.10.4).

- *Acute radiation syndrome* occurs if the radiation dose is high. The dose is usually in excess of 70 Rads but milder symptoms can occur at doses of 30 Rads. At doses between 70 and 1000 Rads, the *hematopoietic syndrome* can occur, which affects the bone marrow and causes bone marrow suppression. Death occurs in 50% of the animals exposed to over 450 Rads.
- The *gastrointestinal syndrome* is next in progression. At doses between 1000 and 10,000 Rads, irreversible damage to the gastrointestinal tract occurs. Survival at this level is very unlikely.
- The *central nervous syndrome* is the last syndrome. Doses greater than 5000 Rads will result in central nervous system signs and survival is not expected.

27.   List the four stages of the acute radiation syndrome.

1. *Prodromal stage*—The prodromal stage consists of nausea, vomiting, and occasional diarrhea. If the vomiting occurs less than 4 hours after exposure, the prognosis is much poorer than after 4 hours.
2. *Latent stage*—In this stage, the patient will feel more normal and look better clinically. This can last from hours to weeks.
3. *Illness stage*—This is where the signs can become more severe and the patient feels much worse. The signs can last up to several months.
4. *Recovery or death stage*—This will occur from weeks up to 2 years following exposure.

28.   Does a cutaneous syndrome result from radiation exposure?

A cutaneous syndrome does occur with exposure to the skin. Localized inflammation, erythema, and hair follicle damage occur. Most of these lesions will heal but may lack hair follicles or the affected areas may become necrotic.

29.   What is an incendiary?

Incendiaries are weapons that produce combustion and fire. The most well-known incendiary is the Molotov cocktail. It is usually a glass bottle filled with gasoline or other flammable liquid. The end of the bottle is stuffed with a rag and ignited. The bottle is thrown or placed into the area that the perpetrator wants to set on fire. Other types of incendiaries can be made by combining chemicals that when combined will produce fire. These do not need an ignition source since the chemical reaction causes heat and fire. On the events of 9/11, the United States witnessed three large incendiaries unleashed on the American people. The three jets loaded with fuel are considered incendiaries where the end result was massive fire, destruction, and death. When compared with chemical, biological, and radiologic terrorism, incendiaries generally do not produce mass fatalities. The events of 9/11 proved that even an incendiary can produce large numbers of fatalities and can definitely produce large-scale panic and terror.

30. What are the major injuries associated with incendiaries?

Because incendiaries produce fire as their primary objective, burn injuries are the major problems encountered by emergency personnel but are not the only concern. Remember that in some cases chemical reactions have occurred to ignite the fire, so attention to other organ systems must be included in the physical examinations. The respiratory system needs to be addressed early on in the care. Inhalation of any of the fumes or smoke from the fire will cause respiratory problems. The ABCs of emergency care must be followed where A is airway, B is breathing, and C is circulation. We must also pay attention to the percentage of the body that is burned.

31. What classifies as a blast injury?

Blast injuries vary greatly depending on the type of blast and the type of material used. There are high-order explosives and low-order explosives. High-order explosives produce an overpressurized shock wave that has some unique characteristics when looking at the injuries produced. High-order explosives include dynamite, C-4, TNT, and other higher-level explosives. Lower-order explosives are generally a less-sophisticated type of explosive such as a pipe bomb and do not have the higher energy to produce the overpressurized shock wave.

32. What are some of the major injuries seen with blasts?

Any organ system can be affected by blasts depending on the mechanism of injury. When dealing with blasts, the mechanism of injury is categorized into primary, secondary, tertiary, and quaternary injuries.

- *Primary injuries* deal with the pressurized shock wave; therefore, these injuries will be seen with the high-order explosives. These injuries concentrate on gas-filled organs and organ systems. The middle ear is a common place for injury, with rupture of the tympanic membrane being a common problem. Gastrointestinal hemorrhage and lung and eye trauma, with possible rupture, can all occur with primary blast injuries.
- *Secondary injuries* are injuries that result from the flying debris from the blast. These tend to be penetrating or concussing types of injuries. Any body system can be affected with these types of injuries.
- *Tertiary injuries* are injuries that result from the body being hurled into something by the blast. Once again, any body system can be affected. Head trauma is common, as well as contusions and fractures.
- *Quaternary injuries* are injuries that do not fit into the other categories. Burns will fall into this category as well as some crushing injuries or respiratory injuries from the fumes or dust. These injuries can also be cardiac in nature if a heart attack occurs after the blast.

Suggested Reading
Belay ED, Maddox RA, Williams ES, Miller MW, Gambetti P, Schonberger LB. Chronic wasting disease and potential transmission to humans. *Emerg Infect Dis* 2004;10:977–983.
CDC, Division of Bacterial and Mycotic Diseases. Brucellosis (*Brucella melitensis, abortus, suis, and canis*). 2005. Available at www.cdc.gov/ndidod/dbm/diseaseinfo/brucellosis_t.htm.

CDC Emergency Preparedness and Response website and associated agent fact sheets for sulfur mustard and nerve agents. Available at http://www.bt.cdc.gov/agent/; http://www.bt.cdc.gov/radiation; www.bt.cdc.gov/masscasualties.

CDC. Fact sheet: Anthrax information for health care providers. March 8, 2002. Available at www.emergency.cdc.gov/agent/anthrax/anthrax-hcp-factsheet.asp.

Department of Agriculture/Department of Defense. Field Manual (FM) 3-11.9, Potential military chemical/biological compounds, multiservice tactics techniques and procedures. January 2005. Available at http://chppm-www.apgea.army.mil/chemicalagent/.

Kingery AF, Allen HE. The environmental fate of organophosphate nerve agents: A review. *Toxicol Environ Chem* 1995;47:155–184.

NRC-COT. *Review of the U.S. Army's Health Risk Assessments for Oral Exposure to Six Chemical-Warfare Agents*. Washington, DC, National Research Council, National Academies Press, 1999. Available at www.nap.edu.

Phillips YY. Primary blast injuries. *Ann Emerg Med* 1986;106:1446–1450.

Shadomy SV, Smith TL. 2008. Zoonosis Update: Anthrax. *J Amer Vet Med Assoc* 233 (1): 63–72.

Watson AP, et al. Development and application of acute exposure guidelines levels for chemical warfare nerve and sulfur mustard agents. *J Toxicol Environ Health* 2006;9(pt B):173–263.

Wightman JM, Gladish SL. Explosions and blast injuries. *Ann Emerg Med* 2001;37:664–678.

CHAPTER 1.11
ZOONOSES AND ZOONOTIC DISEASES

Sherrie L. Nash, MS, DVM, Sally B. Palmer, DVM, and Wayne E. Wingfield, MS, DVM

1. Describe what is meant by the term "zoonosis."

Zoonosis refers to a disease of animals, caused by a variety of biological organisms, that may be transmitted to humans under natural conditions.

2. Why is it important for animal responders to be aware of zoonotic diseases?

In a disaster, animal responders come in contact with a variety of animals, both wild and domestic. It is important to be aware of diseases that these animals could be carrying that may be harmful to you and others.

Some zoonotic disease agents have been developed as biological weapons and are considered weapons of mass destruction. Recognizing certain signs and symptoms in animals may alert one to the possibility of a biological terrorist attack.

3. What types of biological organisms cause zoonotic diseases?

- Bacteria
- Viruses
- Rickettsia
- Protozoa
- Fungi
- Prions
- Biological byproducts (e.g., toxins)
- Internal parasites (worms)
- External parasites (mites, fleas, etc.)

4. Describe the meaning of the term "host."

"Host" refers to the animal (including humans) or plant that harbors another biological organism.

5. Describe the meaning of the term "pathogen."

A pathogen is an organism that produces disease in animals (including humans) and plants.

6. What does the term "normal flora" mean?

"Normal flora" refers to the microorganisms that live upon or within a host in a mutual or commensally symbiotic relationship. Normal flora microorganisms are very important in protecting the host against pathogenic organisms.

7. What are the routes of infection?

Route of infection describes how a microorganism or its byproduct enters the body and includes the following:

- Inhalation
- Ingestion
- Absorption
- Injection (e.g., bite wounds)

8. What is a vector?

A vector is a carrier, usually an *arthropod* (tick, flea, insect, etc.), that transfers an infective agent from one host to another.

9. What is a fomite?

A fomite is an object that in and of itself is not harmful but is able to harbor pathogenic microorganisms and thus may serve as an agent of transmission of an infection. Examples of possible fomites include thermometers, halters, and food and water bowls.

10. What are bacteria?

Bacteria are single-celled organisms. They may be aerobic (requiring oxygen), anaerobic (not requiring the presence of oxygen), or facultative anaerobic (not obligated to an anaerobic environment). They may be motile or nonmotile. Examples of zoonotic bacteria are *Bacillus anthracis* (anthrax) and *Yersinia pestis* (plague).

11. What are viruses?

Viruses are minute infectious agents characterized by a lack of independent metabolism and by their ability to replicate only within living host cells. Examples of zoonotic viral agents include rabies and West Nile virus.

12. What are "rickettsial organisms"?

This is a term used to refer to a specific type of microorganism that does not fit into either a bacterial or a viral grouping. Typically, rickettsial organisms multiply only inside the cells of the host. Zoonotic rickettsial organisms include *Coxiella burnetii* (Q fever) and *Rickettsia rickettsii* (Rocky Mountain spotted fever).

13.   What are protozoal organisms?

Protozoal organisms are unicellular organisms and are the simplest organism of the animal kingdom. They may be free-living or parasitic. Zoonotic protozoal organisms include *Giardia*, *Leishmania*, and *Toxoplasma gondii*.

14.   What is a fungus?

"Fungus" is a general term used to denote organisms that are characterized by the absence of chlorophyll and by the presence of a rigid cell wall, including yeasts, molds, mushrooms, etc. Zoonotic fungal organisms include *Trichophyton* and *Microsporum* species. These are called dermatophytes and are commonly referred to as *ringworm*.

15.   What are prions?

Prions are thought, by some, to be a new kind of infectious agent that is simply an oddly formed protein. A prion has no DNA or RNA and no cell wall or cell membrane. The existence of prions as an infectious agent is not universally accepted. An example of a possible zoonotic prion disease is mad cow disease (bovine spongiform encephalopathy [BSE]).

16.   What are biological toxins?

Toxins are proteins produced by some plants, certain animals, and pathogenic bacteria that are highly toxic for other living organisms. Examples of toxins include staphylococcal enterotoxin B and botulinum toxin (botulism) from the *Clostridium botulinum* bacterium.

17.   What are internal parasites?

"Internal parasite" is the term used to describe a variety of parasites that live within the body. These parasites are commonly referred to as "worms." They may be found inside organs—for example, *Dirofilaria immitus* (heartworm) or *Toxocara canis* (intestinal roundworm)—or they may be found inside tissues. Examples of zoonotic internal parasites include *T. canis* and *Taenia pisiformis* (tapeworms).

18.   Describe what is meant by the term "external parasite."

The term "external parasite" refers to those organisms found on the outside of the body. Most external parasites are organisms from the phylum Arthropoda. Mites, ticks, fleas, lice, other insects, and spiders are included in this group. External parasites not only cause disease by themselves, but they are also major vectors for other disease agents. Since they are on the outside of the body, many can transfer from one animal (including humans) to another relatively easily.

19.   What is an antimicrobial?

An antimicrobial is an agent that kills microorganisms or suppresses their multiplication or growth. Some antimicrobials are effective against more than one type of biological agent. Within any given group of biological agents, no one antimicrobial is effective against all the organisms of that group. Examples of antimicrobials include penicillin and doxycycline.

20. List the factors that contribute to the likelihood of an animal responder encountering a particular zoonotic agent.

- Geographic distribution. While some agents are present essentially worldwide, other agents are very restricted in their geographic distribution.
- Urban versus suburban versus rural environment
- Presence of farm, ranch, or wild animal species
- Environmental conditions. For example, recent or current flooding, summer versus winter, etc.

21. What is the CDC?

The Centers for Disease Control and Prevention (CDC) is a source of information for health professionals, the public, researchers, and others. The CDC was established in 1946 in Atlanta, Georgia, as a result of the Malaria Control in War Areas (MCWA) that was a wartime agency. The original purpose of the CDC was to decrease malaria by destroying mosquitoes. DDT was the weapon of choice to control mosquitoes. The CDC has since evolved into an agency that provides information on issues concerning public health, prevention of disease, health, and preparedness. In addition, they monitor diseases and agents (including bioterrorism) for an increase in incidence, disease control and prevention, and keeping national health statistics.

22. How does the CDC categorize diseases?

The CDC categorizes both diseases and agents according to how effectively the diseases/agents may be spread and cause harm in the United States.

- **Category A** diseases/agents are readily disseminated or transferred from human to human, are readily dispersed, have the potential to cause panic in the public, could cause high mortality rates, have a large impact on the health of the public, and need special attention for public health preparedness.
- **Category B** diseases/agents have moderate morbidity rates, low mortality rates, are reasonably simple to disperse, require disease surveillance, and need specific augmentation of the CDC's diagnostic ability.
- **Category C** diseases/agents involve emerging diseases that have the potential for being produced for mass distribution in the future. They are obtainable, readily produced, have the potential for high morbidity and mortality, are readily dispersed, and would have a key health impact.

23. What is the OIE?

The Office International des Epizooties (OIE) was established in Paris, France, in 1924 as an intergovernment organization. The OIE came about as a result of an outbreak of Rinderpest in Belgium in 1920. Zebus (cattle) were being exported from India, were passed through Antwerp, and were destined for Brazil when the outbreak occurred. The OIE was established to protect and improve animal health throughout the world. In 2003, the OIE became the World Organization for Animal Health, but it is still recognized as the OIE.

24. How does the OIE list diseases?

- An *OIE List A Disease* requires *immediate reporting* to state and federal authorities.
- An *OIE List B Disease* requires reporting to state and federal authorities. There are other diseases that are listed as reportable in the United States, but they do not have an OIE listing. These diseases should always be reported to state and federal authorities.

25. List some of the zoonotic agents.

- Anthrax
- Brucellosis
- Leptospirosis
- Plague
- Psittacosis
- Tuberculosis
- Tularemia
- *Giardia*
- Ringworm
- Toxoplasmosis
- Query (Q) fever
- Hantavirus
- Monkeypox
- Rabies
- West Nile virus
- Viral encephalitis
- Botulism
- *Clostridium perfringens* toxins
- Ricin
- Tetanus
- Bovine spongiform encephalopathy (?)
- Chronic wasting disease (?)

BIOLOGICAL AGENTS AS WEAPONS OF MASS DESTRUCTION

26. Describe what is meant by the term "biological weapon of mass destruction (WMD)."

A "biological weapon of mass destruction" is a living organism or its byproducts that has been purposely produced to be used as a weapon against people, animals, or plants. Many potential bioterrorist agents are zoonotic.

27. List some clues that may indicate a covert assault.

- Unusual number of ill or dead animals (animals are often seen as sentinels of a zoonotic disease)
- Severe disease manifestations in previously healthy people
- Higher than normal number of patients with fever, respiratory, or gastrointestinal complaints
- Multiple persons with similar complaints from a common location or function
- An endemic disease appearing during an unusual time of year
- Unusual number of severe or rapidly fatal cases
- Greater number of patients with severe pneumonia, sepsis, sepsis with coagulopathies, fever with rash, or cranial nerve palsies

28. List a few zoonotic agents that have been identified as possible biological weapons of mass destruction.

- Anthrax (*Bacillus anthrasis*)
- Botulism (*Clostridium botulinum* toxin)

- Brucellosis (*Brucella* spp.)
- Plague (*Yersinia pestis*)
- Q-fever (*Coxiella brunetii*)
- T2 mycotoxins
- Tularemia (*Francisella tularensis*)
- Viral equine encephalitis
- Glanders (*Burkholderia mallei*)
- Nipah virus
- Hantavirus
- Psittacosis (*Chlamydophila psittaci*)
- Ebola virus

29. Describe why it is important for animal responders to be aware of agents that may cause disease in our livestock and poultry industries?

- Disease outbreaks (especially foreign animal diseases), whether naturally occurring or intentionally introduced, have a profound impact on a country's infrastructure, economy, and export markets.
- Most economies are inextricably linked to agriculture (especially the United States):
  - In the United States, agriculture is the largest single sector of the economy at approximately 13% of the Gross Domestic Product.
  - In the United States, agriculture is the single largest employer.
  - The United States is the world's leading exporter of agricultural products.

ANTHRAX (Woolsorter's Disease, Malignant Pustule, Charbon, Malignant Carbuncle, Splenic Fever, Siberian Ulcer, Milzbrand)

30. What is the etiologic agent of anthrax?

Anthrax is caused by the bacterium *Bacillus anthacis* (Fig. 1.11.1).

B. anthracis is a spore-forming bacteria, which means that when discharged from an infected animal or carcass, they form spores that are resistant to heat, low temperatures, chemical disinfectants, and desiccation. *B. anthrasis* persists for a long time in feed, animal byproducts, stored contaminated objects, or soil. Spores revert to the vegetative form when optimal environmental conditions occur. Anthrax may be used as a possible biological weapon.

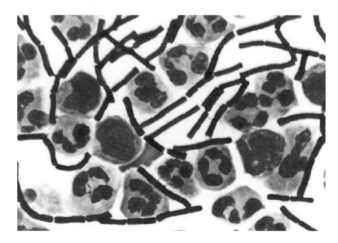

Figure 1.11.1 *Bacillus anthracis* organisms. (Source: Public Domain. http://www.ars.usda.gov/is/AR/archive/jan01/plant0101. htm)

31. What is the disease classification of anthrax?

It is a CDC Category A and OIE List B.

32. What is the geographic distribution of anthrax?

Anthrax occurs worldwide and is enzootic in many areas around the world. In North America, domestic and wild herbivores are affected by anthrax annually.

33. Which species are at risk of infection from anthrax?

Herbivores and raptors are most at risk. Dogs and cats are relatively resistant. Humans are considered accidental hosts.

34. How is anthrax transmitted?

Direct contact, ingestion, or inhalation of the spores may result in infection. In the soil, spores may revert to the vegetative form during warm weather when a heavy rain or flood occurs after a prolonged drought. Animals may become infected when they subsequently graze on this area.

35. What are the three forms of clinical disease?

The three clinical forms of infection are *cutaneous*, *intestinal*, and *inhalation*.

- *Cutaneous anthrax* occurs when the bacterium enters a cut or abrasion on the skin, which may occur when handling contaminated wool or hides. This has been referred to as "woolsorter's disease." Twenty percent of untreated cutaneous anthrax cases may die.
- *Intestinal anthrax* occurs following the consumption of contaminated meat. It results in acute inflammation of the intestinal tract. Up to 60% of untreated intestinal anthrax cases may die.
- *Inhalation anthrax* is very severe, resulting in a mediastinitus (inflammation of the mediastinum), shock, and death in a matter of days. While aggressive treatment is warranted, it may be unrewarding. Antimicrobials including certain tetracyclines, penicillin, and the quinalones are used to treat infection.

36. What are the incubation period and clinical signs of anthrax in animals?

The incubation period may vary from 1 to 20 days (usually 3 to 7 days). Sudden death (peracute) is due to septicemia and is often seen in ruminants. Trembling and convulsions may be observed prior to death or no signs may be seen except death. In acute cases of anthrax, there is rapid onset of fever with excitement followed by depression, dyspnea, stupor, convulsions, and death. Blood may be seen emerging from the mouth, nose, and anus. There is edema, especially around the neck, shoulders, and throat. In horses, illness may be acute with fever and/or chills, colic, septicemia, anorexia, depression, bloody diarrhea, swelling around the neck, shoulders, and thorax. Dogs display depression, fever, weakness, anorexia, and occasionally death.

37. What are the symptoms of anthrax in humans?

Symptoms of ingestion of anthrax may include vomiting, nausea, fever, and anorexia. As the disease progresses, there is diarrhea that may be bloody, extreme abdominal pain, and vomiting with blood. The inhalation route has symptoms of a nonproductive cough, low-grade fever, fatigue, myalgia, malaise, sweating, and chest pain without respiratory symptoms. Most humans are exposed to anthrax by the cutaneous route. Initially there is localized itching and a pimple developing into a dry, ulcerated black scab in 48 to 72 hours. Edema and vesicles appear near the lesion. After about 10 days, the lesion will start to heal and take 2 to 6 weeks to completely heal. Although not typical, cutaneous lesions can lead to more severe disease and death if not treated. Severe symptoms of anthrax include prostration, fever, chills, shock, collapse, and death.

38. What signs may an animal responder encounter suggesting possible anthrax?

Recognizing that animals grazing in an area subjected to periodic or recent flooding and presenting with staggering, difficult breathing, trembling, collapse, and death raises the suspicion of possible anthrax. Animals found dead may have little or no rigor mortis. The classic finding of dark blood oozing from nostrils, mouth, and anus should raise a red flag that an animal responder should not touch the carcass, and the proper authorities **must** be notified.

39. How can the animal responder best protect himself or herself against anthrax?

While there is a vaccine available for humans, it is only given to specific people at high risk of exposure. Therefore, the best protection is an awareness of environmental conditions that support an anthrax outbreak and recognizing signs suggestive of possible infection. Keep a level of suspicion and exercise care (protective clothing, gloves, mask, and eye protection) when handling and caring for sick animals or handling dead animals. If an anthrax exposure is suspected or confirmed, medical attention should be sought immediately. Deep burial or *burning* of infected carcasses is best to eliminate the spores. Disposal of bedding, manure, and other contaminated fomites should also be done. Formaldehyde 5% to 10% is useful in controlling anthrax in the soil. Strong chlorine solutions may be used to destroy the spore.

BRUCELLOSIS (Contagious Abortion, Undulant Fever, Bang's Disease, Enzootic Abortion, Malta Fever, Mediterranean Fever)

40. What is the etiologic agent of brucellosis?

Brucellosis is caused by several species of bacteria known as *Brucella*. *Brucella abortus* is the predominant bacteria to cause disease in cattle, bison, and water buffalo. Sheep are primarily infected by *B. ovis* and *B. melitensis*. Pigs are infected by *B. suis* and goats by *B. melitensis*. Horses can be infected with either *B. abortus* or *B. suis* (also known as fistulous withers). *B. canis* infects dogs, while *B. neotomae* infects rats. Brucellosis is a significant disease because it can potentially infect humans (known as undulant fever or Malta fever). Of all the *Brucella* species, only *B. ovis* and *B. neotomae* do not infect humans. By aerosolizing of these bacteria they may be used as a biological weapon.

41. What is the disease classification of brucellosis?

Brucellosis is CDC Category B and OIE List B.

42. What is the geographic distribution of brucellosis?

Brucellosis occurs in most countries around the world, including the United States.

43. Which species are at risk for brucellosis?

Nearly all animals are susceptible, including cattle, sheep, goats, pigs, wild ruminants, buffalo, bison, elk, horses, dogs, and rats.

44. How is brucellosis transmitted?

Direct contact (requires physical contact between an infected animal and a susceptible animal), ingestion, indirect contact (refers to situations where a susceptible animal is infected from contact with an infected surface or object), and person-to-person (animal-to-animal). All routes are zoonotic. It is a serious public health concern because it is a zoonotic disease.

45. What is the incubation period, and what are the signs of brucellosis in animals?

The incubation period is variable (2 weeks to 5 months in cattle). Cattle will abort and/or have stillborn or weak newborns, inflammation of the placenta or a retained placenta, inflammation of the genitals in the male, arthritis, and lameness. Abortion usually occurs in the second half of pregnancy. Horses have suppurative bursitis, which is also known as poll evil or fistulous withers. This is seen as thick, straw-colored exudates found at the withers. Abortion is rare in mares. Sheep and goats have signs that are similar to cattle. Goats may also have mastitis and lameness. Sheep generally do not have lameness. Abortion occurs late in pregnancy in sheep and during the fourth month of pregnancy in goats. Infertility in rams can also occur. Ewes may abort or shed the organism in the milk. Dogs may be infertile, abort, or have stillbirths. Abortion occurs in the last trimester of pregnancy. A vaginal discharge may be prominent for some time after aborting. Male dogs will have decreased fertility. Abortion can occur any time throughout pregnancy in pigs. Stillborn or weak pigs at birth also occur. Boars will have decreased fertility. Lameness and joint swelling may be seen.

46. What are the symptoms of brucellosis in humans?

Brucellosis in humans occurs 3 to 21 days after exposure. The disease may display a wide range of symptoms. The first symptoms appear as flulike. Headache and body aches are often reported along with fever and chills. Malaise and weight loss can occur. There can be anorexia, back pain, and sweating (night). More serious or long-lasting symptoms include undulant fever, genitourinary problems, neurologic problems, chronic fatigue syndrome, arthritis, and depression.

   Ingestion of unpasteurized milk or milk products, some cured hams, and contact with infected animals are potential sources of infection. Brucellosis in humans tends to be a lifelong illness with periodic symptoms that require medical attention. There is also concern that pregnant women who come in contact with the *Brucella* organism may have a miscarriage.

47. Can brucellosis be treated in animals?

Treatment is generally not recommended in animals because of the zoonotic potential to humans and the cost of treatment. There is a modified live vaccine for cattle that is used to prevent and control brucellosis in this species. It is licensed for use only in female cattle between 4 and 12 months of age.

48. How can the animal responder best protect himself or herself against brucellosis infection?

There is no vaccination for humans. Animal responders can best protect themselves against brucellosis by being aware of the possibility of being exposed. If a brucellosis exposure is suspected or confirmed, medical attention should be sought immediately. Standard decontamination with soap and water is recommended.

GLANDERS (Farcy, Malleus, Droes)

49. What is the etiologic agent of glanders?

Glanders is caused by the bacterium *Burkholderia mallei*. It is a very contagious and often fatal disease in Equidae. It is a zoonotic disease that causes painful nodules in humans and can be fatal. Glanders has the potential to be used as a biological weapon.

50. What is the disease classification of glanders?

Glanders is a CDC Category B and OIE List B.

51. What is the geographic distribution of glanders?

Glanders is found in Mexico, South America, Asia, Africa, the Middle East, and Eastern Europe.

52. Which species are at risk for glanders?

Glanders primarily affects members of the soliped family (i.e., horses, donkeys, mules); however, most mammals are susceptible to experimentally induced infection to some degree. Natural infections in species other than equids are rare, but cats, dogs, camels, goats, and sheep have been affected. Humans are susceptible to glanders, but they are considered accidental hosts.

53. How is glanders transmitted?

Direct contact (zoonotic), indirect contact, or person-to-person. Carnivorous animals are infected by ingesting the infected meat.

54. What is the incubation period and what are the clinical forms of glanders in animals?

The incubation period may be as little as 2 weeks and up to several months. Glanders may be either acute (mules and donkeys) or chronic (nasal, pulmonary, and cutaneous forms). Several forms of the disease may be present in an animal at any one time. In the *acute form*, there is a high fever, septicemia, a viscous mucopurulent discharge from the nose, and respiratory signs. The *nasal form* involves the nasal mucosa with the development of nodules that form into deep ulcers that leave distinctive star-shaped scars. Nasal secretions are yellowish green, and the submaxillary lymph nodes may be inflamed. The *pulmonary form* varies from asymptomatic to obvious respiratory signs of coughing and dyspnea. Calcified or caseous nodules develop in the lungs. The *cutaneous form* is known as "Farcy." Yellowish nodules and ulcers form on the skin, which exude a tacky, contagious pus. There is cutaneous lymphatic involvement, especially on the extremities. These lymphatics swell and fill with a purulent exudate (known as "Farcy pipes").

55. What are the symptoms of glanders in humans?

The incubation period is 1 to 14 days. Symptoms may be varied, depending on the exposure route. Symptoms include headache, fever, muscle stiffness and pain, and chest pain. In addition, there may be diarrhea, light sensitivity, and increased tear production. Localized infections occur through skin abrasions or lesions in 1 to 5 days. There can also be swollen lymph nodes as well as respiratory, ocular, and nasal involvement with increased mucus production. Inhaled or pulmonary infection includes pulmonary abscess formation, pneumonia, and pleural effusion. Systemic involvement is fatal within 7 to 10 days. Chronic infections in humans involve numerous abscesses on the face, arms, legs, nasal mucosa, spleen, or liver. Death occurs in the acute form of the disease in 95% of individuals in about 3 weeks. If antibiotics are used, survival is greatly improved.

56. Is glanders treatable?

Yes. *B. mallei* is susceptible to tetracycline, doxycycline, gentamicin, some sulfa drugs, and ceftrazidime. To prevent spread of disease, animals should be identified, quarantined, and humanely euthanatized.

57. How can the animal responder protect himself or herself against glanders?

Animal responders can protect themselves by being aware of the potential for exposure in areas where glanders is endemic. They should be suspicious of any equidae or other animal with nodules, scars, ulcers, and a fever. In addition, any thick nasal discharges along with respiratory signs may be indicative of glanders. Animal responders should wear protective clothing, gloves, mask, and goggles when handling or caring for sick animals. Most common disinfectants will deactivate the bacteria. Desiccation and sunlight also kill the bacteria.

LEPTOSPIROSIS

58. What is the etiologic agent of leptospirosis?

Leptospirosis is caused by the bacteria *Leptospira* spp.

59. What is the disease classification of leptospirosis?

None is currently listed.

60. What is the geographic distribution of leptospirosis?

Leptospira organisms are found worldwide. They survive in the soil and water, and outbreaks may occur during floods.

61. Which species are susceptible to *Leptospira* infection?

Leptospira infect many wild and domestic animals. Domestically, dogs and cattle are more commonly affected. Certain species of *Leptospira* are more pathogenic for particular hosts.

62. How is the organism transmitted between hosts?

Transmission between animals occurs via direct contact, bite wounds, ingestion of infected meat, venereal, and placental transfer. Organisms may be excreted in urine for months to years, and it is highly infectious. Fomites, for example bedding, may also spread infection. Animals clustered together, as in a sheltering situation, facilitate the spread of infection. The role of vectors in transmission of this disease is not clear. Most human infections are associated with occupational exposure to animals carrying the infection or participation in water activities.

63.   What is the route of infection of leptospirosis?

Leptospira organisms enter the body through mucous membranes or abraded skin.

64.   What are the clinical signs of leptospirosis in animals?

The two major organs damaged are kidneys and liver. Other body systems and organs affected include the nervous system, the reproductive system, and the eyes. Clinical signs vary depending on age, immunity, and species affected. Signs include pyrexia (fever), shivering, generalized muscle tenderness, a reluctance to move, vomiting, dehydration, increased thirst, conjunctivitis, icterus (jaundice), tachypnea (rapid breathing), rapid irregular pulse, and poor capillary perfusion.

65.   What are the symptoms of leptospirosis in humans?

Leptospirosis is also known as Weil's disease. The incubation period is 7 to 10 days (2 to 29 days). Humans have flulike symptoms of headache, fever, chills, vomiting, anemia, jaundice, and a rash (occasionally). If not treated, leptospirosis can cause kidney disease, liver disease, meningitis, respiratory problems, and infrequently death.

66.   Is leptospirosis treatable?

Yes. *Leptospira* bacteria are susceptible to antimicrobials, including penicillin, ampicillin, and doxycycline. Iodine-based disinfectants may be used to treat contaminated areas. Supportive treatment in addition to antibacterial drugs may be necessary to survive this infection.

67.   How can the animal responder best protect himself or herself against leptospirosis?

Animal responders may protect themselves from infection by being aware of the possibility of being exposed, including increased risk during floods, and taking proper precautions (protective clothing, gloves, mask, eye protection) when handling infected animals.

MELIOIDOSIS (Pseudoglanders, Whitmore Disease)

68.   What is the etiologic agent of melioidosis?

The cause of melioidosis is a bacterium known as *Burkholderia pseudomallei* (formerly *Pseudomonas pseudomallei*). It can cause abscess formation in the lymph nodes and viscera in a number of animals. It has been called the "mimic" disease because of the variety of signs of disease. Melioidosis has the potential to be used as a biological weapon.

69.   What is the disease classification of melioidosis?

Melioidosis is a CDC Category B disease.

70. What is the geographic distribution of melioidosis?

Melioidosis is found in Africa, Asia, the Middle East, and Australia. It has occasionally been found in Hawaii and Georgia in the United States and in South America. It is a disease primarily of tropical and subtropical regions.

71. Which animals are susceptible to melioidosis?

Sheep, goats, and pigs are most susceptible, as well as rodents, rabbits, pandas, fish, and nonhuman primates. Dogs, horses, and birds are moderately susceptible, while cattle and cats are only mildly affected.

72. How is melioidosis transmitted?

It is transmitted by direct contact, inhalation, infected body fluids, wound contamination, ingestion, as well as person-to-person. Direct contact with the bacteria in the surroundings (contaminated water, soil, rodents) is the primary route of exposure. Heavy rain, high humidity, flooding, and high temperatures are ideal for infections as a result of contact with soil. Infection through body fluids includes via milk, urine, and nasal discharges. Melioidosis is much less commonly spread person-to-person or zoonotically.

73. What are the incubation period and clinical signs of melioidosis in animals?

The incubation period is variable and may be longer in pigs. Signs vary widely with the site of the lesion. Suppurative or caseous lesions may be found in the lymph nodes, lungs, and viscera. Fever, nasal discharge, inappetence, gastrointestinal involvement, encephalitis, respiratory signs, or lameness may be seen. The prognosis is grave when there is involvement of a crucial organ and abscess formation is widespread. Horses may have neurologic signs as well as having colic, diarrhea, or respiratory signs. If signs are seen in cattle, they are pneumonia-like or neurologic. Sheep and goats have pneumonia-like signs, abscess formation in the lungs, nasal discharge, arthritis, or encephalitis. Mastitis occurs in goats. Pigs may have no symptoms or have chronic symptoms. They may be inappetent and have fever, swollen submandibular lymph nodes, ocular-nasal discharges, or coughing. Reproductive signs of stillbirths, abortion, or orchitis are occasionally seen in pigs.

74. What are the symptoms of melioidosis in humans?

The incubation period in humans is 1 to 21 days, but it may extend for many years. Humans may be asymptomatic or have localized, systemic, pulmonary, or chronic symptoms. Nodules often develop at an exposed skin lesion. There may be fever, muscle pain, chest pain, cough, pneumonia, septic shock, severe headache, shortness of breath, anorexia, diarrhea, disorientation, numerous abscesses, or skin lesions filled with pus. Chronically, there is skin, lymph node, joint, bone, lung, liver, spleen, brain, or visceral involvement. Compromised individuals are more likely to have systemic infections.

75. How is melioidosis treated in animals?

Tetracycline has been used to treat melioidosis. Antibiotics have been used in ruminants, but relapses usually take place when treatment is ended. Vaccines are available but not always effective.

76. How can the animal responder best protect himself or herself against melioidosis?

Animal responders can protect themselves by being aware of the potential for exposure in areas where melioidosis is endemic. They should be suspicious of animals that appear ill and have numerous caseous abscesses present. Animal responders should exercise caution and wear protective clothing, gloves, mask, and goggles when handling or caring for sick animals. *B. pseudomallei* is deactivated by heat (moist 250°F at 15 minutes, dry heat 320° to 338°F for at least 1 hour). In addition, 70% ethanol, 1% sodium hypochlorite, formaldehyde, and glutaraldehyde may be used to deactivate this organism. It is important to recognize that it can survive in water and soil for months.

PLAGUE (Bubonic Plague, Black Death, Pneumonic Plague, Pestis Minor, Septicemic Plague, Peste, Pestis)

77. What is the etiologic agent for plague?

Plague is a disease caused by the bacteria *Yersinia pestis*. It is the agent responsible for the "Black Death" that occurred during the Middle Ages, killing tens of millions of people in Europe and Asia.

78. What is the disease classification of plague?

Plague is a CDC Category A disease and an OIE List B disease.

79. What is the geographic distribution of plague?

In the United States, plague is found in the western half of the country. A significant number of cases occur in Colorado, New Mexico, and California. *Y. pestis* can survive for several weeks to months in infected carcasses, and cold/freezing temperatures may prolong its viability for years.

80. Which species are susceptible to plague infection?

Wild rodents, rabbits, domestic animals (especially cats), and people are host species. There are about 40 rodent species that serve as permanent reservoirs for plague. These species are relatively resistant to plague infections. Prairie dogs, ground squirrels, and rock squirrels are commonly infected wild hosts. Mortality approaches 100% in these species. Many areas are susceptible to rapid expansion of plague because of the presence of amplifying rodent species.

81. How is plague transmitted?

Transmission of plague between hosts occurs by flea bite, by contact of *Y. pestis* with mucous membranes or broken skin, or by inhalation of droplets from animals with pneumonic plague. Prairie dog, ground squirrel, and rock squirrel fleas are effective vectors, while dog and cat fleas are considered poor vectors for the plague (Fig. 1.11.2).

82. What are the three clinical forms of the disease?

The three clinical forms of the disease are *bubonic, septicemic,* and *pneumonic* plague. The most common and least fatal form is bubonic plague. Bubonic refers to enlarged and inflamed lymph nodes, and this form presents

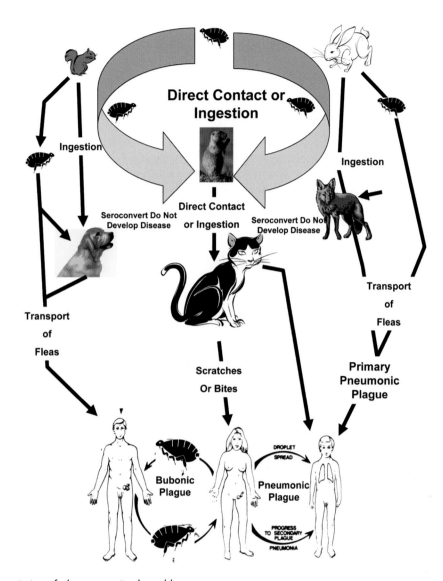

Figure 1.11.2 Transmission of plague to animals and humans.

with high fevers and enlarged, abscessed, lymph nodes. Septicemic plague refers to widespread disease in the body due to the presence and persistence of this pathogenic microorganism and its toxins (endotoxin) in the blood. This form can be rapidly fatal. Pneumonic plague refers to involvement of the lungs and respiratory system. It can develop from the bubonic or septicemic form or as primary pneumonic plague from droplet transmission. In people, untreated pneumonic plague is 100% fatal.

83. What are the incubation period and clinical signs of plague in animals?

The incubation period varies from 1 to 4 days. The bubonic form is most often seen in cats; they will present with a high fever, extremely swollen lymph nodes ("buboes"), lethargy, dehydration, and anorexia. The lymph nodes may form an abscess and drain. Other signs include pneumonia, ataxia, sneezing, and hemoptysis. The pneumonic form usually presents as a severe pneumonia with coughing and is associated with the septicemic form in cats. The septicemic form includes fever, lack of appetite, depression, and sepsis (diarrhea, disseminated intravascular coagulopathy, vomiting, and a weak pulse). Dogs generally do not have clinical signs of plague. When they do, lymphadenopathy, depression, coughing, and high fever may be seen. Horses, cattle, sheep, and pigs have little to no signs.

84. What are the incubation period and symptoms of plague in humans?

The incubation period in humans is usually 1 to 8 days. Humans with the bubonic form have regional lymphade-nopathy (buboes) and this form generally involves 80% to 90% of reported cases. Cervical, axillary, and inguinal lymph nodes are involved. There may be draining at the initial site of the infection. Mortality rates may reach 50% to 60% in untreated individuals. The septicemic form may be seen with the bubonic form or without any lymphadenopathy. In the US, 50% of individuals with this form die. Only 10% of individuals exposed to plague will present with this form. Death occurs as a result of complications associated with meningitis, consumptive coagulopathy, septic shock, and coma. The pneumonic is the most serious and fatal form of plague and it is not routinely seen. Symptoms include an elevated fever, severe pneumonia, dyspnea, and possibly expectoration of blood. If not treated within 18 hours of respiratory symptoms, fatality is almost certain.

85. Is plague treatable in animals?

Yes. *Y. pestis* is susceptible to a wide variety of antibacterial agents including gentamicin, doxycycline, and enro-floxacin. Cats in general *should not be treated* because of the high zoonotic risk, and because 50% of them do not survive infection. If cats are to be treated, the use of parenteral antibiotics and strict isolation must be done. For equipment, instruments, and other fomites, routine disinfectants are effective in killing *Y. pestis*.

86. How can the animal responder best protect himself or herself against plague?

Prophylactic vaccination is available for humans but is only recommended for laboratory workers and field per-sonnel who work with *Y. pestis*. Animal responders can best protect themselves against plague by being aware of the possibility of being exposed. This includes being suspicious of sick and dead prairie dogs or ground squirrels. It is also important to keep a level of suspicion and exercise care (protective clothing, gloves, mask, and eye pro-tection) when handling and caring for sick cats (domestic and wild) with high fever, and enlarged or abscessed lymph nodes or other animals suspected of carrying this disease. If a plague exposure is suspected or confirmed, medical attention should be sought immediately. Routine sanitation of equipment, surfaces, and instruments should deactivate this bacterium.

PSITTACOSIS (Parrot Fever, Avian Chlamydiosis, Ornithosis)

87. What is the etiologic agent of psittacosis?

Psittacosis is caused by *Chlamydophilia psittaci* (formerly *Chlamydia psittaci*).

88. What is the disease classification of psittacosis?

Psittacosis is a CDC Category B disease.

89. What is the geographic distribution of psittacosis?

Worldwide.

90. Which species are susceptible to infection?

Birds such as parakeets, parrots, love birds, doves, mynah birds, and pigeons are susceptible.

91.   How is psittacosis transmitted?

Inhalation of dust from infected bird dander, droppings, or secretions is very common. Respiratory secretions and feces contain elementary bodies that remain infective for months and are resistant to desiccation. Mechanical transfer of infection occurs through mites, biting insects, and lice. Ingestion of infected feed can be a source of disease. It is important to note that some birds are asymptomatic carriers. Humans are most often infected by inhalation or contact with infected birds. Person-to-person transmission is thought to be rare; an acute infection must be present, and only when forcefully coughing directly into another individual's face does spread of infection occur.

92.   What are the incubation period and clinical signs of disease?

The incubation period in birds varies from 3 to 10 days, up to several weeks. Nasal and ocular discharges may be present. Conjunctivitis (inflammation of the eyes), droppings that are yellow-green in appearance, inactivity, ruffled feathers, inappetence, and weight loss can also be seen. There may be a drop in egg production. Pigeons appear temporarily ataxic; ducks tend to have an abnormal gait or may shake. Pet birds display similar signs, but there are also sinusitis, yellow diarrhea, and nervous signs. Some birds may be asymptomatic for psittacosis.

93.   What are the symptoms of psittacosis in humans?

In humans, the incubation period ranges from 4 to 15 days, but is typically 10 days. Symptoms may be mild to severe. Humans may display flulike symptoms that include photophobia, sweating, vomiting, diarrhea, and respiratory symptoms (psittacosis); endocarditis, encephalitis, and myelitis can also occur. Death can occur if left untreated.

94.   Is psittacosis treatable in animals?

Yes. Tetracylines such as doxycycline, oxytetracycline, and chlortetracycline are effective. No vaccine is available. Quarantine of all infectious birds should be done until treatment is complete. When working with suspect or infected birds, one should wear protective clothing, gloves, respiratory protection, and goggles.

95.   How can the animal responder best protect himself or herself against psittacosis?

Animal responders may protect themselves from infection by being aware of the possibility of exposure and taking proper precautions (gloves, mask, eye protection) when handling any sick bird. If a psittacosis exposure is suspected or confirmed, medical attention should be sought immediately. The use of 1:100 sodium hypochlorite, formaldehyde, 80% isopropyl alcohol, chlorophenols, quaternary ammonium compounds, or iodophore disinfectants is effective for deactivating *C. psittaci*.

TUBERCULOSIS (TB)

96.   What is the etiologic agent of tuberculosis?

Mycobacterium spp. *Mycobacterium bovis* causes disease in cattle, *M. tuberculosis* causes disease in humans, and *M. avium* primarily causes disease in birds. *Mycobacterium* spp. may produce infection in species other than their own.

97.   What is the disease classification of tuberculosis?

It is a CDC Category B disease and an OIE List B disease.

98. What is the geographic distribution of tuberculosis?

Worldwide.

99. Which species are most at risk for tuberculosis?

Animals that are known to carry the disease include bison (and related species), sheep, goats, horses, deer, elk, antelope (and related species), elephants, pigs, dogs (and related species), cats (and related species), raccoons, ferrets, rats, badgers, red deer, opossums, Kudu, llamas, camels, rhinoceri, oryx, nonhuman primates, mink, and some cold-blooded animals.

100. How is tuberculosis transmitted?

Tuberculosis is transmitted primarily through the respiratory system. Any tissue in the body can be affected, but most often the lungs, lymph nodes, spleen, liver, and intestines are involved. Large numbers of bacteria are released through coughing and picked up by inhalation of the bacteria. Contact with contaminated feed, water, feces, dust, and dried secretions from infected animals is another source of infection. Infected milk can also be a source of infection.

101. What are the incubation period and clinical signs that are seen with tuberculosis in animals?

The incubation period is variable and it may be chronic. Tuberculosis may not be easily identified until it is in the classic advanced case.

- Cattle have vague to few signs of disease. Coughing and pneumonia are seen early, and with progression of the disease, lymph nodes may become swollen (cattle form nodular granulomas known as tubercles). Swellings are present on the body, especially around the neck and head. Infrequently, the lymph nodes may break open and drain. Signs of intestinal involvement of tuberculosis include diarrhea and constipation, intermittently. In the end stages of tuberculosis, dyspnea and weight loss occur. Female genitalia may often be involved.
- Pigs generally have gastrointestinal lymph node involvement.
- Dogs develop tubercles in the lungs, kidney, peritoneum, liver, and pleura. The nodules are gray with a necrotic center and generally are not calcified. A large amount of a straw-colored fluid may be found in the thorax.
- Horses are generally resistant to tuberculosis. When infected, lesions are found in the lungs, liver, mesenteric lymph nodes, and other regions.
- Cats are infected by consuming infected milk that produces gastrointestinal tract lesions, followed quickly by dissemination to other organs.
- Birds are emaciated and have lameness, diarrhea, pale skin (face, comb, and wattles), and listlessness in the late stages of the disease. Nodules (yellow to gray) are found along the intestines, spleen, liver, and bone marrow. Multiple organs are involved in advanced illness. In general, the lungs remain unaffected or have limited lesions.

102. What are the symptoms of tuberculosis in humans?

In humans, the incubation period is about 15 to 28 weeks. Tuberculosis is seen as pneumonia or a lung infection. Immunocompromised individuals are more likely to have more complications with tuberculosis. Seldom is there involvement of organs such as the intestines, bones, brain, or kidneys.

103. Is tuberculosis treatable in animals?

There is no treatment provided for tuberculosis in animals. Control of the disease is done through test and slaughter of exposed animals. Treatment of animals is usually *not* recommended because of the potential for drug resistance and exposure to humans during the treatment process. Humans, primates, and elephants have had some treatment success with rifampin, isoniazid, and ethambutol.

104. How can the animal responder best protect himself or herself against tuberculosis?

Animal responders can protect themselves against tuberculosis by being aware of the possibility of being exposed. Any animal that has swollen lymph nodes, especially around the neck and head, should be handled with caution. In addition, if respiratory signs are present with lymph node enlargement, precautions should be taken when handling such animals. It is important to keep a level of suspicion and exercise care (protective clothing, gloves, mask, and eye protection) when handling and caring for sick animals. If a tuberculosis exposure is suspected or confirmed, medical attention should be sought immediately. Decontamination is done through thorough cleaning and disinfecting of equipment, troughs, and feeders. It is important to know that *Mycobacterium* is very resistant to moisture, desiccation, cold, heat, many disinfectants, and changes in pH. It remains stable in soil for months.

TULAREMIA (Rabbit Fever, Francis Disease, O'Hara Disease, Deerfly Disease)

105. What is the etiologic agent for tularemia?

Tularemia is caused by the bacteria *Francisella tularensis*. It can survive for a few months in mud, water, or carcasses. It could be used as a biological weapon (aerosol).

106. What is the disease classification of tularemia?

Tularemia is a CDC Category A disease and an OIE List B disease.

107. What is the geographic distribution of *F. tularensis*?

Tularemia occurs in North America, continental Europe, Russia, China, and Japan.

108. What species are affected?

Rodents, rabbits, mink, sheep, cats, hares, beavers, and aquatic animals are the primary species at risk of infection.

109. How is tularemia transmitted?

In animals, infection can be transmitted by arthropod vectors, especially ticks and tabanids (horseflies), and from ingesting infected carcasses. In humans, transmission also may occur directly from handling, skinning, and cleaning infected wildlife or game birds, eating undercooked infected meat, drinking contaminated water, or inhalation. The infectious dose for humans is less than 100 organisms.

110. What are the incubation period and the clinical signs of tularemia in animals?

The incubation period is 1 to 14 days in animals. Signs include a sudden high fever with lethargy, septicemia, stiffness, anorexia, coughing, and diarrhea; prostration, and death occurring within hours to days.

111. What are the incubation period and clinical symptoms in humans infected with tularemia?

The incubation period in humans is 3 to 5 days but can be as long as 14 days. Clinical symptoms include pyrexia, chills, headache, painful joints, stiffness, weakness, tachypnea, coughing, diarrhea, weight loss, ataxia, prostration, and death. Additional signs may include skin ulceration at the portal of infection, associated regional lymph node enlargement, sore throat, mouth ulcers, and painful, swollen eyes. In typhoidal tularemia, pneumonia is most common.

112. Is tularemia treatable?

Yes. Tularemia is susceptible to antimicrobials such as gentamicin, streptomycin, doxycycline, enrofloxacin, tetracyclines, and chloramphenicol. The use of tetracyclines and chloramphenicol in humans has been associated with relapse of infection.

113. How can the animal responder best protect himself or herself against tularemia?

As an animal responder, protection revolves around recognizing and countering the potential risk when handling sick or dead rodents, rabbits, mink, sheep, or other suspected animal. Animal responders can protect themselves against tularemia by being aware of the possibility of being exposed. Suspect animals in endemic areas that have swollen lymph nodes, pneumonia, fever, and appear sick should be handled with caution. It is important to be suspicious of such animals and exercise care (protective clothing, gloves, mask, and eye protection) when handling and caring for them. If a tularemia exposure is suspected or confirmed, medical attention should be sought immediately. In addition, tick and horsefly control is also very important. All foods should be properly cooked to destroy the organism. Drink only from safe sources of water. Frequent hand washing should be done when handling animal carcasses. A live attenuated vaccine is being reviewed by the FDA. Most common disinfectants are effective on tularemia.

GIARDIASIS ("Beaver-fever")

114. What is the etiologic agent for giardiasis?

Giardiasis is an intestinal disease caused by protozoal *Giardia* species. In the environment, *Giardia* survives as resistant, dormant cysts. When ingested, the cyst becomes a fragile motile *trophozoite* that adheres to the mucosa ("the lining") of the intestine.

115. What is the disease classification of giardiasis?

There is currently no disease classification for giardiasis.

116. What is the geographic distribution of giardiasis?

Giardia species are found worldwide.

117. Which species are susceptible to infection from *Giardia*?

Many mammals and birds are susceptible to infection. Young animals and immunocompromised animals are more at risk for developing clinical illness following infection.

118. What is the route of infection for giardiasis?

Ingestion is the route of infection from drinking contaminated water. Most commonly the contaminated water is a stream, river, or lake, but unfiltered municipal water can also be a source of infection.

119. What are the primary clinical signs of *Giardia* infection in animals?

Diarrhea, both acute and chronic, is the primary sign. Vomiting and loss of weight may also be seen. Infection may be present without clinical signs.

120. What are the clinical symptoms of giardiasis in humans?

Symptoms typically appear 1 week (up to 2 weeks) after exposure to *Giardia*. Symptoms include diarrhea, stomach cramps, flatulence, nausea, greasy stools (may float), weight loss, or no symptoms.

121. Is *Giardia* infection treatable?

Yes. Antimicrobials, including fenbendazole and metronidazole (Flagyl), are effective against *Giardia* spp.

122. How can the animal responder best protect himself or herself from *Giardia* infection?

Drinking water only from known safe sources is recommended. Filtration is effective, while some chemical disinfectants (e.g., chlorine) are not. Certain disinfectants (quaternary ammonium compounds) are effective against cysts on premises. Use good hygiene by washing hands completely with soap and water. Wash all fruits and vegetables before eating them. The animal responder should be aware and use caution when any animal is presented with diarrhea. Animal responders should wear protective clothing and gloves when handling or caring for sick animals. Respiratory protection and protective eyewear may also be necessary.

RINGWORM

123. What is the etiologic agent for "ringworm"?

Ringworm, or dermatophytosis, is an infection in the skin caused by a number of fungal species. For dogs and cats, the majority of infections are caused by *Microsporum canis*, *Trichophyton mentagrophytes*, or *M. gypseum*.

124. What is the disease classification of ringworm?

No classification for ringworm is listed at this time.

125.   What is the geographic distribution of ringworm?

Worldwide for the pathogenic fungi.

126.   What animals are susceptible to infection?

Nearly all of the domestic animals are at risk for ringworm.

127.   How is ringworm transmitted?

Transmission occurs by direct contact or contact with infected hair and scale on fomites. Dogs and cats also become exposed and infected by digging in a contaminated environment.

128.   What are the clinical signs in animals?

In animals, clinical signs are variable and include folliculitis, miliary dermatitis, irregular and widespread alopecia (hair loss), scaling, and occasionally a classic ring lesion with central healing. Some animals may show no signs of infection.

129.   What are the symptoms of ringworm infection in humans?

The incubation period is usually 4 to 14 days after contact. In humans, dermatophyte infections occur on the skin. The ringworm lesions usually itch. Humans usually present with a more classic reddened ring lesion, hence the name "ringworm." There is scaling, fissuring, and redness in the affected area. Hair loss may result in areas such as the scalp. Secondary bacterial infections may result if left untreated. Infections are most often seen in humans with suppressed immune systems, participants in contact sports, or those who bathe communally. Healthy humans may also be susceptible to infection. Tinea capitis (an infection of the hair or scalp) is most often seen in school-aged children and rarely seen after puberty.

130.   How can the animal responder best protect himself or herself against ringworm?

Recognizing that the clinical signs of ringworm in animals are variable, animal responders should take care when handling animals with crusting, scaling, pruritic (itchy), alopecia skin lesions. Use of proper protective clothing and disposal of this clothing prior to handling other animals are important. Cleaning of fomites (exam tables, halters, brushes, bedding, etc.) with bleach (1:20 or one-fourth cup bleach to a gallon of water) or 2% chlorhexidine disinfectant should be applied. Items that are washable should be rinsed in hot water and dried with hot air. In addition, separate animals that may be infected from other naïve animals. Vigilant hand washing with chlorhexidine scrub can also help prevent infection in the animal responder.

TOXOPLASMOSIS

131.   What is the etiologic agent of toxoplasmosis?

Toxoplasma gondii is an obligate intracellular coccidian parasite causing toxoplasmosis.

132. What is the disease classification of toxoplasmosis?

There currently is no classification for toxoplasmosis.

133. What is the geographic distribution of toxoplasmosis?

Toxoplasmosis occurs in the majority of regions of the world.

134. What species are infected by toxoplasmosis?

T. gondii infects almost all warm-blooded species, including humans. Domestic and wild cats are the definitive hosts, and all other species are intermediate hosts.

135. How is toxoplasmosis transmitted?

T. gondii is transmitted by ingestion of infected tissues, ingestion of contaminated food or water, congenital infection, transfusion of fluids, or organ transplantation.

136. What are the clinical signs of toxoplasmosis in animals?

Most infections by *Toxoplasma* are latent or asymptomatic. Antibody titers are common in sheep, pigs, and cats; less common in dogs and horses; and even less common in cattle. Clinical infection is relatively uncommon in most species, but sporadic cases and occasional epidemics are seen (particularly in young and stressed animals and congenital infections). Generally, the clinical infection is usually acute and generalized, whereas in adults it is often associated with chronic central nervous system involvement alone. In young animals, particularly puppies, kittens, and piglets, signs include fever, anorexia, cough, dyspnea, jaundice, and central nervous system signs. Congenital toxoplasmosis is an important cause of abortion and stillbirths, particularly in sheep and sometimes pigs and goats.

137. Why is toxoplasmosis of concern for animal responders?

Toxoplasmosis is of greatest concern to pregnant or immunocompromised individuals. First-time *T. gondii* infection during pregnancy causes a placentitis (inflammation of the placenta) and subsequent infection in the fetus. This congenital infection results in severe eye problems (retinochoroiditis). Immunocompromised people are also at risk of developing encephalitis from the infection. In humans, postnatally acquired infections are generally asymptomatic and self-limiting.

138. What are the symptoms of toxoplamosis in humans?

- **Healthy people (nonpregnant).** Healthy people who become infected with T. gondii often do not have symptoms because their immune system usually keeps the parasite from causing illness. When illness occurs, it is usually mild with "flulike" symptoms (e.g., tender lymph nodes, muscle aches, etc.) that last for several weeks and then go away. However, the parasite remains in their body in an inactive state. It can become reactivated if the person becomes immunosuppressed.

- **Mother-to-child (congenital).** Generally if a woman has been infected before becoming pregnant, the unborn child will be protected because the mother has developed immunity. If a woman is pregnant and becomes newly infected with Toxoplasma during or just before pregnancy, she can pass the infection to her unborn baby (congenital transmission). The damage to the unborn child is often more severe the earlier the transmission occurs. Potential results can be:
  - Miscarriage
  - Stillborn child
  - Child born with signs of toxoplasmosis (e.g., abnormal enlargement or smallness of the head)
- Infants infected before birth often show no symptoms at birth but develop them later in life with potential vision loss, mental disability, and seizures.
- **Persons with ocular disease.** Eye disease (most frequently retinochoroiditis) from Toxoplasma infection can result from congenital infection or infection after birth by any of the modes of transmission discussed under epidemiology and risk factors. Eye lesions from congenital infection are often not identified at birth but occur in 2% to 80% of infected persons by adulthood. However, in the United States, less than 2% of persons infected after birth develop eye lesions. Eye infection leads to an acute inflammatory lesion of the retina, which resolves leaving retinochoroidal scarring. Symptoms of acute disease include:
  - Eye pain
  - Sensitivity to light (photophobia)
  - Tearing of the eyes
  - Blurred vision
- The eye disease can reactivate months or years later, each time causing more damage to the retina. If the central structures of the retina are involved there will be a progressive loss of vision that can lead to blindness.
- **Persons with compromised immune systems.** Persons with compromised immune systems may experience severe symptoms if infected with Toxoplasma while immunosuppressed. For example, a person who is HIV infected and who has reactivated Toxoplasma infection can have symptoms that include fever, confusion, headache, seizures, nausea, and poor coordination. Persons who acquire HIV infection and who were not infected previously with Toxoplasma are more likely to develop a severe primary infection.

    Immunocompromised persons who were infected with Toxoplasma at some point before they become immunosuppressed are particularly at risk for developing a relapse of toxoplasmosis. Toxoplasma infection can reactivate in immunocompromised pregnant women who were infected with Toxoplasma before their pregnancy, and this can lead to congenital infection.

139. How can the animal responder best protect himself or herself against toxoplasmosis?

A pregnant or immunocompromised animal responder should avoid contact with cat feces (i.e., litter box and cat cage cleaning in a sheltering/medical situation). Proper hygiene and eating only thoroughly cooked meat will decrease the risk of infection.

QUERY (Q) FEVER

140. What is the etiologic agent of Q fever?

Q fever is caused by the rickettsial organism *Coxiella burnetii*. It is a highly contagious zoonotic disease that can cause flulike signs to chronic endocarditis in humans. Q fever could be used as a biological weapon.

141. What is the disease classification of Q fever?

Q fever is CDC Category B and an OIE List B disease.

142. What is the geographic distribution of Q fever?

Worldwide.

143. What species are susceptible to infection?

Q fever is a zoonotic and humans are most affected by Q fever. Cattle, goats, and sheep are the usual reservoirs for the disease. Rabbits and rodents are the most susceptible, followed by dogs, cats, pigs, pigeons, horses, geese, fowl, wild animals, buffalo, and camels.

144. How is Q fever transmitted?

Q fever is highly communicable by aerosol. Spread of disease is also by direct contact or ticks as a vector. Q fever is commonly transmitted by placental tissues, birth fluids, and excreta of infected animals. It can also be spread by consuming raw milk. Q fever may also be found in urine and feces.

145. What are the clinical signs of Q fever in animals?

The incubation period is variable at 1 to 3 weeks. In most animals the signs are asymptomatic. Fever and pneumonia may be present. Ruminants may have anorexia, infertility, stillbirths, endometritis, and sporadic late abortion. Dogs are usually asymptomatic, but abortions may be seen. Cats have been shown to have anorexia, transient fever, and listlessness experimentally. In animals that abort, they are usually late term.

146. What are the incubation period and the clinical symptoms of Q fever in humans?

In humans the incubation period varies but is generally 2 to 3 weeks. The most common signs in humans are sudden onset and include flulike symptoms of headache, fever (104° to 105°F), chills, sore throat, malaise, nausea, vomiting, diarrhea, and myalgia. Confusion, chest pain, and abdominal pain are also noted. There may be a fever for 7 to 14 days, loss of weight, pneumonia, and hepatitis. In chronic infections, endocarditis occurs. Humans are very susceptible to inhalation of *C. burnetii*. In susceptible individuals, a single inhaled organism is enough to cause disease.

147. Is Q fever treatable?

Tetracycline is used to treat Q fever in dogs and horses.

148. How can the animal responder best protect himself or herself against Q fever?

Animal responders can protect themselves against Q fever by being aware of the possibility of being exposed. Any animal that has had a late-term abortion or retained placenta or appears ill should be handled with caution. It is important to keep a level of suspicion and exercise care (protective clothing, gloves, mask, and eye protection) when handling and caring for sick animals. If a Q fever exposure is suspected or confirmed, medical attention should be sought immediately.

For prevention, heat all foods to destroy the organism. Standard decontamination is done with soap and water. *C. burnetii* is very resistant to heat, drying, and most common disinfectants. It can be deactivated by 0.05% sodium hypochlorite, 1:100 Lysol solution, or 5% peroxide.

TYPHUS FEVER (Epidemic Typhus, Louse-Borne Typhus)

149. What is the etiologic agent of typhus fever?

Typhus fever is caused by *Rickettsia prowazekii*. It is a serious infection in humans and infrequently causes death. Person-to-person contact with body lice has been known to cause large epidemics.

150. What is the disease classification of typhus fever?

Typhus fever is a CDC Category B disease.

151. What is the geographic distribution of typhus fever?

Typhus fever is found in the eastern part of the United States.

152. What species are susceptible to typhus fever infection?

Flying squirrels and humans are the only known reservoirs.

153. How is typhus fever transmitted?

The human body louse, *Pediulus humanus humanus*, is infected by feeding on the blood of a human with an active case of typhus fever. The infected louse is then transferred to a naïve human, whereby the louse eats and defecates on them. Typhus fever is spread through the infective feces left on the naïve host. Humans become susceptible when feces or crushed lice enter wounds or superficial abrasions, such as during scratching. Close person-to-person contact is also a source for typhus fever. Direct contact with flying squirrels or their nests is another source of infection to individuals. Aerosolization of dust or dried feces from either lice or flying squirrels may also serve as a source.

154. What are the clinical signs of typhus fever in animals?

Domestic animals are asymptomatic.

155. What are the incubation period and the clinical symptoms in humans?

The incubation period is 7 to 15 days in humans. Symptoms are flulike with fever, chills, headache, vomiting, and joint pain. Hematuria, abdominal pain, confusion, malaise, anorexia, conjunctivitis, ataxia, and myalgia are also seen. Death can occur in some human infections.

156. Is typhus fever treatable?

Not an important health hazard in animals.

157. How can the animal responder best protect himself or herself against typhus fever?

Animal responders can protect themselves against typhus fever by being aware of the possibility of being exposed. When handling flying squirrels, lice, or working in areas where these species may be present, protective clothing, gloves, mask, and goggles should be worn. To prevent disease, insecticides and good hygiene should be used. Standard decontamination is with soap and water.

AVIAN INFLUENZA, HIGHLY PATHOGENIC (AI, HPAI) (Fowl Plague, H5N1), CANINE INFLUENZA (Dog Flu), AND EQUINE INFLUENZA (Horse Flu)

158. What is the etiologic agent of influenza?

Influenza is a virus in the Orthomyxoviridae family with type A influenza being significant with Avian Influenza (AI). The virus ranges from a mild or even asymptomatic infection to an acute, fatal disease of chickens, turkeys, ducks, guinea fowls, and other avian species. Migratory waterfowl are also affected. The virus is found in the intestinal tract of wild birds. Dogs, cats, mice, ferrets, and horses can also be affected by influenza.

159. What is the disease classification of AI?

AI is an OIE List A Disease.

160. What is the geographic distribution of AI?

Highly pathogenic AI viruses (H5 and H7 subtypes) have been found worldwide. In recent years, it has been found in Australia, Cambodia, China, Korea, Indonesia, Thailand, Vietnam, Malaysia, Mongolia, the Netherlands, England, Ireland, Scotland, Italy, South Africa, Pakistan, Romania, Turkey, Croatia, Russia, Ukraine, Chile, Mexico, and the United States.

161. What species are susceptible to infection?

Most avian species appear to be affected by AI, including imported pet birds, birds at live markets, ratites, and apparently normal sea birds. Ducks appear to have a less virulent form of the disease. Type A influenza viruses will usually have specificity for a particular species (bird virus will infect the same type of birds, human virus infects other humans). Pigs located near turkeys appear to be a reservoir for swine influenza in the turkeys. Humans have also been infected by AI. Avian influenza (H5N1) virus has been shown to be infectious not only for birds but also for humans and mammals such as mice, ferrets, and cats. Carnivorous mammals that are susceptible to subtype H5N1 may contribute to spread of the virus; shedding of influenza (H5N1) by pet carnivores may pose a risk to humans, as well as domestic and large cats, and dogs. Dogs have been infected with highly pathogenic AI by consuming raw meat or carcasses.

Equine influenza is the H3N8 strain of Influenza A, an avian influenza that has mostly affected horses, but has also jumped to dogs, mostly racing greyhounds. Equine influenza was first detected in horses 40 years ago and has never been known to cause illness in humans.

H3N8 flu in dogs is highly infectious causing only mild flu in 80% of dogs it infects, but developing complications in the remaining 20% with an overall mortality rate of 6% to 8%.

162. How is AI transmitted?

Current thought is that waterfowl, sea birds, and shore birds are responsible for introducing the virus into poultry. Most common methods of transmission are aerosol and fecal-oral in birds. Once AI has been introduced to a flock, the virus is easily spread by infected birds, equipment, personnel, feed trucks, flies, and other fomites (Fig. 1.11.3).

Transmission is usually bird-bird, human-to-human, and pig-to-pig, although interspecies transmission is possible. Low pathogenic AI does have the ability to mutate to the high pathogenic form (Fig. 1.11.4).

No studies have been carried out to say with certainty that dogs can transmit H5N1 bird flu to other dogs. Domestic cats have not been known to transmit H5N1 bird flu to other cats in normal situations, but it has been made possible under laboratory conditions. It is thought that dogs infected with H5N1 avian influenza or H3N8 horse flu could pass the flu to other dogs. Both cats and dogs have died as a result of eating infected meat. Dogs in Thailand were thought to have been infected with H5N1 avian flu after eating raw meat from ducks infected with bird flu. Dogs infected with H3N8 "horse" flu were mostly infected at dog racing tracks and their infection had nothing to do with contact with birds or bird derivatives. There is no evidence at present that these infected cats or dogs are contagious to humans, but precautions should be taken because the possibility exists.

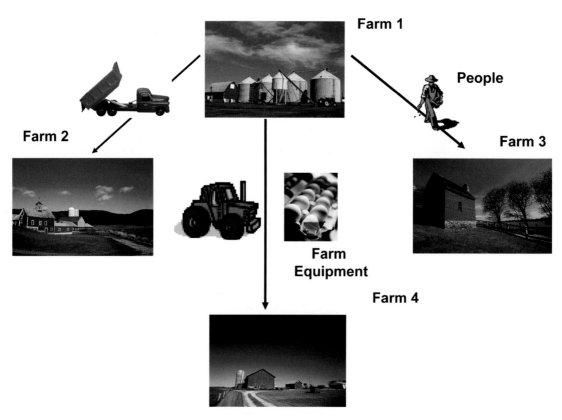

Figure 1.11.3 Transmission of avian influenza occurs via a variety of means.

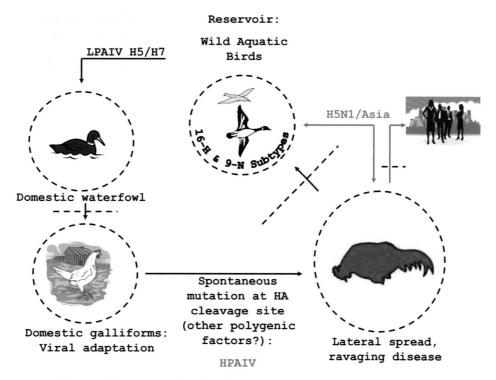

Figure 1.11.4 Avian influenza pathogenesis and epidemiology. LPAIV—low pathogenic avian influenza virus; HPAIV—highly pathogenic avian influenza virus; HA—hemagglutinin protein; dotted lines with arrows represent species barriers.

163. What are the incubation period and the clinical signs of influenza in animals?

A variable incubation period of 1 to 7 days occurs with AI. Signs can be variable with AI from low pathogenicity to high pathogenicity (HP). HPAI is sudden onset and quickly spreads throughout the flock. Mortality is high with the HP form of AI (H5 and H7 subtypes). Depression, inappetence, and respiratory signs are commonly seen. There is often cyanosis and edema of the head, comb, and waddle. Blood-tinged nasal and oral discharges, greenish-to-white diarrhea, and discolored shanks and feet may also be noted. Egg production decreases and eggs may be laid without shells as the disease progresses. Turkeys, ducks, and quail may have sinusitis. Death can occur within 24 hours of the first signs seen, although usually it occurs within 48 hours. Some birds may survive up to 1 week before dying. A few birds may even survive the disease.

   Influenza virus infection of dogs was first reported in 2004, and influenza (H3N8) of equine origin caused outbreaks in greyhounds in Florida and has since been found in dogs in more than 20 states. The course of experimental infection of Specific Pathogen Free (SPF) dogs with subtype H5N1 resembles that of the experimental infection of dogs with the subtype H3N8: all dogs seroconverted, and some excreted virus without obvious disease. In contrast to the experimental outcomes, natural infections with influenza (H3N8) resulted in serious illness, death, and widespread infection for dogs. This finding warrants special attention to the potential course of avian influenza (H5N1) infection in dogs. Therefore, dogs' contact with birds and poultry should be avoided in areas with influenza (H5N1) outbreaks to prevent possible spread of virus and human exposure to influenza (H5N1) virus that might have been adapted to mammals.

164. What are the incubation period and the clinical symptoms of AI in humans?

The incubation period for AI is 2 to 10 days and has been reported to be as long as 17 days. Avian influenza is a type A influenza virus that can potentially mutate and become infective to other mammals, including humans.

The infection and the subsequent deaths of 6 of 18 humans infected with an AI virus in Hong Kong in 1997 have raised the question of the role the avian species plays in influenza in humans. Humans in direct contact with infected birds or contaminated fomites are at risk. Handling of infected meat, such as in cooking, may be another source of infection. Signs in humans include flulike symptoms, respiratory disease, pneumonia, ophthalmia (eye infections), cardiac and renal failure, as well as serious complications, including death.

165. Is AI treatable?

A vaccine is available for birds, but it must be the same strain present in the flock to be effective. The control of secondary bacteria with broad-spectrum antibiotics and raising the temperature of the poultry house may help to reduce losses. The practice of strict sanitation and biosecurity procedures in the raising of poultry is of the utmost importance. Restricting access to the houses is another way to decrease the possibility of introducing disease. The all-in, all-out management of birds is recommended. Areas where waterfowl, shore birds, or sea birds are prevalent should be avoided if possible, since these birds can serve as a source of infection. Cleaning and disinfection procedures are critical. In the face of an outbreak, the best measure may be to test and euthanatize birds on all affected premises.

Just like in humans, dogs can have complications from the flu such as secondary bacterial infections that need to be treated. Isolate dogs with flu from healthy dogs. Keep dogs away from avian flu sources in order to avoid H5N1 bird flu, and do not allow dogs to eat raw poultry suspected of bird flu infection. Dispose of dead birds properly by burying, or use the services of a waste disposal company. To prevent H3N8 "horse" flu, keep your dog away from dog racing tracks and other dogs that may be infected.

166. How can the animal responder protect himself or herself against AI?

Animal responders can protect themselves against AI by being aware of the possibility of being exposed. Birds that have rapid onset of illness with high mortality should be handled with caution. Respiratory depression and any discoloration or swelling of the head, comb, and waddles should raise suspicion of AI. It is important to keep a level of suspicion and exercise care (protective clothing, gloves, mask, and eye protection) when entering facilities that may have sick birds. If an AI exposure is suspected or confirmed, medical attention should be sought immediately. Decontamination is done through thorough cleaning with soap and water. Strict sanitation and restricting access to poultry houses will help in preventing the spread of disease.

HANTAVIRUS (Hanta Virus, Sin Nombre Virus [formerly Muerto Canyon Virus])

167. What etiologic agent causes Hantavirus?

Hantavirus is an RNA virus in the Bunyaviridae family. It is a deadly disease that some rodents can pass on to humans. Initially, it was identified in Korea near the Hantan (Hantaan) river during the Korean War.

168. What is the disease classification of Hantavirus?

Hantavirus is a CDC Category C disease.

169. What is the geographic distribution of hantavirus?

Korea, China, northern and western Europe, Russia, Canada, United States, Chile, Patagonian Argentina, Brazil, and Panama.

170. What species are susceptible to Hantavirus infection?

Deer mice and cotton rats are persistently infected, and they are normally asymptomatic.

171. How is Hantavirus transmitted?

Hantavirus is transmitted through contact with infected rodent urine, feces, or saliva. Fomites contaminated with urine, feces, or saliva can be accidentally introduced through the mouth or nose. Food contaminated with urine, feces, or saliva is another source for disease. Aerosolized dried materials such as nests, saliva, droppings, and urine may also cause disease. Although rodent bites rarely occur, Hantavirus infection can occur.

172. What are the incubation period and clinical signs of Hantavirus infection in rodents?

Rodents appear to be infected while young and remain carriers throughout life. They are asymptomatic carriers.

173. What are the incubation period and the clinical symptoms of Hantavirus infection in humans?

The incubation period in humans is 7 to 39 days, with an average of 14 to 18 days for Hantavirus pulmonary syndrome (HPS). The incubation period for hemorrhagic fever with renal syndrome (HFRS) is 2 to 4 weeks in humans. *HPS* can be fatal in humans if not treated immediately. It is contracted through inhalation of aerosolized rodent urine, feces, and saliva. Nesting material is also a source of infection to humans. *HFRS* begins with flulike symptoms that may last for 3 to 7 days. Renal failure follows, and then recovery.

174. Is Hantavirus treatable?

It is not an important health hazard in animals.

175. How do you control Hantavirus?

Prevention is done by controlling rodents. An experimental vaccine is available.

176. How can the animal responder best protect himself or herself against Hantavirus?

Animal responders can protect themselves against Hantavirus by being aware of the possibility of being exposed. Any area where rats or their feces are present should be handled with caution. Areas that may attract rodents (food, nesting sites) should be cleaned up and kept clean. It is important to keep a level of suspicion and exercise care (protective clothing, gloves, mask, and eye protection) when entering facilities that may have rats. If a Hantaviral exposure is suspected or confirmed, medical attention should be sought immediately. Decontamination is done through thorough cleaning with soap and water. Sodium hypochlorite or other disinfectants may also be used deactivate Hantavirus. Laundering with detergent is also effective.

HENDRA (Equine Morbillivirus Pneumonia, Hendra Virus Disease, Acute Equine Respiratory Syndrome)

177. What is the etiologic agent of Hendra?

The Hendra virus is in the Paramyxoviridae family. It was initially found in Hendra, Australia, where both horses and humans had respiratory and neurologic signs. This virus is closely related to Nipah virus. Hendra is not very contagious, but has a high mortality.

178. What is the disease classification of Hendra?

There is no disease classification.

179. What is the geographic distribution of Hendra?

The disease has only occurred in Australia. Fruit bats (or flying foxes) in Australia and Papua New Guinea were found to have antibodies to Hendra.

180. What species are susceptible to Hendra infection?

Horses and humans are the only animals that are naturally infected with the Hendra virus. Cats and guinea pigs have been infected experimentally. Fruit bats serve as the natural reservoir for the virus.

181. How is Hendra transmitted?

Hendra is spread by direct contact. It is suspected that fruit bats infect horses through either the aborted fetuses or urine of the fruit bat. The fruit bat is asymptomatic for the virus. Horses may become ill after eating feed contaminated by infected fruit bats. The virus has been found in the urine and the oral cavity of horses as well as in cats that have been experimentally infected. In fruit bats, the virus has been found in urine, blood, and fetal tissue. Humans became ill when exposed to excretions and body fluids from infected horses. Handling of infected tissues may also be a source of disease.

182. What are the clinical signs of Hendra in horses and cats?

The incubation period in horses is 6 to 18 days. Experimentally, the incubation period can be as short as 5 to 10 days. Hendra in horses usually causes a fever (up to 106°F), acute respiratory distress, anorexia, depression, nasal discharge (blood tinged or frothy), pneumonia, ataxia, and sweating. Additional signs that may be noted include dependent edema, neurologic signs (head pressing, muscle fasciculations), and jaundiced or cyanotic mucous membranes. Disease is acute in horses and death occurs 1 to 3 days after initial signs are seen. Cats experimentally infected with Hendra usually die within a day after signs of elevated respiration, fever, and serious illness are seen.

183. What are the clinical signs of Hendra in humans?

The incubation period is typically 4 to 18 days and may be up to 3 months. Humans appear to have a severe form of the flu that includes a fever, respiratory illness, and myalgia. Renal failure and pneumonia killed a horse trainer, while another individual came down with meningitis and died as a result of complications from progressive encephalitis. Hendra killed two of three individuals known to be exposed to this virus.

184. Is Hendra treatable?

Unfortunately, treatment for horses would be symptomatic and probably unrewarding. Quarantine and humane euthanasia to control disease are warranted.

185. How can the animal responder best protect himself or herself against Hendra?

Animal responders can protect themselves from Hendra by being aware of the possibility of being exposed. Any horse that appears ill, has respiratory signs, has a nasal discharge, and has had exposure to fruit bats should be handled with caution. It is important to keep a level of suspicion and exercise care (protective clothing, gloves, mask, and eye protection) when handling suspected cases of Hendra. If an exposure to Hendra is suspected or confirmed, medical attention should be sought immediately. No vaccine is available. Identification of infected animals, quarantine, and humane euthanasia were done in Australia to control this disease. Hendra is an enveloped virus that is readily deactivated by formaldehyde, heat, lipid solvents, oxidizing agents, and nonionic detergents.

MONKEYPOX

186. What is the etiologic agent of monkeypox?

Monkeypox is a virus that belongs to the genus *Orthopoxvirus*. This genus also includes the smallpox virus (variola), the virus used in the manufacture of smallpox vaccine (vaccinia), and the cowpox virus. Monkeypox is contagious and looks very similar to smallpox in humans.

187. What is the disease classification of monkeypox?

There is no disease classification for monkeypox.

188. What is the geographic distribution of monkeypox?

Monkeypox infrequently occurs in central and west Africa. It was reported in the United States in 2003 when Gambian rats infected pet prairie dogs. Humans who handled the infected prairie dogs then came down with the disease.

189. What species are susceptible to infection?

Rodents are probably the reservoir for monkeypox. Rodents, prairie dogs, Gambian giant rats, rabbits, squirrels, or nonhuman primates are known to be susceptible. It is likely that other animals may be susceptible to monkeypox, but they are unknown at this time.

190. How is monkeypox transmitted?

It is suspected that animals become infected with monkeypox through the oropharynx and the nasopharynx, by eating infected tissue, or through wounds. Humans are infected through direct contact with body fluids, respiratory droplets (aerosols), wounds, blood, fomites, handling, bites, and handling bedding or cages of infected animals. The monkeypox outbreak in the United States in 2003 was mostly the result of cutaneous exposure to the virus. The spread of monkeypox person-to-person is unusual but does occasionally occur. The virus is spread through contaminated fomites, aerosolization, or body fluids of infected individuals.

191. What are the incubation period and clinical signs in animals?

The incubation period is 6 to 7 days in cynomolgus monkeys that were experimentally infected with a fatal aerosol dose of monkeypox. Current recommendations by the CDC are that any animal exposed to monkeypox is to be quarantined for 6 weeks. Clinical signs of disease in rodents and rabbits include fever, cough, nasal secretions, inappetence, conjunctivitis, depression, and lymphadenopathy. In addition, there is a nodular rash that develops into pustules ("pocks") and patches of hair loss, and pneumonia may be seen. Monkeypox can be fatal in some animals. Gambian rats showed only mild clinical signs when infected. Nonhuman primates typically have a self-limiting rash. Fever and papules are seen first. The papules become pustules that crust (pocks). The pocks generally cover the extremities but may also be found on the rest of the animal. Once the crusts fall off, scars remain. More serious signs of disease include anorexia, dyspnea, coughing, facial edema, nasal secretions, lymphadenopathy, and oral ulcers. Experimental aerosol exposure of monkeypox has been shown to cause pneumonia. Death can occur and is usually more common in infant monkeys.

192. What are the incubation period and the symptoms of monkeypox in humans?

The incubation period is approximately 12 days for humans. Monkeypox is usually a milder disease than smallpox. Initially, fever, swollen lymph nodes, chills, malaise, headache, sore throat, weariness, cough, and myalgia are noted. A rash with papules is seen 1 to 3 days or more after fever develops. The papules turn to pustules, crust, and fall off. More serious signs of monkeypox include respiratory signs and death.

193. Is monkeypox treatable?

Monkeypox is not an important health hazard in most of the domestic animals. Supportive treatment may be done for other animals, although there is *no safe treatment for animals without exposing humans.*

194. How can the animal responder best protect himself or herself against monkeypox?

Animal responders can protect themselves from monkeypox by being aware of the possibility of being exposed. Any rodent or nonhuman primate that appears ill and/or has a fever, rash, or pustules should be handled with caution. It is important to keep a level of suspicion and exercise care (protective clothing, gloves, mask, and eye protection) when handling suspected cases of monkeypox. If an exposure to monkeypox is suspected or confirmed, medical attention should be sought immediately. Vaccination with smallpox in humans may reduce the disease incidence in them. Recommendations by the CDC are to use an Environmental Protection Agency–approved detergent, disinfectant, or sodium hypochlorite solution. Laundering should be done with sodium hypochlorite, if possible. Autoclaving or incineration may be used to deactivate monkeypox. Contaminated objects (clothing, bedding, towels, toys, water and food bowls, etc.) should not be thrown away, disposed of in a landfill, or buried until proper disinfection has been done on them.

NIPAH OR PORCINE RESPIRATORY AND ENCEPHALITIS SYNDROME (PRES) (Barking Pig Syndrome [BPS], Hendra-like Virus, Porcine Respiratory and Neurologic Syndrome)

195. What is the etiologic agent of Nipah?

Nipah virus is in the Paramyxoviridae family. It is a zoonotic disease that causes sickness and death in both humans and pigs.

196. What is the disease classification of Nipah?

It is a CDC Category C disease.

197. What is the geographic distribution of Nipah?

Nipah virus was first recognized in Malaysia. It has also been reported in Singapore, Bangladesh, and India. Workers in Singapore were exposed to infected pigs from Malaysia. It is thought that Nipah virus is endemic in Southeast Asia.

198. What species are susceptible to infection?

Fruit bats serve as a reservoir (infect pigs or humans) and are usually asymptomatic. The fruit bats are found in Malaysia, Indonesia, some Pacific Islands, and Australia. There has been evidence of infection in dogs, cats, horses, and other domestic species.

199. How is the Nipah virus transmitted?

It is transmitted by close direct contact with the secretions (saliva, bronchial, and pharyngeal) or excretions (urine, semen) of infected pigs. Contact with infected pigs can cause disease in humans and other animals. Aerosolization of respiratory or urinary secretions rarely causes disease. Fomites such as equipment and contaminated needles have been implicated in the spread of Nipah. Humans consuming contaminated fresh date palm sap, which is harvested mid-December through mid-February in Bangladesh, have been infected. Fruit bats are readily found in date palm trees. Possible human-to-human cases have occurred recently in Bangladesh and India.

200. What are the incubation period and the clinical signs of Nipah in animals?

The incubation period is as little as 4 days, but typically it is 7 to 14 days in pigs. Pigs often have inapparent infections. If clinical signs are present, they include severe respiratory distress, fever, a harsh "barking" cough, and open mouth breathing in pigs 1 to 6 months of age. Possible neurologic signs such as twitches, trembling, rear leg weakness, muscle spasms, ataxia when forced to move rapidly, and myoclonus have been seen as well as generalized pain and lameness. Mortality in piglets can be as high as 40%. Neurologic disease is more common in older pigs and is seen as head pressing, chomping at the mouth, agitation, seizures, pharyngeal muscle paralysis, and tetanus-like tremors. Older pigs also display fever and respiratory signs as well as a nasal discharge and increased salivation. Abortion has been suspected to occur during the first trimester. Dogs have clinical signs comparable to pigs. One horse was reported with meningitis. Goats can have serious respiratory disease, cough, impaired growth, and death.

201. What are the incubation period and clinical symptoms of Nipah in humans?

In humans, the incubation period is 4 to 18 days. Clinical symptoms include fever, encephalitis, drowsiness, dyspnea, disorientation, severe headaches, myalgia, personality changes, seizures, and death. Severe neurologic signs can have death rates that reach 40% to 60%.

202. Is Nipah virus treatable?

Supportive care and anti-inflammatory drugs may be beneficial. No vaccine is available.

203. How can the animal responder best protect himself or herself against Nipah?

Animal responders can protect themselves from Nipah by being aware of the possibility of being exposed. Any pig that has respiratory distress, has a harsh cough, or has neurologic signs should be handled with caution. It is important to keep a level of suspicion and exercise care (protective clothing, gloves, mask, and eye protection) when handling suspected cases of Nipah virus. If an exposure to Nipah is suspected or confirmed, medical attention should be sought immediately. Cleaning and disinfecting with sodium hypochlorite, detergents, Virkon, Lysol, or iodine solutions will deactivate this virus.

RABIES

204. What is the etiologic agent of rabies?

Rabies is a highly fatal virus that causes acute encephalomyelitis. It is a Lyssavirus in the Rhabdoviridae family that can infect all mammals but primarily carnivores and insectivorous bats. Once clinical signs are seen, it is almost always fatal. Humans are also susceptible to rabies.

205. What is the disease classification of rabies?

Rabies is a reportable disease in the United States and is an OIE List B Disease.

206. What is the geographic distribution of rabies?

Rabies viruses have been isolated worldwide with the exception of some islands and a few countries that have eradicated the disease. It is found in most of Europe, throughout Africa, the Middle East, and most of Asia and the Americas. The United Kingdom, Ireland, parts of Scandinavia, Japan, much of Malaysia, Singapore, Australia, New Zealand, Papua New Guinea, and the Pacific Islands are free of rabies.

207. Describe which animals are susceptible to rabies infection.

All warm-blooded animals are vulnerable to infection with rabies virus, but some species are more susceptible than others, including foxes, coyotes, wolves, jackals, skunks, raccoons, bats, mongooses, cattle, horses, cats, and dogs. All birds have a low susceptibility to the virus. Different areas of the United States may have a higher prevalence in certain species (skunks, bats, raccoons).

208. How is rabies transmitted?

Infections are usually established following introduction of virus-infected saliva into tissues, through either a bite or scratch. Infected tissue fluids in contact with fresh wounds or intact mucous membranes (oral) have the ability to introduce the disease. Animals can also be infected by the nasal (olfactory) route. Bat-infested caves may produce infectious aerosols. Nonbite transmission (aerosols) has been reported in a number of animal species, including humans. The virus often ends up in the salivary glands, so exposure to saliva poses a great risk. Saliva present on the claws of an animal from drooling or licking can transmit rabies by a scratch from an infected animal. Any kind of oral exam on an infected animal will expose the handler to the virus contained in the saliva. Other modes of transmission include ingestion of infected tissue, transplacental, and organ transplantation.

209. What are the incubation period and the clinical signs seen with rabies infection in animals?

The incubation period is variable from 15 days to 6 months but may be less or longer than listed. Clinical signs seen in an infected animal also can be quite variable. The clinical signs of rabies are usually related to a change in behavior. Paralysis of unknown origin is commonly seen. The disease is divided into three phases: prodromal, excitative, and paralytic. Signs are extremely variable in expression and length. The **prodromal phase** (lasting 1 to 3 days) consists of indistinct neurologic signs that become progressively worse. The **excitative phase** or "**furious form**" occurs when sporadic episodes of rage are the primary signs. A normally lively and sociable dog may become anorexic, withdrawn, irritable, or restless. This behavior may suddenly change, with the animal becoming highly affectionate. The dog may try repeatedly to lick the hands and face of its owner or handler. As the disease progresses, the animal appears to have difficulty swallowing, as if a bone were caught in its throat. Any attempt to alleviate the problem manually exposes the handler to considerable risk, either through a bite or the deposition of virus-infected saliva on mucous membranes, or minor scratches. The dog's bark becomes high pitched and hoarse, indicating the onset of paralysis. Saliva drools from the dog's mouth. Convulsive seizures and muscular incoordination become apparent, followed by progressive paralysis, usually terminating in death within 7 to 10 days of the onset of symptoms. In about 25% to 50% of cases, apparently as a result of limbic lobe dysfunction, dogs with rabies develop the furious form of the disease. Affected animals may eat abnormal objects, lose all fear, and during paroxysms of rage attack almost anything. The **paralytic phase** or "**dumb**" **phase** is evidenced as little change in behavior, but there is an early progressive paralysis. The first signs noted are inability to swallow, drooling, and dropped lower jaw, as a result of paralysis of the muscles. Typically, these animals are not vicious and make no attempt to bite. The paralysis progresses, followed by coma and death. Despite the phase or form exhibited from an infected animal, death is invariably the result. Regardless of the species involved, a change in behavior and paralysis of unknown origin are present. There are variations in species infected with rabies. Cattle will attack with the furious form. These animals are overly alert to their surroundings. Bellowing sounds will change and milk production will stop in dairy animals. Horses and mules may appear as if they have colic, may be very agitated, and may attack or bite. Many times they will have self-inflicted wounds. Any horse with neurologic signs should be considered as a possible exposure to rabies. Foxes and coyotes will enter yards and attack people and other animals. Skunks and raccoons generally show no fear of humans and are discovered out during the day despite the fact that they are nocturnal animals. They may or may not show neurologic signs and will readily attack humans and other animals. Bats may be out during the day despite being nocturnal animals. They may be seen flying or found on the ground and may attack humans and animals. Rodents and lagomorphs (rabbits, hares) are not considered a source of rabies but should be handled as any rabies suspect animal is handled until a diagnosis has been confirmed.

210. What are the incubation period and clinical symptoms of rabies in humans?

The incubation period is 14 to 80 days in humans. One man incubated the disease for almost 7 years. Humans with encephalitis, hydrophobia, dysphagia, myelitis, paresis, or paresthesia should be considered suspect for rabies, especially if there has been a nonspecific illness for 3 to 4 days prior to these signs. Neurologic signs gradually worsen with rabies, which is characteristic of the disease. Once other diseases that can cause encephalitis are ruled out through testing, rabies is usually suspected.

211.   How is an exposure to rabies infection treated?

Prophylactic and postexposure vaccines are available for people and domestic animals, and some prophylactic vaccines are being developed for wildlife species. If an exposure to rabies is confirmed or suspected, various postexposure protocols have been developed depending on the species involved (human, domestic animal, wild animal) and the vaccination status. Any animal that receives a bite from a possibly infected bat or infected wildlife is treated as exposed to rabies. In addition, if the rabies status of the biting animal cannot be determined, the bitten animal is to be treated as a possible exposure to rabies. The current recommendation is that **any** unvaccinated cat, dog, stock animal, or ferret that has been exposed to rabies must be euthanatized. If the owner is reluctant to euthanatize their pet, the animal is placed under strict quarantine for 6 months and monitored. Some states may require direct veterinary supervision. The quarantined animal is to have no contact with humans or other animals and must be kept inside a facility that prevents other animals from entering. One month prior to release of the quarantined animal, a rabies vaccination will be given. Some states may require the animal be vaccinated prior to quarantine and 1 month before release from quarantine. All vaccinated animals that have been exposed to rabies should be vaccinated at once and then monitored for the next 45 days. The wound should be thoroughly washed and debrided as necessary to decrease the presence of rabies virus. Animals that are presumed to have rabies should be humanely euthanatized and the brain submitted for testing. The rabies virus is not very stable outside the body for any length of time. It does survive at room temperature in carcasses or refrigerated for up to 48 hours. Rabies is readily inactivated by 45% to 75% ethanol, formaldehyde, 1% sodium hypochlorite, quaternary ammonium compounds, heat, 2% glutaraldehyde, ultraviolet light, and iodine.

212.   How is a rabies infection treated?

There is no specific antiviral agent or specific treatment for rabies. As late as 1990, worldwide, over 27,000 cases of animal rabies were reported annually. While 500 cases of human rabies were reported during that time, the actual number worldwide may have been closer to 20,000. Only a handful of people have survived a rabies infection; therefore, it is considered a fatal disease. Treatment of animals is usually **not** recommended because of the potential for exposure to humans during the treatment process. Once a virulent strain of rabies virus has established itself in the central nervous system of an infected animal or human, the outcome is almost always death. Supportive care is given to humans with rabies. Rarely have humans survived rabies after the onset of clinical disease.

213.   How can the animal responder best protect himself or herself against rabies?

Animal responders can protect themselves against rabies with prophylactic vaccination and by being aware of the possibility of being exposed. They should be suspicious of animals showing abnormal behavioral and/or neurologic signs and should minimize the risk of being bitten, scratched, or exposed to saliva. It is important to keep a level of suspicion and exercise care (protective clothing, gloves, mask, and eye protection) when handling suspected cases of rabies. If an exposure to rabies is suspected or confirmed, *medical attention should be sought immediately*. Prompt, thorough cleansing of any bite or scratch wound is paramount. Rabies vaccination is recommended for dogs and cats. There are several vaccines available: killed, modified-live, and attenuated. Modified-live is not used in the United States. Vaccine for ferrets, horses, cattle, and sheep is also available. Currently, no vaccine is approved in wildlife and is not recommended until efficacy can be demonstrated. An oral vaccine is available for wildlife in Canada and Europe, and it appears to be effective. A vaccinia-rabies glycoprotein recombinant vaccine is under investigation in the United States. Humans who have been exposed to rabies are given a series of vaccinations along with immunoglobulin. Humans who may be exposed to suspect animals should be vaccinated, checked regularly for a rabies titer, and revaccinated as needed. These individuals may still need to be vaccinated after exposure to a rabid animal.

RIFT VALLEY FEVER (RVF) (Infectious Enzootic Hepatitis of Sheep and Cattle)

214. What is the etiologic agent of Rift Valley fever?

Rift Valley fever virus is an RNA virus in the Bunyaviridae family. It is an arthropod-borne disease of sheep, cattle, and goats that is very contagious to humans. RVF could be used as a weapon for bioterrorism (aerosol).

215. What is the disease classification of RVF?

RVF is an OIE List A Disease.

216. What is the geographic distribution of RVF?

RVF is primarily found in Africa, but it has also been found in Yemen and Saudi Arabia.

217. What species of animals are susceptible to RVF infection?

Neonates have almost 100% mortality. Puppies, calves, lambs, kids, kittens, water buffalo, camels, monkeys, gray squirrels, rats, mice, and voles are all susceptible. Morbidity and mortality in adults are variable.

218. How is RVF transmitted?

The *Aedes* mosquito is the reservoir for RVF. The *Aedes lineatopinnis* can remain dormant for 5 to 15 years until heavy rains allow the eggs to hatch. Ruminants serve as the amplifying host; thus other species of mosquitoes become infected and bite naïve animals. Humans become infected through aerosolization of infected tissue during handling (necropsies or slaughtering animals without a mask). RVF in aerosols may be viable for greater than an hour when conditions are optimal. Such conditions include temperatures of 77°F. In addition, at neutral–alkaline pH and combined with protein or serum, RVF survives at 39°F for 4 months and below 32°F for 8 years. RVF is suitable for weaponization. An "animal abortion storm" would be the indication of disease.

219. What are the incubation period and the clinical signs of RVF in animals?

The incubation period is as little as 12 hours in newborns and up to 3 days in adult sheep, goats, cattle, and dogs. Lambs less than a week old have fever (104° to 107°F), weakness, and loss of appetite. Death occurs roughly 36 hours after initial exposure. Adult animals have a fever (104° to 106°F) as well as thick nasal secretions. Vomiting and death may be noted in them. Abortion is frequently the only indication of disease. Calves and adult cattle have a fever (104° to 106°F). Death rates may be high in the calves. Adults may have weakness, foul-smelling diarrhea, anorexia, increased salivation, icterus, and regurgitate. Abortion is frequent in pregnant cows. Horses appear to be viremic only. Newborn puppies and kittens have high death rates due to acute disease. Older dogs and cats are generally viremic without severe disease.

220. What are the incubation period and the clinical symptoms of RVF in humans?

The incubation period for RVF in humans is 4 to 6 days. Humans have signs that range from none to flulike to more serious. Headache, fever (100° to 104° F), nausea, dizziness, photophobia, weakness, muscle pain, back pain, and severe weight loss may occur. Individuals may also display vomiting, photophobia, and a stiff neck. Serious signs of illness (usually less than 1%) with RVF include hemorrhagic fever, ocular disease, hematemesis, encephalitis, melena, and jaundice.

221. Is RVF treatable?

Supportive care for affected animals should be done. A vaccine is available for both animals and humans.

222. How can the animal responder best protect himself or herself against RVF?

Animal responders can protect themselves from rift valley fever by being aware of the possibility of being exposed. Any animals that appear ill, have high death rates among the young, and have unexplained abortions should be handled with caution. It is important to keep a level of suspicion and exercise care (protective clothing, gloves, mask, and eye protection) when handling suspected cases of RVF. If an exposure to RVF is suspected or confirmed, medical attention should be sought immediately. Mosquito control is helpful but is not as efficient as vaccination. Carcasses of diseased animals should be burned or buried. No RVF infected animal should be slaughtered due to potential exposure to humans. Chloroform, ether, and sodium or calcium hypochlorite (chlorine content greater than 5,000 ppm) can be used to deactivate this virus. Most detergents, lipid solvents, and solutions with pH < 6.8 will also deactivate RVF.

VIRAL ENCEPHALITIS (Venezuelan Equine Encephalitis [VEE], Eastern Equine Encephalitis [EEE], and Western Equine Encephalitis [WEE])

223. What is the etiologic agent of viral encephalitis?

VEE, EEE, and WEE are all in the Togaviridae family. These viruses are transmitted by mosquitoes and can cause disease in horses, birds, and humans.

224. What is the disease classification of viral encephalitis?

Viral encephalitis is a CDC Category B disease and an OIE List B disease.

225. What is the geographic distribution of viral encephalitis?

VEE, EEE, and WEE are found only in North, Central, and South America. VEE is not normally seen in the United States or Canada. However, there are some strains of VEE (low virulence) that are considered endemic in the southern part of Florida. VEE is most often found in Central America, the northern part of South America, and Trinidad. Occasionally, there are outbreaks in western and northern South America that extend to Central America and the United States. EEE is found the United States in the east and the north central parts of the country, as well as near the Canadian border. EEE can also be found in the Caribbean Islands and some regions of Central and South America. WEE is found in the central and western United States, some regions of South America, and in Canada.

226. What species of animals are susceptible to viral encephalitis?

Horses and rodents are most affected, followed by birds. EEE also infects amphibians, bats, and reptiles. VEE also infects marsupials and bats.

227. How is viral encephalitis transmitted?

Transmission is through the bite of an infected mosquito. Research and laboratory personnel may be infected through aerosolization of the virus. Human cases typically appear about 2 weeks after horses show signs.

228. What are the incubation period and the clinical signs of viral encephalitis in horses?

The incubation period for EEE and WEE is about 5 to 15 days, while VEE can be as little as 24 hours but is usually 2 to 6 days. Horses have signs that may vary from mild to severe, including death. Signs include neurologic dysfunction, depression, fever, altered mentation, impaired vision, head pressing, circling, inability to swallow, ataxia, paralysis, and convulsions. In the late stage of disease, affected horses may have aggressive movement of the head, limbs, eyes, and mouth. Death can occur.

229. What are the incubation period and clinical symptoms of viral encephalitis in humans?

In humans, the incubation period for EEE is 4 to 10 days, for WEE is 5 to 10 days, and for VEE is 2 to 6 days, but it can be as little as 24 hours. Most individuals are asymptomatic for the disease. Symptoms may include headache, fever, muscle pain, nausea, anorexia, vomiting, malaise, photophobia, cough, diarrhea, sore throat, neurologic involvement (meningitis, altered mental state, disorientation, encephalitis), convulsions, tremors, and coma. Death can occur occasionally. Permanent neurologic deficits have been reported with EEE and WEE. Very young and old individuals have more severe symptoms.

230. Is viral encephalitis treatable?

In horses there is no specific treatment other than supportive (crystalloid fluids, NSAIDS, and the cautious use of dexamethasone sodium phosphate).

231. How do you control viral encephalitis?

There are monovalent (EEE), bivalent (EEE and WEE), and trivalent (EEE, WEE, and VEE) vaccines available for horses. Mosquito control should be done to decrease the adult population as well as decrease breeding grounds for the mosquitoes. In addition, horses should be routinely treated with insecticides effective against mosquitoes and housed with screens or fans to deter the insect. The viruses can be controlled by heat (80°F) for 30 minutes and the use of standard disinfectants.

232. How can the animal responder best protect himself or herself against viral encephalitis?

Animal responders can protect themselves against viral encephalitis by being aware of the possibility of being exposed, wearing protective clothing, and avoiding the times of day (early morning and evenings) when mosquitoes are out. A history of ill or dead birds and/or horses in an area should be handled with caution. It is important to keep a level of suspicion and exercise care (protective clothing, gloves, mask, and eye protection) when handling and caring for sick animals. If a viral encephalitis exposure is suspected or confirmed, medical attention should be sought immediately. Decontamination is done with thorough cleaning with soap and water.

VIRAL HEMORRHAGIC FEVERS (Ebola, Marburg, Lassa, Machupo)

233. What is the etiologic agent of viral hemorrhagic fevers?

Ebola and Marburg viruses are in the Filoviridae family. Lassa and Machupo (Bolivian hemorrhagic fever) viruses are in the Arenaviridae family. All are RNA viruses that cause hemorrhagic disease and possibly death.

234. What is the disease classification for the viral hemorrhagic fever viruses?

They are CDC Category A diseases.

235. What is the geographic distribution of the viral hemorrhagic fever viruses?

Ebola is found in the Sudan, the Democratic Republic of the Congo, the Ivory Coast, Gabon, the Republic of the Congo, and Uganda. One person from Liberia had serologic evidence of exposure without having any disease. Another exposure was reported in England with an accidental needle stick in a lab worker. Monkeys in research facilities in both the United States and Italy had serious illness and death from Ebola. These monkeys originated from the Philippines. Several humans in both of these exposures were infected but did not have any signs of illness. The Marburg virus has been found in Uganda, Europe, western Kenya, the Democratic Republic of the Congo, and Zimbabwe. Regions of West Africa are endemic for Lassa fever. Lassa fever has also been found in Sierra Leone, Nigeria, Liberia, Guinea, and possibly other countries in West Africa. The rodent that carries the Lassa fever virus is found throughout West Africa. Machupo virus (known as Bolivian hemorrhagic fever) is endemic in Bolivia.

236. What species are susceptible to infection?

Nonhuman primates and rodents are most susceptible.

237. How are the hemorrhagic fever viruses transmitted?

Body fluids from infected humans are the main source of infection to other humans. It is initially thought that exposure to an infected animal (unknown for Ebola, primates for Marburg, or rodents for Lassa and Machupo) causes disease in humans. Family members, friends, and hospital personnel become infected when caring for the patient. Rodents are responsible for the spread of the arenavirus (Lassa and Machupo) due to the rodents residing in homes, leaving droppings and urine, or the rodents may be used as a source of food. Contaminated fomites such as needles, syringes, and equipment can also cause disease.

238. What are the clinical signs of hemorrhagic fever viruses in animals?

Flulike symptoms are initially seen in humans and may be sudden for **Ebola**. Vomiting, diarrhea, and stomach discomfort then follow. Bleeding from the orifices, hiccups, red eyes, and a rash may be seen in some patients. A number of cynomolgus monkeys infected with the Ebola virus died in 1989, when they were imported from the Philippines to the United States (to a primate facility in Virginia). **Marburg** is similar to Ebola in that it is also sudden and flulike initially. After about 5 days of illness, a rash may develop on the trunk of the body. Vomiting, diarrhea, chest and/or abdominal pain, nausea, and a sore throat may be noted. Illness may progress to extensive hemorrhaging, organ failure, shock, and weight loss. Signs of **Lassa** virus include fever, sore throat, vomiting, diarrhea, chest, back, and abdominal pain, coughing, swelling of the face, bleeding mucous membranes, and conjunctivitis. Neurological signs (shuddering, hearing loss) may also be seen. **Machupo** can cause mucosal bleeding, fever, epistaxis, tremors, and speech impairment. All of these viral diseases can be fatal.

239. What are the incubation period and the clinical symptoms of hemorrhagic fever viruses in humans?

The incubation period for Ebola is 2 to 21 days, for Marburg it is 5 to 10 days and Lassa it is 1 to 3 weeks. Flulike symptoms are initially seen in humans and may be sudden for Ebola. Vomiting, diarrhea, and stomach discomfort follow. There may be bleeding from the orifices, hiccups, red eyes, and a rash seen in some patients. Marburg is similar to Ebola in that it is sudden and flulike, initially. After about 5 days of illness, a rash may develop on the trunk of the body. Vomiting, diarrhea, chest and/or abdominal pain, nausea, and a sore throat may be noted. Illness may progress to cause extensive hemorrhaging, organ failure, shock, and weight loss. Signs of Lassa virus include fever, sore throat, vomiting, diarrhea, chest, back, and abdominal pain, coughing, swelling of the face, bleeding mucous membranes, and conjunctivitis. Neurologic signs (shuddering, hearing loss) may also occur. Machupo causes mucosal bleeding, fever, epistaxis, tremors, and speech impairment. All of these viral diseases can be fatal.

240. Are the hemorrhagic fever viruses treatable?

These viruses are not an important health hazard in domestic animals. Infected nonhuman primates *should not be treated* because of the high zoonotic risk.

241. How can the animal responder best protect himself or herself against the hemorrhagic fever viruses?

Animal responders can protect themselves from the hemorrhagic fever viruses by being aware of the possibility of being exposed. Any rodent in endemic areas for these viruses or nonhuman primates that appear ill should be handled with caution. It is important to keep a level of suspicion and exercise care (protective clothing, gloves, mask, and eye protection) when handling suspected cases of hemorrhagic fever viruses. If an exposure to any of the hemorrhagic fever viruses is suspected or confirmed, **medical attention should be sought immediately.** No vaccines are available. Sterilization and disinfection of equipment, instruments, and premises where infected animals or humans have been are paramount. Isolation of the infected person is necessary as well as no direct contact with deceased patients. Animals exposed or infected with these viruses should be quarantined, euthanized, and properly disposed of. Proper **sterilization** and disinfection should be done to deactivate the viruses.

WEST NILE VIRUS (WNV) (West Nile Encephalomyelitis, West Nile Encephalitis)

242.   What is the etiologic agent of WNV?

WNV is in the Flaviviridae family. It causes illness in horses, birds, humans, and other animals. WNV was introduced into the United States in 1999.

243.   What is the disease classification of WNV?

There is currently no classification for WNV.

244.   What is the geographic distribution of WNV?

WNV is found in the Middle East, Africa, Asia (central and west), Europe, and North America.

245.   What species are susceptible to infection with WNV?

Horses and birds are most susceptible, followed by many mammals, some reptiles and amphibians, bats, and rabbits. Dogs, cats, cattle, sheep, goats, and pigs are less likely to be susceptible to the disease. WNV remains viable primarily through birds and mosquitoes.

246.   How is WNV transmitted?

The WNV vector is primarily the *Culex* species of mosquito, but ticks and other arthropods may cause infection (Fig. 1.11.5). It is zoonotic in that birds and mosquitoes together serve as a reservoir for WNV. Person-to-person spread is through pregnancy, a mother breastfeeding an infant, organ transplants, or blood transfusions.

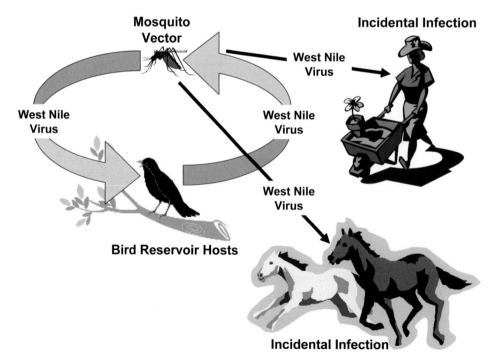

Figure 1.11.5 Transmission cycle of West Nile Virus.

247. What are the incubation period and the clinical signs of WNV in animals?

The incubation period is 3 to 14 days. Nearly all animals that are exposed to WNV show no signs or very few signs of illness. Generally most horses showing illness from WNV will recover. The remaining horses either die from the disease or are euthanized as a result of complications from WNV. Horses with clinical signs tend to have neurologic signs. Some signs include ataxia, sleepiness, facial paralysis, listlessness, difficulty eating, muzzle twitching, weakness or paralysis of the hindlimbs, head pressing, blindness, encephalitis, circling, muscle tremors, seizures, or coma. Fever is occasionally seen in some horses. Many of these horses display a variety of symptoms, so often the unusual presentation of signs is suggestive of WNV.

Crows, magpies, blue jays, and geese seem to be particularly sensitive to WNV. These birds may have depression, weight loss, neurologic signs, or be less active. WNV in chickens and turkeys is inapparent. Often the only sign seen is a dead bird.

Dogs and cats most often are asymptomatic. Dogs have signs comparable to horses, which include depression, fever, weakness, lack of appetite, atypical head posture, tremors, circling, ataxia, flaccid paralysis, inability to stand, hyperesthesia, seizures, diminished or no patellar reflexes, and convulsions. A few cats have shown mild, nonspecific illness through the first 7 days of disease. Signs included some lethargy, a mild fever, nystagmus, ataxia, hyperesthesia, and seizures.

248. What are the incubation period and the clinical symptoms of WNV in humans?

In humans, the incubation period is 3 to 15 days. Illness in humans ranges from asymptomatic to severe. Most humans (80%) will have no symptoms of disease. Less than 20% of exposed humans will have mild symptoms that are flulike and include fever, body aches, headache, vomiting, skin rash, nausea, being very tired, and having swollen lymph nodes.

249. Is WNV treatable?

Treatment in most animals is with supportive care (crystalloid fluids, NSAIDS, cautious use of dexamethasone SP). Mortality rates vary depending on species, age, and general health of the animal.

250. Can WNV be prevented?

There is a vaccine available only for horses. Mosquito control is important in controlling this disease. Avoid dawn and dusk when mosquitoes are most likely to be out. Birds should be removed if living or nesting near animals such as horses. Dead birds should be disposed of properly as dogs and cats become exposed to WNV by consuming the infected birds. In addition, treat or eliminate standing water to decrease mosquitoes. Animals should have mosquito repellants applied to them regularly. Use of fans in barns will help reduce mosquito exposure.

251. How did WNV arrive in the United States?

WNV was once considered a foreign animal disease (i.e., not found in the United States but found in Africa, Asia, and the Middle East). WNV was documented in New York in 1999 but how it arrived here is uncertain. Since that time, the virus has continued to spread west, with some states reporting a relatively high incidence of cases.

252. How can the animal responder best protect himself or herself against WNV infection?

Animal responders can protect themselves from WNV by being aware of the possibility of being exposed. Any sudden deaths in birds or horses that appeared ill or had neurologic signs or unusual presentation of illness should be handled with caution. It is important to keep a level of suspicion and exercise care when handling suspected cases of WNV. If an exposure to WNV is suspected or confirmed, medical attention should be sought. Mosquito bite prevention is very important. Appropriate clothing, tents with mosquito netting, and use of mosquito repellents are helpful. A vaccine is available for horses and has been used in alpacas as well. Standard decontamination can be done with soap and water.

BOTULISM (*Botulinum* Toxins, Limberneck, Shaker Foal Syndrome, Western Duck Sickness, Toxicoinfectious Botulism, Bulbar Paralysis, Loin Disease, Lamziekte)

253. What is the etiologic agent of botulism?

Botulism is caused by a neurotoxin produced by the anaerobic bacterium *Clostridium botulinum*. There are eight types of *C. botulinum* (A, B, C1, C2, D, E, F, and G), and each produces a distinct neurotoxin. The spores of this bacterium are everywhere and they develop into vegetative bacteria that create toxins under anaerobic conditions. There are three naturally occurring forms of botulism: food borne, infantile, and wound. *Botulinum toxin is the most potent neurotoxin known.* It is a possible biological weapon.

254. What is the disease classification of botulism?

Botulism is a CDC Category A disease.

255. What is the geographic distribution of botulism?

C. botulinum is found in the soil worldwide.

256. How potent is botulinum toxin?

It is 15,000 times more toxic than VX (the most toxic of the nerve agents) and 100,000 times more toxic than sarin (a chemical weapon of mass destruction).

257. Which toxins affect humans and animals?

In humans, types A, B, E and F (rarely) may bring about disease. In animals, type C is the most frequent source of botulism. Horses may be affected by type B. Cattle and dogs will occasionally be affected by type D. Birds and mink may be affected by types A and E. Type G toxin has occasionally been noted in animals and humans but apparently does not cause disease. Botulinum toxins all cause the same disease. For effective treatment, it will depend on the use of antiserum for the specific type of toxin.

258. How is botulism contracted?

C. botulinum (in vegetative or spore form) contaminates a food source (raw meat, flesh, silage), decaying vegetation, or infected carcasses (herbivores may ingest feed contaminated by carcasses). The botulinum toxin is not contagious. When botulinum toxin is ingested in the contaminated food source, it has the preformed toxin. The toxin is absorbed from the stomach and upper small bowel into the lymphatic system. Eventually the toxin circulates to the neuromuscular (nerve-muscle) junction, where it prevents the release of a neurotransmitter, thereby blocking the signal for the muscle to contract. The result is a flaccid paralysis. Wound contamination (the toxicoinfectious form) with botulinum toxins results when a wound is anaerobic. Such infections are usually associated with the intestinal tract, deep muscle or skin wounds, navel infections, and lung or liver abscesses. The "shaker foal syndrome" is caused by an endotoxin of *C. botulinum*. In humans, botulinum toxins can enter through wounds that are not properly cleaned or are contaminated with soil (spores are routinely present in soil). Ingestion of the toxins is typically the result of improper handling of food or not heating food thoroughly. Children under 1 year of age are most susceptible to the intestinal form of botulinum. Honey and other foods that may contain spores from soil are a source of infection. The adult colonization form is common in individuals with a history of intestinal illness (inflammatory bowel disease) or recent gastrointestinal surgery. This form of botulinum is extremely rare. Aerosolization of the toxin may be used for weaponization.

259. What are the incubation period and the clinical signs of botulism in animals?

The incubation period ranges from 2 hours to 14 days. Most often illness is seen within 12 to 72 hours. Signs in horses may include incoordination, drooling, paralysis of the tongue, restlessness, and knuckling. Muscle paralysis is common (and is seen in most species of animals). The paralysis is progressive and ascending. These animals lose their ability to swallow or chew, and death results from respiratory or cardiac paralysis. Shaker foal syndrome is seen in very young foals (less than 4 weeks). They are unable to stand for more than a few minutes, muscle tremors are present, and they appear stiff when moving. Often times these foals show no signs before death. Other signs that may be noted include constipation, repeated urination, dysphagia, and dilation of the pupils. Respiratory paralysis is most often the cause of death in these foals in 1 to 3 days. Signs seen in cattle are incoordination, dysphagia, drooling, inability to urinate, restlessness, and sternal recumbency. Sheep display a nasal discharge (serous), incoordination, drooling, and stiffness. The disease can be progressive in ruminants, causing paralysis and death. Birds usually have a flaccid paralysis that involves the neck, legs, eyelids, and wings. Occasionally, diarrhea may be noted with the toxicoinfectious form. Mink and foxes are often found dead. Dyspnea and various stages of paralysis may be seen. Pigs have signs of vomiting, muscle paralysis, anorexia, not wanting to drink, and dilation of the pupils. Pigs are generally resistant to botulinum.

260. What are the incubation period and clinical symptoms of botulism in humans?

In humans, the incubation period is usually 12 to 36 hours after consuming the toxin but can range from 6 hours to 10 days. Humans often display drooping eyelids, altered voice, double vision or blurred vision, difficulty in speaking or swallowing, and dry mouth. Infected individuals may have a descending, symmetrical flaccid paralysis. Other symptoms that may be seen include vomiting, diarrhea, nausea, and abdominal pain. Impaired respiratory function is due to the toxin causing paralysis of the respiratory muscles. Infants will display lack of appetite, constipation, decreased crying and sucking, weakness in the neck and periphery (known as "floppy baby"), and have respiratory failure.

261. Is botulism treatable?

Treatment is primarily supportive: assisting with eating and drinking, intravenous fluid support, assisting urination, changing positions to avoid decubital sores, lubricating the eyes, etc. *C. botulinum* C + D antitoxin may be used to decrease or stop the signs of disease. If botulinum antitoxin can be administered early, it may slow the progression of disease and diminish the symptoms. However, it is not effective against any toxin that has penetrated the nerve endings. The use of antibiotics is questionable and controversial as they have no effect on the already absorbed toxin and may increase toxin release from dying bacteria. In cases of food-borne illness, the levels of toxin in the intestinal tract may be decreased with the use of stomach lavages and enemas. Infected wounds are best treated through debridement and the use of antibiotics. **Antitoxins are used only in the treatment of botulinum toxin and not the prevention of it.**

262.   How can botulism be prevented?

Vaccination with C + D toxoid has proved useful in cattle, sheep, goats, pheasants, and mink.

263.   How can botulinum toxins be destroyed?

Botulinum toxins are proteins that are easily denatured. Toxins that are exposed to sunlight are inactivated within 1 to 3 hours. They can also be deactivated by 0.1% sodium hypochlorite, heating to 176°F for 30 minutes or 212°F for 10 minutes, and 0.1N sodium hydroxide. Water can be treated with chlorine or other disinfectants to deactivate the toxin. The vegetative form of *C. botulinum* is deactivated by 1% sodium hypochlorite, 70% ethanol, and other disinfectants. The spores are deactivated by moist heat at 248°F for a minimum of 15 minutes.

264.   How can the animal responder best protect himself or herself against botulism?

Animal responders can protect themselves from botulism by being aware of the possibility of being exposed. Wounds that become anaerobic (or deep wounds), the presence of intestinal disease, navel infections, and lung and liver abscesses should be monitored closely. Contaminated food, decaying vegetation, improperly cooked food, and infected carcasses are also sources of infection. It is important to keep a level of suspicion and exercise care (protective clothing, gloves, mask, and eye protection) when handling suspected cases of botulism. If an exposure to botulism is suspected or confirmed, medical attention should be sought immediately.

CLOSTRIDIUM PERFRINGENS TOXINS

265.   How does *Clostridium perfringens* result in illnesses?

C. perfringens is a common anaerobic bacillus that produces at least 12 exotoxins. In animals, *C. perfringens* is a normal inhabitant of the intestinal microflora and also found in the soil. Some of the exotoxins produce enterotoxemias (A, B, C, and D), which can cause necrosis and death of the host. It is uncertain if type E plays a role in disease in animals.

266.   What is the disease classification of *C. perfringens*?

The epsilon toxin of *C. perfringens* is a CDC Category B disease.

267.   What is the geographic distribution of *C. perfringens*?

Worldwide.

268.   What species are susceptible to infection?

Domestic mammals, birds, and nonhuman primates are affected by *C. perfringens*. Some toxins are more potent in some species versus others.

269. How is *C. perfringens* transmitted?

C. perfringens is in the soil and the intestinal tract of normal healthy animals and people. Most cases of enterotox-emia in animals are the result of food contaminated with these bacteria or spores. The bacteria can also proliferate suddenly in the altered intestinal tract, which allows for production of toxin. In humans, the route of transmission is through improperly cooked food or food that is not adequately stored or kept at proper temperature.

270. What are the incubation period and the clinical signs of *C. perfringens* in animals?

The incubation period is 1 to 6 hours, but one may only find dead animals. Young animals appear more severely affected, and often it is the animal on full feed. In lambs, calves, and pigs, the clinical sign is of a healthy animal that died suddenly and for no apparent reason. There is often abdominal pain, depression, inappetence, bloody or nonbloody diarrhea, recumbency, convulsions, and opisthotonus. There is septicemia prior to an acute death. A necrotic enteritis, excitement, and incoordination may also be noted.

271. What are the incubation period and the clinical symptoms in humans for *C. perfringens*?

In humans, the incubation is usually 10 to 12 hours but ranges from 6 to 24 hours. *C. perfringens* is also called the "food service germ." It results from raw food that is not properly cooked, food that is not heated and main-tained at proper temperature, or food that is not properly cooled. Most often, food poisoning is the result of food served in large quantities and left out either at room temperature or on steam tables for several hours. The typical history is a large number of individuals displaying the same symptoms after eating a particular food. Clinical signs are most often sudden and include cramping, abdominal pain, and gas, as well as watery diarrhea. Fever, dehydra-tion, and vomiting may occur in a few cases. The duration of illness is usually less than 1 day and is not serious in most healthy individuals.

272. Is *C. perfringens* treatable?

In animals with severe clinical signs, it may be too late to treat. Supportive care should be provided along with *C. perfringens* antitoxin and large doses of penicillin.

273. Can *C. perfringens* be prevented?

C. perfringens antitoxin is given to very young animals (if mothers are unprotected) for immediate protection, followed with the toxoid product when older. Reduce the amount of concentrate and increase the roughage pro-vided to animals in feedlot situations.

274. How can the animal responder best protect himself or herself against *C. perfringens*?

Animal responders can protect themselves from *C. perfringens* by being aware of the possibility of being exposed. Sudden death in animals should be handled with caution (protective clothing, gloves, mask, and goggles). Most important, animal responders need to be aware of how their food has been prepared, if it has been properly cooked, and if it has been maintained at the correct temperature (hot foods kept hot, cold foods kept cold). It is

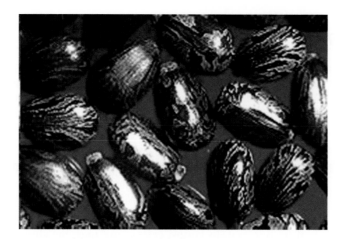

Figure 1.11.6 Castor beans are the source of ricin. Source: Public Domain. http://www.ars.usda.gov/is/AR/archive/jan01/plant 0101.htm

important to keep a level of suspicion and exercise care when responding to any incident where the animal responder is not familiar with the surroundings. The consumption of food should only be from a reliable and trustworthy source. If an exposure to *C. perfringens* is suspected or confirmed, medical attention should be sought. Standard decontamination is with soap and water.

RICIN

275. What is the source of ricin?

Ricin is a potent cytotoxin derived from the beans of the castor plant (*Ricinus communis*) (Fig. 1.11.6). The ricin toxins are potent inhibitors of DNA replication and protein synthesis. Ricin may be used as a biological weapon.

276. What is the disease classification of ricin?

Ricin is a CDC Category B disease.

277. What is the geographic distribution of ricin?

Worldwide. Castor oil is processed from castor beans with ricin being in the "mash," which is a waste product.

278. What species are susceptible to ricin exposure?

Domestic animals, birds, nonhuman primates—most, if not all, species of animals are susceptible to ricin toxicity.

279. What is the route of transmission for ricin?

Ricin is found in the castor bean plant, and the seeds contain the highest concentration of this toxin. Large quantities of the plant or bean must be consumed to cause illness. It is not very palatable, so animals will eat it if hungry, if fed as castor bean meal, or if it has been accidentally introduced into feed. Transmission by inhalation occurs during industrial operations (extraction of oils from the plant). Ricin has been used as a terrorist weapon in humans when the product was injected via a modified umbrella into an individual in Great Britain.

280. What is the mechanism of action of ricin?

Ricin enters the cells of the body (ingestion, inhalation, or injection) and inhibits the production of necessary proteins in the cell. Cell death occurs, which leads to the death of the animal or human who was exposed.

281. What are the incubation period and the clinical signs of ricin toxicity in animals?

The incubation period in animals is a few hours up to 48 hours. Animals may exhibit a fever, abdominal pain, muscular twitching, vomiting, diarrhea, convulsions, coma, and death. Shock and anaphylaxis (allergic reaction) can occur due to ricin being a cytotoxin. Horses may die within 24 to 36 hours after ingestion of ricin.

282. What are the incubation period and the clinical symptoms of ricin toxicity in humans?

In humans, the incubation period is less than 6 hours if ingested and 8 hours if inhaled. Accidental exposure may happen through the consumption of castor beans. Exposure to ricin usually results from the deliberate use of it as a poison. Violent vomiting and diarrhea are initially seen and may contain blood. Dehydration, flulike symptoms, hypovolemic shock, weakness, seizures, hallucinations, and multiorgan system failure occur. Inhaled exposure of ricin is not well documented. A few symptoms that may be seen or all may occur and include flulike symptoms, respiratory distress, cough, bronchial constriction, pulmonary edema, nausea, weakness, multiple organ failure, cyanosis, respiratory failure, and death. Individuals exposed to dust from the castor bean can have an allergic reaction, hives, tightness in the chest, watery itchy eyes, or wheezing. Information on exposure to ricin by injection is limited. Symptoms vary some but include flulike symptoms, dizziness, nausea, weakness, vomiting, anorexia, pain at the injection site, myalgia, shock, and death. If the individual survives 3 to 5 days, he or she generally recovers. There are only four reported cases to date, and two of the individuals died.

283. Is ricin exposure treatable?

Supportive care, laxatives, antihistamines, and gastrointestinal protectants (fats or oils are best) may be tried with an exposure to ricin. Sedatives may be used to control the signs. There is currently no vaccine or prophylactic antitoxin available.

284. How can the animal responder best protect himself or herself against ricin exposure?

Animal responders can protect themselves from ricin exposure by being aware of the possibility of being exposed. Sudden death in any animal, feeds that may contain castor bean or its products, or an environment that is hostile to responders should be cautiously approached. It is important to keep a level of suspicion and exercise care (protective clothing, gloves, mask, and eye protection) when handling suspected cases of ricin exposure or when present in hostile environments where ricin may be available. **If an exposure to ricin is suspected or confirmed, medical attention should be sought immediately.** The use of copious amounts of soap and water is used to rinse ricin off of the skin. All clothing and personal belongings should be removed, double bagged, and sealed for proper disposal. Environmental decontamination should be accomplished with soap and water and deactivated with 0.1% hypochlorite solutions (0.1%) or EPA-registered disinfectants.

STAPHYLOCCAL ENTEROTOXIN B (SEB) (Staph Enterotoxicosis)

285.   What is the etiologic agent of SEB?

Staphylococcus aureus can produce seven types of toxin that exert their effects on the intestinal tract and is most often the source of food poisoning. It may also be used as a biological weapon (aerosol).

286.   What is the disease classification of SEB?

It is a CDC Category B disease.

287.   What is the geographic distribution of SEB?

Worldwide.

288.   What species are susceptible to SEB?

Domestic animals, birds, humans, and nonhuman primates are susceptible to SEB.

289.   How is SEB transmitted?

The usual route of SEB transmission is through food that is not properly handled. Direct contact with infected animals (mastitis in cattle and sheep, rodents as a reservoir) may also result in SEB infection. Humans do not transmit the disease to other humans. Aerosolization of SEB (used as a weapon) was done by the United States in the 1960s.

290.   What are the incubation period and the clinical signs in animals?

The incubation period in animals, if ingested, is typically 2 to 4 hours, but may range from 30 minutes to 12 hours. The incubation period for inhalation is 3 to 4 hours, and 8 to 20 hours in nonhuman primates. When contaminated food is ingested, signs include vomiting, abdominal pain, nausea, weakness, hypotension, a drop in body temperature, and diarrhea. Nonhuman primates that were exposed by inhalation of nonlethal SEB have abdominal pain in less than 24 hours, with signs beginning in about 8 to 20 hours. Fever is seen only with inhalation of SEB. In addition, sudden hypotension, nonproductive cough (for up to 4 weeks), and myalgia are noted. The primates are ill for 3 to 4 days. If SEB is inhaled at a lethal dose, signs are noted within 2 days. Signs of pulmonary edema, dyspnea, and gastrointestinal distress are seen. Death within 3 to 4 days results from multiorgan failure.

291.   What are the incubation period and the clinical symptoms in humans exposed to SEB?

Humans may experience symptoms 30 minutes to 6 hours after consuming contaminated food. When SEB is inhaled by humans, the incubation period is 3 to 12 hours. Clinical signs of SEB food poisoning include vomiting, abdominal pain, diarrhea, and nausea. Symptoms of SEB usually last 1 to 3 days and are generally mild in humans.

Symptoms of inhalation exposure to SEB include dyspnea, fever, nonproductive cough, acute respiratory difficulty, myalgia, vomiting, diarrhea, nausea, headache, anorexia, hypotension, and pulmonary edema. Illness may last up to 14 days in humans.

292. Is SEB exposure treatable?

Supportive care for ingestion of SEB includes fluids, electrolytes, and medications to ease abdominal discomfort. Inhalation SEB exposure may require oxygen, mechanical ventilation, atropine, antihistamines, and cough suppressants.

293. How can the animal responder best protect himself or herself against SEB exposure?

Animal responders can protect themselves from SEB by being aware of the possibility of being exposed. Rodents, mastitis in cows or ewes, and food that is not properly cooked should be handled with caution. It is important to keep a level of suspicion and exercise care (protective clothing, gloves, mask, and eye protection) when handling suspected cases of SEB. Consumed food should only be from a reliable and trustworthy source. Most important, animal responders need to be aware of how their food has been prepared, if it has been properly cooked, and if it has been maintained at the correct temperature (hot foods kept hot, cold foods kept cold). If an exposure to SEB is suspected or confirmed, medical attention should be sought. Prevention is by keeping foods at proper temperature. The use of good hygiene will help prevent food poisoning. No vaccine is currently available. A toxoid vaccine and a vaccine with toxins have or are being developed, respectively. Decontaminate with soap and water. Sodium hypochlorite 5% can be used to deactivate SEB on surfaces. When handling dead carcasses, use protective clothing, mask, gloves, and goggles. Dispose of carcasses by incineration or deep burial.

TRICHOTHECENE (T-2) MYCOTOXINS

294. What is the etiologic agent of T-2 mycotoxin?

Fusarium is a fungus that produces the trichothecene (T-2) mycotoxins and is often found on grain products. These mycotoxins are unique in that they are dermally active. T-2 mycotoxins must be suspected when any aerosol occurs in the form of "yellow rain." The yellow rain will contain droplets of pigmented oily fluids that contaminate hair coats of animals and the surrounding environment. T-2 mycotoxin has been used as a biological weapon.

295. What is the disease classification of T-2 mycotoxin?

There is no disease classification.

296. What is the geographic distribution of T-2 mycotoxin?

Worldwide.

297. What species are susceptible to infection?

Horses, cattle, pigs, birds (poultry), fish, humans, and invertebrates are susceptible. It is highly likely that dogs, sheep, goats, cats, and other mammals are also susceptible.

298.   How is T-2 mycotoxin transmitted?

In domestic animals, ingestion is most often through moldy food such as corn, corn silage, wheat, legumes, sorghum grain, barley, pelleted feed, rice meal, groundnuts, cottonseed meal, tall fescue grass, standing corn, and maize. Humans may be infected by consuming contaminated cereals and grains. A terrorist event would result in the spraying of the oily agent that could affect the hair coat and skin.

299.   What are the clinical signs of T-2 mycotoxin exposure in animals?

Signs of ingestion of T-2 mycotoxins in animals include inappetence, decreased milk and egg production, hypotension, staggering, diarrhea, shock, vomiting, and lesions in the mouth and upper gastrointestinal tract. There may be deaths of some animals. Dermal exposure causes inflammation and cutaneous necrosis, while eye exposure may result in damage to the cornea.

300.   What are the incubation period and the clinical symptoms of T-2 mycotoxin exposure in humans?

The oral incubation period is 3 to 12 hours; respiratory route, less than 1 hour; dermally, 6 to 12 hours; and ocular exposure, less than 5 minutes. Ingestion results in vomiting and diarrhea relatively quickly. Skin exposure results in redness, pain, pruritus, necrosis, blisters, and sloughing. Blurred vision is often the result of ocular exposure. Inhalation causes nasal secretions, itching, irritation in the nose and throat, blindness, coughing, bleeding, sneezing, chest pain, and seizures. High levels of T-2 mycotoxins cause ataxia, weakness, shock, prostration, and death.

301.   Is T-2 mycotoxin exposure treatable?

Supportive care should be given to the affected animal. Bathe the dermally exposed animal with soap and water. Activated charcoal given within an hour of ingestion may help. Animals being fed contaminated feed or grazed on affected pastures should be immediately removed from the source. Flush eyes with copious amounts of water if there has been ocular exposure. Prevent mold contamination of feed. No vaccine is available.

302.   How can the animal responder best protect himself or herself against T-2 mycotoxin exposure?

Animal responders can protect themselves from T-2 mycotoxins by being aware of the possibility of being exposed. Any animal with skin lesions, skin necrosis, or ocular lesions; moldy feed or food; and oily residues on animals or fomites (objects) should be handled with caution. It is important to keep a level of suspicion and exercise care (protective clothing, gloves, mask, and eye protection) when handling suspected cases of T-2 mycotoxin. Be aware when present in hostile environments where T-2 mycotoxin may be available that it can be placed in food, beverages, or weaponized as an aerosol. **If an exposure to T-2 mycotoxin is suspected or confirmed, medical attention should be sought immediately.** Decontaminate with soap and water. Environmental decontamination can be done with 5% sodium hypochlorite to deactivate contaminated equipment. T-2 mycotoxins are deactivated by heating at 900° For 10 minutes or 500° For 30 minutes. Dermal lesions can result if contaminated clothing is touched.

BOVINE SPONGIFORM ENCEPHALOPATHY (BSE) (Mad Cow Disease)

303.   What is the etiologic agent of BSE?

BSE is a fatal, nonfebrile, progressive disease of cattle most likely caused by a prion protein. The BSE outbreak is responsible for FSE in cats and spongiform encephalopathy in exotic ruminants. A variant of Creutzfeldt-Jakob disease (CJD) that occurs in humans is apparently related to BSE.

304.   What is the disease classification of BSE?

It is an OIE List B Disease.

305.   What is the geographic distribution of BSE?

BSE has been found in Great Britain (initial occurrence of the disease), many countries in Europe, Canada, the United States, Japan, Israel, Oman, and the Falkland Islands. To date, it has not been found in New Zealand, Australia, South America, or Central America.

306.   What species are susceptible to BSE infection?

Cattle are most susceptible. Experimentally, sheep, goats, pigs, cats, mink, cynomolgus monkeys, mice, and marmosets have been infected (Fig. 1.11.7). It is possible, but not proved, that dogs may also be infected.

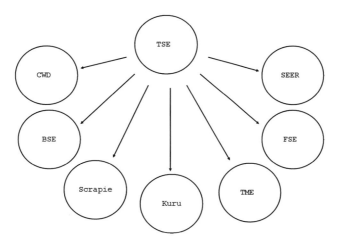

Figure 1.11.7 Transmissible Spongiform Encephalopathies (TSE) affect cattle (Bovine spongiform encephalopathy, BSE, mad cow disease); sheep, goats, Moufflon, rodents, monkeys (Scrapie); white-tailed deer, black-tailed deer, mule deer, elk, moose (Chronic wasting disease, CWD); mink (Transmissible mink encephalopathy, TME); cats (Feline spongiform encephalopathy, FSE); humans (Kuru); and exotic ruminants (Spongiform encephalopathy of exotic ruminants, SEER).

307. How is BSE transmitted?

BSE is transmitted through the ingestion of nervous tissue. There are several theories as to how BSE was introduced into cattle. It may be a genetic mutation that occurred as early as the 1970s, it may be a mutation of scrapie in sheep (cattle were fed infected sheep tissue), or it possibly is a human TSE mutation. BSE was noted in Great Britain during the 1980s. In November 1986, scientists became aware of the problem in cattle. At this time period, cattle were being fed meat-and-bone meal (MBM) that had been added to their rations. The MBM came from animal carcasses that were in all probability infected with the BSE agent. Cattle that acquire BSE through natural means have this agent in the spinal cord, brain, and retina. Experimentally, it can also be found in the distal ileum of infected calves. Cows infected with BSE are more likely to produce calves that are at increased risk of having BSE. At present, the mode of transmission of the agent to these higher-risk calves is unknown.

308. What are the incubation period and the clinical signs of BSE in animals?

The incubation period of BSE in cattle is longer than a year to a number of years (usually 2 years) . Typically, cattle are affected at 4 to 5 years of age. BSE in cattle is progressive and insidious. Once clinical signs become evident, the disease progresses fairly rapidly. Death usually occurs 3 months after signs are initially noted. Neurologic signs are predominant in this disease. At the outset, these animals demonstrate sneezing, rubbing and tossing of the head, decreased rumination, increased licking of the nose or crinkling it, and bruxism. As the disease progresses, they may have hyperesthesia, head shyness, kicking, ataxia of the hindlimbs, or tremors; be easily startled; fall down; and appear nervous. Animals with advanced disease tend to have a fixed facial appearance, standing with a lowered head for extended periods of time; lose weight; have reduced milk production; become recumbent; lose consciousness; and then die. Unlike scrapie, there is no pruritus in BSE-infected cattle.

309. What are the incubation period and the clinical symptoms of BSE exposure in humans?

The incubation period is unknown in humans (it may be years to decades). Symptoms are only seen in some individuals, and it appears to be a variant of Creutzfeldt-Jakob disease (vCJD). The disease is seen in young individuals (about 28 to 29 years of age); symptoms persist for about 14 months; and it is probably linked to food contaminated with the BSE agent. CJD is more common in humans 65 years and older, and illness lasts about 4.5 years. Initial clinical presentation of vCJD involves sensory or behavioral changes. Neurologic symptoms follow weeks to months later. Neurologic symptoms are ataxia, dementia, and myoclonus. The final, fatal progression of vCJD is the inability to speak or move, followed by death.

310. Is BSE treatable?

There is no treatment other than supportive. Humane euthanasia is recommended when illness incapacitates the animal.

311. Can BSE be prevented?

No vaccine is available for BSE. Humane euthanasia is recommended for any adult bovine demonstrating neurologic signs. Animals with neurologic signs that die on the owner's premises and are negative for rabies should not enter the food chain. A ban of all ruminant animals and their products from countries known to have BSE has been used to control the disease. In addition, the "animal feed rule" was implemented, which forbids feeding animal proteins or animal protein products, especially spinal cord, brain, and eyes, to domestic ruminants. Once BSE has been identified in an animal, the herd is quarantined, and tracebacks are performed by the USDA to identify all animals that are related to or had contact with the positive animal.

312. How can the animal responder best protect himself or herself against BSE exposure?

Animal responders can protect themselves from BSE by being aware of the possibility of being exposed. Ruminants or other animals exhibiting neurologic signs should be handled with caution until a diagnosis of the disease can be made. Meat and meat byproducts from countries that have BSE should also be handled with caution. It is important to keep a level of suspicion and exercise care (protective clothing, gloves, mask, and eye protection) when handling suspected cases of BSE. If an exposure to BSE is suspected or confirmed, medical attention should be sought.

313. How is BSE decontaminated?

BSE appears to be resistant to heating at normal cooking temperatures, pasteurization, freezing, sterilization, and drying. Scrapie, which is a similar disease, is very resistant to heat, ionizing radiation, disinfectants, formalin, and ultraviolet radiation. Scrapie is also very resistant to destruction if it is in desiccated organic material or tissue. Autoclaving with a minimum temperature of 273° to 80°F for 18 minutes may deactivate this abnormal prion protein. Incineration or autoclaving contaminated tissue is recommended. Disinfectants that may be used to deactivate BSE include sodium hydroxide, sodium hypochlorite, and sodium hypochlorite with 2N sodium hydroxide or 2% available chlorine for at least 1 hour at 68°F (overnight for equipment) is recommended. It is unclear if these procedures will completely deactivate this prion, but they may reduce the titer of this agent. Great Britain disposes of contaminated carcasses by heating to 271°F at 3 bar pressure for at least 20 minutes. The prevailing thought in the medical field of neurosurgery is to use disposable instruments if CJD is highly suspicious in a patient. In Great Britain, equipment that is used in brain biopsies is quarantined until a final diagnosis has been made. This is due to the high risk for CJD in that country.

CHRONIC WASTING DISEASE (CWD)

314. What is the etiologic agent of CWD?

CWD is a contagious, fatal disease of deer and elk, which are the only known animals to serve as a natural host for this disease. In 1967, it was identified as a "wasting" syndrome in mule deer at a wildlife research facility in northern Colorado. It has subsequently been recognized as a transmissible spongiform encephalopathy (TSE or prion) in 1978.

315. What is the disease classification of CWD?

It is an OIE List B Disease.

316. What is the geographic distribution of CWD?

CWD is endemic in Colorado, Nebraska, and Wyoming. The disease has also been found in other regions of the United States.

317.   What species are susceptible to CWD infection?

Cervids such as mule deer, white-tailed deer, and elk are susceptible. Moose are also reported with CWD. Experimentally, mice, squirrel monkeys, mink, domestic ferrets, and hamsters have been infected.

318.   How is CWD transmitted?

Lateral transmission (animal-to-animal) appears to be the main source of CWD infection. Maternal transmission may also occur but is not significant. It is suspected that the naïve animal may ingest the protein through contaminated food and water. To date, it has not been proved that there is a risk in humans, and it would be considered low if there is one. A few cases possibly suggest that eating venison in endemic areas may increase the risk of CJD.

319.   What are the incubation period and the clinical signs of CWD in animals?

The incubation period ranges from 1.5 to 3 years. Most animals are older than 16 months, and it has been found in animals older than 15 years. In cervids, CWD is progressive and fatal in adult animals. Initially, there may be subtle loss of weight and changes in behavior. As the disease becomes more obvious, there may be persistent walking and change in interactions with other animals (and toward caregivers), and the animals become less wary and show head tremors, polydipsia, polyuria, difficulty swallowing, ataxia, and drowsiness. In the final stages of disease, there may be excess salivation, bruxism, fixed gaze, droopy ears, and lowered head. *Aspiration pneumonitis should always raise the suspicion of CWD in adult cervids.* The most prevalent and consistent sign of CWD is weight loss. Elk may also display hyperexcitability and nervousness. Some affected animals may not show any weight loss. Death usually results from debilitation, stress, or cold weather.

320.   What are the clinical symptoms of CWD exposure in humans?

Information is limited and has not been confirmed that CWD can cause disease in humans. There have been just a few cases to date that suggest CJD or a prion disease in humans with no family history of CJD and with a history of consuming venison. Symptoms seen in these humans included seizures, depression, fatigue, memory loss, speech abnormalities, headaches, social withdrawal, combative behavior, anger outbursts, vision problems, photophobia, confusion, ataxia, incontinence, and coma. Documented illness lasted from 5 to 6 months up to 22 months prior to death. Death was due to a degenerative neurologic disorder or a prion disease.

321.   Is CWD treatable?

There is no treatment other than supportive. Humane euthanasia is recommended when illness incapacitates the animal.

322.   How is CWD prevented?

There is no vaccine available for CWD. Humans should avoid tissues that are known to contain CWD (brain, spinal cord, eyes, tonsils, lymph nodes, and spleen) from deer, moose, or elk in areas endemic with the disease.

Any animal that is suspicious for the CWD disease or is abnormal should be avoided for consumption by animals and humans. All utensils (knives, tables, saws) used to butcher a cervid carcass should be disinfected with 50% sodium hypochlorite. The animal should then be tested for CWD prior to consuming the meat. Humans should wear protective clothing, mask, gloves, and goggles when any cervid is being harvested for the meat.

323. How can the animal responder best protect himself or herself from CWD exposure?

Animal responders can protect themselves from CWD by being aware of the possibility of being exposed. Any cervid that displays unusual behavior, neurologic signs, or has significant weight loss should be handled with caution (protective clothing, mask, gloves, and goggles). If an exposure to CWD is suspected or confirmed, medical attention should be sought.

324. How is CWD decontaminated?

There are limited methods for deactivating prion proteins. The use of 50% sodium hypochlorite for at least 30 to 60 minutes is beneficial in deactivating CWD. There may be other disinfectants that may prove useful for deactivating CWD, but they are not known at this time. Alkaline digestion and incineration may be done to dispose of carcasses and infected tissue. It has been suggested to dispose of these remains in landfills, but this may not be practical as scavenger animals will seek these tissues.

Suggested Reading

Avian Disease Manual. 2nd ed. The American Association of Avian Pathologists, 1995.

Belay ED, Maddox RA, Williams ES, Miller MW, Gambetti P, Schonberger LB. *Emerg Infect Dis* 2004;10:977–983.

Butler D. Thai dogs carry bird-flu virus, but will they spread it? *Nature* 2006;439:773.

Crawford PC, Dubovi EJ, Castleman WL, Stephenson I, Gibbs EP, Chen L, et al. Transmission of equine influenza virus to dogs. *Science* 2005;310:482–485.

Foreign Animal Diseases, "The Gray Book." 1998. Committee on Foreign Animal Diseases of the United States Animal Health Association, P.O. Box K227, Richmond, VA 23288.

Glaser A. West Nile encephalitis: A new differential for neurological illness in dogs and cats. *DVM Newsmagazine* 2003;June:16–19.

Howard JL, ed. *Current Veterinary Therapy 2: Food Animal Practice.* Philadelphia, WB Saunders, 1999.

http://emergency.cdc.gov/agent/Botulism/clinicians/Background.asp, Botulism: Background Information for Clinicians, 2006.

http://emergency.cdc.gov/agent/ricin/clinicians/clindesc.asp, Ricin: Clinical Description, Emergency Preparedness and Response, 2008.

http://emergency.cdc.gov/agent/ricin/clinicians/control.asp, Ricin: Control Measures Overview for Clinicians, Emergency Preparedness and Response, 2006.

http://emergency.cdc.gov/agent/ricin/clinicians/treatment.asp, Ricin: Treatment Overview for Clinicians, Emergency Preparedness and Response, 2006.

http://emergency.cdc.gov/agent/ricin/facts.asp, Facts about Ricin, 2008.

http://emergency.cdc.gov/agent/ricin/han_022008.asp, Official CDC Health Advisory, Emergency Preparedness and Response, 2008.

http://emergency.cdc.gov/agent/trichothecene/casedef.asp, Case Definition: Trichothecene Mycotoxin, Emergency Preparedness and Response, 2006.

http://emergency.cdc.gov/coca/pdf/avianflu_062206.pdf, Avian Influenza, 2006.

http://en.wikipedia.org/wiki/Clostridium_perfringens, Clostridium perfringens.

http://en.wikipedia.org/wiki/Hantavirus, Hantavirus.

http://en.wikipedia.org/wiki/Henipavirus, Henipavirus.

http://en/wikipedia.org/wiki/T-2_mycotoxin, T-2 mycotoxin.

http://nabc.ksu.edu, Rift Valley Fever, National Agricultural Biosecurity Center.

http://ohioline.osu.edu/hyg-fact/5000/5568.html, *Clostridium perfringens:* Not the 24 hour flu, 1998.

Hulbert LC, Oehme FW. 1981. *Plants Poisonous to Livestock.* 3d ed. Manhattan, KS, Kansas State University Printing Service.

Kuiken T, Rimmelzwaan G, van Riel D, van Amerongen G, Baars M, Fouchier R, et al. Avian H5N1 influenza in cats. *Science* 2004;306:241.

Matrosovich M, Zhou N, Kawaoka Y, Webster R. The surface glycoproteins of H5 influenza viruses isolated from humans, chickens, and wild aquatic birds have distinguishable properties. *J Virol* 1999;73:1146–1155.

Orriss GD. Animal diseases of public health importance. *Emerg Infect Dis* 1997;3:497–502.

Shadomy SV, Smith TL. Anthrax. *J Am Vet Med Assoc* 2008;233:63–72.

Songserm T, Amonsin A, Jam-on R, Sae-Heng N, Pariyothorn N, Payungporn S, et al. Fatal avian influenza H5N1 in a dog. *Emerg Infect Dis* 2006;12:1744–1747.

Spicler AR, Roth JA. *Emerging and Exotic Diseases of Animals.* 3rd ed. Ames, IA, Iowa State University, 2006.

Ten Asbroek, AH, Borgdorff MW, Nagelkerke NJ, Sebek MM, Deville W, van Embden JD, van Soolingen D. Estimation of serial interval and incubation period of tuberculosis using DNA fingerprinting. *Int J Tuberc Lung Dis* 1999;3:414–420.

The Merck Veterinary Manual. Rahway, NJ, Merck and Company, 2007.

Tremayne J. Canine flu confirmed in 22 states. *DVM Newsmagazine* August 1, 2006 [cited 2007 May 22]. Available from http://www.dvmnews.com/dvm/article/articledetail.jsp?id=363966

van Riel D, Munster VJ, de Wit E, Rimmelzwaan GF, Fouchier RA, Osterhaus AD, et al. H5N1 virus attachment to lower respiratory tract. *Science* 2006;312:399.

Vial, PA, Valdivieso F, Mertz G, Castillo C, Belmar E, Delgado I, Tapia M, Ferres M. Incubation period of hantavirus cardiopulmonary syndrome. *Emerg Infect Dis* 2006;12:1271–1273.

www.aphis.usda.gov/vs/ceah/cei/taf/emergingdiseasenotice_files/nipahupd.htm, Center for Emerging Issues, Emerging Disease Notice Update Nipah Virus, Malaysia, 1999.

www.aphis.usda.gov/vs/ceah/cei/taf/emergingdiseasenotice_files/nipah.htm, Center for Emerging Issues, Nipah Virus, Malaysia, May 1999, Emerging Disease Notice, 1999.

www.azdhs.gov, Typhus fever—Frequently asked questions, Bureau of Emergency Preparedness and Response Home Page, 2005.

www.azdhs.gov, Venezuelan equine encephalitis (profile for healthcare workers), 2005.

www.azdhs.gov, Western equine encephalitis (profile for healthcare workers), 2005.

www.ccohs.ca/oshanswers/diseases/psittacosis.html, Psittacosis, Canadian Centre for Occupational Health and Safety, 1998.

www.cdc.gov, *Emerging Infectious Diseases*, Volume 3, Number 4, Animal diseases of public health importance, Orriss GD, 1997.

www.cdc.gov, *Emerging Infectious Diseases*, Volume 9 Number 10, Flying squirrel–associated typhus, United States, Reynolds MG, Krebs JW, Comer JA, Sumner JW, Rushton TC, Lopez CE, Nicholson WL, Rooney JA, Lance-Parker SE, McQuiston JH, Paddock CD, Childs JE, 2003.

www.cdc.gov, International Notes Bolivian hemorrhagic fever—El Beni Department, Bolivia, *MMWR Weekly* (December 23, 1994) 43(50):943–946.

www.cdc.gov, Rift Valley fever fact sheet.

www.cdc.gov.nczved/dfbmd/disease-listing/glanders_gi.html, Glanders (*Burkholderia mallei*), 2008.

www.cdc.gov/eid, *Emerging and Infectious Diseases*, Volume 12, Number 11, Possible typhoon-related melioidosis epidemic, Taiwan 2005. Su HP, Chou CY, Tzeng SC, Ferng T, Chen YL, Chen YS, Chung TC, 2006.

www.cdc.gov/eid, *Emerging Infectious Diseases*, Volume 11, Number 8, Laboratory exposures to Brucellae and implications for bioterrorism, Yagupsky P, Baron EJ, 2005.

www.cdc.gov/mmwr/PDF/rr/rr5606.pdf, Compendium of measures to prevent disease associated with animals in public settings, 2007. *MMWR Recommend Rep* (July 6, 2007) 56(RR-5):5.

www.cdc.gov/mmwr/preview/mmwrhtml/00001512.htm, Ebola virus infection in imported primates—Virginia, 1989, *MMWR Weekly* (December 08, 1989) 38:831–832, 837–838.

www.cdc.gov/mmwr/preview/mmwrhtml/00024911.htm, Brucellosis outbreak at a pork processing plant—North Carolina, 1992. *MMWR Weekly* (February 25, 1994) 43:113–116.

www.cdc.gov/mmwr/preview/mmwrhtml/00044836.htm, Prevention of Plague: Recommendations of the Advisory Committee on Immunization Practices (ACIP). *MMWR Recommend Rep* (December 13, 1996) 45(RR-14):1–15.

www.cdc.gov/mmwr/preview/mmwrhtml/mm4924a3.htm, Laboratory–acquired human glanders—Maryland, May 2000. *MMWR Weekly* (June 23, 2000) 49:532–535.

www.cdc.gov/mmwr/preview/mmwrhtml/su5501a2.htm, Investigation of avian influenza (H5N1) outbreak in humans—Thailand, 2004, *MMWR Weekly* (April 23, 2006) 55(SUP01):3–6.

www.cdc.gov/ncidod/dbmd/diseaseinfo/staphlococcus_food_g.htm, Staphylococcal food poisoning, 2006.

www.cdc.gov/ncidod/dfmd/diseaseinfo/leptospirosis_t.htm, Leptospirosis, 2005.

www.cdc.gov/ncidod/diseases/hanta/hps/noframes/FAQ.htm, Hantavirus pulmonary syndrome (HPS): What you need to know, 2006.

www.cdc.gov/ncidod/diseases/hanta/hps/noframes/transmit.htm, All about hantaviruses, Special Pathogens Branch, 2004.

www.cdc.gov/ncidod/dpd/parasites/giardiasis/2004_PDF_Giradiasis.pdf, Giardia infection.

www.cdc.gov/ncidod/dvbid/westnile/qa/wnv_dogs_cats.htm, West Nile virus and dogs and cats, 2003.

www.cdc.gov/ncidod/dvbid/westnile/wnv_factsheet.htm, WNV fact sheet, 2005.

www.cdc.gov/ncidod/dvrd/mnpages/dispages/arena.htm, Arenavirus fact sheet, 2005.

www.cdc.gov/ncidod/dvrd/qfever, Q fever, 2003.

www.cdc.gov/ncidod/dvrd/spb/mnpages/dispages/fact_sheets/ebola_fact_booklet.pdf, Ebola hemorrhagic fever information packet, 2002.

www.cdc.gov/ncidod/dvrd/spb/mnpages/dispages/lassaf.htm, Lassa fever fact sheet, 2004.

www.cdc.gov/ncidod/dvrd/spb/mnpages/dispages/marburg.qa.htm, Marburg hemorrhagic fever fact sheet, 2007.

www.cdc.gov/ncidod/dvrd/spb/mnpages/dispages/nipah.htm, Hendra virus disease and Nipah virus encephalitis, 2007.

www.cdc.gov/ncidod/eid/vol12no12/pdfs/06-0732.pdf, *Emerging Infectious Diseases* Volume 12, Number 12, Foodborne transmission of Nipah Virus, Bangladesh, 2006.

www.cdc.gov/ncidod/eid/vol5no2/schmitt.htm, *Emerging Infectious Diseases* Volume 5, Number 2, Bacterial Toxins: Friends or Foes? Schmitt CK, Meysick KC, O'Brien AD, 1999.

www.cdc.gov/ncidod/monkeypox/animalhandlers.htm, Monkeypox infections in animals: Updated interim guidance for veterinarians, 2003.

www.cdc.gov/ncidod/monkeypox/factsheet.htm, Basic information about monkeypox, 2003.

www.cdc.gov/ncidod/monkeypox/factsheet2.htm, What you should know about monkeypox, 2003.

www.cdc.gov/nczved/dfbmd/disease_listing.html, Dermatophytes (ringworm), 2008.

www.cdc.gov/nczved/dfbmd/disease_listing/melioidosis_gi.html, Melioidosis, Division of Foodborne, Bacterial and Mycotic Diseases (DFBMD), 2008.

www.cdc.gov/ndidod/dbm/diseaseinfo/brucellosis_t.htm, Brucellosis (*Brucella melitensis, abortus, suis, and canis*), Division of Bacterial and Mycotic Diseases, 2005.

www.cdc.gov/ndidod/ddvrd/qfever/, Q fever, Viral and Rickettsial Zoonoses Branch, 2003.

www.cdc.gov/ndidod/dvbid/arbor/arbdet.htm, CDC Information on arboviral encephalitides, 2005.

www.cdc.gov/rabies/healthcare.html, Information for health care professionals, 2007.

www.cdc.gov/toxoplasmosis/factsheet.html, Toxoplasmosis fact sheet, 2008.

www.cfsph.iastate.edu/Factsheets/pdfs/nipah.pdf, Nipah, 2004.

www.dhs.ca.gov, Guidelines for conducting surveillance for hantavirus in rodents in California, 2004.

www.emergency.cdc.gov/agent/anthrax/anthrax-hcp-factsheet.asp Fact sheet: Anthrax information for health care providers, March 8, 2002

www.emergency.cdc.gov/agent/tularemia/facts.asp, Key facts about tularemia, 2003.

www.fsis.usda.gov/OPHS/tbbroch.htm, Tuberculosis: What you need to know, 1997.

www.hantaviru.net, 2000.

www.health.state.ny.us/diseases/communicable/leptospirosis/docs/fact_sheet.pdf, Leptospirosis (Weil's disease), 2004.

www.health.state.ny.us/diseases/communicable/, Psittacosis (ornithosis, parrot fever, chlamydiosis), 2006.

www.health.vic.gov.au/ideas/bluebook/hendra, Hendra and Nipah viruses.

www.healthpet.com, West Nile virus.

www.johnson-county.com, Fact sheet *Clostridium perfringens* food poisoning, 1998.

www.mda.state.md.us/pdf/animlimp.pdf, Bioterrorism agents: Implications for animals.

www.michigan.gov/documents/MDA_WNVHorses_8938_7.pdf, West Nile virus in horses, diagnosis and prevention tips.

www.nsc.org/resources/Factsheets/environment/west_nile_ virus.aspx, West Nile virus.

www.ohioline.osu.edu/wnv-fact/1007.html, What horse owners should know about West Nile virus, 2006.

www.searo.who.int/en/Section10/Section372_13452.htm, *Communicable Diseases Department Newsletters* June 2007, Volume 4, Issue 2, Nipah outbreak in India and Bangladesh, Krishanan S, Biswas K.

www.who.int/mediacentre/factsheets/fs113/en/print.html, Bovine spongiform encephalopathy, 2002.

Yagupsky P, Baron EJ. Laboratory exposures to Brucellae and implications for bioterrorism. *Emerging Infectious Diseases* (www.cdc.gov/eid) 2005;11:1180–1184.

Young JC, Hansen GR, Graves TK, Deasy MP, Humphreys JG, Fritz CL, Gorham KL, Kan AS, Ksiazek TG, Metzger KB, Peters CJ. The incubation period of hantavirus pulmonary syndrome. *Am J Trop Med Hygiene* 2000;62:714–717.

CHAPTER 1.12
PUBLIC HEALTH

William R. Ray, BS

1. What determines whether there is a public health issue?

Any incident, whether man-made or natural, that either will, can, or immediately does cause harm to the general health and well-being of the community should be considered as a public health issue. These public health issues can harm either humans or animals, or both. Disease investigations are handled the same regardless of whether they apply to humans or animals.

2. How do natural disasters affect public health concerns?

A natural disaster, depending on the scope of the disaster, will cause a widespread breakdown of services that are generally taken for granted by the general populace. Some of the resulting concerns could be contamination of food and water, community loss, increased prevalence of disease due to decreased sanitation, and loss of psychological well-being. Further, disaster plans seldom take into account how the individual will provide care for his or her animals. The realm of care could extend to the inability of the owner to take the animal(s) with him or her during the disaster or the inability to provide adequate shelter, food, and water for the animal.

3. What are the disease entry routes that would pose a threat in a disaster?

There are five routes of disease transmission that should be of concern—respiratory tract, digestive tract, urogenital tract, transdermal, and other mucosa. In any disaster with the breakdown of services due to the disaster process itself, the general population is rendered unable to be self-sufficient for a sustained time. Because of this, disease or contamination may enter the body by any of the above-mentioned routes.

4. What are the modes of infectious disease transmission? Give an example of each.

- **Animal-to-human**—arthropod acts as a vector or as a vehicle (mosquito: malaria, West Nile virus, Dengue fever), mammal directly infects (cats: pneumonic plague), avian (psittacosis), and others
- **Object-to-person**—food harboring pathogenic bacteria (raw eggs: *Salmonella*), contaminated water system (leptospirosis), unclean housing (*Escherichia coli* enteritis, salmonellosis, *Klebsiella* spp. pneumonia)
- **Animal-to-animal**—airborne (distemper, pneumonic plague), contact (parvovirus enteritis, sexually transmitted diseases)
- **Person-to-animal**—plague, sarcoptic mange

5. What are the routes that an organism may use to exit the body?

An organism may leave the body via six routes: respiration, urination, defecation, exudates, coughing, and other body fluids. Control of these processes will control the spread of any infectious agent.

6. What diseases pose the greatest public health concern?

Any disease is of concern in a disaster; however, diseases that are spread either through the air or through the food and water supply would be of primary concern. The primary places of concern are the animal shelters and refuge centers; the victims are in very close proximity and their hygiene is quite variable. Those victims not in shelters will have the same problems, but these problems will be contained within the "family units."

7. What contributing factors can precipitate a public health concern?

Loss of food, water, housing, illness, and continuity exacerbated by the disaster can all contribute to precipitation of a public health concern. Many of today's routine services for on-demand electricity, roads, water, food, and veterinary/medical care are taken for granted. Only those victims experiencing the total realm of a natural disaster can fully appreciate the loss of these services.

8. What are the steps to follow when a public health concern arises?

To adequately and efficiently handle public health issues, there are certain steps that the investigators (field epidemiologists) follow. These steps are generally referred to as "case management" and apply to any disease investigation.

Case management is the systematic pursuit, documentation, and analysis of the medical and epidemiologic information about a case to develop a priority of disease intervention actions. In other words, *Develop a case definition and stick to it unless relevant information proves differently.* A case definition is a set of parameters set arbitrarily by the epidemiologist to constrain the activities in the investigation. As an example, for the disease "pertussis," a patient must have a paroxysmal cough longer than 14 days and either a whoop, apnea, or posttussive vomiting, or a combination of the three. If a patient does not meet these parameters, then he or she is not a case and it is not worked. What defines the index case? The **index case** is that individual animal that precipitates the investigation of an outbreak. Simply put, it is Case No. 1—the very first case.

9. What are the objectives of a disease-control program?

- Reduce the incidence of communicable diseases
- Reduce the spread of communicable disease in outbreak situations
- Educate the population on how diseases are spread and controlled
- Educate the medical community on prompt reporting of communicable diseases

10. What are the components of a disease-control program?

- Surveillance: active surveillance—actively looking for the disease; passive surveillance—waiting for someone to call you
- Treatment

- Control of the environment
- Case follow-up
- Case detection through screening
- Education

11. List the major responsibilities of a field epidemiologist.

- Interview the owners of infected patients (original patient, index case)
- Locate infected patients from the interview (contact spread)
- Locate unknown infected patients (clustering)
- Look for patterns, associations, and occurrences out of the norm

12. List items needed in an investigator's Epi-Kit.

- Pens and pencils—Pens are excellent for making a permanent record; however, in cold weather they do not work.
- Notepads—A standard steno pad works well for note taking and does not take up much room.
- GPS and compass—These are used to locate the patient/farm geographically so GIS mapping may be done at a future date.
- High-intensity, yet small, flashlight—It is surprising how often there is not enough light when examining a patient, taking notes, or completing environmental examinations.
- The appropriate sampling equipment for the biological agent that is being investigated.
- Tyvek®, latex gloves, booties, duct tape, N-100 face mask, insect repellent, knife, bottled water, snacks, garbage bags, biohazard bags, and personal first aid kit
- Clothing for the mission—whether hot, cold, rainy, sunny

13. What might be the recommended personal protective equipment (PPE) for animal/human decon?

Listen to the safety officer on-site. They will know what the agent is (hopefully!) and will inform you what the appropriate PPE of the day should be. It may be as simple as the N-100 face mask or as complex as having to don level A, B or C protective equipment.

14. What other agencies are involved in public health issues?

This will depend on what type of incident has transpired. The major responders will be fire, police, and emergency medical services (EMS) personnel. In the majority of incidents, public health personnel are not first responders. Other agencies that may be involved depending on the scope of the incident include the state department of agriculture, wildlife agencies, private agencies (Red Cross, Salvation Army), and mirror agencies at the county and federal levels.

15. Should the general public be notified of a public health concern?

The general public should be kept well informed on the issues involving a public health incident. Some issues will be withheld from the public if it is not necessary for their general health and it could constitute a violation of human privacy acts.

16. How should notification of the public be accomplished?

The lead agency should be the primary designee in the promulgating of all information going to the public. Notification can be done through the press (radio, television, and print), Internet postings, flyers/handouts, billboards, etc.

17. Who releases the information?

The public information officer (PIO) or designee should be the only individual speaking to the press. The PIO should review all information going out to make sure that the same message is being distributed in all formats of information release.

18. Discuss some of the problems with agency cooperation during a disaster.

There are numerous agencies from city to federal levels that have the ability to assist in an event. The primary problem with requesting help is that many times individuals on the political level, who are the ones responsible for requesting the help, fail to recognize that their local agencies cannot handle the task. Commonly, the event has escalated to the point of being out of control before the help is requested. Many times, the pressure of the local population's complaints about the event is what precipitates the request for help.

19. What are the divisions within most public health departments?

- Nursing services
- Environmental health services
- Emergency preparedness
- Health education
- Administration

20. Where are the public health agencies located?

These agencies are located in cities, counties, districts, and state levels. Depending on the size of the county, it may range from a small solo nursing service to a large fully operational health department. Some counties have consolidated to make health districts. Large metropolitan areas have their own health departments. On the state level, there is the state department of health and environment.

21. Which agency usually takes the lead in handling an incident?

In most states, the lead is usually taken by the local agency.

22.   As a responder you will be deployed to a disaster. List some of the public health awareness actions you should consider.

- What personal hygiene measures should you take for your own safety?
  - Wash your hands frequently.
  - Wash/change your clothes as often as possible.
  - Shower as frequently as possible.
  - Rest and acclimate as best as possible when moving into the area.
  - Depending on the season, situation, and location, you should have a daily leech and/or tick check. It is best to buddy up to do this, as there are areas of the body you cannot see.
  - Wash or change, if possible, your bedding at least once a week. If this is not possible, sunning the sleeping bag or linen for an hour or two will freshen them and remove excess moisture.
- Approximately how much water will you use daily?
  - Drinking: 1 gallon per day; in hot weather or if you are wearing protective clothing (PPE), 1 quart or more per hour
  - Hygiene: 1 gallon per day
  - Laundry and dishwashing: 2 gallons per day
- What precautions should you take to avoid water or food-borne illness?
  - Practice good personal hygiene
  - Do not eat contaminated food.
  - Decontaminate canned foods before use. Peel off the label and disinfect with a freshly made 1:10 bleach solution.
- Discard the following items:
  - Screw top bottles
  - Snap lid cans
  - Crimp lid cans
  - Twist top bottles
  - Be very careful with home-canned foods.
  - Do not eat any donated foods.
- What can you do for vector control in the base area?
  - Keep your personal area clean and free of food and trash.
  - If you see unsanitary situations, report it to your safety officer.
  - Remind your team members to do the same.
  - Use mosquito netting around your sleeping area.
  - Use personal insect repellent with DEET according to the manufacturer's recommendations.

23.   There may be a time when it is necessary for an individual to make field expedient guesses on where a downwind spread may occur. How would you do this?

- Place a "+" on the site of contamination.
- Draw a circle around the site using either a 500- or 1000-yard radius. This will depend on whether the agent being investigated or released has been identified. They will most likely know the identity of the agent. Err on the side of caution.
- From the source, draw a line downwind and draw two parallel lines on either side of the hot zone with the downwind line.
- Where the + would have crossed the circle at 0 and 180 degrees, draw an angle outward from the parallel lines at 20 degrees.
- Knowing how long the agent was present and how fast the wind was blowing, multiply the two to come up with an estimate of downwind spread inside the cone.

This may also be done with a line source. Use the same procedure except your cone will start at the beginning and end of the line. All other calculations are the same (Figs. 1.12.1, 1.12.2, and 1.12.3).

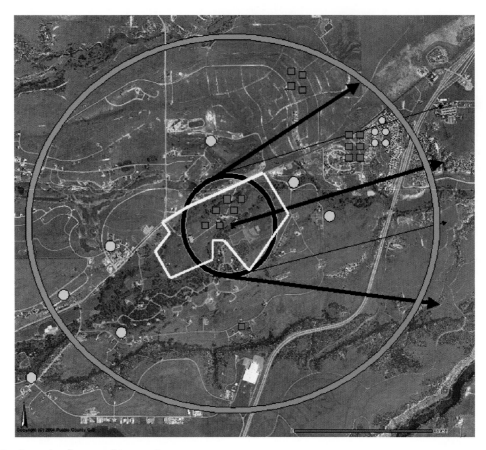

Figure 1.12.1 Example of geographic mapping.
• yellow dots—cases found after community-wide testing
• red squares—original infected cases
• green circle—1 mile radius of hot zone
• white outline—property line of index case
• black circle—¼ mile hot zone around index case
• black east/northeast arrows—prevailing winds indicating possible downwind clusters of airborne agent
(Used with permission from the Pueblo County GIS.)

Down wind hazard distance = Wind speed (kph, mph) X Source (cloud) duration

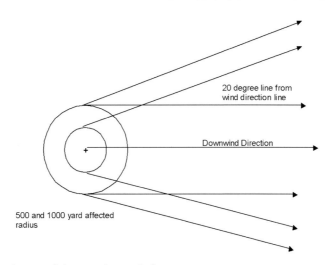

20 degree line from
wind direction line

Downwind Direction

500 and 1000 yard affected
radius

Figure 1.12.2 Estimating the rate of downwind spread of an agent using point-source emissions. (Based on FM-21-40, NBC Defense, United States Army.)

• <u>Ground Source</u>: Down wind hazard distance =
Wind speed (kph, mph) X Source (cloud) duration.

• <u>Air Source</u>: Down wind hazard distance = Wind
speed (kph, mph) X Source (cloud) duration X 4

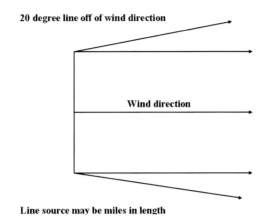

20 degree line off of wind direction

Wind direction

Line source may be miles in length

Figure 1.12.3 Estimating downwind spread of an agent using line source emissions. (Based on FM-21-40, NBC Defense, United States Army.)

Acknowledgments

The author would like to thank the following individuals for their assistance in preparing this chapter: John Pape, CDPHE; Mark Korbitz, PCCHD; Barbara Ray; and Robert Kellner.

Suggested Reading
Visit your local county health departments or nursing services websites.

Colorado Department of Health and Environment
www.cdphe.state.co.us/cdphehom

State of Colorado
www.colorado.gov

Centers for Disease Control
www.cdc.gov

American Veterinary Medical Association
www.avma.org

CHAPTER 1.13
HAZARDOUS MATERIALS

Lori A. Swenson, BSME, EMT-P

1. What is a hazardous material?

A *hazardous material* is defined as any substance that, when released or contacted, has the potential to damage health (human or animal), the environment, or property.

2. What is the *Emergency Response Guidebook* (ERG)?

This is the manual that a responder uses to identify hazardous materials. It provides guidelines for initial response such as evacuation instructions, mitigating health risks, and evaluating fire or explosion potential. This free book is available at the following website: http://hazmat.dot.gov/pubs/erg/gydebook.htm.

3. Describe the five sections found in the ERG.

- Yellow—Numerical Index (UN/ID)
- Blue—Alphabetical Index (by product name)
- Orange—Emergency Guides
- Green—Initial Isolation/Protective Action Distances
- White—Information/Criminal/Terrorist Use of Weapons of Mass Destruction (WMD)

4. What does it mean if an entry in the blue or yellow sections is highlighted?

Any material or substance that is highlighted under these sections is a "Toxic Inhalation Hazard" (TIH).

5. List the nine different U.S. Department of Transportation (DOT) classes of hazards (Table 1.13.1 and Figures 1.13.1 and 1.13.2).

The following placards correspond to the hazard class. Look in the lower corner for the hazard class number. The numbers in the circle next to the placard indicate the guide number you should look at in the ERG.

205

Table 1.13.1 The Nine Different Department of Transportation (DOT) Classes of Hazards

Class	Explanation	Examples
1	Explosives	Dynamite, TNT, grenades, ammonium nitrate/fuel
2	Gases	Propane, anhydrous ammonia, phosgene, chlorine
3	Flammable or Combustible Liquids	Gasoline, methyl alcohol, acetone
4	Flammable Solids	Matches, potassium, phosphorus, charcoal briquets
5	Oxidizers and Organic Peroxides	Ammonium nitrate, oxygen, benzoyl peroxide
6	Toxic Materials and Infectious Substances	Carbon tetrachloride, anthrax, botulism
7	Radioactive Materials	Cobalt, uranium, iodine-131
8	Corrosive Materials	Sulfuric acid, mercury, lime
9	Misc. Materials	PCBs, dry ice

6. List the WMD hazards.

- Chemical
- Biological
- Radiologic
- Nuclear
- Explosive

7. Describe an acronym to help you recall the WMD hazards.

The acronym CBRNE (Chemical, Biological, Radiological, Nuclear, Explosive) is often used to describe the WMD hazards. Another acronym you often see is BNICE (Biological, Nuclear, Incendiary, Chemical, Explosive).

8. Describe an acronym that will help you recall the hazard class and explanation.

- Every (1 = Explosives)
- Good (2 = Gases)
- Fire (3 = Flammable Liquids)
- Fighter (4 = Flammable Solids)
- Ought (5 = Oxidizers)
- To (6 = Toxins and Infectious Substances)
- Read (7 = Radioactive Materials)
- Cooking (8 = Corrosive Materials)
- Manuals (9 = Miscellaneous Materials)

9. What are some sources of hazardous materials in your home?

Cleaning agents, automotive fluids, chemicals for the hot tub, and lawn and garden products are examples of hazardous substances commonly found around the average house.

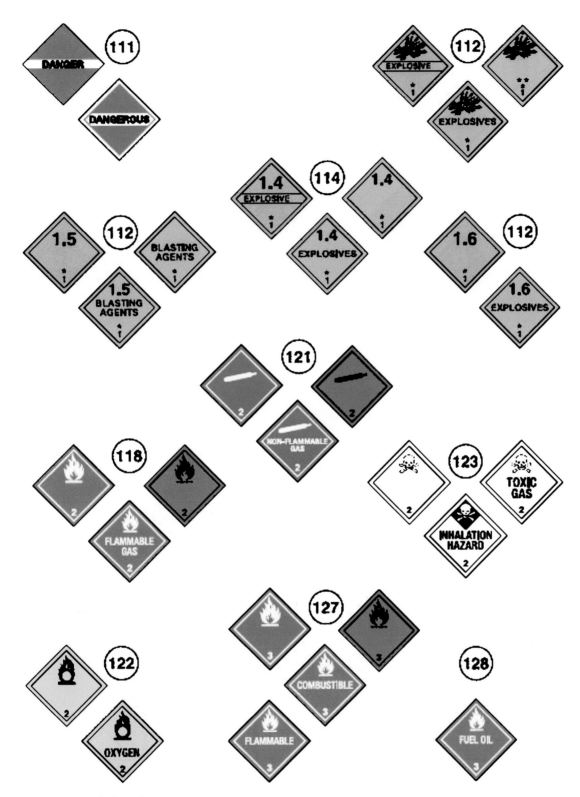

Figure 1.13.1 Hazard placards part 1.

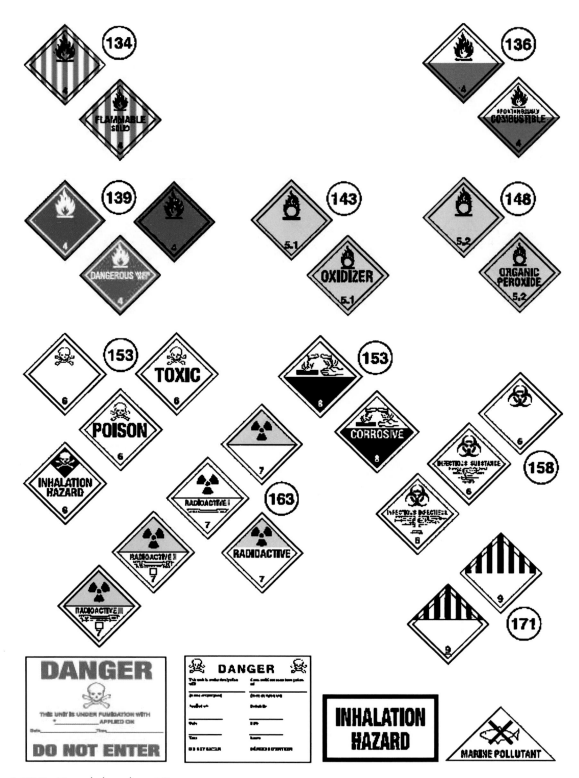

Figure 1.13.2 Hazard placards part 2.

208

10. Describe some hazardous materials you encounter in everyday life, outside of your home.

Gasoline or fuel, trucks or vehicles carrying materials or chemicals, and workplace chemicals including those used in the heating or cooling (ammonia) of facilities are commonly found hazardous materials.

11. List the three basic control zones in a hazardous materials incident (Fig. 1.13.3).

- Exclusion zone (formerly known as the "hot zone")
- Contamination (containment) or reduction zone (formerly known as the "warm zone")
- Support zone (formerly called the "cold zone")

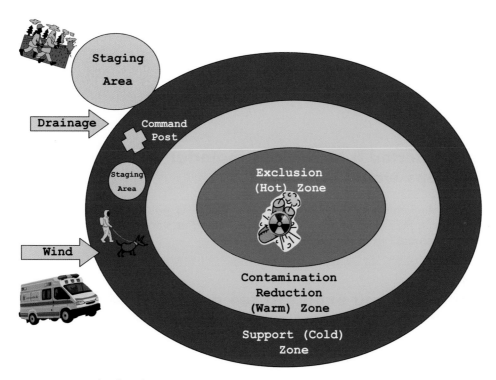

Figure 1.13.3 Zones associated with a disaster.

12. What is the "exclusion zone" at a hazmat incident?

The exclusion zone is the area immediately surrounding the hazardous material where responders will be harmed by the material if protective measures are not taken.

13. What is a "security perimeter"?

The security perimeter serves as a barrier between the general public and the cold zone. It helps control large crowds, those with prying eyes, and those with cameras and keeps them from interfering with operations.

14. List the common symptoms of a hazmat poisoning.

- Difficulty breathing
- Skin, eye or throat irritation
- Headache, dizziness or blurred vision
- Difficulties with coordination and motor skills
- Sweating, vomiting and/or intestinal disturbances.
- Confusion or changes in mental status

15. Describe the signs and symptoms of organophosphate poisoning.

The acronym "SLUDGEM" is used to remember the signs and symptoms of organophosphate poisoning.

- Salivation
- Lacrimation
- Urination
- Diarrhea
- Gastrointestinal distress
- Emesis
- Miosis

16. If you suspected a hazardous material is present at a scene, what initial steps would you take?

Remove yourself from the immediate vicinity of the scene. Whenever possible, retreat to a place that is *upwind* and *uphill* of the incident. Stay clear of any vapors, spills, fumes, or smoke. Attempt to identify the hazardous material, and request assistance from the incident commander.

17. Where would you expect to see a placard like the one in Figure 1.13.4?

This is a National Fire Protection Association (NFPA) placard and it is found on the side of a building or structure containing hazardous materials.

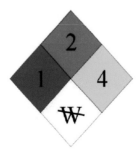

Figure 1.13.4 NFPA placard.

18. What is the meaning of the colors on the placard in question No. 17?

- Red indicates the Fire Hazard of a material.
- Blue indicates the Health Hazard.
- Yellow indicates Physical Hazard.
- White indicates Personal Protection information.

19. Explain what the numbers mean on the placard in Figure 1.13.4?

- In general, hazard levels are numbered from 0 to 4, with 4 being the most hazardous.
- The 2 in the red diamond indicates a fire flash point above 100° F but not exceeding 200° F.
- The 3 in the blue diamond means there is an extreme health danger present.
- The 0 in the yellow position indicates that the chemical is stable in regard to reactivity.
- The W̶ in the white diamond indicates that water SHOULD NOT be applied to the hazard.

20. How would you determine the safe distance from a chemical spill due to a tractor-trailer highway rollover?

First, you would try to identify the chemical from the placard information on the truck. Look up the UN identification number in the yellow pages of the ERG, then turn to the corresponding guide number in the orange pages. If the entry in the yellow pages is highlighted, you can go to the green pages of the ERG. This section will provide "Initial Isolation and Protective Action Distances."

If there is no UN number visible but you can see a DOT placard, use the "Table of Placards" at the front of the book. This section has the placards and the associated guide number in a circle next to the placard graphic. In the orange section of the ERG you can find the guide numbers, which will help determine the safe distance.

21. How might you confirm the presence of a hazardous material at an outdoor scene while remaining a safe distance from the scene?

Use binoculars to visualize a placard or UN identification number if possible. If not, you can still use the binoculars to describe the scene to your incident commander or 911 contact. Try to obtain as much information as possible about the material without placing yourself in danger.

22. What is a "secondary hazard"?

Terrorists also target rescuers. It is not uncommon to find secondary explosives or hazards meant to kill and injure those trying to help. Be aware of this fact when you are surveying a scene of a hazardous materials incident.

23. What do the numbers mean on the symbol in Figure 1.13.5?

These are the UN identification numbers. Using the yellow pages of the ERG you can determine that 1219 is the chemical *isopropyl alcohol*.

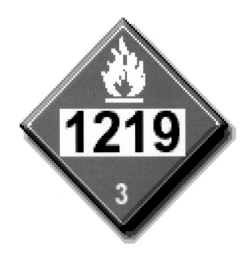

Figure 1.13.5 UN identification number.

 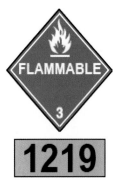

Figure 1.13.6 UN ID–DOT class.

24. Name the different routes of entry by which a poison or hazardous material can enter an animal.

- Inhalation
- Ingestion
- Injection
- Absorption

25. Describe the difference between the two placard configurations in Figure 1.13.6.

There is no difference as far as information displayed. The four-digit number on both the signs is called the UN identification number. The red sign is the DOT hazard class placard. Red placards with the number 3 on the bottom indicate that the chemical present is flammable.

26. In question No. 25, where would you expect to see signs of this type?

These will be on moving vehicles such as cars, trucks, railroad cars, etc.

27. What does the symbol in Figure 1.13.7 indicate to you?

Figure 1.13.7 Biohazard placard.

This placard indicates the presence of a biohazard such as anthrax, smallpox, etc.

28. How should you respond if you believe you have a hazardous material incident but cannot find a means to identify the material?

Go immediately to guide 111 (Orange Section) of the ERG and follow the directions there until more information can be obtained about the nature of the material.

29. What is the meaning of the placard in Figure 1.13.8?

Figure 1.13.8 Radioactive placard.

This placard indicates the presence of radioactive material(s).

30. You are on scene of a cattle truck rollover. You have found barrels of an unknown substance in the same trailer as the cattle. Where would you look to try and identify the substance in the barrels?

Manifests or bills of lading will be found either with the driver, on the seat of the vehicle, or in a pouch on the inside of the vehicle door.

31. Identify the various types of personal protective equipment available during a response to a hazardous material incident (Table 1.13.2).

Table 1.13.2 Types of Personal Protective Equipment Available during a Response to a Hazardous Material Incident

Level	Expected Protection
Level A	Maximum respiratory protection Maximum skin protection Required in unknown environments
Level B	Maximum respiratory protection Moderate skin protection Minimum required for entering an unknown environment
Level C	Moderate respiratory protection Moderate skin protection
Level D	Minimum respiratory protection Minimum skin protection

32. Describe three ways that will enhance one's safety in the presence of a hazardous material.

- Time, distance, and shielding
- The buddy system
- Backup personnel

33. You are part of a field team that is rescuing animals from homes after a disaster. As you arrive at one of the houses on your list, you see the fence has been damaged and the backyard is now open. Bags of cat litter and Sterno cans are visibly piled in the yard. What precautions should you take?

Cat litter and Sterno are items commonly found in meth labs. Finding these things should raise your level of suspicion that you have located a neighborhood hazmat site. You should notify your team leader of your findings and not enter the property. Any animals taken from this property will require decontamination.

Suggested Reading
National Fire Protection Agency. 2008. Available at http://www.nfpa.org/index.asp.
Partnership for a Drug-Free America. Meth360. 2008. Available at http://www.drugfree.org/meth360/onlineLearningCourse.aspx.
Pipeline and Hazardous Materials Safety Administration. 2008. Available at http://hazmat.dot.gov/pubs/erg/gydebook.htm.

CHAPTER 1.14
PERSONAL PROTECTIVE EQUIPMENT

Thomas F. Pedigo, MSc, PA-C

1. What is personal protective equipment (PPE), and why is it necessary?

PPE consists of the protective barriers used to keep health care providers from being exposed to hazardous substances. These substances can include routine illnesses (e.g., skin infections), biological hazards (e.g., anthrax), chemical hazards (e.g., oil spills, organophosphates, chlorine), radiological hazards (e.g., alpha, beta or neutron particles), or other particles that may damage the body if inhaled or ingested (e.g., asbestos). PPE helps reduce the chances of such substances being introduced into the body.

2. What are the four routes of introducing hazards into the body?

The four routes of introducing hazards or toxins into the body are inhalation, ingestion, injection, and absorption. With most agents, inhalation and ingestion are the primary concerns because most of their effects on the body occur once they become internalized. However, some agents (and particularly manufactured chemical weapons) are surreptitiously designed to be absorbed through the skin. Injection remains a concern when working with sharp tools, removal of shrapnel from injured victims, animal bites, or kicks that break protection barriers.

3. What are the five basic points of coverage that need to be addressed by all levels of PPE?

The five basic points of coverage include:

- *Skin*
- *Airway*—The airway includes consideration of inhalational exposures.
- *Mucous membranes*—This includes exposure to the eyes in instances where airway protection does not include a full-faced mask.
- *Hands*
- *Feet*

Some suits are built to protect more than one of these points of coverage. All five must be addressed in any instance in which PPE is required.

4. What are the available options for airway protection, and how do they differ?

There are six basic types of airway protection.

- The first is a basic mask for *large-particle filtration* (Fig. 1.14.1). This mask is useful when operating in an area of large-particle dust (e.g., Ground Zero at the World Trade Center, 9/11). It does not filter out smaller aerosolized viral particles like influenza.

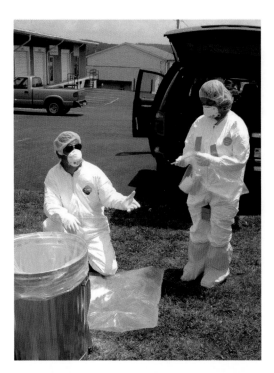

Figure 1.14.1 Large particulate mask.

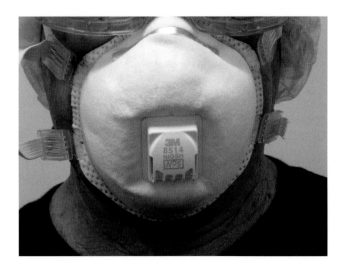

Figure 1.14.2 N-95 particulate filter.

• The second type is a *particulate mask*, such as the N-95 or N-100 (Fig. 1.14.2). These masks provide fitted protection of the mouth and nose from large particles and smaller bacterial and viral particles. The "N-95" and "N-100" designations have a particular meaning that is useful to know for the responder/care provider. N-95, N-99, and N-100 masks are considered HEPA masks, meaning that they are high-efficiency particulate air filters. To be qualified with one of these designations, masks must meet the guidelines as established by the National Institute for Occupational Safety and Health (NIOSH). All masks are required to filter particles down to 0.3 micron ([mu]m) in size. The number assigned indicates the efficiency (95%, 99%, or 100%) of filtering these particles. The "N" designation stands for "Not resistant to oil." A "P100" mask, by comparison, is 100% effective in filtering out particles to 0.3 [mu]m and is oil Proof. For the purposes of filtering out bacteria and

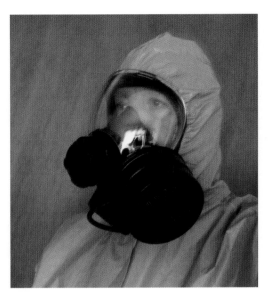

Figure 1.14.3 Air-purifying respirator.

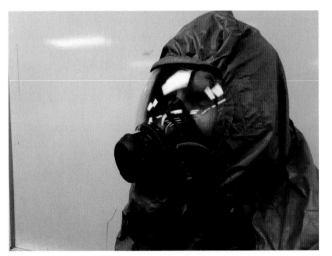
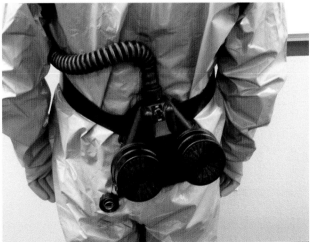

Figure 1.14.4 **A,** Powered air-purifying respirator, fitted to face (PAPR attached to belt on the back of the provider pictured, see B.) **B,** Powered unit with filters attached.

viral particles, typically a filtration of down to 0.5 [mu]m is all that is needed. Therefore, the N95, N99, and N100 are all adequate choices for the provider.
- The third type is an air-purifying respirator (APR) (Fig. 1.14.3). This mask provides an advanced level of filtration by using agent-specific filter cartridges screwed into a fitted face mask.

The next three types of airway protection require additional hardware.

- A powered air-purifying respirator (PAPR) may be attached to a fitted face mask (Fig. 1.14.4, A and B, Figure 1.14.5) or may be attached to a one-size-fits-most overhead hood. The fitted PAPR may be assigned to one individual and can function as a basic APR if the battery fails, while the overhead hood may be used by most providers and can be handed off to others as decontamination operations require but is dependent upon battery power for positive-pressure air to ensure airborne particles cannot enter the airway. Both of these

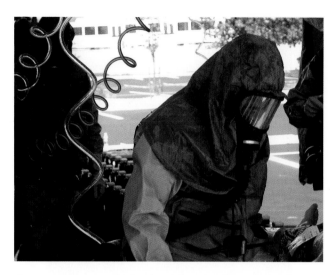

Figure 1.14.5 Powered air-purifying respirator, attached to hood. (Used with permission from Dennis "Duff" Dyer.)

variations are considered to be the same basic type of airway protection and are generally referred to as PAPRs. All of these preceding four types of airway protection *filter existing air* and require a normal level of oxygen in the surrounding air to be useful. The last two types of airway protection allow the provider to supply his or her own air in an environment where the surrounding air does not have a normal level of oxygen or has a disproportionate level of toxic gases that cannot be effectively filtered.

- Self-contained breathing apparatus (SCBAs) permit the provider to carry fresh air on his or her back and supply it through a fitted face mask.
- The last type is the supplied airline (SAL), which provides air through an airline attached to the provider's fitted face mask. The airline is supplied from outside the exposed area and requires regular exchange of bottled air by an assistant. Users of an SAL often carry a 5-minute "escape bottle" on their hip.

5. What are the available options for skin protection, and how do they differ?

There are three basic types of skin protection available.

- The first type is basic skin coverage with clothing, known as *permeable skin protection*. Examples of this include basic scrubs, long-sleeve shirts, and full-length pants and surgical "bunny suits" (Fig. 1.14.6). These are used when spills are not anticipated, primarily to minimize any scrapes or cuts in the integumentary system.
- The second type is the *chemical protective suit*, which provides splash protection from a liquid (Fig. 1.14.7). While it may be used for incidents other than chemical exposures, it is usually a combination of materials that are rated for a specific duration of time to protect the provider from certain chemicals. There are a multitude of these types of suits provided from a wide range of manufacturers, to meet a wide range of chemical exposures. Use of these suits requires some expertise at the site to determine which type of suit is appropriate to the situation. Recently, some suits have been advertised as an all-purpose weapon of mass destruction (WMD) type of suit. These are usually appropriate for decontamination operations at a receiving facility.
- The third type of protection is the highest level and is an *airtight suit*, commonly referred to as a Level A suit. These combine a level of splash protection for a specific duration of time with an airtight seal to prevent gas fumes and particles from permeating the edges of the suit (Fig. 1.14.8). These suits trap exhaled air within the suit and require the use of an SCBA to ensure full encapsulation and protection from gas fumes.

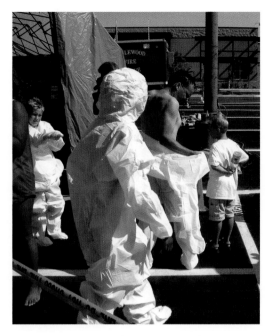

Figure 1.14.6 Surgical "bunny suit". (Used with permission from Dennis "Duff" Dyer.)

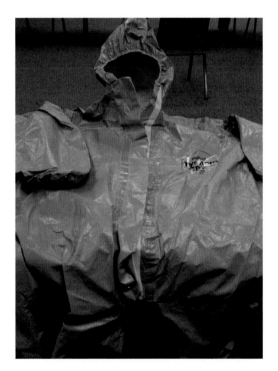

Figure 1.14.7 Chemical protective suit.

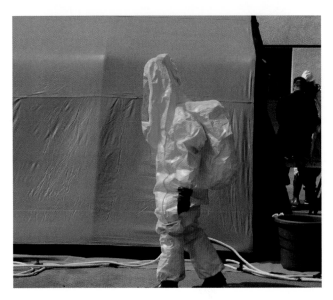

Figure 1.14.8 Level A airtight suit.

6. What are the available options for foot protection, and how do they differ?

The most difficult aspect of foot protection is understanding the difference between protection from trauma (e.g., thick soles, steel-toed boots, etc.) and protection from a contaminant. The feet are the only portion of the body constantly in direct contact with the environment, increasing the likelihood of both contamination and trauma. As a result, foot protection must be identified relative to its ability to provide protection from both of these dangers.

- The first basic type is the use of *standard footwear*, such as tennis shoes or work boots. The more durable the standard footwear, the less exposed to trauma the feet will be. Any type of standard footwear requires the addition of a protective layer, preferably one that is sewn into the chemical suit being used.
- The second type is the use of *hazard-protective footwear*, such as fire-resistant boots (a.k.a. "bunker boots") worn in the structural firefighting service (Fig. 1.14.9), or durable chemical boots (Figs. 1.14.10 and 1.14.11). These generally provide an enhanced barrier from traumatic punctures, as well as a degree of environmental protection. They may or may not require the addition of a protective layer, depending on how they are used. For instance, fire-resistant boots may be worn inside a level A suit. Alternatively, durable chemical boots may be applied outside of standard footwear and taped to the chemical protection suit. Each method has its uses, specific to the situation that the responder is facing and the equipment available.

Care must be taken to ensure that the seals between protective footwear and protective suits are well sealed when the situation dictates.

7. What are the available options for mucous membrane protection, and how do they differ?

There are three basic types of mucous membrane protection available.

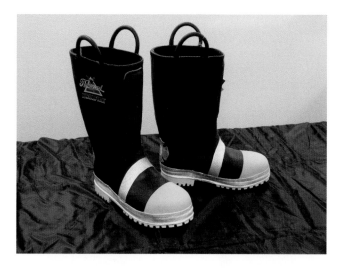

Figure 1.14.9 Bunker boots.

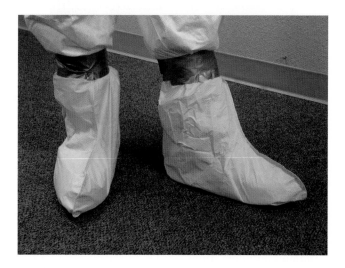

Figure 1.14.10 Lightweight chemical protective booties.

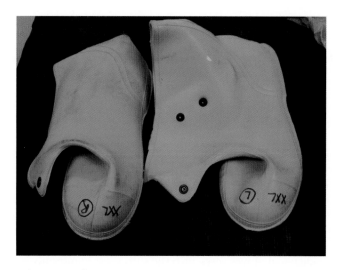

Figure 1.14.11 Durable chemical protective boots.

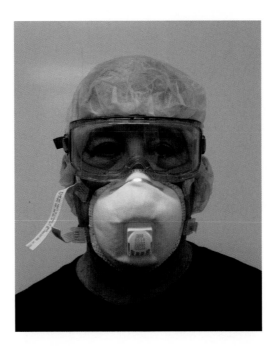

Figure 1.14.12 Goggles.

- The first is a mask with an open face shield. This *splash-protective mask* may or may not have a particulate mask, such as an N-95, attached. It provides basic protection from the initial splash of body fluids while working over a patient.
- The second type is a *PAPR*. Recall from question No. 4 that a PAPR may be attached to a fitted mask or an overhead hood, providing full protection to the mucous membranes of the mouth, nose, and eyes. This option carries the advantage of providing airway protection and mucous membrane protection, making it the most commonly used tool in decontamination operations.
- The third type of mucous membrane protection only provides protection for the eyes when the mouth and nose are already covered by airway protection. *Goggles* (Fig. 1.14.12) fitted to cover the eyes are the most common example of this type of protection.

8. What are the available options for hand protection, and how do they differ?

Gloves are the standard of protection for the hands in any scenario. However, the type of glove used can make a notable difference in the level of protection.

- *Work gloves* are commonly used to protect skin surfaces from friction injuries, puncture trauma, and burns. These may be worn under chemical clothing to help protect the hands from thermal burns or friction.
- *Biohazard gloves* (Fig. 1.14.13) are typically thin and relatively nonporous, to protect from bodily fluid exposure. They are commonly used in decontamination operations as the *initial layer* in Level C PPE.
- *Chemical gloves* are thicker, usually 7 mil or greater, and resemble the thick gloves used to wash very hot dishes (Fig. 1.14.14). These are often placed over biohazard gloves and serve as the *second layer*, providing protection from the contaminant during decontamination operations.
- *Suit-encapsulated gloves* are chemical gloves sewn into the suit, most commonly seen with the *airtight suits* used for Level A (Fig. 1.14.15). If the gloves are not sewn into the suit, then the breaks between the suit and the gloves must be addressed.

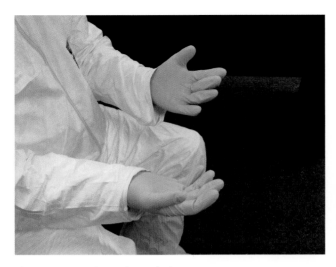

Figure 1.14.13 Biohazard gloves.

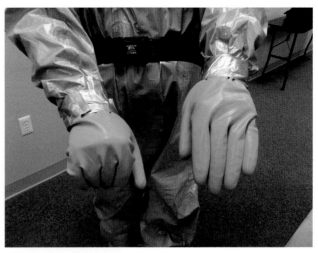

Figure 1.14.14 Chemical gloves.

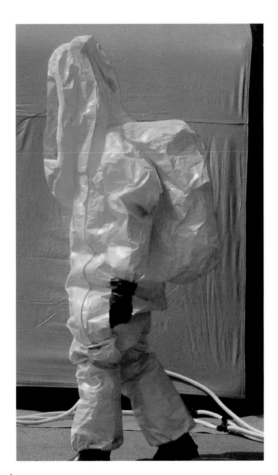

Figure 1.14.15 Suit-encapsulated gloves.

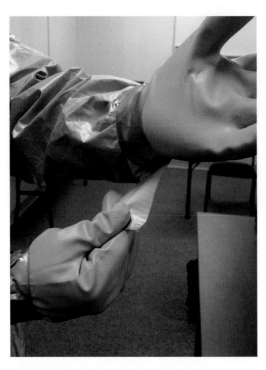

Figure 1.14.16 Using duct tape to secure the sleeve of a protective suit to chemical gloves.

9. How are breaks between gloves and suits or boots and suits addressed?

Sealing tape is the most appropriate way to ensure there are no openings between the extremities of the suit and the respective glove/boot. Rolling, tucking or intertwining sleeves with gloves or suit legs with boots may smooth out surfaces and reduce the chance of a large amount of fluid contaminant, yet these methods are insufficient without some type of adhesive sealing tape to cover any potential gaps.

For decontamination operations, the most widely accepted methods involve tucking the top of the gloves/boots under the edge of the suit and wrapping them with sealing tape starting from the inner aspect of the extremity moving outward, with at least a *50% to 75% overwrap* from one layer to the next.

- *Chemical sealing tape* is the gold standard for this type of seal, although it is costly and can be agent specific.
- Duct tape has been used in some decontamination operations and can be a reasonable alternative when using Level C PPE in a receiving-facility type of decontamination operation (Fig. 1.14.16). *It is imperative to wrap from the proximal area of the extremity moving toward the hand/feet*, as decontamination operations frequently expose the responder to water flowing from overhead and down the body. Such a wrap allows the water, if mixed with contaminant, to flow down and off the extremity instead of pooling at the cuffs and gradually soaking through the material.

10. What is the difference between the four levels of PPE known as Levels A, B, C, and D?

The four levels of PPE are designated for the levels of exposure, with A corresponding to the most immediately dangerous operations, and D corresponding to the least. Typically, they correlate as follows:

- Level A—Hazardous Materials Intervention (entering an area of active contamination in an attempt to neutralize or stop the spread of agent and/or to recover contaminated people)
- Level B—Hazardous Materials Defensive Operations (preventing the spread of an area of contamination, with the potential to come in contact with a high concentration of the contaminant)
- Level C—Hazardous Materials Decontamination Operations (removing contamination from people, animals, or objects that have been removed from the area of contamination, operating in the "warm zone")
- Level D—Infectious Disease Operations (working with patients that are victims of a contagious disease and do not require decontamination)

It is worthy to recognize that while an infectious disease may be lethal, the environment in which the responder is working is not Immediately Dangerous to Life and/or Health within the next 30 to 60 minutes (referred to as an IDLH environment) and therefore is rated as Level D within the context of decontamination principles. However, that is not to say that trained responders would not use higher levels of PPE in the event they are working in a more hazardous environment, for example, while disposing of dead animals.

11. What level of training is required for each level of PPE use?

- Level A requires an expert level of knowledge with all levels of equipment, environmental monitoring devices, and in-depth knowledge of the contaminants the responder may be dealing with. Individuals using this level of PPE should be well-trained, knowledgeable and certified in a number of hazmat, WMD, and environmental chemistry areas. It can take months to years to acquire the necessary training for this level.
- Level B requires an advanced level of knowledge with all levels of equipment (except the airtight suit), environmental monitoring devices, and in-depth knowledge of the contaminants the responder may be working in and around. Structural firefighters are an example of one profession that routinely uses this level of equipment. It takes many months and regular, routine training to maintain this level of capability.
- Level C requires a solid foundation of the use of chemical protective clothing, routine training, and an awareness of the types of contaminants that may be encountered through decontamination operations. This type of training can be completed with roughly 40 hours of didactic and skills preparation, reinforced with intensive monthly or quarterly training sessions. This level is typical of most modern, metropolitan hospital decontamination systems.
- Level D requires a foundation in blood-borne pathogens and is typically indoctrinated throughout all formal health care provider training coursework.

12. In what circumstances should Level D PPE be used, and what type of protection for each of the five basic points of protection should be included?

Level D is appropriate for instances where basic splash protection is needed from bodily fluids, where airborne viral or bacterial particles may be encountered, and in instances where gross decontamination is not indicated (Fig. 1.14.17). Examples of this would be when addressing an influenza outbreak or pneumonic plague.

An example of Level D coverage includes the use of *permeable skin protection* plus a surgical gown, *biohazard gloves*, *standard footwear* and a *particulate mask* with *goggles*.

13. In what circumstances should Level C PPE be used, and what type of protection for each of the five basic points of protection should be included?

Level C is the minimum standard level for decontamination operations. Examples would include a veterinary facility receiving injured animals or prestaged decontamination operations removed from the "hot zone" through

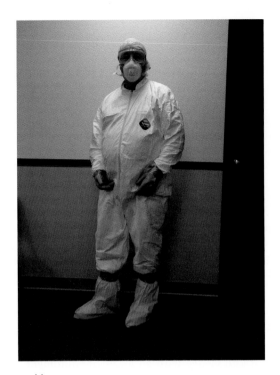

Figure 1.14.17 Level D protective ensemble.

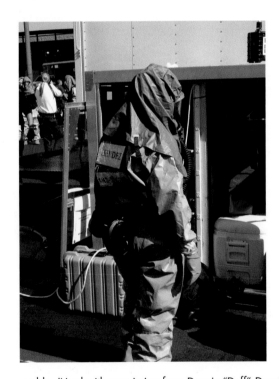

Figure 1.14.18 Level C protective ensemble. (Used with permission from Dennis "Duff" Dyer.)

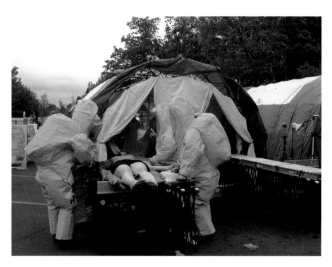

Figure 1.14.19 Level A protective ensemble. (Used with permission from Dennis "Duff" Dyer.)

a decontamination corridor in the "warm zone." Examples of agents that might require this protection include alpha/beta radiological particles, ricin, and mustard gas.

An example of Level C includes the use of a *chemical protective suit*, *a PAPR with hood* (including the requisite air filter cartridges), *hazard-protective footwear*, an inner layer of *biohazard gloves* with an outer layer of *chemical protective gloves*, and *chemical sealing tape* used to seal the suit-glove and suit-boot interfaces (Fig. 1.14.18).

14. In what circumstances should Level B PPE be used, and what type of protection for each of the five basic points of protection should be included?

Level B is the minimum standard level for working in an environment requiring the use of supplied air, via either SCBA or SAL. Examples include structural firefighting and removal of patients from an area contaminated with a pulmonary agent such as ammonia or chlorine.

An example of Level B includes the use of a *chemical protective suit*, an *SCBA*, *hazard-protective footwear*, an inner layer of *biohazard gloves* with an outer layer of *chemical protective gloves*, and *chemical sealing tape* (if the suit does not encapsulate the outer layer of gloves).

15. In what circumstances should Level A PPE be used, and what type of protection for each of the five basic points of protection should be included?

Level A is the minimum standard level for working in an IDLH environment that requires protection from vapor fumes. One example would be entering an area contaminated with VX nerve agent. Level A gear includes an *airtight suit*, *SCBA*, *hazard-protective footwear*, and an inner layer of *work gloves* or *biohazard gloves* (the suit provides the outer layer) (Fig. 1.14.19).

Note: It requires a great deal of expertise and training to be proficient with the tasks that are performed in a Level A suit and the environment in which it is likely to be used.

16. If I am receiving casualties from an incident at a veterinary facility, what level of PPE is appropriate?

In accordance with the *OHSA Guidelines for Hospital First-Receivers Decontamination Operations*, providers should be prepared to use Level C PPE. Any provider using the Level C PPE should have the appropriate 40 hours of didactic and skill preparation, with documented, routine training on the equipment they are most likely to use during such an event. Various biohazard situations may make the use of Level D PPE appropriate, depending on the biological agent, in instances where decontamination is not indicated.

17. What are the concerns that need to be addressed with each level of PPE?

- Level A—Are the personnel using this PPE properly trained, capable of the requisite expertise, and knowledgeable about the environmental monitoring they will need in a hazardous environment? Are the personnel physically fit enough to maintain operations in these enclosed, humid, and hot suits they will be using? Have the suits been certified, checked, rechecked, and routinely tested by certified technicians to ensure they remain airtight? Are there enough personnel to "rotate 'n rehab" enough team members to successfully accomplish the Level A objectives of the operation? Is Level A necessary for this operation?
- Level B—Are the personnel using this PPE properly trained, capable of the requisite expertise, and knowledgeable about the environmental monitoring they will need in a hazardous environment? Are the personnel physically fit enough to maintain operations in these enclosed, warm suits and SCBA they will be using? Have the suits been certified and checked by the appropriate safety personnel to ensure they remain intact? Are there enough personnel to "rotate 'n rehab" enough team members to successfully accomplish the Level B objectives of the operation? Is Level B necessary for this operation?
- Level C—Are the personnel using this PPE properly trained and knowledgeable of the equipment and decontamination operations? Do you have available expertise to assist with clarification of unanticipated PPE concerns? Are the personnel physically fit enough to maintain operations in these enclosed, warm suits, and the PAPRs they will be using? Have the suits been certified and checked by the appropriate safety personnel to ensure they remain intact? Are there enough personnel to "rotate 'n rehab" enough team members to successfully accomplish the decontamination operation? Do you have a practiced, predetermined decontamination operations plan in place? Is a higher level of protection necessary for this operation? Is decontamination necessary for this incident?
- Level D—Are the personnel using this PPE properly trained and knowledgeable of its limitations? Do you have available expertise to assist with clarification of unanticipated PPE concerns? Have all personnel been fit-tested on any particulate masks provided? Is a higher level of protection necessary for this operation? Is decontamination necessary for this incident?

18. How does the type of PPE selected affect the decontamination operation conducted at a facility?

A standing facility has a variety of unique needs that may require an adaptable arsenal of PPE. For one, most standing facilities have frequent three-times-a-day rotation of staff, with reduction of manpower at night and an increase in administrative staff during the day. Standing facilities must meet standard health care regulations, ordinances, and rules for day-to-day operations.

The type of PPE selected should take into consideration the following questions:

- Will your staff need to share equipment, necessitating a one-size-fits-most approach to PPE?
- What type of technical expertise will you have available within your staff?
- What is the size of your decontamination operation (how many can you decontaminate in an hour)?

- Can you sustain a 24-hour operation? If so, for how long? Do you have the equipment to support it?
- Will your staff be expected to respond out to an actively contaminated site?
- What type of storage capability do you have for your PPE? How much PPE do you have stockpiled? Is it regularly inspected and updated, with expired items replaced in an efficient manner?

In general, a standing facility or a small decontamination response team should focus on having these items on the top of their list:

- Multipurpose chemical protective suits (one suit fits many contaminants)
- PAPRs, either hooded (for standing facilities that rotate staff) or fitted (for a small response team with dedicated members), with multipurpose filter cartridges
- Biohazard gloves for an inner layer, and chemical protective gloves for an outer layer
- Chemical sealing tape or duct tape
- Hazard-protective footwear fitting over a suit that has encapsulated booties; the footwear should have traction-enabling soles
- A safety officer, trained to a high level of expertise in various types of PPE, environmental hazards, contaminants, and matching of the PPE to the likely contaminant
- A decontamination officer, trained to a high level of expertise in the decon operation, including rotation and rehabilitation of team members using PPE

19. How is PPE removed, and what needs to be done before "doffing" the PPE?

Putting PPE on correctly is referred to as "donning" PPE. Taking it off is often referred to as "doffing" the PPE. Prior to doffing, the individual in PPE must first go through responder decontamination. This is a process by which contaminated tools are set aside in the warm zone where they can be used by the next shift. The individual is then scrubbed from head to toe by another provider, as they slowly rotate 360 degrees, with arms elevated to 90%. The same decontamination solution is used for the responder's PPE as for the victims. Last, each boot is decontaminated as the responder steps out of the pool of decon solution at their feet, stepping onto a clean surface after the soles are scrubbed and rinsed.

Of utmost importance in the doffing procedure—it must be emphasized that the airway protection (PAPR, SCBA, etc.) is the last piece to be removed. Typical doffing procedures follow these steps:

- First, chemical tape is removed at the boots and outer gloves.
- The power supply/air bottle pack is removed and handed to a partner who holds it away from the responder as he or she doffs remaining equipment. The face mask is left in place. This protects the airway without undue exposure to any remaining contaminant.
- The outer boots are removed, followed by the outer suit. The suit is grabbed by the shoulders and pulled off the shoulders. Arms are then pulled through the sleeves, inverting them to keep contaminant folded inside the suit.
- The outer gloves are removed using standard biohazard degloving technique.
- With the inner gloves remaining, the suit is then rolled from the inside to the out, rolling it down to the feet.
- As each foot is removed from the suit, the responder steps away from the suit to avoid contact with any remnants of contaminant.
- Finally, the face piece is removed by leaning forward, and loosening the straps/hood. After pulling it up and away from the face, it is handed to the partner.
- Last, the inner gloves are removed using standard biohazard degloving technique.

Responders must first practice these procedures in the presence of experienced hazmat technicians/experts and should do so with the specific equipment they will be using. Doffing procedures should not be attempted the first time during an actual response—*prior practice is essential* to avoid cross-contamination onto the responder!

Suggested Reading

Centers for Disease Control and Prevention. Emergency Preparedness Against Biological, Chemical and Radiological Emergencies. Available at http://emergency.cdc.gov/.

Currance PL. *Medical Response to Weapons of Mass Destruction.* St. Louis, Mosby Elsevier, 2005.

NIOSH. Establishing protective requirements for CBRN air-purifying respirators and SCBAs. Available at http://www.cdc.gov/niosh/npptl/standardsdev/cbrn/.

Oak Ridge Institute for Science and Education. Publications and radiation resources for management of radiation accidents and hospital triage. Available at http://orise.orau.gov/reacts/pubs-resources.htm.

Occupational Safety and Health Administration. Best practices for hospital first receivers, guidelines for personal protective equipment and decontamination operations. Available at http://www.osha.gov/dts/osta/bestpractices/html/hospital_firstreceivers.html.

Occupational Safety and Health Administration, Department of Labor. Resources for emergency preparedness standards. Available at http://osha.gov/SLTC/emergencypreparedness/index.html.

CHAPTER 1.15
BASIC VETERINARY DECONTAMINATION: WHO, WHAT, WHY?

Lisa A. Murphy, VMD

1. What is the purpose of decontamination?

Due to dangerous materials that may be present in their environment, animals affected by disasters are at risk of developing significant adverse health effects. Decontamination will limit exposure time to potentially harmful substances and minimize further spread and distribution of chemical hazards through the movement of contaminated animals.

2. What kinds of harmful substances may animals be exposed to following disasters?

Countless numbers of solids, liquids, and gases may be released into the environment during a disaster. Common examples include detergents, cleaning agents, solvents, automotive fluids, pesticides, hydrocarbons, asbestos, mold spores, and even drugs and medications. Floodwaters may contain high levels of fecal coliforms, heavy metals, and various mixtures of organic chemicals. Biological warfare agents may be encountered in a terrorist event. Gases that are lighter than air (e.g., hydrogen cyanide, carbon monoxide) will dissipate outside, but gases that are heavier than air (e.g., carbon dioxide, hydrogen sulfide, nerve agents) may pose a risk to both humans and animals as they settle in pockets close to the ground. It will be important to work with on-site authorities to determine the presence of potentially-hazardous substances that may pose a risk to both animals and the human personnel handling them.

3. What others hazards may also be present?

Physical injury may also be caused by glass, particulates, and other debris dispersed during a disaster. Prevalence of infectious disease agents, including zoonoses, may also be increased.

4. Under what circumstances will decontamination of animals be performed?

Animal decontamination should only occur if it is possible to minimize the potential for injury to *both* the affected animals and the human personnel performing the decontamination.

5. Who can perform animal decontamination?

Only personnel with appropriate hazardous materials training should be allowed to participate in animal decontamination operations. In many situations, this may be local hazardous materials response teams or fire departments. Some state and federal veterinary response teams have veterinary personnel with hazardous materials training, but local first responders should identify veterinarians, animal control, agricultural agents, and other

231

animal personnel who may respond within their communities during a disaster and help them to obtain the training and certifications that will enable them to participate in animal decontamination operations.

In situations where veterinary or other animal-care personnel are unable to enter the disaster site, communication technologies may allow a veterinarian or other qualified personnel to remotely assist on-scene responders with animal management, decontamination, and triage from an appropriate distance.

6. Can animal owners decontaminate their own animals?

In general, animal owners should not decontaminate their own animals. If the owner is also contaminated, it is important that they themselves are effectively decontaminated, something that is less likely to occur if they are instead participating in the decontamination of their animals. To provide comfort and reassurance to an animal owner who does not want to become separated from his or her animal, the owner and animal(s) should be commonly identified before proceeding through the respective decontamination lines so they can be more easily reunited afterward.

Working animals may be one exception to this general rule. Working dogs are sometimes not safely separately from their handlers, and search-and-rescue or other detection dogs (bombs, arson, etc.) may belong to handlers who are themselves hazmat-trained, emergency first responders. Prior training in both animal and self-decontamination should be encouraged for this group of animal owners. Personal assistance dogs are service animals, and removing them from their owner may not be possible due to the severe distress this may cause both individuals in an already stressful situation. In these cases, normal human decontamination procedures will need to be altered to accommodate them.

7. When is dermal decontamination of animals needed?

Skin can serve as both a target of toxicity and a source of absorption of chemicals into the body. Systemic effects may develop from exposure to agents that are able to penetrate through the layers of the skin.

Animals may also act as fomites. As they move from place to place, hazardous substances on their feet, skin, or hair coat contaminate objects, people, and animals with which they come in contact. Another indication for the dermal decontamination of animals is to prevent their ingestion of potentially toxic substances as they groom themselves.

8. What are the possible side effects of dermal exposures to toxic substances following a disaster?

Dermal exposures to chemicals may cause signs ranging from mild redness, irritation, and hair loss to severe corrosive injury that may result in full thickness burns, systemic shock, eventual sloughing and scarring, and even death.

9. What can be used to perform dermal decontamination?

Large quantities of clean water are vitally important for dermal decontamination of animals. Flushing or flooding contaminated skin with water can remove or dilute significant amounts of hazardous agents that may be present. For species that are *not* well accustomed to being sprayed with water, such as cats, immersing the animal up to its neck in a bucket of warm water instead may better facilitate washing. Gentle use of scrub brushes or towels can help allow penetration of water and soap to the skin without causing abrasions or other injuries. If animals will tolerate it, gauze, cotton swabs, or even a soft toothbrush can be used to remove debris from the nostrils and ears. Repeated bathing may be required for heavily contaminated animals. Radiation cannot be neutralized but may be removed in this manner. Do not forget that large bodies of water (ponds, lakes, oceans, etc.) may have to serve as a decontamination site in a mass casualty event.

Many soaps and detergents have been recommended for the decontamination of humans and animals, but perhaps the safest, most effective, and readily available cleaning agents are *liquid* dishwashing detergent and baby shampoo. Green soap is commonly used in human decontamination, although due to its ethanol content, proper dilution and use according to the manufacturer's instructions (especially with concentrated tinctures) must be strictly adhered to before applying it to animals, and its use on very small or debilitated patients is probably not advisable. In contrast, automatic, dry dishwashing *detergents* are highly alkaline and should *always be avoided* to prevent injuries due to either contact with skin or ingestion.

10. Is it important to dry animals after bathing?

Preventing thermoregulatory problems is more important for animals after bathing rather than whether they are actually wet or not, although towel drying after bathing is recommended in animals that will easily tolerate it. To prevent chilling, wet animals should be protected from wind and drafts. To prevent overheating, ventilation and shade should be provided, especially since some dark-colored animals may actually absorb more solar radiation when wet. Regardless of the ambient temperature, animals should be monitored for signs of hypothermia or hyperthermia before, during, and after decontamination.

11. Can all harmful substances be removed using soap and water?

Some dried or tarry substances are not easily removed with water, so other techniques may be needed. If time permits, powdered or clumped materials may be removed from animal hair by combing or brushing. Dry materials may be removed by vacuuming if animals will tolerate it. Sticky materials may be scraped off using tongue depressors or similar wooden tools. Loosening tacky or sticky substances by rubbing them with edible oily substances such as mineral oil, vegetable oil, mayonnaise, or peanut butter may facilitate their removal. Chemical solvents should never be used due to their potential for damaging skin and mucous membranes and causing aspiration or other complications if ingested. Some persistent substances (e.g., dried paint, tar, tree sap) may need to be removed by shaving or clipping, although this can be very time consuming, can lead to accidental abrasions and lacerations of personal protective equipment (PPE) and human or animal skin and may compromise an animal's normal thermoregulatory mechanisms.

Due to time constraints imposed by either the circumstances of the disaster situation or the number of animals needing decontamination, many of these techniques may not be practical on a large scale, and instead a general gross decontamination with soap and water may be all that is performed initially, with a more thorough decontamination and monitoring to follow later.

12. Do animals' eyes need to be decontaminated in disasters?

Yes. In addition to flying debris and heavy dust that may cause irritation and physical trauma to animals' eyes, exposures to harmful or corrosive chemicals can occur. Ocular signs can range from mild conjunctivitis and blepharospasm to corneal ulcerations, perforations, severe pain, and permanent loss of vision.

13. How is ocular decontamination performed?

Eyes should be flushed with tepid water or saline solution. Ideally, this should be performed for 20 to 30 minutes, but many animals will tolerate this for only a few minutes at a time. Eyedroppers can be used for small animals such as birds. For animals with very large eyes, such as horses, slowly pouring fluid over the ocular area with a disposable cup may be less startling to the animal and more easily performed than flushing the eyes with a direct stream. Do not use Visine or other similar products due to the systemic pharmacologic effects that may be caused by their active ingredients. Do not forget to also gently flush the nostrils.

Fluorescein staining of the corneas should be performed after flushing if injury or significant ocular exposures are suspected, and repeated 12 to 24 hours later. Treatment with lubricant ophthalmic ointments can follow staining.

14. When is gastrointestinal decontamination used?

Puddles of liquids, solid deposits, and inhaled particulates that are later coughed up and swallowed are all potential sources of oral chemical exposures that may require intervention. Ingestion of chemical agents may also result from normal grooming behaviors. Preventing or minimizing oral absorption of harmful substances may help prevent severe neurologic, hepatic, renal, cardiovascular, reproductive, and other acute and chronic systemic effects.

15. What are the most common methods of gastrointestinal decontamination?

Emesis, inducing vomiting, is used to remove substances from the stomach and is most useful within 30 to 90 minutes of the ingestion. In general, complete stomach emptying is not expected. Dogs vomit only 40% to 60% of their stomach contents. Hydrogen peroxide (3%) acts as a local gastrointestinal irritant to induce vomiting. One tablespoon is administered orally per 10 pounds of body weight, with a maximum dose of 3 to 4 tablespoons. Hydrogen peroxide 3% works best if given after a small amount of food and can be repeated once. Apomorphine can be used under veterinary supervision, although its sedative side effects may be undesirable under disaster conditions. Due to their inconsistent effectiveness and potential for causing severe adverse effects, salt, liquid dishwashing detergent, xylazine, syrup of ipecac, and powdered mustard should not be used as emetics in animals.

Other alternatives to inducing vomiting are diluents, adsorbents, and cathartics. Diluting chemical compounds with small amounts of liquids such as milk, water, milk of magnesia, or kaopectate can render them less irritating. Activated charcoal, administered orally at 1 to 3 grams per kilogram of body weight, is an adsorbent that binds most organic compounds and facilitates their excretion in the feces. Saline, osmotic, and bulk cathartics are used to enhance elimination of substances, including activated charcoal, by moving them through the gastrointestinal tract. Enemas can be helpful in eliminating toxicants from the lower gastrointestinal tract.

Gastric lavage is an advanced gastrointestinal decontamination technique that requires general anesthesia and a cuffed endotracheal tube and should not be used to remove caustic substances or hydrocarbons.

16. Can all toxic ingestions be treated using gastrointestinal decontamination?

Vomiting should not be induced if caustic substances or petroleum distillates have been ingested, if the animal is already exhibiting symptoms (especially neurologic, cardiovascular, or respiratory abnormalities), or if the animal has known underlying seizure or cardiovascular disorders.

17. What are the possible complications of toxic oral exposures?

Many chemical agents can be strong local irritants. Mild gastrointestinal effects may include hypersalivation, vomiting, and diarrhea. Severe gastrointestinal effects are mucosal ulcerations and perforations, hemorrhage, and eventual esophageal strictures. Extreme pain, shock, and other systemic effects leading to death are also possible. An important risk associated with hydrocarbons such as oils, greases, kerosene, turpentine, and gasoline is aspiration, leading to potentially life-threatening respiratory signs.

18. How are animals decontaminated following exposures to toxic gases?

The most effective treatment for exposure to toxic gases or vapors is removal of the animal to fresh air. As long as the animal is able to breathe normally, the gas will be rapidly eliminated by exhalation, although dermal decontamination may still be warranted to remove any solid residues that could potentially endanger the animal or emergency responders. Some gases with irritant (e.g., chlorine) or systemic (e.g., hydrogen cyanide) toxic effects can cause life-threatening signs and will require further antidotal treatment or supportive care such as supplemental oxygen support. Animals displaying severe or prolonged symptoms due to toxic gas exposures may not survive the decontamination process; humane euthanasia may need to be considered.

VETERINARY DECONTAMINATION DECISION MAKING AND TRIAGE

19. Will animals always be decontaminated following a disaster?

No. Especially if a zoonotic disease or highly toxic chemical is involved, risks to human health may be deemed too great to allow for an animal decontamination operation.

20. What initial animal information is needed when making the decision of whether to decontaminate?

Initial assessments should communicate information about what species are involved and the number of live and dead animals present. It should also be determined if adequate veterinary resources are available to support triage, stabilization, decontamination, and supportive care, particularly for injured animals. Availability of appropriate means of animal transportation must also be considered.

21. What are the financial considerations for the decontamination of animals?

Finances may be an important issue, especially when food-producing animals are involved. If exposure to hazardous materials during a disaster results in animals that will not be marketable due to residue issues, consultation with the animal owners/producers and agricultural officials is indicated to determine the best course of action. Some situations may dictate the euthanasia of healthy animals rather than decontamination, such as when the cost of decontamination exceeds the market value of the animals.

22. What is the best way to keep animals from leaving the hot zone until they can be decontaminated?

If animals are free-ranging, they should ideally be moved to a single containment point prior to being brought to the decontamination area. Animals in unsafe structures, vehicles, and other compromised or dangerous locations may need to be similarly relocated to a containment area. Animals adequately confined to intact structures, fenced pastures, and other similar locations may be able to be at least temporarily left in place to minimize human exposure to hazardous agents if disaster conditions have stabilized and safe food, water, and shelter are present or can be provided.

In some cases where animals are either inaccessible or cannot be confined, making removal for decontamination impossible, euthanasia may be considered if the animals are at high risk for injury, dehydration, or starvation, or pose a significant human safety or public health risk.

23. Are some kinds of animals more likely to be decontaminated than others?

Yes. Working and service animals may be given special preference and priority over other animals, including pets. Restraint may be either highly specialized or even impossible in an emergency situation for exotic companion animals, laboratory animals, and wild and feral animals, decreasing the likelihood that they will be able to be decontaminated, although in certain situations, animal decontamination plans will need to be prepared to address culturally valuable animals, wildlife, zoo animals, and threatened and endangered species.

24. Can sick and injured animals be decontaminated?

Triage should be performed to identify animals with mild, moderate, and major injury or illness. Although it would be ideal to stabilize all animals prior to decontamination, resources for this may be limited following a disaster, especially if the presence of highly dangerous substances or conditions limits the number of personnel and time spent in the hot zone. With people, decontamination is typically performed before any medical treatments are administered. Similarly, it is doubtful that much medical intervention for animals would be performed in the hot zone either. Euthanasia should be considered for life-threatening conditions and animals too severely debilitated to withstand the stress of decontamination. In incidents involving large numbers of animals, treatment should be reserved for those deemed most likely to survive, while those with life-threatening conditions should be euthanized for humane reasons. Arrangements should be made for continued care of ill or injured animals following their decontamination.

25. Should dead animals be decontaminated?

Due to the variety of potentially hazardous agents that may be present in disaster situations, environmental authorities should be consulted to determine whether decontamination and/or removal of animal carcasses is required. Animals euthanized with barbiturate-containing euthanasia solutions are potentially lethal to scavengers that feed on the carcasses, so these should be removed or deeply buried. Decontamination of carcasses should only be instituted after all live animals have been decontaminated.

PREPARING FOR VETERINARY DECONTAMINATION

26. What equipment and supplies are needed to perform animal decontamination?

Supplies for the detailed written or electronic identification and documentation of animals should be acquired before beginning their decontamination. Since many uniquely identifying items, such as collars and halters, may be either lost during a disaster or discarded during the decontamination process, it is important that these unique items also be documented to later assist in the reunion of animals with their rightful owners.

Animal restraint equipment that can be either effectively decontaminated after use or discarded should be easily accessible. Depending on the types of animals involved, this could include halters, leashes, muzzles, crates, and cages. Another clean set of similar equipment should also be designated for wherever the animals will be staged or housed following their decontamination.

27. Should sedatives be used to facilitate the decontamination of animals that are difficult to handle?

Tranquilizers and other forms of chemical restraint, used under the direct guidance and supervision of a licensed veterinarian, may also be warranted under certain circumstances. Individual animals that are dangerous or frightened, especially those unaccustomed to be handled by people, can increase the risk of injury to themselves and others and delay their timely decontamination. All pharmacologic agents have the potential for adverse effects, especially during a disaster situation where access to advanced veterinary care may be limited. For this reason, chemical restraint should not be considered a routine component of animal decontamination and would not be practical for severely injured or debilitated animals or large animal groups or herds.

28. What protection should be worn by the responder while performing animal decontamination?

In addition to protecting against oral, dermal, ocular, and respiratory exposures to hazardous substances, PPE worn during the decontamination of animals should ideally also protect against bites, scratches, punctures, and exposure to bodily fluids. It is important to remember that personnel wearing PPE may appear quite frightening to animals. This, in combination with the general loss of agility and dexterity experienced by people wearing PPE, may increase the risk of animal escape along with injury to animals, people, equipment, and the PPE itself. Ultimately, the Incident Commander, in consultation with the appropriate environmental and hazardous materials specialists, will determine the type of PPE (including respiratory protection and other safety equipment) to be used by all on-scene responders.

29. What happens to the dirty water and other waste products after decontaminating animals?

Contaminated run-off water produced by decontamination operations should ideally be contained in such way as to prevent animals in the decontamination line from ingesting it and to keep from further dispersing hazardous substances it may contain into the surrounding area. Environmental officials should be consulted about wastewater issues prior to setting up and commencing decontamination operations, and also prior to leaving the area after decontamination has been finished. The Environmental Protection Agency has provided a waiver to wastewater containment during mass casualty events. Proper methods of disposal for contaminated collars, leashes, and similar items should be predetermined, along with how to handle accumulated urine, feces, hair, and other biological materials.

VETERINARY DECONTAMINATION TECHNIQUES

30. What special techniques should be used to decontaminate large animals such as horses and livestock?

Human safety should always be the primary goal when decontaminating animals, particularly when working with large animal species. Efforts to limit direct contact with the animals will minimize the potential for both physical injury and contamination of personnel. Large animals are often wary of doorways and low-roofed structures and are unlikely to be safely led into a tent or other enclosed area for decontamination; so instead, if available, portable fencing panels or something similar can be used to form a chute or alleyway for large animals to move through. This kind of handling and movement technique is already familiar and readily acceptable to many large animal species and so can better facilitate their decontamination while also minimizing the need for contact with the decontamination team. As the animals move through the chute, water can be applied from the sides and above and personnel can use long-handled brushes for washing. Two stationary lines of fire vehicles or other large trucks with the animals being moved in between them could also be used in this manner. Most large animals will not voluntarily walk onto slick or unstable surfaces or gratings. If dirt or another natural surface cannot be provided, rubber mats or indoor-outdoor carpet may provide more secure footing.

If large animals are found already confined to a secure field or structure and circumstances of the disaster allow it, it may be most appropriate to minimize the potential for escape and human injury by bringing the decontamination operation to the animals rather than moving them to another location.

31. Can large exotic pets or zoo animals be decontaminated in the same way?

Variations on large animal decontamination techniques will be needed for the safe movement and decontamination of large exotic species or zoo animals. Individuals with species-specific animal husbandry or handling expertise should be consulted, including a veterinarian familiar with chemical restraint of nondomestic animals.

32. Can the decontamination of wildlife species be accomplished following a disaster?

Due to the high likelihood of adverse complications associated with the capture and restraint that would be needed for the decontamination of native wildlife, it may be worthwhile to start by examining a small number of individuals to better assess the extent of contamination of wildlife within the affected area. If the animals are unlikely to further spread significant contamination through their movements, leaving them undisturbed may be a better strategy than attempting their decontamination.

If the decision is made to decontaminate wildlife species with minimal risk to human personnel, appropriate experts should be consulted to ensure that adequate quantities of necessary equipment and trained individuals are available. Handling and movement of rabies target species (raccoons, skunks, foxes, bats) in endemic areas is generally prohibited, although their euthanasia or quarantine may be appropriate during a disaster response.

33. What should be done with wildlife after decontamination?

Whether to hold wildlife or immediately release them after decontamination should also be carefully considered. Release at the animal's exact point of origin is ideal although it may not be possible following a disaster, so identification of a suitable alternate location and the necessary transportation equipment is required. If environmental contamination prevents releasing wildlife to or near the capture location and another release site is not available, removal to a remote site may be the only option, although this may limit the ability to ever return the animal to a natural habitat in future.

34. What postdecontamination surveillance is recommended?

Even healthy animals will require monitoring and supportive care following decontamination, and arrangements should be made for adequate feeding, housing, and sanitation. Ill or injured animals may require more specific veterinary care and support. In addition to a complete physical examination, blood work, thoracic radiographs, and other screening tests may be warranted depending on the hazardous substances to which the animal may have been exposed.

Dosimetry badges and other detection and monitoring instrumentation will be needed after events involving radiation. Animal wastes should be handled and monitored appropriately to prevent environmental contamination with radioactive materials. Although there are no dosing recommendations for nonhuman animals, potassium iodide (KI) is recommended as a thyroid blocking agent following radiation emergencies (*KI will only be effective if I-131 is the radiation contaminant*). Calcium supplementation may prevent strontium deposition in bones.

Suggested Reading

DeClementi C. Prevention and treatment of poisoning. In Gupta RC, ed. *Veterinary Toxicology*. New York, Academic Press, 2007, pp. 1139–1158.

Murphy LA, Gwaltney-Brant SM, Albretsen JC, et al. Toxicologic agents of concern for search-and-rescue dogs responding to urban disasters. *J Am Vet Med Assoc* 2003;222:296–304.

Wenzel JGW. Awareness-level information for veterinarians on control zones, personal protective equipment, and decontamination. *J Am Vet Med Assoc* 2007;231:48–51.

Wismer TA, Murphy LA, Gwaltney-Brant SM. Management and prevention of toxicoses in search-and-rescue dogs responding to urban disasters. *J Am Vet Med Assoc* 2003;222:305–310.

CHAPTER 1.16
WILDLIFE HANDLING

Sally B. Palmer, DVM

There is a school of thought that believes humans should not intervene when incidents and disasters, especially natural disasters, affect wildlife as this is Nature's way of managing wild populations. Another school of thought concedes that it may be Nature's way, but humans have significantly affected and eliminated some options wildlife once had to avoid or react to disasters. As such, our interference is not so much attempting to control or supersede Nature's way as it is recognizing the impact we have and accepting our role and responsibility to mitigate loss.

Handling wildlife in rescue, emergency, and disaster situations is fraught with challenges. The wide variety of animal species and almost limitless emergency scenarios make it difficult to write a complete reference. This chapter should be considered as a primer highlighting some general handling techniques and concepts to be used when responding to emergencies involving wildlife. For more information, a few suggested readings and additional resources are included at the end of this chapter.

GENERAL PRINCIPLES

1. What is the most important consideration when dealing with wildlife?

Safety! One must take into consideration your own safety, the safety of those assisting you, the safety of bystanders, and the safety of the animal.

2. What is meant by "primary hazards" of an animal?

Primary hazards describe the parts of that species that are most dangerous to a handler or animal responder. These include antlers, claws, teeth, hooves, etc.

3. What are some things that can be done to optimize safety?

- Learn about behaviors and hazards of the different species to facilitate movement, capture, handling, and transport, thereby minimizing stress and risk of injury.
- Do a risk/benefit analysis. Is what you are trying to accomplish worth the risk of injury or death to the animal or handler?
- Develop a plan of operation and communicate the plan to *everyone* involved in the operation. (See Question No. 4.)
- Before starting a rescue operation, have the proper equipment, drugs, and personnel ready and available.
- Create an environment that is as calm and quiet as possible.
- If possible, try to handle animals at risk of developing capture myopathy (see Question No. 12) during the cooler hours of the day.
- Expect the unexpected and plan for contingencies.

4. When working with wildlife, what are things to consider when developing an operational plan?

- Establish a leader for the operation.
- Evaluate the scene and situation. This is sometimes referred to as a *"Size up,"* and includes the following:
  - Is the scene safe?
  - What things on scene could become an obstacles? For example, irrigation ditches, bodies of water, roads, or fence lines may be obstacles.
  - What things on scene could be useful? For example, a fence line or alleyway might be useful to direct the animals into confinement.
  - Identify the specie(s) involved.
  - How many animals are involved?
  - Do any of the animals have any apparent medical issues? (Visual triage; see Chapter 1.9.)
  - What time of day is it? For example, could there be heat-related problems such as hyperthermia or increased risk of capture myopathy?
  - What kind of weather is expected throughout the anticipated time of operation? For example, wind will affect the use of tarps.
- Inventory available equipment, drugs, and personnel.
- Check that the equipment functions properly.
- Develop a drug plan for each species that includes:
  - List drugs that may be used and make notes of their proper dosing. A separate listing of drugs that are *contraindicated* (should NOT be used) can also be helpful.
  - Estimate the quantity of drugs needed, and confirm the quantities of drugs available and their expiration dates.
  - Confirm, where applicable, reversal agents are available.
  - Confirm that emergency life support drugs, such as epinephrine, are available.
  - Confirm that you have proper drug storage containers, such as coolers with ice packs for those drugs that require refrigeration.
- Make ready access to equipment and drugs.
- Confirm the capabilities of personnel.
- Brief *everyone* who will be involved in the plan of operation, and convey all pertinent information.
- Assign specific job duties. For example, name the person(s) responsible for monitoring the captured animal(s) and assign one individual to obtain temperature, pulse rate and quality, and respiratory rate (TPR).
- Establish signals, both verbal and hand, that will be used, and any communication phrases.
- Establish escape routes for personnel, should they be needed. For example, if the bear comes out of anesthesia unexpectedly, all personnel should know their route of escape.
- Establish a plan for managing injured personnel.
- Establish how an animal will be released from capture. For example, what happens first: complete or partial removal of the muzzle or release from lateral restraint?
- Anticipate the NEXT step after the animal is successfully moved, contained, or captured. Confirm that the next step is ready to go. For example, as part of the Technical Animal Rescue Team, before you capture the animal, confirm that the Evacuation Team is ready to transport that animal and the Sheltering Team is ready to receive that animal.
- Anticipate what could go wrong and make contingency plans. Of note, chemical restraint can be very unpredictable in wild animals.
- Inventory equipment and drugs postoperation.
- Following an operation, debrief *as soon as possible*. Review what went right, what went wrong, and what to do differently next time. This will significantly improve outcomes in future operations.

5. Are operational plans only for complicated large-scale incidents?

No. The parts of an effective operational plan are applicable whether you are working alone capturing an injured goose, in a small group of two to six people tasked with rescuing waterfowl from an oil-slick shore, or on a large-scale operation as part of a team responding to an animal welfare case involving the seizure of numerous large carnivores.

6. Describe what is meant by "fight or flight."

When an animal perceives a threat, real or imagined, the instinct is to either flee from the threat (flight) or fight the threat. There is very little reasoned thought; rather the limbic (primal instinct) part of the brain and the animal's sympathetic autonomic nervous system take over. Catacholamines, including epinephrine (adrenalin), are released, which create the physiologic changes that facilitate the fight-or-flight response. Almost always, animals prefer to flee and will only fight when flight is not an option. When handling wildlife, it may be possible to move them where you want them to go by allowing them "flight." It is also important to recognize that if you remove the flight option, by cornering them or physically restraining them, then their remaining option may be to fight. While fight or flight is a physiologic survival mechanism, it can have detrimental consequences contributing to the development of capture myopathy. (See Questions Nos. 12 through 18.)

7. What are some general techniques that can be used to keep wild animals calm?

- Minimize shouting and sudden loud noises.
- Avoid making direct eye contact.
- Minimize threatening gestures, such as grabbing the antlers or horns.
- Avoid creating a perception of "stalking." While it is important to speak quietly and move slowly and deliberately, do not overdo this and create an environment that resembles stalking to a wild animal.
- Use visual barriers such as tarps, plywood panels, etc. to direct animals.
- Some species may calm with properly implemented physical or chemical restraint.
- Once an animal is restrained (physical and/or chemical), the use of a blindfold or hood can be helpful for some species.
- In sedated or anesthetized (larger) animals, cotton balls in panty hose may be used safely as noise reduction ear plugs.
- If you are dealing with multiple species, recognize that one species may be a "prey" animal to another species, so visual, auditory (hearing), or olfactory (smell) cues may trigger a fight-or-flight response. Whenever possible, do not handle predator species and then attempt to handle prey species.

8. What is the goal of restraint?

The goal of restraint is to minimize the risk of injury to both handler and animal.

9. What are the two main types of restraint?

The two main types of restraint are physical and chemical.

10. List some limitations of physical restraint.

- Using physical restraint requires training to properly operate certain equipment and become familiar with certain holding techniques.
- Physical restraint poses the risk of injury to, or death of, the animal or handler.
- Physical restraint is associated with the risk of initiating the development of capture myopathy in certain species.
- Not all animals are amenable to physical restraint alone.

11.   List some limitations of chemical restraint.

- Chemical restraint requires a tremendous breadth of knowledge of drugs and dosages for many species.
- Chemical restraint requires proper training on various delivery systems.
- There are specific drawbacks with each of the delivery systems, such as how close to an animal one must be when using a pole syringe, or how predictable is the flight of a projectile dart.
- Maintaining control of the animal after the drugs are administered is vital.
- There can be an unpredictable response to a drug, such as from an anxiety override or from having little knowledge of the drug response in a given species.
- Some drugs are not reversible, so once administered there is no way to counteract the drug.
- Chemical restraint does expose an animal to the risk of injury from the delivery system or drugs and the risk of death as a direct result of the drugs or as a consequence of having their faculties impaired.
- Chemical restraint is associated with the risk of contributing to the development of capture myopathy.
- Special licensing (Veterinary and Drug Enforcement Agency [DEA]) is required to obtain and administer most restraint drugs.
- Maintaining security of Schedule (DEA regulated) drugs from theft and unlawful use
- Maintaining accurate records of the use of Schedule (DEA regulated) drugs
- Inadvertent exposure of humans to the drugs

12.   What is capture myopathy?

Capture myopathy is a muscle disease associated with the stress of capture, restraint, and/or transport. The disease is characterized by the degeneration and necrosis (death) of skeletal and cardiac (heart) muscle.

13.   What is the disease process of capture myopathy?

The pathophysiology is complex, but an overview notes that the activated sympathetic nervous system causes an increase in metabolic activity resulting in a switch from aerobic metabolism to anaerobic metabolism and the subsequent production of lactic acid. The buildup of lactic acid eventually creates a systemic (whole body) acidosis. In addition, when muscles remain in a steady state of contraction, perfusion of the muscle is compromised and hypoxia (lack of oxygen) in the tissue quickly develops. Hyperthermia (high body temperature) also develops. Tranquilization may exacerbate these problems as blood pressure drops and perfusion of tissues is further compromised. As muscle tissue dies, the breakdown products damage the kidneys during clearance, leading to kidney failure.

14.   Which species are susceptible to capture myopathy?

Numerous species of birds and mammals are susceptible to capture myopathy. It has not been documented in reptiles. Prey animals appear to be more susceptible, but young and submissive predator animals are also at risk of developing capture myopathy when exposed to the increased stress of capture and restraint. Bighorn sheep appear to be especially susceptible to developing capture myopathy.

15.   What factors predispose an animal to developing capture myopathy?

Predisposing factors include fear, anxiety, over-exertion, repeated handling, failure to allow an exhausted animal to rest before transporting, and constant muscle tension such as during restraint or transport. It can occur with either physical or chemical restraint. While it is generally seen in animals that maximally exert themselves it can also occur in animals that appear relatively quiet.

16. How quickly does capture myopathy develop?

The disease can develop immediately, in a matter of hours, or many days post-stress. Death can occur suddenly during capture or restraint, usually as the result of factors affecting cardiac muscle, or weeks later often as a result of renal (kidney) failure.

17. Is there any treatment for capture myopathy?

There is no specific treatment to reverse the disease process. Therapy is primarily supportive including IV fluid therapy, sodium bicarbonate, vitamin-E, selenium, calcium channel blockers, and antibiotics.

18. How can animal responders minimize the risk of capture myopathy?

Prevention is most important since development of capture myopathy often results in the death of the animal. Things that can be done to help prevent capture myopathy from developing include the following:

* Perform a risk/benefit analysis. Is what you are trying to accomplish worth the risk that an animal may develop capture myopathy as a direct result of your actions.
* An operational plan should be developed and all involved personnel briefed.
* Equipment and drugs should be inventoried and made ready for easy access.
* Only properly trained personnel should use the equipment and/or participate in manual restraint.
* If possible, handling, immobilization, and transport should be done during the cool hours of the day to minimize the association of heat stress.
* While restraining or transporting animals, minimize overheating by providing a shade environment and good air flow.
* Avoid making any unnecessary noise or conversation.
* Blindfolds may be used to decrease visual stimulation.
* Cotton balls placed in panty hose can be utilized as ear plugs for noise reduction.
* If using chemical restraint, use appropriate doses of drugs and reverse them when possible.
* If a capture was stressful, consider prophylactic IV fluids with sodium bicarbonate added, and add vitamin E and selenium to feed. Avoid putting the sodium bicarbonate in Lactated Ringers or Normosol-R as precipitates form and can lead to kidney failure.
* Chemical restraint should not last longer than 1–2 hours.
* With ungulates (hoofed animals), monitor their TPR every 15–30 minutes. Reverse the chemical immobilization if their body temperature goes above 104° F (40° C).

19. What are some things that you can do to better prepare yourself to respond to emergencies or disasters involving wildlife?

* Identify the wildlife species that are found in your area or in areas where you may respond. If you have a particular interest, focus on that animal or group of animals and learn as much as you can about them, including hazards, normal vital signs (TPR), lifestyles, behaviors, nutritional requirements, zoonotic disease risks, etc.
* Attend classes or workshops to learn, maintain, or improve your skills of restraining wild animals.
* Ahead of time, for each wildlife species in your area, research and compile a list of drugs and dosages that can be used. This information can be difficult to come by and in an emergency there will not be time to acquire it. Even if *you* are not able to obtain or administer drugs, having accurate drugs and dosage information available to someone who can is invaluable.

AVIANS

20. To avoid compromising a bird's respiration during manual restraint, what is an important consideration?

Birds do NOT have a diaphragm. They move their sternum (breast bone) to draw air into their lungs, much like a bellows. Therefore, it is important to limit compression of the chest and avoid restricting the movement of the sternum.

21. What primary hazards are posed by waterfowl (swans, geese, pelicans, etc.)?

The primary hazard is the wings which are quite powerful and are used to strike forward. Secondarily their head and bill can also deliver a hearty blow. For larger waterfowl (pelicans, swans, geese) safety goggles are recommended.

22. How should one physically restrain waterfowl?

Gain control of the wings first and the head second. Fold the wings to the body; a towel may facilitate this. With the wings folded in, hold the bird using one arm over the back, and use your other hand to restrain the head. A hood over the eyes may help calm the bird. A large pole net may facilitate capture, and then the responder can gain control of the wings.

23. What types of containers work well to transport waterfowl?

Cardboard boxes can work as a temporary container for transporting smaller waterfowl. Dog and cat carriers are more durable and can accommodate different sized birds, with the larger crates being suitable for geese and swans. Placing pieces of scrap carpet in the bottom of the crate will provide good footing and a less abrasive surface for when they sit down, but care must be taken to not have any unraveling fibers that could cause injury or be ingested. A crate that is not large enough to allow the bird to stand up and stretch its wings is only suitable for short periods of time such as during transport.

   If a cloth or nylon bag mesh bag is used, care must be taken to avoid having any loose threads entangle the bird.

   As with all birds, covering the crate with a breathable towel or blanket can reduce stress by decreasing visual stimuli.

24. What is the primary hazard of large wading birds (herons, egrets, cranes, etc.)?

These birds have spear-like beaks and they can strike with lightning speed. These birds will often strike at the responder's head placing the handler's eyes at great risk for injury.

25. How should one physically restrain large wading birds?

Two people may be needed to restrain these birds safely. Safety goggles are **strongly** recommended. Full face shields may also work, but be aware that a bird may be able to strike underneath the shield.

Gain control of the beak and head first. Grasp the beak as close to the head as possible, or grasp the head at the base of the skull where it joins the neck. Once the beak and head are controlled, placing a beak tip cover, such as a Styrofoam block, will increase the safety. Even with a beak cover, always maintain control of the beak and head. A bird should <u>NEVER</u> be left unattended if a tip cover is used. As with any type of muzzling device, there is risk of aspiration should the animal vomit, and these birds may use vomiting as a defense mechanism.

While maintaining control of the beak and head, fold both wings and legs into the bird's body. With one hand controlling the beak and head, place your other arm over the bird's back thereby holding the wings into the body, and with this arm's hand, grasp the legs near the feet to allow flexion of the legs up into the body. One may use a large towel to wrap the whole body, but it must be wrapped loosely enough to allow movement of the sternum and respiration. Gently face the bird's head and beak towards the back of the handler to increase the safety for the handler.

26. What type of container works well to transport large wading birds?

Since many of these birds stand close to 4 feet (1.25m) tall; consider a livestock trailer for transport.

27. What hazards are posed by raptors (eagles, hawks, owls, etc.)?

The primary hazard of raptors is their talons (the nails on their feet). Raptors will attempt to grab things with their talons, and will then lock their feet/talons in contraction.

The beak of some raptors can also be a hazard, although it is secondary to the risk of injury from the talons. Owls can rotate their head quite far (approximately 270°) and very quickly, so extra caution is warranted.

28. How should one physically restrain raptors?

Heavy leather safety or welding gloves are strongly recommended. Quickly grasp both legs to gain control of the talons first. For some birds, a towel or blanket thrown over the top of the bird, while allowing the handler to see the legs, may help a handler to grasp both legs. To maintain control of the legs, interdigitate the lower legs, above the feet, with your fingers.

Gain control of the head and beak by gently grasping the base of the skull. Again, a towel may be used to throw over the bird to help wrap the wings into the body and gain control of the head. Care must be taken to not restrict the movement of the sternum. A towel or a hood or mask should be used to cover the bird's eyes and help calm the bird.

Once the bird is controlled, an assistant can place small leather balls (such as hacky sacks), or balls of tape against the bottom of the bird's feet. This will stimulate the talons to grasp these objects, providing a little extra, though not guaranteed, safety.

29. What type of container works well to transport raptors?

Dog crates of the appropriate size can work well. Branches and scrap carpet can provide good footing and comfortable perching. Covering the crate with a towel or blanket to decrease visual stimuli can be helpful, though one must be cognizant of airflow and temperature.

30. What is the primary hazard of Psitticines (parrots, macaws, cockatiels, etc.)?

The beak is the primary hazard of Psitticines. Some of the larger species of Psitticines are capable of removing a human's finger!

31. How should one physically restrain Psitticines?

A towel may be used to throw over the bird to decrease the body movement and allow one to gain control of the head and body together. Continue to hold the body and maintain control of the head by gently grasping it around the base of the skull.

32. What type of container works well to transport Psitticines?

Bird cages or dog crates work well with branches and carpet scraps on the bottom to provide perching and good footing. As with other birds, covering the crate to decrease visual stimuli can be helpful.

33. What are ratites?

Ratites are ostriches, emus, and cassowaries.

34. What is the primary hazard of ratites?

Ratites can be extremely dangerous. The primary hazard of ratites is their feet. Ratites strike high and forward with their feet, but they can also reach back over their "shoulders." A handler's head and face are at risk if standing over the body of the bird from the rear or side. Humans have been disemboweled by the strike of a ratite.

   The beak is a secondary hazard. Though blunt, it can be wielded with quite a bit of force by their strong necks.

35. How should one approach a ratite?

One should approach from the rear or side only. Do NOT approach from the front.

36. What is the safest way to move ratites?

The safest way to move ratites is to get behind them and use push boards to drive them forward in an alleyway, chute, or along a fence. Shaking a broom or stick with plastic strips or a bag on the end can also be helpful.

   For smaller ratites, once they are forced into a corner, the operator behind the push board can grab the neck and pull a hood over the head. Hoods can be made from the legs of sweatpants.

37. What type of container works well to transport ratites?

Livestock trailers.

MAMMALS

38. If your goal is to examine or handle a large mammal (as opposed to trying to move or drive it in a given direction), what is the safest way to approach it?

Most of the larger mammals that you would be approaching will be either injured or sedated. The safest way to approach most mammals is from the front quarter, the side, or the rear quarter. Avoid approaching an animal head on as this is very challenging and threatening to animals. Avoid approaching directly from the rear as most animals have a blind spot directly behind them and this is very frightening and startling.

39. What is the safest way to approach a mammal in lateral recumbency (i.e., lying on its side)?

One should approach from the dorsum (back) to avoid hooves and claws.

40. What is the safest way to approach a mammal in sternal recumbency (i.e., lying on its chest)?

One should approach from the side or rear quarter. Do NOT approach from the front, and avoid approaching ungulates (see Question #41) from the rear as they are apt to startle and can deliver a dangerous kick.

41. What are ungulates?

Ungulates are hoofed mammals. The ungulate grouping includes elk, deer, cows, antelope, horses, zebras, pigs, sheep, and rhinoceros, among others. Because of the tremendous variety of species in this group it is difficult to summarize behaviors and handling techniques. Most of this discussion will be oriented towards deer, elk, antelope, big horn sheep, mountain goats, moose, etc. Again, I encourage the reader to learn about the wildlife in their region or area of interest and consider how one would assist those animals in a disaster response.

42. What are the primary hazards of ungulates?

The primary hazards of ungulates are antlers, horns, hooves, and strength. When threatened, these animals charge, kick, and strike (a kick with the front feet).

While not an injury inducing or life-threatening hazard, Camelidae (camels, llamas, alpacas) can regurgitate and spit foul stomach juices, which are quite unpleasant.

43. When working or moving deer, antelope, or elk in a larger pen or paddock (or adjacent to a highway barrier fence, etc.), of what behavioral trait must you be aware?

The flight instinct is extremely strong in many ungulate species, especially deer, antelope, and elk. In larger pens, or open areas, as they attempt to get away from you they will frequently run and/or jump full force into the enclosure barrier, seriously injuring or killing themselves. This "blind" flight response can be even more pronounced the fewer animals present, as these herd prey animals do not like to feel separated or left behind.

There are times when it is safer and ultimately more efficient to leave the enclosure and allow the animals to settle, before attempting to move them again. If along a highway barrier fence, try to position responders to encourage animals to move *away* from them and *along* the fence.

44. In smaller pens, corrals, or alleyways what challenges do these same species pose to responders attempting to move or handle them?

In smaller enclosures these animals perceive no escape or flight option and often resort to the aggressive fight behaviors of charging, striking, and kicking.

45. What techniques can help move ungulates?

Because these animals prefer the flight option whenever possible, they will try to increase the distance between you and them. If you approach them from the front, they will turn and run away. If you approach from the side they will turn and run; if you approach them from behind they will run away from you. While this is basic herding many people will inadvertently position themselves such that an animal moves off in an undesired direction. Recognize what an animal perceives as a threat and anticipate how they might respond to your actions.

Employing visual or physical barriers, such as plywood sheets, corral panels, tarps, or rolls of webbed plastic snow/construction fencing, etc., to *encourage* a direction of movement can be helpful. When using long rolls of fencing to push or direct animals, it is best to divide these rolls into shorter lengths and have people holding the ends to create a longer barrier. Should an animal double back and try to run through this fencing the shorter length is more manageable and less likely to cause injury to the animal or responders.

These animals are extremely athletic and can jump quite tall barriers if they so choose. Oftentimes an animal will move *along* a barrier as the easiest way to get away from a perceived threat, but when pressed too much (for example responders moving in too quickly) that is when they will expend the extra energy to cross a barrier and move in a different direction in an attempt to take flight from the threat. Because wild ungulates can and will jump barriers, consider this a distinct possibility and develop contingency plans. Of note, antelope can jump over fences, but many prefer to crawl under them. Recognize that an antelope may see a flight option under a barrier.

Lighting strategies can also encourage movement in a desired direction. Ungulates will often perceive (day) light and lighted areas as an escape path. Lighting an area such as an alleyway, enclosure, or trailer may help encourage an animal to enter it. Sometimes opening a doorway to reveal daylight or lighting an area outside may help you move an animal through a darker area. Conversely, it is difficult to move an animal into a dark enclosure, trailer, alleyway, or chute.

One must also be aware that an animal may see (day) light and perceive an escape path which is not suitable, such as a gap in a visual barrier, or through a window (if trapped in a building) or through too small an opening. Anticipate this and cover these areas while lighting or revealing daylight in acceptable openings.

Broomsticks or poles with plastic strips or bags on the end can help direct an animal by scaring it away from you and toward a desired direction.

In more confined spaces, a responder should have a push board to herd an animal from behind. This is partly a visual barrier but primarily offers some protection to the responder. Common sense must prevail in appreciating the size and strength of these animals and recognizing that not all animals can be handled this way.

46. What techniques can help restrain an ungulate?

In terms of physical restraint, for some of the moderately-sized wild ungulates, specially designed squeeze chutes which apply gentle pressure to the sides of the animal are the gold standard. Obviously, access to one of these in a disaster is highly unlikely. However, recognizing that these animals calm in response to pressure against their sides and not from trapping and restricting the head can be useful. Smaller ungulates can be pushed up against a solid barrier with side pressure, with most of the restraint being applied to the trunk and little to the neck or head. (As an aside, this is very effective for llamas and alpacas, and they respond much more favorably to this type of restraint than trying to control their head or neck.)

Especially important is to avoid grabbing the antlers or horns for restraint. This is a challenging and threatening move to an animal and will create more fight than calm and cooperation. If you must handle the antlers, hold them at their base.

Once restrained, applying a blindfold can help decrease the visual stimuli and reduce stress. Large soft stretchable fleece "neck gators" work well as they can be pulled up quickly over and past the nose, thereby covering the eyes while not interfering with respiration. If an animal gets away with this blindfold on, it will fall off on its own almost immediately.

Placing cotton ball–stuffed panty hose for noise reduction ear plugs can help decrease the auditory stimuli.

For many wild ungulates, chemical restraint will be required. Blindfolds and ear plugs should still be utilized in these sedated or anesthetized animals.

47. List risks associated with chemical restraint in ungulates.

- Regurgitation and aspiration
- Bloat
- Capture myopathy

48. Can you use a halter on wild ungulates?

ONLY if the animal is confined and restrained in some other way, AND you can be sure to get the halter off before losing control of the animal.

49. What are some additional risks when dealing with bison or moose?

Bison, (also referred to as American Buffalo or just Buffalo), and moose can be very dangerous. When trying to move or push them in a certain direction, they may not opt for flight and move away from you, rather some, especially cow moose with calves, may be quite aggressive. Do not be foolish and think you can direct these animals away from you with a push board or broomstick and plastic bag.

Another concern with bison is when they do become panicked and take flight they may not run away from you. While most animals tend to run away or at least shy away and run around you, frightened bison may stampede right over you! In addition, panicked bison also have a tendency to run "blindly" into enclosure walls which can result in injury or death.

50. What are the primary hazards of large carnivores (bears, cats, wolves, etc.)?

The primary hazards are claws, teeth, and strength.

51. If a large carnivore must be handled what type of restraint will most likely be needed?

Chemical restraint.

52. Should an anesthetized large carnivore be physically restrained also?

Yes. This is to avoid an unexpected waking animal from causing injury. The operational plan must take into account this contingency and should include personnel escape routes, methods to regain control of the animal, and removal of any physical restraint devices should re-anesthetizing not be an option.

53. What are the primary hazards of the smaller mammals?

Primary hazards for the smaller mammals are teeth, claws, and for porcupines—quills. While a skunk's spray is mostly an assault on the nose and is not fatal, it can be very irritating to the eyes and should be flushed as soon as possible with copious amounts of water or saline. Zoonotic diseases including rabies, plague, and tularemia should also be considered a potential hazard of smaller mammals. It has been estimated that 40–50% of raccoons carry a zoonotic intestinal parasite called *Baylisascaris procyonis* (raccoon roundworm). This parasite can be extremely harmful or deadly in humans.

54. What are some techniques that can be used to move and capture small mammals?

Most small mammals prefer dark close spaces. To counter the fear of being out in the open, use or place physical barriers such as walls, panels, or boards for the animal to run along. Create darker pathways and provide dark containers such as trash cans, crates, boxes, etc. for them to move into for capture. Brooms may be used to direct or "haze" an animal into a container. Washtubs, buckets etc., can be dropped over an animal and a piece of plywood slid carefully under.

55. List some techniques for handling small mammals.

- Heavy leather gloves are recommended. A note of caution, quills and teeth will penetrate leather gloves.
- Muzzles may be used on foxes and coyotes (see Question #56).
- Except for larger coyotes, catch poles should not be placed around the neck alone. They should be placed over the head AND under one arm. This is to prevent a fatal neck injury or strangulation.
- Scruffing the nape of the neck with one hand, and holding the rear legs with the other hand can effectively restrain some small mammals.
- Coyotes and foxes can be physically restrained using similar techniques to those used on dogs. These include restraining an animal in lateral recumbency, and gaining control of the head. Grabbing an animal's legs is very threatening and these animals will try to bite. Therefore, it is important to neutralize this hazard (i.e., muzzle or chemical restraint) before using certain physical restraint techniques. To restrain an animal in lateral recumbency, stand or kneel at the animal's back; with one arm reach OVER the neck and grab the DOWN front leg; with the other arm reach OVER the flank area of the body and grab the DOWN rear leg. This prevents the animal from being able to roll up into a sternal position and have any leverage to stand. To control the head of a fox or coyote, place yourself to the side or behind a standing/sitting/sternally recumbent animal or along the back of a laterally recumbent animal. Firmly grasp the thick haircoat on either side of the neck.

56. What are some important considerations for using a muzzle?

Every effort should be made to avoid placing a handler/responder in a position where they could be bitten. If a person is bitten, aside from the obvious injury to the responder, that animal (coyotes, foxes, raccoons, skunks, etc.) will likely be euthanatized and tested for rabies; even in circumstances where an animal has reacted appropriately and is simply defending itself. If responders must handle and restrain these animals the use of a muzzle is an added precaution to assure both the responder's and animal's safety. There are certain requirements when using muzzles which include the following:

- An animal should NEVER be muzzled if there is a possibility that the animal could escape and not be recaptured.
- A muzzled animal should NEVER be left unattended.
- If an animal is in respiratory distress or heat stress the ONLY type of muzzle that may be used is an open cage (wire) muzzle. Cloth, leather, or strap muzzles should not be used in these situations.
- Proper sizing of muzzles is important.
- A temporary "field" muzzle may be fashioned out of 2"–4" (5–10 cm) roll gauze, a quick release tourniquet, or a leash.
- Muzzles must be removed immediately if an animal vomits or develops signs of respiratory distress or heat stress. An open cage muzzle may allow an animal to vomit or pant, but common sense must prevail in these situations.

REPTILES, CHELONIA, AND AMPHIBIANS

57. What are Chelonia?

Chelonia are turtles and tortoises. The taxonomy of turtles and tortoises used to have them grouped in with other reptiles such as snakes, lizards, and geckos, but since 2002 they have been separated into their own taxonomic class, Class Chelonia.

58. What are the primary hazards of reptiles, chelonia, and amphibians?

Depending upon the species, primary hazards include venom, constriction, claws, teeth, mouth (chelonia), poisonous or irritating slime, and potential zoonotic disease concerns such as *Salmonella*.

59. Describe what is meant by *ectothermia*, and why is it important to an animal responder?

Reptiles, chelonia, and amphibians rely on the outside temperature to determine their body temperature hence the term *ecto-* referring to outside and *thermia-* referring to temperature. A common phrase used to describe these animals is "cold blooded animals." The term "cold blooded animals" is a misnomer because some of these animals may raise their body temperatures as high as or higher than endothermic animals. Birds and mammals are able to generate heat internally allowing them to maintain a relatively constant body temperature, and are referred to as *endothermic*. (*endo-* meaning "inside"). A common phrase used to describe these animals is "warm blooded animals."

Even though the outside temperature dictates the body temperature of ectothermic animals, this does not mean that they can live in any temperature. In other words, they still must manage their body temperature within a temperature range and they accomplish this by moving into warmer or colder situations as needed. For example snakes, turtles, and lizards will often warm themselves by sunning on a warm rock or log, or cool themselves by moving into the shade or a den during the heat of the day.

This is important to responders as they must consider thermoregulation when handling, containing, and transporting these animals. Hot vehicles, direct sunlight on containers, etc. are hazardous.

60.   What techniques may be used to capture reptiles, turtles, and tortoises?

Many reptiles prefer dark close spaces. A physical barrier such as a panel or board can be used to minimize the exposed "out in the open" feeling and direct their movement. A broom can be used to push the animal along the barrier and effectively haze it into a container. Once in, the container should be quickly covered.

A snake hook can be used to briefly pick up a snake and place it in a container. Snake hooks are sticks approximately 4–5 feet (1.2–1.5 m) long, with a blunt hook on the end. The technique is to place the hook under the middle of the body, and lift the snake quickly off the ground. The snake will balance on the stick for a short period of time. The snake hook can also be used to briefly pin the head of the snake to the ground thereby allowing you to grasp the snake just behind the head. Special long-handled snake tongs with wide flat grips can also be used. Once you have control of the head, your other hand, or someone else, can lift and support the body of the snake. The body should be supported in multiple places to avoid damaging the vertebrae.

Handling venomous species requires special considerations. **Only** experts should participate in the capturing and handling of these animals. A minimum of two people should work together. Antivenin should be on hand and readily available. A medical transport plan to a facility capable of managing an envenomation incident should be in place.

Lizards move very fast, and many species have tails that "break away" when grabbed. Although loss of the tail is not life threatening, it can influence future growth and reproduction by depriving the animal of fat stores. It may also affect the behavior of the animal, and expends one of their lifesaving defense mechanisms. A towel can be used to cover a lizard; allowing you to gently grasp around the body of the lizard.

All turtles and tortoises can bite. Snapping turtles can reach 30–60 pounds (13–27 kg) and can easily remove a finger. Their long necks can reach half-way back along their sides. Most chelonia can be picked up by their shells. Shovels may be useful for scooping up and moving smaller turtles or tortoises. Placing a dark cloth or hood over the eyes of some turtles can help calm them.

61.   What types of containers work well for reptiles and chelonia?

Lizards, snakes, land turtles, and tortoises can be transported in appropriate hard sided containers including trash cans with lids, buckets with lids, or dog and cat carriers for the larger animals. With the exception of venomous species, these animals can also be carried in breathable cloth bags or pillow cases. Venomous species can be placed in cloth bags but the bag must then be placed inside an additional hard sided carrier which is appropriately labeled. Cloth bags can be lightly sprayed with water if needed to help with temperature regulation. Fresh water turtles can be transported in wet bags. Water turtles can be transported in containers that have water with perches, and obviously must have air access.

62.   Discuss the handling and transport of amphibians.

Amphibians, including frogs, toads, and salamanders, have very delicate skin that is easily traumatized from handling. The heat of human hands can be stressful and handling time also has a negative influence on hormone balance. Therefore, any handling of these animals should be kept to a minimum. Skin lotions, insect repellent, sunscreen lotions, etc. are harmful and readily absorbed across the skin of amphibians. If you must handle these animals bare-handed, make sure your hands are clean and wet before touching the animals. In addition to the risk of the handler damaging their skin, amphibians may produce excretions that are irritating or even poisonous to the handler. The wearing of exam gloves when handling amphibians can protect both animal and handler. These gloves should be talc-free and thoroughly rinsed free of all powders. Wet all gloves prior to handling animals to decrease the risk of harming these delicate creatures. Gloves should be changed between species, or between groups of the same species, to prevent inadvertent contamination of individuals.

Because of the delicate nature of their skin, capture of amphibians can be challenging. Nets made of very soft materials are a good choice. Care must be taken to not grasp larval and neotenic salamanders around the head and neck because their gills can be easily damaged. ("*Neotenic*" refers to the prolongation of the larval form in a sexually mature organism.)

Amphibians need to be kept moist with access to air, so transport containers must take this into consideration. For transport, small amphibians can be placed inside a sealed plastic bag with a small amount of water and blown full of air. This also provides some protective cushioning for these small young animals. For larger more mature amphibians, placing damp moss or moistened paper towels in a secure hard sided container, such as a smooth plastic bucket, can work well. Avoid any containers that could be abrasive to their skin. Soft sided wet bags carry the risk of smothering a small amphibian from the weight of the wet cloth. In all cases, these bags and containers must be kept cool and out of direct sunlight.

63. How should one manage Crocodylia (alligators, crocodiles)?

The best way to manage a situation involving Crocodylia is to use a phone and call the experts. . . . "Hello, is this the zoo? . . ."

64. What are special considerations regarding zoo animals impacted by disasters?

Different states have language written into their state disaster response plans that addresses the management of wildlife, zoo, and exotic animals in a disaster. Beyond these official documents outlining disaster response for zoos, and like facilities (such as private wildlife or exotic animal "ranches"), it is important for these individual entities to develop and maintain their own disaster preparedness and response plan, as they are best able to develop detailed plans pertinent to their situation, and can best direct a disaster response that involves them.

Obvious key points regarding zoos (and like facilities), are that they house and contain a wide variety of wild animals in separate enclosures, and different types of disasters impact zoos in different ways. Certain types of disasters may affect some or all of the *animals only,* such as disease outbreaks. Other types of disasters may affect the infrastructure of the zoo resulting in a release of some or all of the animals. We will focus on the latter for discussions here.

All zoos should have in place various plans to manage their most likely disasters. These plans are part of the *preparedness* phase of disasters and do NOT supplant an *operational plan* during a response. Experts should contribute to these plans detailing the capturing, handling, and transporting of all the different species. Options for transport and evacuation destinations should be established. The possibility of sheltering in place and plans to secure and deliver feed and water should also be included. Planning for the disposition of escaped animals might include the following: 1) Under what circumstances would re-capture be an option? 2) What type of equipment, personnel, and drugs might be needed to re-capture different animals? 3) For those animals where re-capture is not an option, standard operating procedures should be established that allow for safe and humane euthanasia.

It is important to have a communication plan that includes not only details regarding communication protocols for the response personnel, but also how information will be disseminated quickly and efficiently to the public both within the zoo and in the surrounding community. These plans should take into consideration variables that could affect the ability to communicate, such as significant damage to the public address equipment, or the possibility of a prolonged loss of power and electricity.

Table-top training exercises and hands-on training exercises should be done periodically, and personnel should do their best to enhance their skills.

65. What governmental act directs response to disasters involving marine mammals?

The Marine Mammal Health and Stranding Response Act addresses unusual mortality events that 1) are unexpected, 2) involve a significant die-off of any marine mammal population, and 3) demands an immediate response.

The National Marine Fisheries Service (NMFS) is responsible for mortality events involving cetaceans (whales and dolphins), and pinnipeds (seals and sea lions, but not walrus), and the U.S. Fish and Wildlife Service (FWS) have responsibility for sea otters, walrus, manatees, and polar bears.

Aside from incidents involving significant numbers of marine mammal deaths within a short period of time, this act also governs response to a (mass) stranding of species of cetaceans, or when an endangered marine mammal species is affected. The contingency plan includes provisions for detecting and responding to these conditions.

66. Who are the first line marine mammal responders?

Networks of volunteers have been authorized by NMFS and FWS to respond to events involving cetaceans, pinnipeds, manatees, and sea otters. In order to participate, members of the Stranding Networks are issued Letters of Authorization by the NMFS Regional Offices. Network members are the first line of response to any marine mammal stranding. (For those who have an interest in participating as a member, these volunteer networks are based out of different areas of the country and are most easily identified by entering "Marine Mammal Stranding Networks" in your computer search engine.)

67. What type of event does NOT follow procedures laid out in the Marine Mammal Health and Stranding Response Act?

According to Summary of the National Contingency Plan for Response to Unusual Marine Mammal Mortality Events (Wilkerson, Dean M., 1996, U.S. Dept. of Commerce, NOAA Tech. Memo, NMFS-OPR-9):

"There is one type of unusual mortality event during which procedures laid out in the Act including responsibilities, appointment of Onsite Coordinators, and funding will not be followed. Responses to oil discharges or releases of hazardous substances are governed by either the Clean Water Act, as amended, the Oil Pollution Act of 1990, or the Comprehensive Environmental Response Compensation and Liability Act. The U.S. Coast Guard has primary responsibility for response to spills and releases within or threatening the coastal zone.

Many of the resources identified for response under the Marine Mammal Health and Stranding Response Act also will be utilized in spill emergencies."

68. What can be done to care for animals affected by oil spills?

Unfortunately oil spills occur all too frequently from mega-disasters like the Exxon Valdez in Alaska, to contamination of land and waterways from tractor/trailer and auto accidents. While we tend to think of oil spills as ocean and coastal events animals living inland may also be exposed to this hazard. Animals contaminated by oil suffer from both external contamination and internal contamination.

Aside from being unable to fly, feathers coated in oil also lose their insulating property placing birds at risk of dying from hypothermia. Animals that rely on a haircoat for insulation such as sea otters, river otters, etc. are also at risk of developing hypothermia when oil coats and destroys the insulating loft. Animals which rely on fat insulation rather than haircoat, such as seals, may not have as great a risk of becoming hypothermic, but like other animals they are vulnerable to the other external effects such as eye irritation, skin irritation, and toxin absorption of oil contamination as well.

Internal contamination can occur through aspiration of the volatile hydrocarbons, and from ingestion, (especially prevalent as these animals attempt to groom themselves clean of the oil, eat their food source contaminated with oil, or nurse on mothers contaminated with oil).

These animals are obviously stressed and debilitated. Treatment and rehabilitation techniques have improved over the last few decades. A mild soap, (Dawn® Dishwashing Liquid is preferred by many), is used to thoroughly clean feathers and haircoat while minimizing additional irritation and trauma to the skin. Activated charcoal is administered orally to absorb ingested toxins, and nutritional support is started as soon as possible. Additional treatment and supportive care for pneumonia, anemia, etc. is implemented as well. Proper holding facilities that minimize additional stress and trauma are vital to the rehabilitation process.

CONTROVERSIES

69. Should individual animals affected by major oil spills be treated?

Some people think that treating individual animals affected by oil disasters is too labor intensive and cost prohibitive to be justified. They believe that the success rate of treating individuals in terms of numbers surviving to be released back to the wild, survival time after release in the wild, and successful reproduction are too low to be considered a viable option. They believe this money and effort would be better spent in other conservation efforts directed towards species as a whole—such as control of introduced species, or banning gill nets, etc. They also argue that rescue, treatment, and rehabilitation efforts create an illusion that these animals are being saved primarily for the purposes of publicity and to appease the public.

Others disagree and support efforts to treat individual animals which have been affected by oil spills. Aside from there being a moral obligation to care for animals affected by our actions or negligence, treating individuals does positively impact conservation efforts. These situations may draw a lot of attention and publicity which in turn helps inform the public and stimulate interest in conservation efforts. In addition, success rates have been improving as techniques improve and this becomes more cost effective over time. Lessons learned in caring for these animals also benefits care of animals in other situations. When endangered species are affected by these disasters saving every individual is important to conservation of that species as a whole.

Recognizing the devastating widespread and long-term consequences of oil spills, it is apparent that implementing conservation principles in support of *both* the individual and the "herd" is important.

70. Should venomous species automatically be euthanatized by animal responders?

Some people feel these animals should be euthanatized whenever they are encountered. Others support euthanasia in a disaster response due to the complexities of dealing with them. Because of the recommendation that only people trained and experienced in handling these animals should interact with them there may be a lack of qualified personnel available to safely capture and transport these animals out of harms way and to a suitable new location.

The other side of the argument is that emergency animal responders are there to help all animals impacted by the disaster. Venomous species are a part of their ecosystem and play an important role in the web of life. If properly trained personnel are available these animals are worthy of our efforts. While the logistics are complicated, the situation should be evaluated before a euthanasia policy is mandated.

71. Is placing snakes in a refrigerator or freezer to cool them down a viable immobilization technique?

This is definitely *not* recommended. However, people very experienced with snakes have used this technique on extremely aggressive individuals that are already captured and in a container, in order to then handle the snake. Placing the container with the snake in a refrigerator, for an appropriate length of time, slows the snake down, thereby enabling a handler to use other techniques (tongs, manual restraint, tubes, or chemical restraint) to secure control of the snake.

Cooling a snake—or any ectotherm—is NOT a substitute for appropriate analgesia and/or anesthesia.

Suggested Reading

American Veterinary Medical Association. The AVMA *Disaster Preparedness and Response Guide* can be accessed via their website at http://avma.org and clicking the link "Disaster Preparedness" under *Public Resources—Animal Health,* and then the link AVMA Disaster Preparedness and Response Guide.

Fowler M. *Restraint and Handling of Wild and Domestic Animals,* 3rd ed. Ames, IA, Wiley-Blackwell, 2008.

Global Wildlife Resources, Inc., PO Box 10248, Bozeman, MT 59719–0248; 406–586–4624; http://www.wildliferesources.org/index.html. This is a company that teaches hands-on courses in chemical restraint for wildlife.

Mullineaux E, Best R, Cooper J. *British Small Animal Veterinary Association Manual of Wildlife Casualties.* Ames, IA, Blackwell Publishing, 2003.

National Marine Fisheries Service. Available at http://www.nmfs.noaa.gov.

National Wildlife Health Center; 608–270–2400; http://www.nwhc.usgs.gov.

Safe-Capture International, Inc., PO Box 206, Mount Horeb, WI 53572; 608–767–3071; email: safecaptur@aol.com; www.safecapture.com. This company teaches hands-on courses in chemical immobilization of animals.

U.S. Fish and Wildlife Service. Available at http://www.fws.gov.

West G, Heard D, Caulkett N. *Zoo Animal and Wildlife Immobilization and Anesthesia.* Ames, IA, Blackwell Publishing, 2007.

CHAPTER 1.17
DOMESTIC ANIMAL HANDLING

Sally B. Palmer, DVM

Many different types of domestic animals are encountered in a disaster response. From an agricultural perspective in the United States, there are 90 million beef cattle, 10 million dairy cattle, 10 million sheep, 60 million hogs, and 8 billion poultry. This industry translates into 13% of our gross domestic product and 17% of all employment. In terms of companion animals, it is estimated that there are 72 million pet dogs and 82 million pet cats in the United States. It is clear from these numbers that when disasters affect our domestic animals, they affect not only our food sources and economy but also vital "members of the family." Animal disaster responders must have a solid understanding and comfort level in dealing with a wide variety of domestic animals that may be encountered in an emergency or disaster response.

1. What is the most important consideration when handling animals?

The most important consideration is *safety*. When handling animals, the safety of the responder/handler, the owner, any assistants, all bystanders, AND the safety of the animals is paramount. Understanding the behavior of a species and recognizing their primary hazards (teeth, claws, hooves, horns, strength, etc.) can contribute greatly to the safety of a situation.

It goes without saying that there is an inherent risk of injury when working with animals. Whenever discussions or recommendations are made with regard to handling, moving, or restraining animals, it is worth stating that different people have different talents, instincts, and levels of experience. Recommendations suitable for one person may not work for someone else, or what works in one setting may not work in another setting. In other words, recognize your limitations and use your *own* best judgment when dealing with animals, as you are ultimately responsible for your own safety.

2. How does understanding the behavior of different species facilitate their handling and improve safety?

Understanding the behavior of a species is the cornerstone to moving, capturing, and handling different groups of animals safely and effectively. Operations can be planned and executed based on how animals are likely to react. Once engaged with an animal or group of animals, responders with a good grasp of behavior will recognize behavioral cues and be able to anticipate an animal's reaction. Behavioral clues include facial expressions (lips tight or pulled back, teeth barred, fearful dilated eyes, etc.), ear positions, head and body position, vocalizations, and body movement. Having an appreciation for how an animal perceives your actions, and the likely reaction, allows a responder to alter his or her approach or plan if need be so as to not endanger the animal or himself or herself (Fig. 1.17.1).

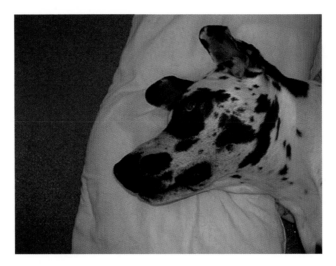

Figure 1.17.1 Note how this dog is keeping a wary eye on you as you move to assist him. Be careful and move slowly.

3. What is the "fight or flight" reaction?

As discussed in Chapter 1.16, when an animal perceives a threat, real or imagined, the instinct is to either flee from the threat (flight) or fight the threat. The sympathetic nervous system releases various catacholamines, such as epinephrine (adrenalin), to kick in a booster of strength, speed, and quickened reaction times. This instinct is not restricted to wild animals but is present in domestic animals (and people) as well. Most animals will flee from a threat if given the option, but some animals—especially some domestic animals (dogs or mothers with young)—are more apt to fight.

4. How might different domestic animals be categorized?

Domestic animals may be divided into categories in any number of ways. For our purposes, these categories are not meant to be absolute and definitive; rather they are simply one way to organize and discuss domestic animal handling. Two broad categories that we will start with are *companion animals* and *livestock animals*. Again, these designations are not absolute and certainly many "livestock" animals can be "companion" animals, and in different cultures some "companion" animals are considered "livestock." Some designations do have legal implications, so proper terminology may be more that just a matter of semantics. As an example, horses are legally/technically livestock animals, but many people relate to them as companion animals. For our discussion, companion animals include the following:

- Dogs
- Cats
- Pocket pets such as rabbits, guinea pigs, hamsters, ferrets, gerbils, mice, rats, sugar gliders, hedgehogs, etc.
- Birds such as Psitticines (parakeets, cockatiels, cockatoos, parrots, macaws, etc.) and passerines (canaries, finches, etc.) (see also Chapter 1.16)
- Reptiles, Chelonia (turtles and tortoises), and Amphibians (see also Wildlife Handling Chapter)
- Fish

Livestock animals include the following:

- Cattle
- Sheep

- Goats
- Swine
- Horses
- Llamas and alpacas
- Poultry (chickens, turkeys, ducks, pheasant, quail, etc.)
- Emus and ostriches (see Chapter 1.16)

5. List some types of equipment that may be helpful to capture, handle, or transport companion animals.

- Leashes
- Catch poles
- Nets (various sizes of poles and mesh); fishnets work well
- Gloves
- Carriers/kennels
- Muzzles
- Blankets or towels
- Sturdy cloth or mesh bags
- Long-handled (cat) tongs
- Specially designed "cat bags" that encompass the trunk and legs but allow access to parts of the cat as needed
- Stretchers
- Snake hooks or snake tongs
- Food treats
- Polyethylene/plastic bags for transporting fish
- Coolers for transporting fish
- Ice packs to help maintain proper temperature
- Oxygen cylinders and regulators for transporting fish

6. List some types of equipment that may be helpful to handle or transport livestock animals.

- Halters
- Lead ropes
- Stud chains
- Twitches
- Lariats
- Soft cotton ropes
- Nose tongs
- Swine snout snares
- Push boards—partial sheets of plywood
- Sorting sticks (4–5-feet/1.2–1.5-m long poles that "extend" your reach and assist in guiding animals to move in a desired direction)
- Tarps or web fencing
- Corral panels (can be used to create an enclosure or an alley way or a temporary squeeze chute)
- Cattle chutes (squeeze chutes and head catch)
- Stock trailers
- Food treats, salt blocks
- Cattle prods are frequently misused and therefore NOT recommended.
- A WELL TRAINED dog can be invaluable. (Needless to say, a poorly trained dog is less than helpful.)

7. What are some general principles that can help calm animals and decrease their stress levels?

- Speak in calm, relaxed tones and avoid shouting or loud noises. This is important whether you are speaking to a particular animal or talking with other people in the vicinity of animals. In a hectic disaster or sheltering environment, responders and handlers know the animals around them are anxious and stressed and will usually speak quietly to them, but they may inadvertently raise their voices to shout something to a coworker, forgetting that the animals are taking in the whole environment.
- Avoid prolonged direct eye contact, as this is very threatening. You do not like a stranger staring at you, and neither do animals.
- Avoid cornering or backing an animal into a space where he or she feels trapped. If possible, allow the animal to come to you. Sometimes pausing in your approach or maybe even taking a step back will settle an animal so that the animal will come to you.
- When a flight option is NOT available, avoid facing an animal head-on. In a situation where they feel cornered or trapped, even if you are not actively moving towards them but simply facing them directly, this is still very threatening. Standing face on also tends to result in making more direct eye contact (or appearing to make direct eye contact) creating an even more threatening situation for the animal. Aside from possibly triggering a fight response, it significantly raises their overall level of stress.

    Changing your body position so that your side is to them is much less threatening. This holds true if you kneel down to encourage a small animal to come to you; kneel so more of your side is exposed to them rather than facing the animal directly.
- If you must corner an animal to capture him, recognize that the animal may take drastic measures to escape from you, such as attempting to jump a barrier or bolting over you. The other response may be one of fight and aggression, including biting, clawing, turning to kick, or striking (kicking with front feet). In these situations, a risk-to-benefit analysis should be done to assess whether the benefit of the capture is worth the risk of injury or death to the animal or responder.
- Whenever possible, approach animals from the side, front quarter, or rear quarter. Avoid approaching an animal head-on as this is generally threatening and tends to result in the animal turning or pulling away. In an open field, you may walk toward the front of an animal, and then change your direction so that before you breach his personal space ("safety zone"), you are then approaching him from his front quarter. In this situation, even though you are facing him head-on as you approach, as you get closer you have changed your path to one that is less threatening and challenging to the animal.

    Because most animals have a blind spot directly behind them, approaching directly from the rear can be very frightening to them; it also places the handler at risk of being kicked.
- Talk to an animal as you approach and periodically pause to allow an animal to adjust to your presence.
- Avoid bringing your hand over the top of the head of some animals (dogs especially) as this is a threatening gesture. If possible, bring your hand up from below.
- It is important to move quietly and calmly, yet deliberately. Just as important is to not overdo this and give an impression of stalking. Stalking is very unsettling to animals.
- Not infrequently, in an effort to move a herd of animals more quickly (especially in an alleyway or corral and pens, or even when trying to load a reluctant animal in a trailer), people will begin to raise their voices and become more aggressive in their actions, *excessively* poking, prodding, and slapping animals to push them. This is frequently where cattle prods are misused. *Overly* aggressive shouting, poking, etc., is often counterproductive as animals become more stressed and more agitated and reluctant to move. If a situation appears to be escalating and the temperament of the herd (or in the case of trailer loading, the individual animal) is changing, it is best to regroup the team of responders, allow the animal(s) to calm if possible, and/or reassign those individuals who cannot appreciate the subtleties of working with livestock.
- Recognize that herd animals like to be in a herd, meaning that individuals do not want to be separated or isolated from the herd. Having one or more herd-mates nearby is calming and frequently makes handling a single individual much easier.
- Mothers tend to be very protective of their young. As a matter of safety, responders must be aware that a mother may be more aggressive than normal.
- Responders can also use a mother's devotion to her young to move these animals. Often it is easier to move a mother by moving her young. Directing foals and calves, or picking up the young and carrying them (such as

lambs, kids, and puppies, or even placing calves in a trailer and driving slowly), frequently results in the mothers following. This is a two-fold benefit: the babies and the mothers are being moved. To facilitate the loading of mares and foals or cows and calves into a trailer, it is often easiest to load the foals/calves, and the mares/cows will readily follow.

Trying to do the opposite—move babies by moving mothers—is usually *much* more difficult and stressful. Most mothers do not want to leave their young, so they will not move the way you want them to if it means leaving their baby or babies, and some babies are not very good at following their mothers. The end result is that the babies are not moving in the desired direction and the mother is trying to get to her baby and is not moving in the desired direction.

- Understanding basic herding principles can decrease stress levels. Animals tend to move away from you, so changing your position relative to theirs will guide and direct them. While this is a very basic principle, many people will inadvertently place themselves in the wrong position or move into an inappropriate position. Understanding this basic principle also allows responders to anticipate the animals' movement.

8. What are some different types of muzzles?

Muzzles can be made out of cloth, leather, metal (thick wire), or plastic cages. In addition to cloth muzzles specifically designed to fit the face of a cat, there is an Air Muzzle Restraint device, which is a clear plastic globe that encircles the cat's (or small brachycephalic [short-nosed] dog's) head. While technically not a muzzle, Elizabethan collars (E-collars), which are thick plastic cones placed over an animal's head, may offer some protection from being bitten.

"Field" muzzles can be fashioned out of leashes wrapped around a dog's muzzle, quick-release rubber tourniquets tightened around a muzzle, or 2- to 4-inch (5- to 10-cm) roll gauze (Figs. 1.17.2 through 1.17.4). A length of gauze approximately 6 feet (1.8 m) long is doubled in half for added strength. An overhand knot is made in the middle of this gauze to hold the lengths of gauze together, and this adds just a bit of weight to what will be the bottom of the loop. Another overhand knot creates a loop that is a couple of inches (5 cm) larger in diameter than the diameter of the dog's muzzle. This loop is slipped over the muzzle and tightened. It should be tight enough that the dog cannot open his mouth to bite you, but not overly tight as this becomes very painful very quickly. The lengths of gauze now pass under the muzzle and another overhand knot is placed here under the jaw; finally, the ends are brought around the back of the neck and tied in a bow to allow for a quick release.

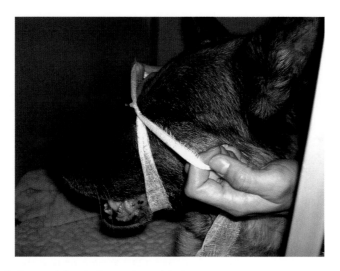

Figure 1.17.2 Gauze is applied around the dog's muzzle and tied.

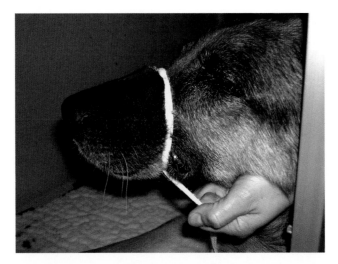

Figure 1.17.3 Gauze is then wrapped under the muzzle and again tied snuggly.

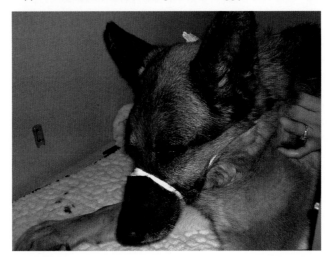

Figure 1.17.4 The gauze strip is then brought behind the ears and tied in a bow knot that can be quickly undone should the dog begin to vomit and the muzzle needs to be quickly removed.

9. What should be considered when using a muzzle?

- Muzzles are frequently used on aggressive dogs and cats. A muzzle may also be placed when moving or examining an injured animal, even a docile or friendly one, as pain or anticipation of pain may cause that animal to bite.
- Animals should NEVER be muzzled if there is a possibility that they could escape and not be recaptured.
- The muzzled animal should NEVER be left unattended.
- Muzzles should NOT be left in place for extended periods of time. Muzzles are to be used to allow animals to be handled and then they should be removed. Wire-cage muzzles are sometimes left in place for longer periods, but the caveat remains that a muzzled animal should never be left unattended.
- If it is hot, dogs and cats need to open-mouth breathe to cool themselves; therefore, do **NOT** place muzzles that restrict their ability to do this; for dogs, a wire cage muzzle is preferred. If another type of muzzle must be placed on an animal in these conditions it should be for an extremely short period of time only—to lift them, draw blood, etc., and then promptly removed.
- If an animal is in respiratory distress or heat stress, the **ONLY** type of muzzle that may be used is one that allows the animal to open-mouth pant and breathe. Again, a wire cage muzzle is preferred as there is better

airflow than plastic cage muzzles. The Air Muzzle Restraint may also work for small dogs, brachycephalic dogs, or cats, but because it wraps around the face, it may not allow the necessary airflow for these distressed animals. These animals need to be monitored closely, and the muzzles removed if necessary.
- Cloth and leather muzzles should be properly sized.
- Muzzles should be removed **IMMEDIATELY** if an animal vomits.

DOGS

10. What is the primary hazard of dogs?

The primary hazard is their teeth, but claws and strength should be considered (secondary) hazards as well (Fig. 1.17.5).

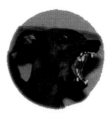

Figure 1.17.5 The teeth of an angry or scared dog can cause serious injury.

11. What are some behavioral characteristics of dogs of which an animal responder should be aware?

Many dogs behave as protectors of their "territory"—home, yard, ranch, vehicle, etc. Dogs may so aggressively defend an area that rescuing a dog from their environment can be difficult, especially when an owner is not present.

In disaster/rescue situations, many dogs are stressed and afraid, and they may perceive a responder as just one more threat. Often, stress and fear manifest as aggression.

Responders who understand why a dog may be behaving aggressively can try different techniques to calm, reassure, and secure a dog from the scene. Since the first rule of animal handling is safety, some techniques are *not* appropriate (such as kneeling down with an aggressive 150-lb [70-kg] Presa Canario) if they place you at risk for injury. Each situation is different and a responder must decide what attempts are reasonable. Techniques may include the following: speaking calmly; positioning yourself with the dog off of your side rather than facing them directly; kneeling down, again oriented such that the dog is off to your side; using the dog's name; offering food treats; and avoiding trapping him in a corner or small area.

12. If a dog remains aggressive, what options are available to a responder?

If an animal remains aggressive, then a responder may have to proceed with a capture and restraint using a catch pole or net (depending on the size of the dog), gloves, and muzzles. Capture or catch poles are approximately 6 feet (1.8 m) long with a loop of cable or rope on the end. This pole allows the handler to place the loop around the dog's neck and tighten this "collar." The pole maintains this safe distance from the animal and allows the handler to move and direct the dog (Fig. 1.17.6). Care must be taken to not choke the animal. Animals should NOT be lifted with the catch pole. For very large dogs, two catch poles may be needed (one person on each side) to overcome the dog's strength and effectively direct his movement.

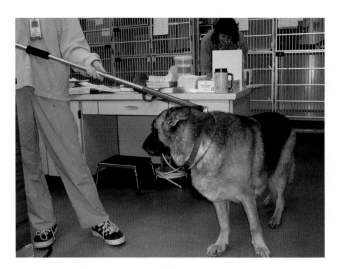

Figure 1.17.6 Use of a catch pole to handle a large dog.

13. How should dogs be lifted?

Proper lifting techniques vary with the size and temperament of the dog. Dogs that are apt to bite (afraid, aggressive, or injured) should have a muzzle placed prior to lifting. If a muzzle is not an option (heat stress, respiratory distress, vomiting, head or facial trauma, etc.), then the head should be controlled in such a way as to protect the face of the handler. A second or third person may be needed to control the head.

For smaller dogs, the person lifting may be able to scruff the back of the neck with one hand and reach *over* the dog with the other hand so as to lift primarily with this hand under the chest and body.

Slightly bigger dogs can also be lifted by one person scruffing the neck, but rather than reaching *over* the dog, the handler uses their other arm to scoop and lift under the abdomen while picking up the front end with the scruff. There is a bit of momentum used in this lift with the scoop.

Medium-size and large dogs can be cradled with one arm around the front of the chest and the other around behind the haunches. An alternative to this lift is to place one arm around the front of the chest and the other arm under the abdomen. For some dogs with degenerative joint disease of the hips and spine, this may be a more comfortable lift for them. With either of these lifts, the hand cradling the front can reach around and hold the back of the neck in order to control the head somewhat, but recognize that the handler's face is still at risk of being bitten. To further minimize the risk, the handler should turn his/her head to face the tail and move his/her head closer to the spine of the dog. While doing these things may decrease the risk of being bitten, it must be noted that the handler's head and face are still in danger (Fig. 1.17.7).

If two people are available, one person can control the head by grasping the thick fur or skin on either side of the neck while the other person lifts the dog.

For large and giant breed dogs, two people should lift, with a third person controlling the head as above. When two people lift, it is best for them to both be on the same side. One person lifts the chest with one arm around the front and the other arm scooping underneath the chest (again, this person's head and face is at risk of being bitten). The other person lifts the rear with one arm scooping under the abdomen and the other arm wrapped around behind the haunches. If a third person is available to control the head, they will be on the opposite side of the dog. The lift should be coordinated with ONE person giving the count. Clarify how the count relates to the lift—in other words, if you say "lift on 3," does this mean "1–2–3–lift" or "1–2–lift"?

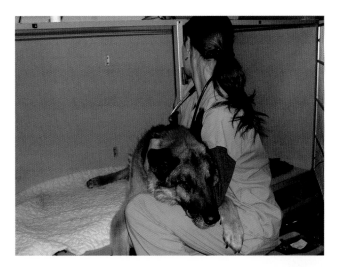

Figure 1.17.7 When preparing to lift a large breed dog, turn your face away from the dog's head to protect yourself from being bitten.

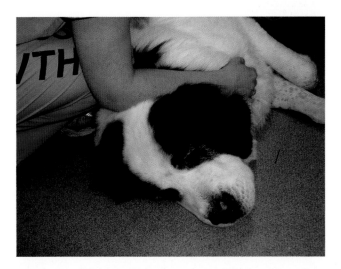

Figure 1.17.8 Restraining a large dog in a lateral position is best done by placing your forearm over the dog's neck and grasping the lower (down) fore- and hindlimb.

14. What are some methods to manually restrain dogs?

Manually restraining a dog that is standing may be as simple as holding his collar (or snubbing up on the leash) to prevent him from moving off and using your other hand along the side or under the abdomen to keep him standing and in place. For a dog in sternal recumbency (lying on his chest), holding his collar with one hand and placing your other hand on his lumbar spine area may be all that is needed.

To restrain a dog's head in a standing, sitting, or sternally recumbent position, stand to the side or behind him facing the *same* direction as the dog. Grasp the thick fur (or loose skin) on either side of the neck. The hold should be firm and capable of holding tightly if the dog tries to bite, but not so tight as to cause pain that would stimulate the dog to bite.

To manually restrain a dog in lateral recumbancy (lying on the dog's side), place yourself on the dorsal side of the dog (on the side of the dog's back). Place one arm OVER the shoulder/neck and take hold of the DOWN front leg; place your other arm OVER the flank and take hold of the DOWN rear leg. This restraint hold takes away his leverage by preventing the animal from rolling into a sternal position and being able to get his legs underneath himself to stand (Fig. 1.17.8).

266   Domestic Animal Handling

CATS

15. What are the primary hazards of cats?

The primary hazards are teeth and claws (Figs. 1.17.9 and 1.17.10).

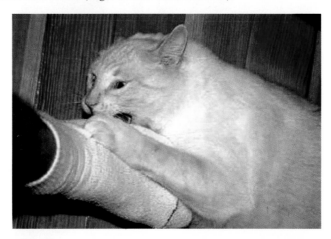

Figure 1.17.9 Cats often use both teeth and claws to protect themselves.

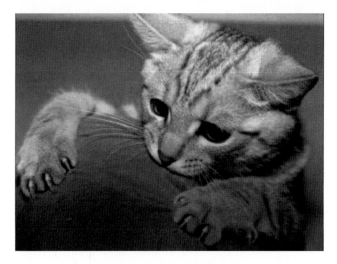

Figure 1.17.10 Cat claws are sharp and can be used as weapons of self-defense.

16. How can one minimize the risk of being bitten and/or scratched?

Maintain a calm quiet environment. Avoid handling a cat if there are loud disruptive noises such as shouting, sirens, barking dogs, etc. Avoid trying to handle cats where they can see (unfamiliar) dogs or other (unfamiliar) cats.

Unlike many dogs, which will calm in the presence of their owner, a fractious cat is unlikely to settle down until left alone in a secure quiet environment.

Whenever possible, allow the cat to come to you, whether coming out of a carrier, in a building, or outside. "Ignoring" a kitty is sometimes an effective technique to get him to come to you (although he will never admit to falling for this reverse psychology!).

Reaching into a carrier can be very threatening, triggering the "fight" response of a cornered animal. Some cat-carriers have a top zipper or door, and many cats (and other animals as well) prefer to be removed from a carrier this way. Some carriers can be taken apart, and the top half removed. Although this takes extra time, it may be well worth it and more efficient in the long run.

Wearing heavy leather or Kevlar gloves or throwing a blanket over the cat can help protect your hands and forearms from being bitten and scratched but know that cats can bite through these protective barriers, so care should still be exercised (Fig. 1.17.11).

Muzzles specifically designed for cats can protect a handler from being bitten (Fig. 1.17.12).

Long-handled tongs can be used to grasp a cat around the torso. These cat tongs are best used as a pinning device to allow a handler to get hold of the cat, or they can be used to pull the cat on a smooth surface toward the handler. They should not be used for picking up a cat.

Breathable cloth or mesh bags can be used to hold a cat for transport.

A fishnet can be an excellent tool to capture a fractious cat. Those who are good with a net are quite adept at catching cats and "flipping" the net to keep the cat inside, carrying them safely, and then transferring them to a more secure carrier.

A catch pole can be used on cats but is less than ideal and should be considered **as a last resort**. Cats do not react well to this type of restraint and are at risk of breaking their necks. If a catch pole is used, it should be looped behind *one* front leg; you do not want the loop to encircle just the neck or just the trunk. Again, this is not a lifting device. It should be used to briefly restrain the cat, allowing another handler to move in and gain control. This should ONLY be used by someone very skilled with a catch pole and knowledgeable about cats and cat behavior.

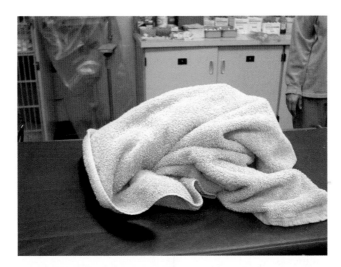

Figure 1.17.11 Throwing a blanket or towel over a cat will sometimes calm the cat enough to allow one to apply restraint. Be careful. Cat teeth and claws can still penetrate these items.

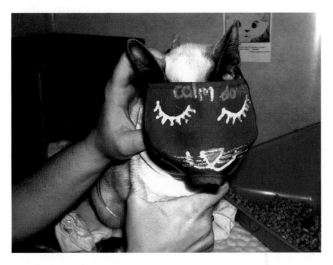

Figure 1.17.12 A cloth muzzle applied to a fractious cat.

17. What is a good secure way to hold and carry a cat?

A good way to hold and carry a cat that is comfortable and easy on the cat, but is also safe and secure, is to pick up the cat with one arm supporting the chest and holding the cat's body into your side. Your upper arm crosses the flank and helps trap the cat's body to yours with the hind legs "free." The hand of this arm holds the two front feet by interdigitating the fingers with the cat's forearms. Your other hand rests lightly on the scruff but can grab the scruff if needed. Many cats relax completely in this position, and for those who become a little fractious this hold will also safely restrain them.

If a cat becomes explosively fractious, this hold can quickly be modified to a more severe temporary hold that "stretches" the cat, effectively immobilizing him long enough to place him in some type of cage, carrier, or enclosed room. The one hand is in position to scruff the neck and lift from this point and the body support arm changes from supporting the trunk and holding the front legs to grasping and controlling the rear legs, again interdigitating your fingers with the legs at the level of the hock.

There is a tendency to hold cats by scooping them up primarily around the chest and then holding their body against the front of your body without taking proper control of the front legs. In this position, the cat may roll and get his claws into your clothing, which gives him the leverage to climb and push away from you. Often the handler is left grasping the middle of the cat's body and holding them out in space while trying to detach the claws from their clothes and not get scratched or bitten.

18. What are some behavioral characteristics of cats that make them challenging for disaster responders?

Cats are very sensitive and cautious animals. They will most often hide when frightened. It can be very challenging to find where a cat may be hiding in a home or building. They will not come when called and are less food oriented than some other animals. Hiding places tend to be dark and/or difficult for a human to access, such as under furniture or even up in furniture (box springs being a popular hideaway), behind appliances, in closets, etc. In addition, cats that move from their hiding space when confronted tend to flee to another equally difficult place for a human to access. Cats that do not take flight often feel trapped and may resort to the fight response.

Another challenge for responders is caring for these rescued cats. Cats tend to be very routine-oriented animals, and when their lives are disrupted they can suffer medically as well. Cats that are stressed may not eat, placing them at risk for developing a serious liver condition called hepatic lipidosis; other cats, when stressed, may groom excessively, causing significant skin irritation. Responders must have an appreciation for the nature of cats and strive to provide a calm environment.

POCKET PETS

19. What is a pocket pet?

Pocket pets tend to be small mammals. This grouping can include rats, mice, guinea pigs, gerbils, and rabbits, as well as ferrets, sugar gliders, hedgehogs, and other exotics.

20. What are some behavioral generalities of pocket pets?

Most pocket pets prefer to be within enclosed spaces, or have ready access to a secure "den." Many of these animals are "prey" animals so they prefer to not be exposed out in the open.

Responders can use this to their advantage if they have to capture loose pocket pets. Containers can be placed at the end of walls or boards and an animal hazed along the security of the barrier into the container. A towel can be dropped over a small mammal to facilitate capture, and nets can also be used.

21. What is the best way to transport and handle pocket pets?

Moving these animals in their own cage is best. The cage is familiar to them and will have needed items such as water bottles and "den" shelters. Taking them in their own cage also minimizes the risk of escape during transfer to another cage.

If you must transfer them, make sure that they are awake so as not to startle them upon handling. Many of these small mammals are nocturnal, so waking them gently will help minimize stress.

Leather gloves can be worn to protect one's hands from their primary hazard, which are teeth, and in the case of hedgehogs—spines.

For the smaller pocket pets (gerbils, hamsters, mice, rats, etc.), it is best to hold and support the body with one hand while cupping your other hand over the head to prevent him from wiggling or jumping out of your grasp. Do **NOT** pick up rats by their tails.

Mice may be caught and lifted by their tails (hold between the midpoint and base of the tail) for a short transfer to another surface or container. Heavy or pregnant mice should not be lifted by their tails alone but should have their bodies supported as well. Mice should not be dropped into a cage, as they may suffer spinal fractures. Mice placed on a surface may be restrained by holding their tails. For the more talented handler, the head can be restrained by scruffing the skin on the neck and shoulders between thumb and index (with or without middle) finger (done quickly to avoid being bitten), and restraining the tail and rear legs with the third and little finger of the same hand.

Rabbits can be scruffed like a cat, but they must have their back legs fully supported into their body and restrained from kicking. Rabbits can kick out so explosively that they will break their back. Rabbits should NEVER be lifted by their ears.

Relaxed, frequently handled ferrets can be picked up with one hand supporting under their chest and the other cradling the back legs. Scruffing a ferret can be an effective technique to immobilize a ferret; many will completely relax when picked up by the scruff of the neck.

Chinchillas are very quick and skitterish and can administer a bad bite. They can be scruffed to decrease the bite risk, while supporting their body with the other hand.

BIRDS

22. What type of pet birds may be encountered by disaster responders?

The two main groups of pet birds are passerines and psitticines. Passerines are songbirds such as canaries and finches, and psitticines include parakeets, cockatiels, cockatoos, lovebirds, conures, parrots, macaws, etc. (For a more complete discussion on capture and restraint techniques of psitticines, see the avian section of Chapter 1.16.)

23. List things a responder should be aware of when handling, housing, or transporting passerines and psitticines.

- Birds do not have a diaphragm; rather they move their sternum (breast bone) to draw air into their lungs, much like a bellows. When handling and restraining birds, one must be careful to not restrict this movement or a bird will suffocate.
- Birds can stress very easily, and some will die suddenly from this stress. This sudden death has been attributed to a condition called *capture myopathy.* (See Chapter 1.16 for a more thorough discussion of capture myopathy.) It is important for responders to be aware of this possibility when handling, holding, and transporting birds and to minimize stress. This includes gentle and appropriate restraint, housing birds out of sight (and sound, if possible) of other animals, transporting and housing birds in a proper temperature. Even though many of these birds are tropical birds, *they can heat stress very easily* if in too warm a vehicle or placed in direct sunlight on hot days. Be aware of the changing position of the sun in sheltering situations.

- The primary hazard of psitticines is their beak. The larger birds can deliver a severe bite. When placing your hand near a psittacine, it is best to make a fist with your thumb tucked inside. It is difficult to gently and properly restrain these birds wearing gloves, and the bite of larger birds can still be very crushing even through a glove. A towel is usually more helpful.
- Passerine song birds really do not have any primary hazards that could be dangerous to responders (other than perhaps possible zoonotic diseases). When handling these birds, there is no need to protect yourself against physical injury, so the primary focus is to not stress or injure them. A lightweight towel thrown over these birds or a net may be used for the initial capture. Holding these delicate birds can be difficult because they are very nimble but fragile. People trained in banding birds use specific holds to secure these birds while working on their legs. Most responders will be engaged in trying to capture a loose bird and/or move it a short distance into a carrier. One general type of hold that works well is to very gently wrap one hand around the body from the back, to prevent the wings from flapping, and lightly encircle the neck with thumb and index finger to prevent it from jumping forward out of your hand. Simultaneously, as you lift the bird, your other hand is cupped over the head and supports the bird from underneath. Basically, your hands are a mini-cage restraining the bird rather than holding the bird.
- Whenever possible, transport a bird in its own cage. Moving the entire cage is ideal, but bird cages that house birds appropriately tend to be quite large (a minimum of five times their wing span) and may not be moveable. If a travel cage is available, this can be used for transport and as temporary housing.
- It is important to realize that all these different birds are truly different species with different nutritional requirements and different reactions to medications and drugs. While we readily grasp that mammalian species are very different in this regard, we must raise our awareness that avian species are, too.

FISH

24. What is the best way to transport fish?

You may be able to transport fish in their own tank if the container is small enough; it is not uncommon for people to keep goldfish or betas in smaller tanks, bowls, or "vases." Remember that fresh water weighs 8 lb (3.6 kg)/gal and 62.4 lb (28.4 kg)/cubic foot, and salt water weighs 64 lb (29 kg)/cubic foot, so be aware of how heavy these aquariums may be. These tanks should be placed inside a protective box (a cardboard box reinforced with packing tape will work) or a cooler to avoid breakage and to decrease light. The tanks or bowls may need a temporary cover during transport to prevent spillage. Because oxygen diffuses into the water at the surface, temporary tank covers should not be left in place for any length of time, and if transport times are extended, they may need to be removed periodically.

If it is not feasible to move the entire tank, the fish will need to be transferred into plastic bags and placed in a protective box or cooler for transport. Polyethylene bags are used to ship koi and are available from koi dealers. Pet stores that sell fish will also have plastic transport bags, but Ziplocs will work in an emergency. Equipment for capture and transport of fish includes the following: appropriately sized clear plastic bags; cup, pitcher, or bucket; rubber bands; nets; protective containers such as cardboard boxes reinforced with shipping tape or coolers; ice packs; and, ideally, an E-cylinder oxygen tank with a regulator and hose.

It is best to use the water from the fishes' tank or pond. Netting fish frequently stimulates bowel evacuation and stirs up debris, which diminishes the water quality, so whenever possible transfer water from the tank or pond into all the bags *first*, before attempting to net the fish. A cup or pitcher can be used to carefully transfer the water, or the bags can be lowered into the water for filling. Either way, it is important to minimize clouding the water. The water and fish should take up approximately 20% of the bag with the remaining volume filled with air. Because these bags do not have the benefit of a tank aerator, they rely on oxygen diffusion at the surface. It would be ideal to replace the air (21% oxygen) with 100% oxygen, but this may not be feasible in a disaster situation. However, small portable oxygen "E" cylinders are available (home medical equipment/service companies, etc.), so it may be possible to secure this equipment. Remember to also have a regulator for the cylinder. As an aside, a wrench may be needed to open the tank valve when secured to the regulator. Once the bag is filled with air (oxygen), secure the top with a thick rubber band. For added safety, these bags should be double-bagged and placed in a protective container to decrease light, temperature, and trauma. Fish are ectotherms ("cold-blooded"), relying on environmental temperature to control their body temperature; thus, water temperatures during transport must be closely monitored. Ice packs, car air conditioners, or other cooling devices should be used to maintain the appropriate temperature of the water.

Minimizing time and stress in capture and transport is important. Working in teams is ideal and allows for two nets to facilitate capture, with another team member standing ready with the bags. An additional team member should be assigned to take the bags to the vehicle to place in the protective carrier.

25. What is the best way to capture fish?

The best way to capture fish is with a net. Depending on the size of the tank/pond and fish, two nets may be used: one to calmly shepherd a fish into the other. Fish should be netted head first as they are much too quick to scoop them from behind. "Chasing" a fish from behind not only adds greatly to their stress but also can result in the fish jumping out of the water and possibly the tank or pond, leading to injury. If fish are bagged after a prolonged chase, their increased respiratory rate will decrease the oxygen content of the water very quickly. Note on the bags if this is a risk. In general, bigger fish are easier to net than are smaller fish, and the fewer fish that remain in a tank or pond, the more room they have to evade capture.

Once fish are captured and readied for transport, the next consideration is destination. Appropriate tank/pond systems need to be in place with attention to water quality, filtration systems, temperature, etc. Floating the bags in the new system to acclimatize the water temperatures is important, and finally, rolling down the edge of the bag to mix the two waters further readies the fish for release. As fish are added, the water quality and filtration need to be closely monitored to avoid overwhelming the new system.

REPTILES, CHELONIA (TURTLES AND TORTOISES), AND AMPHIBIANS

(Also see Chapter 1.16.)

26. What are some special considerations when handling and transporting these animals?

These animals are *ectotherms*, meaning they rely on the outside temperature to control their body temperature. While these animals rely on the outside temperature, this does not mean that they can survive in any temperature. Maintaining a proper temperature range is very important. Different species have different temperature requirements. As a general rule, avoid placing containers in direct sunlight and be cognizant of overheating in cars, closed buildings, etc.

27. What is the best way to transport pet reptiles, chelonia, and amphibians?

Whenever possible, transport them in their own cages. If this is not possible, transfer them to a container appropriate for the species. (See Chapter 1.16 for capture, handling, and transport details.)

CATTLE, SHEEP, AND GOATS

28. What are the primary hazards of cattle, sheep, and goats?

The primary hazards of cattle are horns, head, feet, and strength. With or without horns, cattle will use their heads to knock down a handler. Their necks are very strong and they can swing their heads to the side or up into a handler, or lower their head to charge. Cattle can kick backward and are quite good at kicking out to the side, sometimes referred to as "cow kicking." They tend to bring their rear leg up to their belly and then sweep it out to the side, so if you are examining an animal from the side, be aware of this talent. From a standing position, cattle may not kick as high out behind as a horse, but they can kick high enough. Cattle are very strong. Do not place your hands or arms between the animal and a solid object such as a head catch or coral panel. If your limb is caught between hard horn, bone, or hoof and solid wood or metal, serious injury may occur.

The primary hazards of sheep and goats tend to be the horns of the rams and bucks. These animals may charge, usually when a handler is not paying attention, and while not usually life-threatening they can cause serious injury. While not as serious as the bite from some other animals, goats will also bite.

29. What are some behavioral characteristics or cattle, sheep, and goats?

Cattle, sheep, and goats are herd/flock animals, and as such will generally respond to the basic principles of herding in that when approached they will move away from you. They move best as a herd/flock and do not like to be separated. Trying to capture a single individual can be quite challenging. If a herd becomes too scattered, they may not move well in a desired direction as groups of individuals may wander. Keeping them somewhat bunched together will make it easier to move a herd/flock. Sometimes a dominant animal can be identified, usually an older female, and moving this animal in the desired direction may facilitate moving the herd/flock. Many of these animals have a strong maternal instinct. Taking the time to keep mothers and young together will also facilitate moving the animals. Recognize that this strong maternal instinct can change the typical herd/flock animal behavior from one that prefers to move away from a "threat" (i.e., a responder) to one that is more aggressive in protecting their young.

Bulls prefer flight over fight. They tend to be more aggressive and may prefer to confront a threat. As the "No Trespassing" sign on the ranch property said: "If you choose to trespass I hope you can run 100 yards in under 8 seconds . . . my bull can!" This is especially true for dairy bulls. Places that maintain herds of breeding bulls (such as those collecting semen for artificial insemination) recognize the difficulties and dangers in working with these animals. Some places have found the only way to round up and move the bulls is with a very fast, tough, smart, fearless, well-trained cattle dog, such as a Heeler.

Remember, too, that sheep and goats can crawl under many bottom rails and jump unexpectantly high and may readily escape from corrals or pens meant for cattle. Kid goats and lambs are very gregarious and love to climb and stand on top of things, so be aware that pens may need to be modified to contain these animals.

Even though we do not tend to think of these animals as athletes, do not underestimate their abilities!

30. Describe some techniques for moving and handling cattle, sheep, and goats.

Basic herding techniques are the foundation for this group of livestock. When you approach them from the rear, they will move away from you; approach from the side or come up along side their head, and they turn away; approach from the front, and they will turn and move away from you. Sorting poles can help separate and direct animals. Whenever possible, pre-place barriers such as corral panels or gates to direct the animals' movement. Moving these animals along an effective barrier such as a fence line or paddock wall works well. If moving animals through a fence opening or gate, plan the direction of movement such that the herd will move along a fence line and then be turned by another barrier to go through the opening, rather then having to negotiate around a barrier and then through. These animals work much better when calm. If the herd starts to get excited and begins to run and bolt away, it is best to back off, regroup, and try to move them more slowly to keep them calm. Responders holding tarps or webbed fencing can be used to direct animals, although the lengths of webbed fencing should be short enough so responders are holding the ends of sections and not holding long lengths of fencing. This is to minimize the risk of injury, to both responder and animal, should an animal run back through the fencing. Holding the ends of short sections allows the responder to let go if necessary.

Cattle are best restrained in a narrow alleyway or chute. Other means of restraint include roping, but before you do this, you should decide if this will afford you enough restraint for your intended mission. When roping cattle (even young calves), you must have a way to secure the rope to a relatively immoveable object to prevent being dragged and receiving rope burns. A trained horse or snubbing post will work. Another caution is that a lariat can tighten and strangle an animal—especially an animal that is on the fight. It can be very difficult to loosen or release the loop on the neck. A lariat should be a temporary restraining device allowing you to get a halter or some other restraint in place, and then promptly release the loop. Do not rope an animal (unless in a corral or pen) if you do not have a means of retrieving your rope should that animal get away from you.

Sheep and goats are easier to restrain because of their more manageable size. Resist grabbing the horns of rams and bucks as this is a move challenging the animal and will be met with more resistance. Sheep and goats can be restrained in the standing position, and for animals that are less docile, applying side pressure to the body and gently pushing them against a barrier can have a calming effect. To examine the underside of sheep, the animal can be tipped up into a sitting position such that the animal is resting on its haunches with its back leaning against the handler's legs.

HORSES

31. What are the primary hazards of horses?

The primary hazards of horses are hooves, teeth, size, and strength. The risk of injury includes being kicked, struck (kicked with a front foot), stepped on, jumped on, knocked down, and bitten.

32. What are some behavioral characteristics of horses?

Horses have a strong herd instinct. There is a familiarity within a herd but also a very strong pecking order, or social hierarchy. Introducing new horses into a herd should be done with care to allow the animals to adjust to each other and work out the new animal's position in the herd. This can be important if you are moving horses or holding horses in close proximity that are not familiar with one another.

Animals may inadvertently injure you as they attempt to get away from another horse higher in the pecking order, or they may be reluctant to load in a trailer if placed next to a horse that establishes his position in the hierarchy.

Separating an individual from the herd can be very unsettling for some horses. If you are trying to examine or treat a horse, it may be easier to keep the horse near the herd, or if you must take him away, sometimes taking two horses instead of one can have a significant calming effect.

Another interesting characteristic of horses is that the two halves of their brain are not well connected. The nerve fibers of the *corpus callosum*, which relay information back and forth between the two hemispheres, are poorly developed. This means that a horse may get used to something on one side of his body, but when that same something happens on the other side of his body, it is a completely new experience. (*Vuja dé*, or "never seen that before"!) This is one reason why when moving around a horse it is important to maintain some sort of contact with him as this provides him with "real-time information" as to where you are. Most horses are worked from *their* left side, so a horse will likely have "experience" when you approach and handle them from this side.

Horses are sensitive creatures that can easily become nervous and excitable in unfamiliar situations. Maintaining a calm demeanor and a calm environment is very important around horses.

When placing horses in a pen, do not put stallions with stallions, stallions with mares or geldings with stallions. Invariably, you will have a major disagreement between these animals, and serious injuries almost always will result.

One challenge responders will face is working with other "horse people." It seems that many of these people think they know more about horses and are better with horses than anyone else, and they usually want to prove it!

33. Describe some techniques and equipment that may be helpful when handling and restraining horses.

When holding a haltered or bridled horse, do not loop the excess lead or reins around your hand. Rather, fold or flake the excess; this will allow you to let out slack if needed while minimizing the risk of serious injury to your hands.

Stud chains are a type of lead rope with approximately 20 inches (50 cm) of small link chain on the clip end. This chain is attached to the halter in various ways (over the nose, in the mouth, or across the gums) as a more severe method of restraint. Stud chains are best used by an experienced handler.

Twitches are another device which can be helpful in restraining a horse for examination or treatment. There are various twitch designs, but all are applied to the upper lip of a horse as a method of acupressure and distraction. It has been suggested that this acupressure triggers the release of endorphins. The person handling the twitch must stay to the side of the horse and apply just the right amount of pressure. Twitches should not be used for extended periods of time. As with stud chains this device is best used by an experienced handler. Ear and neck twitches are hand holds that should not be used.

The use of ropes, to incapacitate a leg or restrict its motion, is not an appropriate method of restraint in a disaster setting. Scotch hobbling, tying a leg up, single side line, etc. should not be used.

Horse stocks may also be used as a method of physical restraint, but are unlikely to be available in a disaster setting.

Talking and maintaining some sort of physical contact with a horse are two of the most effective and reassuring things you can do when handling horses.

Horses respond well to touch, so maintaining some sort of contact with a horse while you are examining or moving around an individual is helpful. Most animals are sensitive to having their legs and feet handled, so touching a leg or foot "out of the blue" can be startling. Animals respond better if your touch starts on the back or trunk and then your hand slides down the leg.

Being kicked by a horse will cause serious injury. When passing around behind a horse, either give plenty of clearance such that you are well out of reach of a full extension kick or stay in very close and maintain body contact with the horse as you move around his hind end.

Many horses are halter trained and will lead. For young or untrained horses that do not know how to lead, these animals may be moved by leading other individuals and hoping they will follow. If trying to lead a horse forward that does not want to move, pulling on their head is generally unrewarding. Most horses do not like to feel this pressure on their head and they will resist (oppositional reflex) rather then go forward. You can cue a horse with a slight short pull on their head, but then the pressure should be released. Horses who refuse to move forward may be cued from behind by an assistant, or if you are by yourself you can try to push them off at a 45-degree angle for a few steps and them turn them back 90 degrees for a few steps and so forth, basically "tacking" to move forward. Another means to move young horses is to place a loop over the rear quarters and gently apply pressure as you walk forward.

Groups of horses can be herded by riders, but because of their athletic ability this can get out of hand. If trying to evacuate a small enough herd, and no other transportation or personnel resources are available, a last resort option would be to identify the leader of the herd and then lead or ride this animal, relying on the other horses to follow in a general direction.

It can be difficult to move horses away from their comfort zone of home. In times of crisis, chaos compounds this problem. Handlers and responders must strive to remain calm and confident and implement strategies to foster a controlled calm environment.

SWINE

34. What are the primary hazards of swine?

Teeth and strength are the primary hazards, but responders should have ear protection available as the squeal of a pig can be extremely loud.

35. What are some behavioral characteristics of swine?

Swine are quite intelligent and curious animals. They have had a reputation for being aggressive and dangerous animals, but thankfully much of that temperament has been bred from of them. This is not to say that all domestic swine are docile and gentle, because certain individuals can be aggressive. As with other species, some sows will be very protective of their young. Swine tend to be herd animals and free-range pigs prefer to congregate in groups. Of note, pigs will squeal quite loudly whenever they are handled or restrained.

When sheltering piglets of different ages, separate them based on size and age. Older, larger piglets will injure or kill younger, smaller piglets.

36. What techniques work well for moving and handling pigs?

The easiest way to move pigs is to herd them using a sorting pole or push board. A handler can walk behind them, push them along, and tap their shoulder or side of head with a sorting pole to turn them. More aggressive individuals can be pushed using a push board. Most subadult and adult pigs are quite strong, but not necessarily in good aerobic condition. If you have to herd pigs very far (for some, this might be more than 100 meters!), recognize that they may need to rest frequently. This is especially true for breeding sows.

Pig snares are mini–catch poles where the cable loops around the upper maxillae. The loop goes in the mouth, behind the canine teeth, and around the snout. Pig snares are used for restraint to hold an animal in place. Be aware that pigs squeal very loudly when a snare is placed. Pig snares may be helpful should you need to euthanatize a pig by shooting him in the head. The snare will help steady the head in a position to allow someone to properly place the shot, thereby minimizing any suffering.

POULTRY

37. When handling domestic poultry, what must you be aware of?

Birds do not have a diaphragm; rather they use their sternum (breast bone) like a bellows to draw air into their lungs. When holding birds, it is important that you not compromise this movement or the bird may suffocate.

38. Describe the primary hazards of poultry.

The term *poultry* refers to different types of domesticated birds raised for meat, eggs, and feathers, so primary hazards will vary depending on the species.

Spurs are bony projections found on the caudomedial (back/inside) aspect of the legs of sexually mature male birds belonging to the order Galliformes. Galliformes include roosters, tom turkeys, pheasants, partridges, and guinea fowl. The spur is an outgrowth of the tarsometatarsal bone and is surrounded by a horny keratinized material. This spur grows, hardens, and curves as a bird matures. It is used as a weapon, and some birds can be quite aggressive.

Geese have powerful wings used to strike forward. Their bill can be considered a secondary hazard, and they will use it to strike. Some domestic geese are protectors of property and can be fairly aggressive.

Zoonotic diseases (diseases that may be transmitted from animals to humans) may be considered a hazard when working with poultry. One zoonotic example includes avian chlamydiosis (also referred to as psittacosis) or parrot fever. This is an obligate intracellular bacterium that can affect people following airborne exposure from infected birds. This disease affects other types of birds as well, but among poultry, turkeys and ducks are most often affected. Chickens are *infrequently* infected. Other examples of zoonotic diseases are *Salmonella* and *Campylobacter* bacterial infections.

39.   What is the proper way to hold a chicken?

For those new to handling chickens, place one hand on the middle of the chicken's back, securing the wings as much as possible with this hand. (Expert poultry handlers do not need to secure the wings or place this hand on the back.) With your other hand, support the chicken under the breast, and place your index finger back between the legs. This allows you to secure one leg between thumb and index finger and the other leg between index finger and middle finger. Tilt the bird slightly so the chest is lower than the tail as this is calming, and hold them close to your body to minimize struggling.

40.   What is the proper way to hold ducks and geese?

Some domestic geese are protectors of property, and you may need to capture these geese much the same as wild geese. The proper way to hold ducks and geese is to get control of their wings first and the head second. A towel draped over the bird or a net can be used to allow the handler a chance to fold the wings into the bird's body and then gain control of the head by grasping it near the base of the skull.

41.   Describe some concerns when dealing with poultry.

These birds heat stress very easily. As birds are unable to sweat, they must pant to cool themselves, and hot weather (or even more so, hot *and* humid weather) can be very dangerous for them. Attention must be paid to temperatures inside buildings, and cooling options should be implemented. Holding and transport carriers *must* be kept out of direct sunlight. An appropriate number of birds per carrier to allow good airflow should be considered. Access to water is very important for these birds to prevent dehydration from panting. One-half inch to 1 inch (1 to 2 cm) of clean water in a trough or pan works well. Typically, the water is kept outside the crate with a window available for the birds to lean through and drink. This helps keep the water clean from contamination. As this may not be practical in a disaster response, care must be taken to ensure clean water is available inside the carriers. Nipple waterers, which are less prone to contamination and spilling inside a container, can be used, but birds may not drink as much as they should from these devices. As feed is digested, heat is produced from the increase in metabolism. In very hot areas, one strategy is to feed poultry in the first 2 to 3 hours of sunlight, and again after sunset. This minimizes the amount of body heat generated during the hottest part of the day.

LLAMAS AND ALPACAS

42.   Describe the primary hazards of llamas and alpacas.

The primary hazard of llamas and alpacas is the fighting teeth of adult males. There are three fighting teeth on each side of the mouth. These teeth, two upper and one lower, are behind the incisors and in front of the molars. The fighting teeth are more rudimentary in females. Fighting teeth erupt at about 2 to 2½ years of age (but can be later) and are very sharp and pointed. Most owners will have these teeth cut, but some may not. For llamas used as protectors in sheep herds against coyotes and other predators, an owner may opt to *not* have the fighting teeth cut. Responders may also encounter males with fighting teeth because of an owner's poor husbandry.

Another hazard of llamas is their size and strength. Some llamas, typically intact males or females with a cria (baby), can be quite aggressive. A syndrome seen when these animals first became popular in the United States in the 1980s was termed "berserk male syndrome" (interesting that this is not just a phrase describing fans of professional wrestling entertainment!). Since that time, this term has been modified to "aberrant behavioral syndrome," which may apply to females as well as males. However, there is much discussion as to whether these animals have a truly aberrant behavior or are just poorly trained. Regardless, suffice it to say that there are some aggressive individuals and their size and strength make them a hazard to responders.

Another hazard which is not life threatening but pretty unpleasant is their ability to regurgitate the contents of the first compartment of the stomach (essentially the rumen fermenting vat) and spit.

43. What are some techniques for moving and handling llamas and alpacas?

As a generalization, llamas and alpacas can be herded fairly well, although individuals tend to scatter a bit more than other herd animals. On the other hand, they can be quite sensible, and something as simple as a length of rope held between two people can be used effectively to guide and direct their movement.

Many llamas and alpacas are trained to lead, but the technique for placing a halter is slightly different than that for other animals. Unlike horses, which respond well and tend to settle when their necks are restrained, allowing you to place a halter, llamas and alpacas do NOT like to have their necks held. If you must grab the neck for that initial moment of restraint, grab very low near the thorax. Llamas and alpacas respond well to side pressure against the trunk of their body. The fiber in the shoulder region can be grasped to counter forward movement, or an arm can be wrapped around the front of their chest. If you are alone, using your body to gently push them sideways against a barrier will tend to hold them still and allows you to use both hands (one on either side of the neck, but not touching the neck) in order to raise the halter up to the face and slip it over the nose. If you are out in the open, you may need someone else on the other side to (1) mildly push against the animal and (2) to place the halter (again, they should come up from below with an arm on either side of the neck), while you hold the animal in place.

Most llamas and alpacas do not like to have their legs or feet touched. If you must handle the feet or legs for examination, wound treatment, etc., you should recognize they will resist by pulling the leg away or possibly kicking.

Crias (babies) can be picked up by cradling them with your arms wrapped around the front of the chest and behind the haunches. Alpacas and smaller subadult llamas can be restrained in the standing position with this hold as well.

OSTRICHES AND EMUS

See this section in Chapter 1.16.

44. Why should you be especially cautious when handling ostriches or emus?

These are very large birds that make extremely quick movements. Their legs and feet are so powerful the responder can sustain a very serious injury. Be extremely cautious around these birds.

Suggested Reading and References
American Veterinary Medical Association. Available at http://avma.org. A booklet titled *Saving the Whole Family* is available through the AVMA website via their Public Resources and Disaster Preparedness links. This website has other timely, accurate, and helpful information as well.
Fowler M. *Restraint and Handling of Wild and Domestic Animals.* 3rd ed. Ames, IA, Wiley-Blackwell, 2008.
http://www.canadianpoultry.ca. This website has a lot of good information on poultry husbandry.
http://www.ithaca.edu/staff/jhenderson/chooks/chlinks. This website lists a number of other resources for poultry education.
http://www.national4-hheadquarters.gov. This website is the homepage for 4-H. 4-H provides a lot of information on raising a variety of domestic animals.

Much can be learned from the many magazines and journals available that cater to specific animals. While the articles may not be scientifically based or peer reviewed, they may contain appropriate tips and information that can be helpful to an animal responder.

CHAPTER 1.18
SMALL ANIMAL FIRST AID

Wayne E. Wingfield, MS, DVM

1. Who needs to learn first aid for animals?

Everyone should have a basic understanding of first aid. This is especially true of disaster responders, search and rescue personnel, firemen, police officers, families with small children, pet owners, breeders, and individuals who travel.

2. What are the four basic steps in an emergency?

- *Recognize* that an emergency exists.
  - ○ Unusual noises
  - ○ Unusual sights
  - ○ Unusual odors
  - ○ Unusual appearances or behaviors
- *Decide* to act.
- There are many ways to help in an emergency. In order to help, you must act!
- *Call* for help. Who do you call?
  1. 911
  2. Veterinarian
     (   ) —
  3. Veterinary Emergency Clinic
     (   ) —
  4. County Humane Society or Animal Control
     (   ) —
- *Provide care* until help arrives.
  - ○ Always care for life-threatening emergencies first!

3. It is not uncommon for people to avoid becoming involved in first-aid care. List some of the reasons people do not act in an emergency.

- Presence of other people
- Uncertainty about the victim and fear of self-injury
- Type of injury or illness
- Fear of catching a disease
- Fear of doing something wrong
- Fear of litigation

4. Once you have decided to act, what are some of the first things to consider?

- *Check* the scene and the victim.
  - ○ Is the scene safe?
  - ○ What happened?
  - ○ How many victims are there?
  - ○ Can bystanders help?
- *Call* for help.
- *Care* for the victim.

5. Veterinary first aid is the immediate care given a companion animal that has been injured or suddenly taken ill. The immediate care includes first the primary survey. What is the primary survey?

- Airway
- Breathing
- Circulation
- Disability
- Examination

6. What are some of the important questions to ask when assessing the airway?

- Is the animal having difficulty with breathing (dyspnea)?
- Is the airway clear?
- Are there bite wounds to the trachea or larynx?
- Is there subcutaneous emphysema present? (Passing your hand over the body will feel like crepe paper under the skin.)

7. What are some of the important questions to ask when assessing breathing? See Appendix 1.18.1 for normal values.

- Is the animal showing respiratory distress (dyspnea)?
- What is the color of the mucous membranes?
- Does changing position worsen the dyspnea?
- Is there evidence of a thoracic wound?
- Are the peripheral veins distended?

8. What are some of the important questions to ask when assessing the circulation? See Appendix 1.18.1 for normal values.

- Is there evidence of hemorrhage?
- How large is the swelling associated with a limb fracture?
- Are the mucous membranes pale, cold, and tacky?
- What is the duration of the capillary refill time (discussed below)?
- Are the femoral pulses rapid and weak?
- Are the extremities cold?

9.   What are some of the important questions to be asked when assessing for disability?

- Is there evidence of neurological injury?
- What is the behavioral posture of the animal? (comatose, aggressive, alert)
- What is the motor posture of the animal? (discussed below)
- Is the animal bright, alert, and responsive?
- Does the animal respond to painful stimuli?
- Are the pupils dilated, constricted, of equal size, and responsive to light?
- Is there an extremity fracture that might threaten a peripheral nerve?

10.   What are some of the important questions to ask during your examination?

- Are there lacerations?
- Where is the bruising and is it getting worse?
- Are there multiple fractures?
- Is the abdomen painful?
- Is there evidence of debilitation or intercurrent disease?
- Is there evidence of a fever? (See Appendix 1.18.1 for normal values.)

LIFE-THREATENING EMERGENCIES: WHEN SECONDS COUNT

11.   List some of the common causes leading to breathing emergencies.

- Trauma
- Chemical inhalation
- Upper airway obstruction
- Airway diseases (asthma, pneumonia)
- Near-drowning
- Choking

12.   List some of the important causes of injuries to companion animals.

- Tornados
- Hurricanes
- Wildfires
- Motor vehicle
- Animal bites
- Physical abuse
- Weapons
- Terrorist event
- Explosions
- Sharp objects
- House fires
- Falls
- Near-drowning

13. List some of the other emergencies that will benefit from first-aid care.

- Seizures
- Chemical injuries
- Sudden illnesses
  - Urethral obstruction
  - Gastric-dilatation volvulus
  - Hemorrhagic diarrhea
  - Vomiting
- Poisonings
- Radiation exposure
- Paralysis
- Heatstroke (hyperthermia)
- Frostbite and hypothermia
- Difficult birth (dystocia)
- Bites and stings

14. List some of the important causes of poisonings in pet animals.

- Antifreeze
- Rodenticides
- Malicious poisonings (including terrorist events)
- Eating poisonous or harmful plants
- Ingestion of contaminated carcasses
- Insecticides
- Bioterrorism
- Ingestion of onions, raisins, certain mushrooms, lead paint, or coins containing lead or zinc (pennies)

15. List some of the important environmental causes that might require first-aid care.

- Terrorism
- Heatstroke
- Frostbite and hypothermia
- Chemical injury
- Dehydration
- Radiation exposure

PREPARING FOR AN EMERGENCY

16. List items that should be included in a pet's evacuation first-aid kit.

- Activated charcoal (liquid)
- Adhesive tape (1 and 2 inches)
- Antidiarrheal (liquid/tablets)—Caution: Pepto-Bismol contains salicylates (aspirin) which can be toxic to certain animals, especially if dehydrated 2° to diarrhea.

- Antibiotic ointment (wounds)
- Antibiotic eye ointment
- Bandage scissors
- Bandage tape
- Betadine or Nolvasan (scrub and solution)
- Bulb syringe
- Cotton balls or pledgets
- Cotton bandage rolls
- Elastic bandage rolls
- Eye rinse (sterile)
- Flea and tick prevention/treatment
- Gauze pads and rolls
- Hemostats
- Hydrogen peroxide
- Ice cream sticks (for splints)
- Ice pack
- Isopropyl alcohol/alcohol prep pads
- Kling gauze
- Latex gloves/nonallergenic gloves
- Liquid dish detergent (mild wound/body cleanser)
- Measuring spoons
- Medications and preventatives with clearly labeled instructions (heartworm, flea, etc.)
- Newspaper
- Nonadherent bandage pads
- Petroleum or K-Y Jelly
- Plastic food wrap (SeranWrap)
- Rectal thermometer
- Rope or leash
- Saline solution (for rinsing wounds)
- Scissors
- Styptic powder (clotting agent)
- Syringes (3, 12, and 35 mL)
- Sunscreen (SPF >40)
- Suture (absorbable and nonabsorbable (2-0, 3-0, 4-0)
- Syringe/eyedropper
- Thermometer (digital)
- Tourniquet
- Towel and washcloth
- Tongue depressors
- Tweezers

17. How can you decrease chances of being bitten by an injured animal?

It is not unusual to be bitten by an injured animal if you are not extremely careful. The animal is usually afraid and often in pain. Be careful if you plan to proceed with first-aid care. The best way to handle the injured animal is to first try to gain the animal's confidence through a gentle, soothing voice. If there is no evidence of a neurological problem, a blanket or coat placed gently over the animal may help you gain control. If at all possible, place a muzzle on animals with long noses (Fig. 1.18.1).

- Take precautions in muzzling animals.
- Don't get bitten!
- Immediately remove the muzzle if the animal begins to retch or vomit.
- Do not apply a muzzle to an animal showing respiratory distress.

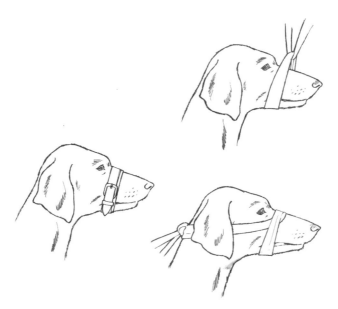

Figure 1.18.1 A muzzle on a dog will help protect against an accidental bite. (Based on Gfeller RW, Thomas MW. *First Aid: Emergency Care for Dogs and Cats.* Available at http://www.veterinarypartner.com/Content.plx?P=A&A=294&S=1&SourceID=20.)

CARDIOPULMONARY RESUSCITATION IN SMALL ANIMALS

18. What is cardiopulmonary resuscitation?

Cardiopulmonary resuscitation (CPR) is the treatment required to save a life when an animal has no respiratory or cardiac function.

19. What are the two means to provide CPR to an animal suffering respiratory or cardiopulmonary arrest?

- Rescue breathing
- Chest compressions

20. Describe the approach required to perform CPR to an animal.

- First, establish that the animal is actually in arrest. Talk to the animal, gently shake the animal, and finally, make a loud noise. If there is no response, use the following criteria to confirm that the animal is in arrest.
  - There are four criteria for recognition of cardiopulmonary arrest:
    - Absence of breathing and development of cyanosis
    - Absence of heart beat (the heart sounds will cease when the systolic pressure is <50 mm Hg)
    - Absence of pulse (the pulse will not be palpable when systolic pressure is <60 mm Hg)
    - Dilation of the pupils (remember that some drugs will lead to an unresponsive pupil [e.g., atropine sulfate])

- Second, ensure an open airway by carefully extending the head and neck and looking into the mouth for evidence of a foreign body, vomitus, or anything obstructing the airway (Fig. 1.18.2). Notice the tongue can be used to open the mouth by gently pulling down on the mandibles as you pull up on the maxillae. Be careful not to injure the tongue or the teeth.
- Third, observe the animal's chest for evidence of breathing. If no chest wall motion is observed within 5 to 7 seconds, begin rescue breathing.
- Give two long breaths (1.5 to 2 seconds in duration) (Fig. 1.18.3). Look for the chest rise as you give the breath to confirm effectiveness and aid in determining the appropriate volume of air to give.
- Observe the chest to see if the animal's chest begins to move indicating it is breathing on its own.
- If there is a pulse but no chest wall motion is observed, breathe into the animal's nose at a rate of 12 to 20 times each minute. Stop every 2 minutes to see if there is any evidence of spontaneous breathing. At this stage, it is extremely important to feel for a heartbeat or pulse. If there is no heartbeat or pulse, the animal is in cardiopulmonary arrest! Begin chest compressions immediately.

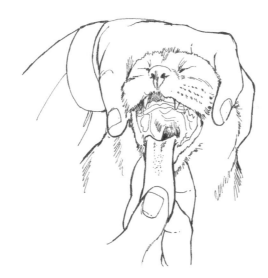

Figure 1.18.2 Checking the oropharynx for evidence of obstruction, vomitus, or foreign material(s). (Based on Gfeller RW, Thomas MW. *First Aid: Emergency Care for Dogs and Cats.* Available at http://www.veterinarypartner.com/Content.plx?P=A&A=294&S=1&SourceID=20.)

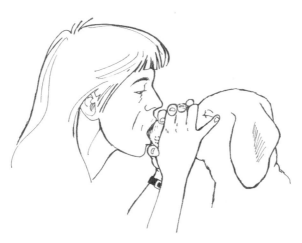

Figure 1.18.3 Mouth to nose breathing in an unconscious dog. (Based on Gfeller RW, Thomas MW. *First Aid: Emergency Care for Dogs and Cats.* Available at http://www.veterinarypartner.com/Content.plx?P=A&A=294&S=1&SourceID=20.)

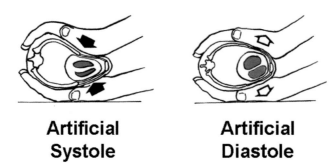

**Artificial   Artificial
Systole   Diastole**

Figure 1.18.4 The cardiac pump theory suggests blood is physically moved from the cardiac chambers during artificial systole. During artificial diastole, the ventricular chambers are passively refilled with blood.

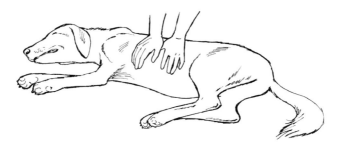

Figure 1.18.5 External cardiac compression in large dogs (>15 pounds [7 kg]) is accomplished by pressing on the ribs behind the heart. Blood is theorized to move forward by the thoracic pump. Whenever one presses down on the thorax, the intrathoracic pressure increases and moves blood forward. Releasing the compression allows a passive refill of blood to the ventricular chambers. (Based on Gfeller RW, Thomas MW. *First Aid: Emergency Care for Dogs and Cats.* Available at http://www.veterinarypartner.com/Content.plx?P=A&A=294&S=1&SourceID=20.)

21. How do you administer chest compressions during CPR?

- In cats and dogs weighing less than 15 pounds, apply chest compressions at a rate of 120 times each minute over the heart. Blood is believed to flow during CPR in small patients via the cardiac pump theory.
  - The cardiac pump theory implies you are pressing over the heart and physically moving the blood from the ventricular chambers in a forward direction (i.e., right ventricle pushes its blood into the pulmonary artery; left ventricle pushes its blood into the aorta) (Fig. 1.18.4).
- In dogs over 15 pounds, place a fist or sandbag under the chest and apply compression just *behind the heart* at a rate of 80 to 100 times each minute. Pressing behind the heart will increase intrathoracic pressure. Increased intrathoracic pressure is believed to be responsible for forward blood flow via the thoracic pump theory (Fig. 1.18.5).

22. Is rescue breathing required during chest compressions?

Interestingly, new research shows that CPR with only chest compressions provides the same survival rate in dogs as compared to standard CPR with chest compressions and ventilation. When one stops thoracic compression, myocardial and cerebral blood flow also stops. It is these two factors that lead to the unsuccessful resuscitation. Therefore, do not stop chest compressions in order to provide an artificial breath. As the chest is compressed, you will hear air leaving the mouth and nose. When the chest is not being compressed, there will be some passive refill of air into the lungs. If oxygen is available, use either a face mask or endotracheal tube to provide a increased oxygen availability.

23. How long should you continue with CPR?

This is a very controversial question. In all likelihood, if there is no return of spontaneous ventilation or heartbeat/pulses after 20 minutes, the animal is dead.

24. What should you do when the animal is resuscitated?

Take the animal directly to the nearest veterinarian's office. The biggest problem seen following arrest is a second arrest. Regardless, the animal's brain and tissues will be suffering from the effects of decreased oxygen and perfusion and the pet needs aggressive medical therapy that can only be administered by your veterinarian.

ABNORMAL BLEEDING

25. What should you do if your animal is bleeding?

Importantly, you need to provide first-aid control of bleeding and then transport your pet to a veterinarian.

26. What is the best means for controlling bleeding?

Direct pressure over the wound is the preferable way to control bleeding. If possible, place a clean cloth or gauze sponge over the bleeding and then apply a piece of tape around the limb to apply pressure and hold the cloth/sponge in place. The tape should be applied snugly but don't apply it so tightly as to cut off all blood flow.

27. Where are the pressure points located in the dog and cat?

The following figure shows the pressure points for the femoral artery (rear legs), brachial artery (front legs), and caudate artery (tail) (Fig. 1.18.6).

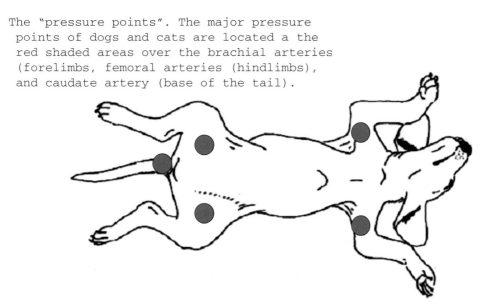

The "pressure points". The major pressure points of dogs and cats are located a the red shaded areas over the brachial arteries (forelimbs, femoral arteries (hindlimbs), and caudate artery (base of the tail).

Figure 1.18.6 Pressure points in the dog and cat are located at positions marked by the red dots.

28. Should you apply a tourniquet to control bleeding?

Tourniquets are dangerous if applied too tightly or too long. If you do not know what you are doing in applying a tourniquet, err on the side of safety and use direct pressure and pressure points.

29. How do you identify internal bleeding?

Internal bleeding is not obvious on inspection of an animal. If there is a fracture, internal bleeding is what causes the swollen leg. If the animal has bleeding into its abdomen, you will see clinical signs of shock (pale mucous membranes (gums), cool extremities, increased heart rate, increased pulse rate, and either an excited or subdued behavior). Other clues to possible internal bleeding include the presence of severe bruising on the abdomen or chest.

30. What should you do if you suspect internal bleeding?

You can wrap 4-inch Kling around the abdomen from the last rib to the ileum of the pelvis. The wrap should be snug but you should still be able to insert two fingers under the bandage. The idea is to compress abdominal contents in hopes of getting a clot to form and the bleeding to cease. Should your animal have respiratory distress prior to placing this abdominal compression bandage, DO NOT apply the bandage. The animal could have a diaphragmatic hernia and you would be forcing additional abdominal organs into the thorax. Should the animal's breathing become more labored after applying the bandage, it is advisable to either remove or loosen the bandage. Take your animal to the veterinarian as soon as possible!

DIFFICULTY WITH BREATHING (DYSPNEA)

31. How do you know if your animal is having difficulty with breathing?

A dog or cat that is open-mouth breathing, has pale or bluish (cyanotic) mucous membranes (gums), prefers to sit instead of laying down, postures his/her elbows away from the chest wall (orthopnea), and often makes loud respiratory noises with each breath is in severe respiratory distress.

32. What are some of the common causes of respiratory distress in the dog and cat?

- Trauma (pneumothorax, pulmonary contusions, broken ribs, diaphragmatic hernia, hemothorax)
- Hazardous chemicals
- Pneumonia
- Aspiration pneumonitis (may follow an episode of vomiting)
- Heartworm disease (dirofilariasis)
- Collapsing trachea
- Brachiocephalic syndrome (Pugs, Boxers, Bulldogs, Pekinese, Boston Terriers)—These breeds "normally" are very noisy breathers and their breed makes them more susceptible to extreme heat and exercise-induced respiratory distress.
- Laryngeal paralysis (Golden Retrievers, Labrador Retrievers, German Shepherds, Eskimo breeds, Saint Bernards)

- Asthma (especially in cats)
- Allergies
- Pyothorax (cats and hunting breed dogs)
- Others

33. What should you do if your pet is in respiratory distress?

First, *do not stress* the animal! Keep the animal as calm as possible and do not force the animal to walk, move, or change positions. The best thing you can do is transport the animal to a veterinarian as soon and quickly as possible. Upon arrival at the veterinarian's office, supplemental oxygen will be administered and the cause of the respiratory distress identified and treated.

CARDIOVASCULAR PROBLEMS

34. What sort of cardiovascular problems develop in dogs and cats?

There are many cardiovascular problems in the dog and cat. The problem may be with the heart or it may be other problems where the heart and blood volume are severely affected (shock). Heart problems arise from congenital problems where the animal is born with the defect or there may be an acquired disease that occurs from parasites (heartworms), diseases of the heart valves, or of the heart muscle. Interestingly, dogs and cats do not commonly develop coronary artery disease as is seen in humans.

35. How would you recognize heart disease in a dog or cat?

When the heart is diseased, the animal is usually incapable of strenuous exercise. In many cases, one of the first clinical findings noted is a *cough*. Although coughing is commonly recognized as a sign of pulmonary disease, it also is common with cardiac disease. Other signs suggestive of heart diseases include the following: weight loss or gain, muscle atrophy, weakness, fainting (syncope), weak pulses, an enlarging abdominal girth (ascites), open-mouthed breathing with the elbows moved away from the chest wall, and mucous membranes of the gums often appearing pale or even slightly bluish color (cyanosis). If there is a severe problem there is usually a heart murmur that can be auscultated. When you lay your hand over the heart (left sixth intercostal space = apex beat), you can sometimes feel a buzzing sensation over the heart, which may be the result of abnormal blood flow associated with the cardiac murmur.

36. Do certain heart diseases appear in families of a dog or cat breed?

Yes! Many congenital heart diseases are passed from one generation to the next. If your pet has a heart disease, talk with your veterinarian before you consider breeding this pet. Offspring of this pet will likely also have the same heart disease when they are born.

37. What is shock?

Shock is defined as "abnormal tissue perfusion leading to abnormal cellular metabolism." There are many causes of shock, which have led to the following etiologic classification:

- Hypovolemic shock (dehydration), blood loss
- Cardiogenic shock (heart diseases and arrhythmias)
- Traumatic shock (bomb blasts, tornados, hit by a car, kicked by a horse)
- Septic shock (parvovirus enteritis, pyometritis, gastric dilatation-volvulus)

38.   What are some of the common clinical signs of shock?

The classic signs of an animal in shock include the presence of a weak pulse, pale mucous membranes (gums), increased heart, pulse, and respiratory rate and cold extremities (feet and ears) (Fig. 1.18.7).

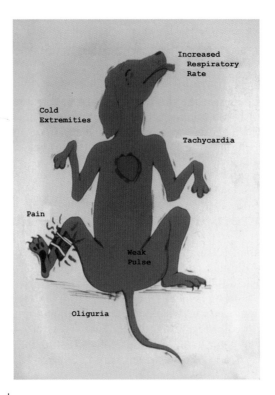

Figure 1.18.7 Clinical signs of shock.

39.   What are the first-aid procedures for a small animal in shock?

- Be careful! The pet is often painful, possibly excited, and may bite or claw you.
- Check the airway and be sure the animal is breathing.
- Apply a pressure bandage to any obvious hemorrhage
- Keep the animal warm and try to calm the animal.
- If there is evidence of a neurological injury, immobilize the pet on a solid surface such as a piece of plywood. Be very careful when moving the animal!
- If a fracture involves a lower part of the extremity, apply a temporary splint.
- Transport the animal to a veterinarian's hospital as soon and quickly as possible.

40. What should you do if you suspect the animal is in heart failure as the cause of shock?

- Do not stress the animal!
- Make sure the animal has a clear airway and is breathing.
- Transport the animal to your veterinarian's hospital as soon and quickly as possible.

ACUTE GASTRIC DILATATION-VOLVULUS (CANINE BLOAT)

41. What is acute gastric dilatation-volvulus?

Gastric dilatation-volvulus (GDV) is a periacute condition predominantly affecting large breed, deep-chested dogs (Fig. 1.18.8). It results from an abnormal, acute accumulation of air in the dog's stomach. The source of this air is believed to be from abnormal swallowing of air (aerophagia).

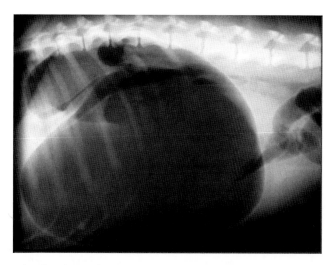

Figure 1.18.8 Lateral radiograph of a dog with acute gastric dilatation-volvulus results in the stomach twisting upon itself and passively dragging the spleen along. This twisting leads to severe cardiovascular compromise and shock.

42. What causes GDV in the dog?

- Diet has been implicated in the etiology of canine bloat but thus far there is no evidence to support this theory.
- Most clinically affected GDV dogs have gas-filled stomachs and analysis of the gas has shown it to be consistent with room air.
- GDV does appear most commonly in the nervous and hyperactive dogs.

43. What are the clinical signs of GDV in the dog?

- The classic picture of a GDV dog is described with the following three characteristics:
  - ○ Retching with the inability to vomit (dry-heaves).
  - ○ Abdominal distention with tympany. Using one's index finger and thumping on the right side near the last rib will result in a very tympanic (drumlike) sound.
  - ○ The inability to pass an orogastric tube. Passing an orogastric tube relieves the gaseous accumulations but *does not* rule out the presence of gastric volvulus (twisting of the esophagus and stomach).

- The GDV dog will exhibit abdominal discomfort and will often pace and whine due to pain.
- There are usually clinical signs of shock, with the heart and pulse rates being elevated and pulse pressure being decreased.
- The capillary refill time is quite variable. If the dog is in the hyperdynamic phase of shock, the capillary refill time may be accelerated or normal. If the shock is hypodynamic, the capillary refill time may be prolonged or normal.
- When viewed over the dog's back looking forward, the abdomen tends to protrude unevenly to the right.

44. What is the emergency treatment for GDV in the dog?

- Gastric decompression.
  - Most commonly involves the passage of a large-bore (colt-sized) orogastric tube.
  - Measure the length of the tube by measuring from the tip of the dog's nose to the last rib. This is the distance the tube will travel to enter the stomach. Make a mark or place a piece of tape on the tube to alert you when the stomach lumen has been entered.
  - As the tube is passed, never push the tube too vigorously as this might result in a ruptured esophagus.
  - If obstruction is encountered, stop and either let a more experienced person pass the tube or, as an alternative, you may need to trocarize the stomach through the abdominal wall.
    - Using a 10- to 14-gauge, 1.5-inch, sterile hypodermic needle, first percuss the abdomen on the **right side**. You are seeking an area that is quite resonant. If you do not have a resonant sound, it may be due to the fact that the spleen has also been rotated with the stomach. Do NOT trocarize through the spleen!
    - Once you have found that resonant area (usually located on the right and at lower half of the abdomen, quickly insert the needle all the way to the hub. Foul smelling gas will escape the needle.
    - Leave the needle in place and as the stomach decompresses, gently press on the cranial abdomen to release even more gas.
    - Once you have trocarized the stomach it is usually possible to now pass the orogastric tube.
  - Do not think the stomach has rotated back to its normal position even though you were able to pass the stomach tube.
- Transport the dog quickly to a veterinary hospital, where they will begin intravenous fluid therapy for shock.

45. What is the definitive treatment for GDV in the dog?

- Treatment of shock
- Definitive treatment of GDV involves surgery.
  - Surgical replacement of the stomach into its normal position
  - Surgical prevention of future rotation of the stomach

NEUROLOGICAL EMERGENCIES

46. What are some of the causes for a neurological emergency?

- Seizures
- Inability to use the front or rear legs
- Trauma (brain and/or spinal cord)
- Abnormal behavior
- Fainting
- Muscle weakness or incoordination
- Lameness in the front or rear legs
- Uneven sizes to the pupils of the eyes

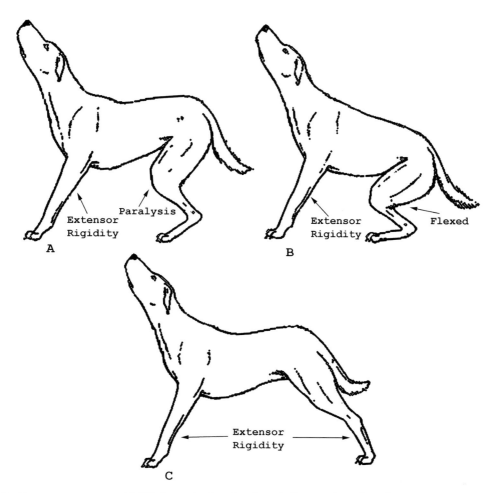

Figure 1.18.9 Motor postures seen with (**A**) thoracolumbar, (**B**) decerebellate, and (**C**) decerebrate injury. See description of each.

47. Describe three important motor postures identified with neurological injuries (Fig. 1.18.9).

1. **Shiff-Sherington Posture:** Usually associated with a fractured thoracolumbar vertebrae. Most commonly the fracture is between the second thoracic and fourth lumbar vertebrae. The prognosis is severe to grave.
2. **Decerebellate Rigidity:** Injury to the cerebellum of the brain. This is serious, but the animal would have a fair prognosis.
3. **Decerebrate Rigidity:** Severe injury to the brain and carries a grave prognosis for recovery.

48. What should you do if your animal is found seizuring?

- Be careful and don't get bitten! The animal is not in control of its faculties and it is possible to be injured severely.
- Be especially careful if you believe the seizure may have been caused by exposure to poisons and chemicals. These agents will contaminate you when you contact or pick up the animal for transport. Err on the side of caution and either be protected by wearing personal protective gear or have a barrier between you and the animal when moving it (i.e., blue tarp, raincoat, etc.).
- Try to prevent the animal from injuring itself (falling down stairs, into water, into the street, etc.).
- Remove other pets from the scene. It is not uncommon that another dog may actually attack the seizuring animal!

- Record the duration of the seizure. If it is longer than 1½–2 minutes, contact and proceed to a veterinarian immediately.
- Check the animal's rectal temperature when the seizuring ceases. A seizure is a sudden and uncontrolled spastic type of movement of the animal's body. This muscle activity can generate increases in body temperature. If the animal's temperature is >106°F, place a wet towel over the animal and quickly transport the animal to your veterinarian's office.
- If your pet loses consciousness and is not breathing, begin basic life support.
- Take your pet to the veterinarian's office for a diagnosis and treatment. Many poisons and chemicals can cause seizures so check around for evidence of poisons, protect yourself from being exposed, and bring along the container so the veterinarian can accurately determine the potential cause of the seizure.

49. What should you do if you find your pet recumbent or dragging itself around and unable to use the back legs?

- There are many potential causes for an inability to use the rear legs. Most commonly, this occurs in some of the long-backed dogs (Dachshunds, Bassett Hounds, Pekingese, Poodles, etc.). In these breeds, it is likely the dog has ruptured a disk located between the spinal vertebrae. Dogs and cats that rupture a disk require immediate professional attention.
- A dog with a broken back will also be unable to use its rear legs. Before transporting the dog to the veterinarian's office, place the dog on a solid surface (i.e., sheet of plywood, old door) and tape the dog to the board to prevent further injuries to the spinal cord.
- Fractures of the pelvis or bones of the rear legs will also prevent the animal from using its legs.
- A "spinal stroke" (fibrocartilagenous emboli) may cause paresis, paralysis, or hemiplegia, but has a more favorable prognosis.

50. What should you do if your animal seems to have a significant change in behavior or personality?

- Sudden behavior changes are cause for concern and your animal should be examined by a veterinarian.
- Some of the causes for behavior changes include a stroke, tumor, poisoning, seizures, rabies, etc.

CUTS, LACERATIONS, AND FRACTURES

51. Wounds commonly occur in pets. How should you manage a wound?

- Clean the wound of dried blood, dirt, and debris using a mild soap and warm water.
- If possible, clip the hair away from the wound to prevent further contamination.
- Apply a bandage to the wound. Generally antibiotics are not applied to a wound.
- Check bandages frequently for any signs of swelling, odor, contamination, or wetness to the bandage. If any of these are present, the bandage must be changed.
- All bandages should be changed once every 24 hours.

52. If you suspect a fracture, when should you apply a temporary splint?

Only splint a fracture if it occurs below the elbow or below the knee (stifle) joint. Fractures of the upper foreleg or rear leg are not easily amenable to placement of a temporary splint.

53. How do you apply a temporary splint?

- Front leg (Fig. 1.18.10)
  - Plan to immobilize the joint above and below the fracture.
  - A newspaper or magazine can be used for a temporary splint.
  - Roll the newspaper and form a "U" shape.
  - Gently place the leg in the splint and tape around the leg to hold the limb in place.
  - If the upper forelimb (humerus or scapula) is fractured, it is best to not attempt a temporary splint.
  - Transport the dog/cat to the veterinarian's hospital as soon as possible.
- Rear leg
  - Plan to immobilize the joint above and below the fracture.
  - Splints for the rear leg are more difficult to apply due to the conformation of the bones.
  - If the fracture is below the knee (stifle), it is probably best to attempt to place a splint with the limb in extension.
  - As for the forelimb, a newspaper, magazine, or a bent coathanger can be used as a temporary splint. An alternative approach would be using two to four boards or sticks applied around the extended limb and then taped in place (Fig. 1.18.11).
- When the upper leg (femur) is broken, it is best to transport the animal to the veterinarian's office without attempting to splint.

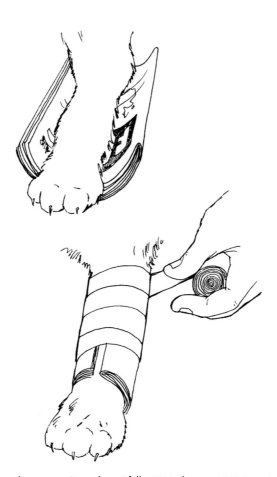

Figure 1.18.10 Forelimb splint for a dog or cat. (Based on Gfeller RW, Thomas MW. *First Aid: Emergency Care for Dogs and Cats.* Available at http://www.veterinarypartner.com/Content.plx?P=A&A=294&S=1&SourceID=20.)

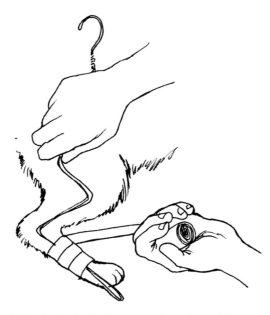

Figure 1.18.11 Splinting a fracture below the hock of a dog or cat. (Based on Gfeller RW, Thomas MW. *First Aid: Emergency Care for Dogs and Cats.* Available at http://www.veterinarypartner.com/Content.plx?P=A&A=294&S=1&SourceID=20.)

RATTLESNAKE BITES

54. Which rattlesnake do we need to worry about in Colorado (Fig. 1.18.12)?

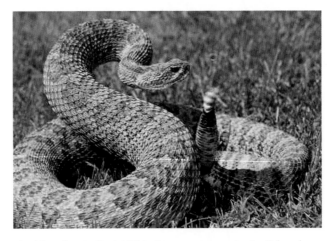

Figure 1.18.12 Prairie rattlesnake (*Crotalus viridis viridis*) is the common species in Colorado.

55. What should you do if your dog/cat is bitten by a rattlesnake?

- Check the scene to be sure the snake has vacated the area.
- Most bite wounds occur on the head, lower leg, or nose of the dog.
- If the animal is bitten on the leg, try and immobilize the leg with a splint (described above).
- Keep the pet as calm as possible.

- Ideally, it would be best to carry the animal and not allow movement of the affected area. This decreases the likelihood of spreading the venom more rapidly.
- Apply a tourniquet only if you are aware of proper usage. Obviously, you will not apply a tourniquet if the bite is on the head or nose!
- Transport the pet to the veterinarian's hospital as quickly as possible.

56. List procedures you should AVOID when your pet has been bitten by a rattlesnake:

- Do *NOT* cut the skin over the fang marks and attempt to suck the venom from the wound.
- Do *NOT* apply ice to the wound.
- Do *NOT* apply electrical shock from a car battery to the wound.
- Do *NOT* give the pet medications without specific directions from your veterinarian.
- Do **NOT** *delay* seeking medical assistance from your veterinarian as quickly as possible.

FIRST AID FOR POISONING

57. List some of the poisons that dogs and cats may encounter:

- Antifreeze (ethylene glycol)
- Acetaminophen (Tylenol), especially cats!
- Rat and mouse poisons
- Plants
- Insecticides, herbicides, lawn fertilizers
- Terrorist chemicals
- Over-the-counter medications
- Other malicious poisons (strychnine, arsenic, lead)
- Illicit drugs

58. If you suspect your pet has been exposed to a poison, what should you do?

Call your veterinarian and the poison control center.

- ASPCA National Animal Poison Control Center
  888-426-4435 ($50/case; no charge for follow-up calls)
- Pet Poison HELPLINE
  800-213-6680 ($35/case; no charge for follow-up calls)

59. How should you induce vomiting if the animal has ingested a poison?

- Hydrogen peroxide (1 tablespoon per 15 pounds body weight).
- Table salt (1 teaspoon) placed in the back of the mouth
- DO NOT use syrup of Ipecac as it may enhance absorption of ingested poisons.

60. When should you AVOID inducing vomiting?

- If the dog or cat is unconscious, semi-conscious, or seizuring.
- If any one of the following was ingested:

- ○ ASPCA National Animal Poison Control Center
  888-426-4435 ($50/case; no charge for follow-up calls)
- ○ Pet Poison HELPLINE
  800-213-6680 ($35/case; no charge for follow-up calls)
- ○ Strong acids
- ○ Alkali (bleach)
- ○ Gasoline
- ○ Cleaning products
- ○ If the ingestion was more than 2 hours earlier

CONCLUSIONS

61. Are all the emergencies in dogs and cats listed?

Of course not! The purpose for this presentation was to provide principles in first aid. If you have a question about your pet, your veterinarian is prepared to help you with an answer. Don't hesitate to call if you think you have an emergency. It is best to seek veterinary assistance rather than experience the disappointment of not taking your pet into the hospital soon enough to save its life!

Everybody should know what to do in an emergency. . . .
Everybody should know first aid!

Suggested Reading

Glickman LT, Lantz GC, Schellenberg DB, et al. A prospective study of survival and recurrence following the acute gastric dilatation-volvulus syndrome in 136 dogs. *J Am Animal Hosp Assoc* 1998;34:253–259.

Hackett TB, Wingfield WE, Mazzaferro EM, Benedetti JS. Clinical findings associated with prairie rattlesnake bites in dogs: 100 cases (1989–1998). *J Am Vet Med Assoc* 2002;220:1675–1680.

Plunkett SJ, McMichael M. Cardiopulmonary resuscitation in small animal medicine: An update. *J Vet Intern Med* 2008;22:9–25.

Wingfield WE. *Veterinary Emergency Medicine Secrets.* 2nd ed. Philadelphia, Hanley and Belfus, 2001.

Wingfield WE, Raffe MR. *The Veterinary ICU Book.* Jackson, WY, Teton New Media, 2002.

APPENDIX 1.18.1
NORMAL TEMPERATURE, PULSE, AND RESPIRATIONS OF SMALL ANIMALS

RECTAL TEMPERATURE OF HEALTHY AND RESTING ANIMALS

Species of Animal	Temperature (° Celsius)	Temperature (° Fahrenheit)
Dog	37.5–39.0 C	99.5–102.2 F
Cat	38.0–39.5 C	100.4–103.1 F
Rabbit	38.5–39.5 C	101.3–103.1 F
Guinea pig	37.8–39.5 C	100.0–103.1 F
Mink	39.7–40.8 C	103.5–105.4 F
Ferret	37.8–40.0 C	100.0–104.0 F
Silver Fox, up to ½ year	39.5–40.5 C	103.1–104.9 F
Silver Fox, adult	39.0–40.0 C	102.2–104.0 F
Coypu (nutria)	36.8–38.1 C	98.2–100.6 F
Rhesus monkey	37.5–38.5 C	99.5–101.3 F
Domestic Fowl	40.5–43.0 C	104.9–109.4 F
Domestic Fowl (average)	40.8 C	105.4 F
Pigeon	41.0–44.1 C	105.8–111.4 F
Pigeon (average)	41.8 C	107.2 F
Duck (average)	40.7 C	105.3 F
Other aquatic birds, average	42.2 C	108.0 F

PULSE RATE OF HEALTHY AND RESTING ANIMALS

Species of Animal	Pulse Rate per Minute
Young dog	110–120
Dog of large breed, adult	60–80
Dog of small breed, adult	80–120
Cat, young	130–140
Cat, old	100–120
Rabbit	120–150
Mink	80–300
Coypu (nutria)	125–175
Silver fox	80–140
Rhesus monkey	60–70
Domestic fowl	180–440 Average 312
Pigeon	140–400 Average 244

RESPIRATORY RATE OF HEALTHY AND RESTING ANIMALS

Species of Animal	Respiratory Rate per Minute
Dog, young	20–22
Dog, old	14–16
Cat	20–30
Rabbit	50–60
Guinea pig	100–150
Mink	35–160
Ferret	30
Silver fox	12–60
Coypu (nutria)	32–120
Rhesus monkey	15–30
Domestic fowl	15–30
Turkey	12–16
Pigeon	20–40
Duck	16–28
Goose	12–30

CHAPTER 1.19
LARGE ANIMAL FIRST AID

Sally B. Palmer, DVM

Frequently in disasters, animals will be sick or injured and in need of medical care. Animal responders may be called on to administer first aid while awaiting more definitive veterinary medical care. While most of this discussion will reference horses and cattle, many of these principles are applicable to any livestock specie.

1. What is the most important consideration when rendering first aid to an animal?

Safety is the most important consideration; taking into account your safety, the safety of those assisting you, the safety of bystanders, and the safety of the animal. Before initiating aid, evaluate the area and minimize hazards. Clear away obstacles, move away from potentially dangerous objects or structures, decrease the number of bystanders, or move to a quieter more secure location if possible.

2. What are the two main methods of restraint?

An important aspect of safety is to make sure that an animal is properly restrained for examination and treatment. The two main methods of restraint are physical and chemical restraint. Chemical restraint is beyond the scope of first aid, but handlers and responders should recognize when chemical restraint may be required to proceed with caring for an animal. For a discussion on physical restraint, please see Chapter 1.17.

Of note, when working with horses the horse should be held by a capable assistant rather than tied, and this assistant assumes a critical role in securing everyone's safety. The assistant holding the horse should be on the same side of the horse as the medic. If the medic changes sides the assistant should also change sides. Ideally everyone including by-standers should be on the same side of the horse. Because this is not always practical, it is the medic and assistant's responsibility to maintain an awareness of by-standers and warn them to move out of a danger zone.

3. What are normal vital signs for horses (Table 1.19.1)?

- Temperature (T): 99°–100.5°F (37.2°–38°C)
  A rectal thermometer is most accurate, and should be lubricated to ease insertion. One should hold on to the thermometer or attach a lanyard to it that can be clipped to the tail to prevent the thermometer from being sucked into the rectum (Fig. 1.19.1).

- Pulse/heart rate (P/HR)
  Normal resting heart rate is in the range of 35 to 45 beats per minute (bpm). The easiest place to auscultate the heart in a standing horse is low down on the side of the chest wall just up under the elbow (Fig. 1.19.2) When listening for the heartbeat, recognize that it is quite a bit slower than a human's, so move your stethoscope around slowly to find the point of maximum intensity.
  Readily accessible arteries to assess pulse rate and pulse pressure include the facial artery (Fig. 1.19.3), the transverse facial artery (Fig. 1.19.4), and the medial and lateral digital arteries (Figs. 1.19.5 and 1.19.6).

Table 1.19.1 Expected Normal Values for the Resting Healthy Horse

Horses	Value
Rectal Temperature	
Foal during first few days	Up to 102.7°F (39.3°C)
Foal to 4th year	99.5°–101.3°F (37.5°–38.5°C)
Horses, adult	99.5°–101.3°F (37.5°–38.5°C)
Horse, over 5 years	99.5°–101.4°F (37.5°–38.0°C)
Pulse/Heart Rate	
Foals, Newborn	128 bpm
Foals, 1–2 days	100–120 bpm
Foals, up to 2 weeks	80–120 bpm
Foals, 3–6 months	64–76 bpm
Foals, >6–12 months	48–72 bpm
Foals, 1–2 years	40–56 bpm
Adult Horses	
Stallion	28–32 bpm
Gelding	33–39 bpm
Mare	40–56 bpm
Respiratory Rate	
Foal	14–15 bpm
Horse, adult	9–10 bpm

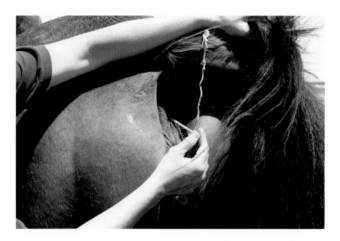

Figure 1.19.1 Rectal thermometer, lubed to ease insertion, and lanyard attached for safety.

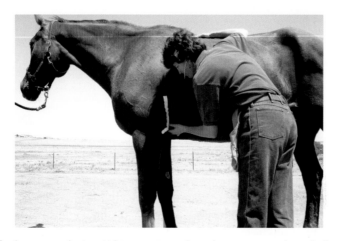

Figure 1.19.2 Location for heart auscultation. White tape is marking the triceps muscle and elbow. The bell of the stethoscope is on the chest wall just up under the elbow.

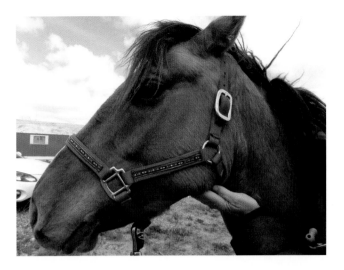

Figure 1.19.3 Facial artery.

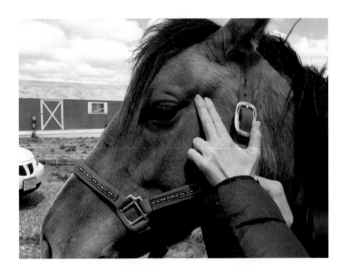

Figure 1.19.4 Transverse facial artery.

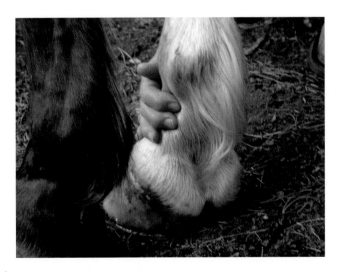

Figure 1.19.5 Medial digital artery.

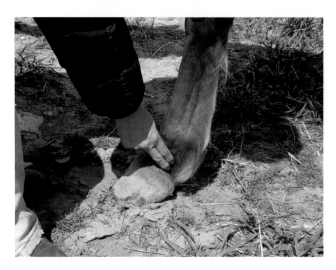

Figure 1.19.6 Lateral digital artery.

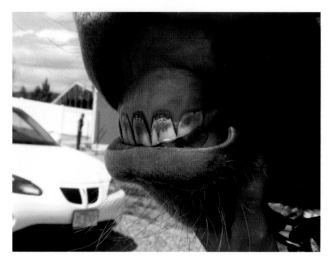

Figure 1.19.7 Mucous membranes in the horse.

- Respiratory rate (R)
  Normal resting respiratory rate is in the range of 10 to 14 breaths per minute (bpm).

- Mucous membranes (MM)
  Normal mucous membranes are pink and moist. The gums are the easiest location to assess mucous membranes (Fig. 1.19.7). Mucous membrane color aids in the subjective assessment of perfusion, oxygenation, and shock. Pale, cyanotic (blue tinged color), hyperemic (red color), injected (deep dark red color), or muddy mucous membranes suggest cardiovascular and/or respiratory pathology.

- Capillary refill time (CRT)
  Normal capillary refill time is 1 to 2 seconds. CRT aids in the subjective assessment of perfusion and shock. To assess CRT, press your finger into the gum to blanch it white and then remove your finger and observe the time for color to return.

- Blood pressure (BP)
  Objective BP measurement on horses in the field is not practical. Pulse quality and pressure give a subjective assessment of BP.

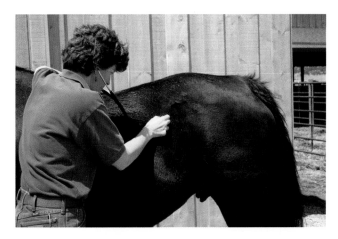

Figure 1.19.8 Dorsal flank auscultation.

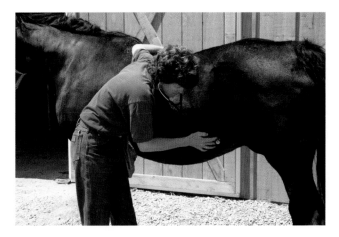

Figure 1.19.9 Ventral flank auscultation.

- Intestinal motility
  Gut motility is very important and can be subjectively assessed by auscultation of the upper (dorsal flank) and lower (ventral flank) quadrant on both the left and right side of the horse (Figs. 1.19.8 and 1.19.9). Normal gut sounds resemble distant rumbling thunder and occur approximately 2 or 3 times per minute, with lighter gurgling sounds interspersed.

4. What are normal vital signs for cattle and other livestock (Table 1.19.2)?

Methods for assessing the vital signs in these animals are very similar to those used for horses.

For ruminants (cattle, sheep, goats, llamas, and alpacas), the first compartment of the stomach is a large fermenting vat called the rumen (in first compartment in llamas and alpacas) and it is on the left side of the abdomen. Pigs have a simple stomach similar in shape to horses and dogs.

Accessible arteries for palpating pulse rate, quality, and pressure are as follows:

Table 1.19.2 Rectal Temperature, Pulse/Heart Rate, and Respiratory Rate of Healthy Resting Animals by Large Animal Species

Species	Rectal Temperature
Ass	99.5°–101.3°F (37.5°–38.5°C)
Mule	101.8°–102.2°F (38.8°–39.0°C)
Calf, young	101.3°–104.9°F (38.5°–40.5°C)
Young cattle up to 1 year	101.3°–104.0°F (38.5°–40.0°C)
Cattle, over 1 year	99.5°–103.1°F (37.5°–39.5°C)
Bison	99.5°–102.2°F (37.5°–39.0°C)
Camel	95.0°–101.5°F (35.0°–38.5°C)
Lamb (sheep)	101.3°–104.9°F (38.5°–40.5°C)
Sheep over 1 year	101.3°–104.0°F (38.5°–40.0°C)
Kid (goat)	101.3°–105.8°F (38.5°–41.0°C)
Goat, adult	101.3°–104.9°F (39.5°–40.5°C)
Piglet	101.2°–104.9°F (39.0°–40.5°C)
Pig, adult	100.4°–104.0°F (39.0°–40.0°C)
Dolphin (Atlantic Bottlenose)	98.5°F (98.5°C)

Species	Pulse/Heart Rate (bpm)
Ass, mule, adult	45–60
Ass, mule, young	65–75
Calf during the first days after birth	116–141
Calf 8–14 days old	108
Calf 1 month old	105
Calf 2 months	101
Calf 3 months	99
Calf 6 months	96
Young cattle up to 12 months	91
Cow, adult	70–90
Ox, adult	70–90
Lamb (sheep)	115
Yearling (sheep)	85–95
Sheep, adult	70–80
Sheep, old	55–60
Ram	68–81
Kid (goat)	100–120
Yearling (goat)	80–110
Goat, adult	70–80
Billy goat	70
Piglets up to 2 weeks	38
Porkers, 12–14 weeks	112
Adult pig, boar	63–68
Adult pig, sow	88–92
Camel	30–50
Elephant	25–28
Dolphin (Atlantic Bottlenose)	50–120

Species	Respiratory Rate (bpm)
Calf, 4 days	56
Calf, 14 days	50
Calf, 5 weeks	37
Young cattle, 6 months	30
Young cattle, 1 year	27
Cattle, adult	12–16
Sheep (lamb)	15–18
Sheep, adult	12–15
Sheep, old	9–12
Kid (goat)	12–20
Goat, adult	12–15
Goat, old	9–12
Pig	10–20
Camel	5–12
Whale	4–5

- **Cattle:** the middle coccygeal artery (in the middle on the underside of the tail near the base) may be used.
- **Sheep, goats, and small pigs:** the femoral artery (inside the back leg up near the groin) is readily accessible. For large pigs finding a palpable artery may be difficult; the coccygeal artery (in the tail) may be available.
- **Llamas and alpacas:** they tend to resent having their legs touched, and palpating the femoral artery in the groin may be difficult. The carotid artery (sometimes) can be palpated in the groove on the side of the neck just below the jaw.

FIRST-AID WOUND CARE PRINCIPLES

5. Why is proper wound care so important?

Wound infection is a serious complication that contributes significantly to delayed wound healing. Different species have different "strategies" for dealing with infection; horses tend to mount a response to clear an infection, while cattle try to isolate the infection from the rest of the body by walling it off. Regardless of the strategy, minimizing the risk of infection developing or progressing is an important goal of wound care.

Appropriate first aid including wound cleansing, lavage (fluid irrigation of a wound), antiseptics, antimicrobial ointments, and where appropriate, bandaging can decrease contamination and facilitate wound healing. When feasible, using basic aseptic (preventing contact with microorganisms) techniques of hand washing and/or wearing exam or surgical gloves can help minimize additional contamination.

6. What is the most effective way to irrigate a wound?

Irrigation agents delivered at an oblique angle under pressure between 7 and 15 pounds per square inch (PSI) are more effective at cleansing wounds and decreasing bacterial load. This pressure lavage can be accomplished using a 35-mL or 60-mL syringe with a 19-gauge needle and is superior to irrigation with a bulb syringe. For added safety to both animal and responder/medic, a 35-mL or 60-mL syringe with a soft flexible 18-gauge intravenous catheter (stylet removed) can be used to deliver pressure lavage. Care must be taken to not drive contaminates into the tissues and to stop the irrigation before tissue swelling occurs.

Water delivered via a hose at the appropriate flow with a nozzle (or thumb) can provide the fluid pressure that aids in the removal of debris. Some animals are not conditioned to being sprayed with a hose and may become quite excited. Directing the hose stream to the ground adjacent to the animal and then moving it onto the foot and leg and on up to the trunk, neck, head, or rump may greatly reduce the animal's anxiety.

7. Discuss different lavage (meaning: to wash out or irrigate) and antiseptic agents.

There are many irrigation and antiseptic agents available for cleaning wounds. Some of these may be used safely in a variety of wounds and wound locations, but others are more restricted in their use (Table 1.19.3).

- Water
  Water can be used on external surfaces to remove gross contamination such as dirt, gravel, plant material, etc. Because of water's hypotonicity (i.e., it has less osmotic pressure than tissue and vascular fluids of the body; essentially this means it is more "dilute" than serum and fluid inside cells), care must be taken to not overuse water as it causes tissues to swell. It is a good choice for removal of large amounts of contamination, or contamination from a large area. Following this preliminary decontamination a more detailed decontamination can be done with an isotonic (i.e., same osmotic pressure as tissue and vascular fluids) irrigation agent, or an appropriate antiseptic solution.

Table 1.19.3 Wound Irrigation and Antiseptic Agents

	Water	Crystalloid Fluids	Chlorhexidine Diacetate, 2% Solution*	Povidone Iodine, 10% Solution*	Hydrogen Peroxide
Further Dilution Required			Yes (Water)	Yes (Water or Saline)	No
External Soft Tissues	Yes	Yes	Yes	Yes	
Simple Puncture Wound		Yes	Yes	Yes	Yes
Eye/Ocular Adnexa	Yes	Yes	No	Yes	No
Bone		Yes	Yes	Yes	No
Exposed Joint		Yes	No	Yes	No
Cautions	Imbibe Tissues		Imbibe Tissues	Imbibe Tissues	Limit Use to 1–2X

*These are "solutions"; do not use "scrub" agents.

- Saline solution (physiologic sterile saline [PSS], 0.9% NaCl), Normosol-R, and Lactated Ringer's solution (LRS)

  Saline solution (PSS, 0.9% NaCl), Normosol-R, and LRS are all nearly isotonic fluids. Normosol-R, LRS, and 0.9% NaCl are used for IV (intravenous) fluid therapy, so these products may be readily available from an ambulance or field hospital. Because they are nearly isotonic, a large volume can be used to aid in the removal of foreign debris.

- Chlorhexidine Diacetate Solution 2%

  Chlorhexidine diacetate solution 2% is an antiseptic solution that has a good spectrum of activity against a variety of bacteria. It also maintains this activity in the presence of organic matter (i.e., really dirty wounds) and it has good residual activity meaning that it stays around to help minimize further contamination.

  This 2% stock solution must be diluted in water to avoid damaging tissues. Mixing 25 mL (5 teaspoons) of chlorhexidine diacetate 2% into 1000 mL (1.06 quarts) of water is a 1:40 dilution that results in a 0.05% solution, which is the recommended strength for wound lavage. Concentrations stronger than 1:40 are detrimental to tissues. When chlorhexidine diacetate is diluted in saline, it forms precipitates. Because of this, water is the recommended diluent even though the precipitates do not effect wound healing.

  Chlorhexidine diacetate solution is an excellent antiseptic that decreases bacterial concentrations on the surface of soft tissues and bone but it should NOT be used in or around the eye and is not suitable if a joint is exposed.

  It is important to note that for wound treatment, this discussion refers to Chlorhexidine diacetate SOLUTION and not Chlorhexidine diacetate SCRUB. "Scrub" agents are detergents for use on intact skin in which the normal protective barriers are in place. Detergents and alcohols are damaging to tissues exposed in wounds.

- Povidone-Iodine Solutions (Betadine Solution)

  Povidone-iodine solutions (10%) are a tamed iodine solution containing 1.0% iodine combined with a carrier and are NOT to be confused with tincture of iodine (7%), which contains 7% elemental iodine.

  Povidone-iodine solution (10%) should be diluted in water or saline to an "iced tea/weak iced tea" color. This dilution with water (or saline) releases the iodine thereby increasing its antiseptic properties. Failure to dilute this solution is not only more irritating to tissues it is also less effective.

  Povidone-iodine solution is the antiseptic of choice when wounds involve joints or eyes and their surrounding structures (i.e., eyelids, etc.). For these wounds, povidone-iodine solutions (10%) diluted to a "weak iced tea" color that is approximately a 1:50 dilution is an effective antiseptic that is not irritating to these tissues.

  Again, it is important to note that this discussion is referring to povidone-iodine SOLUTION and not povidone-iodine SCRUB. As previously mentioned, "scrub" agents are detergents for use on intact skin and they are damaging to tissues exposed in wounds.

- Hydrogen Peroxide (H_2O_2)

When hydrogen peroxide comes in contact with an enzyme found in cells, oxygen is released, which has a germ-killing effect. In addition, this effervescent action mechanically helps remove contamination.

Some wounds, such as puncture wounds, are prone to developing an anaerobic (without oxygen) environment within the wound. Bacteria that thrive in this type of environment are termed *anaerobic bacteria,* some of which can cause deadly infections. When oxygen is released from the hydrogen peroxide, this helps to create a less hospitable environment for these anaerobic bacteria.

Hydrogen peroxide's mode of action makes it a good choice for the initial treatment of simple puncture wounds that do not involve a joint or tendon sheath (or eye structures). It should NOT be used repeatedly, however, as it injures capillary beds and is damaging to healthy tissues.

- Dakin's Solution 0.5%

Dakin's solution 0.5% is a 1 : 10 dilution of stock laundry bleach; it is more commonly used in human medicine. It is further diluted in water to one-quarter to one-half strength. Its germ-killing activity results from the release of chlorine and oxygen. Because it is also toxic to healing cells of the body, its application is limited to dissolving dead tissue and is not recommended as a topical disinfectant for wound lavage.

8.   Discuss antimicrobial ointments and their proper use.

There are a variety of over-the-counter and prescription antimicrobial ointments and creams that are applied to wounds to decrease bacterial contamination or control infection. They should not be used on exposed joints, and in the first aid setting, these ointments and creams should NOT be used if a wound will receive more definitive veterinary medical care *imminently* because of the difficulty in clearing them from the tissues. During the healing process, once a wound is considered "clean" they should be discontinued.

Two main "types" of antimicrobial ointments are those suitable for most wounds on the body, and ophthalmic (eye) preparations. A third grouping of miscellaneous antimicrobial preparations would include the insect repellent ointments, such as Swat, which are important as they decrease the risk of fly-strike and maggot infestation, and other liquid preparations such as Blu-Kote.

Examples of ointments suitable for general wound use include Neosporin and other triple antibiotic preparations, povidone-iodine ointment, and chlorhexidine ointment.

As a guideline, ophthalmic ointments will contain the word "ophthalmic" (or some variation thereof: "ocu," "opti") in the product name or label, and ophthalmic preparations ONLY should be used in or around the eye. These preparations can also be used on the rest of the body, but this tends to be cost prohibitive.

Some ophthalmic preparations contain corticosteroids with or without antibiotics. Corticosteroids are anti-inflammatory drugs with very specific uses. Ophthalmic preparations containing corticosteroids, such as dexamethasone, prednisone, or prednisolone, etc., should NOT be used when corneal wounds or ulcers are present. Do not use an ophthalmic preparation containing a corticosteroid until a veterinarian has performed a thorough ophthalmic exam. Always read the label carefully before placing any ointment in the eye.

FIRST-AID BANDAGING PRINCIPLES

9.   What are some basic bandaging principles?

In terms of first aid, the purpose of a bandage is to control hemorrhage, prevent further contamination of a wound, and provide comfort in stabilizing a wound until definitive veterinary medical treatment can be obtained. There are a variety of bandaging protocols, techniques, and preferences which are acceptable. Understanding the purpose of various layers and types of bandage materials and the various anatomical pitfalls of bandaging certain areas can help minimize adverse effects from bandaging.

10. What are the basic layers of a first-aid bandage?

- Tape "stirrups"
- No-stick tad (Telfa)
- Roll Cotton
- 2- to 6-inch (5- to 15-cm) conforming roll gauze
- 2- to 4-inch (5- to 10-cm) adhesive elastic wrap (VetWrap, PetFlex, Flex Wrap, Coban, etc.)
- 2- to 4-inch (5- to 10-m) Elastikon tape®

Choose the appropriate width of roll gauze, adhesive elastic wrap, and Elastikon tape based on the size of animal and the body part being bandaged (Fig. 1.19.10).

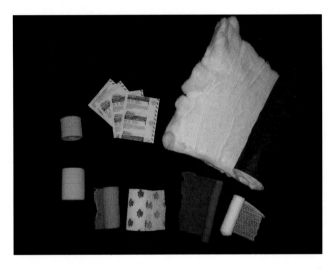

Figure 1.19.10   Bandage materials include Telfa pads, brown gauze, Kling gauze, Elasticon, roll cotton, and tape.

11. Describe the purpose of these various layers and how to apply a proper first-aid bandage.

Tape stirrups are used to prevent a bandage from sliding down. They need not be placed for every bandage, but should be considered if bandage slippage could be a problem. Tape stirrups are placed on opposite sides of the limb, avoiding any wounds, and extend approximately 6 inches (15 cm) beyond what will be the bottom of the bandage (Fig. 1.19.11). This extension will be doubled back onto the bandage and incorporated into the bandage on the (outer) roll gauze layer or the adhesive elastic wrap layer, thus creating the tape stirrup that helps hold the bandage in place (see Fig. 1.19.15).

No-stick pads are placed over the wound to prevent the exposed tissues of a wound from adhering to the dressing and to help prevent the disruption of any clot formation (Fig. 1.19.11).

Some prefer to wrap conforming roll gauze as the next bandage layer to hold the no-stick pad in place. Because of the risk of wrapping this layer too tightly, or having a crease or fold present that can become a pressure point, or having it shift from bandage motion and inadvertently creating a tourniquet-type effect, I prefer to place rolled cotton as the next layer.

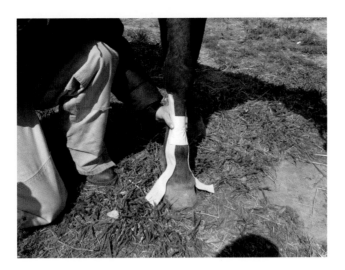

Figure 1.19.11 Stirrups and no-stick pad.

Rolled cotton will hold the no-stick pad in place, conforms well, can be absorbent, and provides cushioning. This bulky layer allows the subsequent layers to be applied fairly tightly while minimizing the risk of crushing or constricting the tissues leading to compromised circulation (Fig. 1.19.12).

After the rolled cotton layer, 2- to 6-inch (5- to 15-cm) conforming roll gauze is used to compact and hold the cotton layer in place (Fig. 1.19.13). The 2-inch size is more appropriate for the limbs of young lambs, kids, cria (baby llamas/alpacas), etc.; 3- to 4-inch (7- to 10-cm) width is suitable for adult sheep, goats, young horses, and cattle; and 4- to 6-inch (10- to 15-cm) width is ideal for adult horses and cattle.

The conforming roll gauze is wrapped moderately tight from *distal to proximal*. *Distal to proximal* means that this layer is wrapped from the end of the limb back up *toward* the body. In doing so, bandage compression is applied in the direction of venous and lymphatic return helping to minimize the "trapping" of return circulatory flow.

The tape stirrups can be folded back against either this layer or the next layer.

Adhesive elastic wrap is the outer layer, again wrapping from *distal to proximal*. This layer affords the bandage some protection from the elements and debris (Fig. 1.19.14).

As an alternative, a reuseable elastic wrap such as an Ace Bandage, may be used for this layer. These reuseable wraps do not have the mild adhesive property that adhesive elastic wraps have, and therefore have a tendency to slide down. Folding the tape stirrups back onto this layer and taping the top and bottom of the bandage will help counter this slipping, but these reusable elastic bandage wraps need extra monitoring.

The conforming roll gauze and elastic wrap layers should not exceed the top or bottom edges of the rolled cotton (Fig. 1.19.15).

Elastikon tape is used at the top and bottom of the bandage extending from the bandage onto the skin/hair as a seal to keep debris from getting in under the bandage and also to hold the tape stirrup ends if placed on the outer layer (Fig. 1.19.16).

Each layer of a bandage should be wrapped in the same direction (Figs. 1.19.12 through 1.19.14). In horses, to avoid causing tendonitis (inflammation of the tendon, commonly referred to as a "bowed tendon"), the direction of wrap should be counterclockwise on the left-side legs and clockwise on the right-side legs.

The accessory carpal bone protrudes from the back of the carpus ("knee" on the front legs) and when bandaging this area is at risk to develop a severe pressure sore (Fig. 1.19.17). To prevent this, a "donut hole" should be cut into any bandage over the accessory carpal bone (Fig. 1.19.18).

When bandaging the hoof or heel bulbs, it is best to incorporate the whole foot into the bandage. A disposable baby diaper can be used in place of roll cotton and fits nicely around the foot (Fig. 1.19.19). As an additional layer added to the outside, duct tape crisscrossed in strips to cover the bottom of the bandage will make it more durable and decrease water on the ground from soaking into the bandage (Fig. 1.19.20).

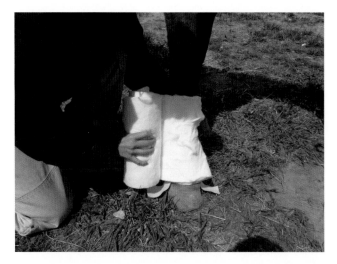

Figure 1.19.12 Rolled cotton.

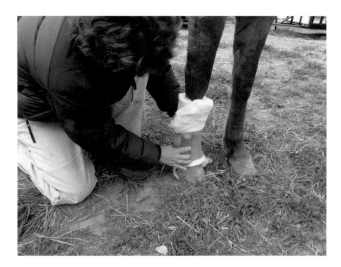

Figure 1.19.13 Rolled cotton being held in place with brown gauze.

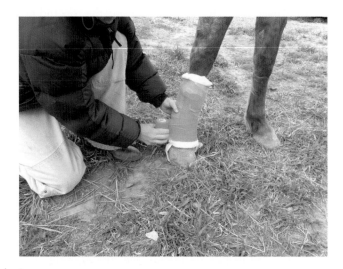

Figure 1.19.14 Adhesive elastic wrap.

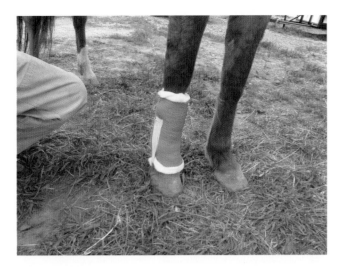

Figure 1.19.15 Taped stirrup ends on VetWrap.

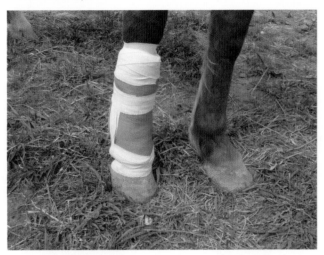

Figure 1.19.16 Elastikon and tape to complete the bandage.

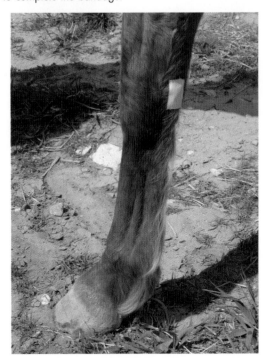

Figure 1.19.17 Tape marking accessory carpal bone.

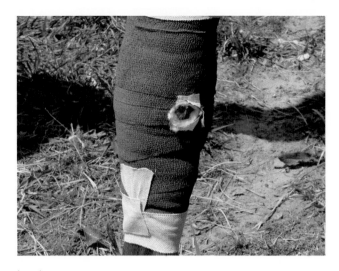

Figure 1.19.18 Donut hole in bandage.

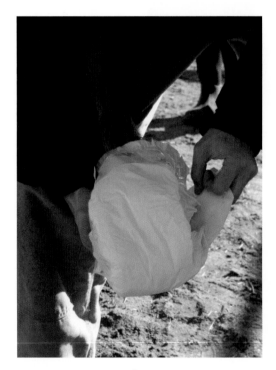

Figure 1.19.19 Diaper on foot.

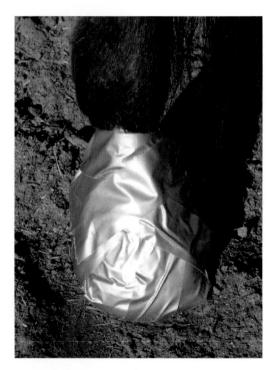

Figure 1.19.20 Duct-taped foot bandage.

FIRST AID FOR COMMON INJURIES AND CONDITIONS

12. How should lacerations and abrasions be managed in the first-aid setting?

- Assess the lacerations and abrasions for depth, severity, and involved structures including tendons, joints, nerves, vessels, or ocular (eye) injury.
- Control hemorrhage with direct pressure, bandage, or pressure bandage. A *pressure bandage* places padding (gauze sponges, towels, sanitary napkins/menstrual pads, etc) over the hemorrhaging area to create additional compression or pressure on that area. Its purpose is to control hemorrhage and as such is a temporary bandage. If you are unable to control the bleeding, continue direct pressure, apply a pressure bandage, or add pressure bandaging to a bandage already in place, and seek definitive veterinary medical treatment as soon as possible.
- When bleeding has been controlled, clean the wound with an appropriate lavage or antiseptic agent. (Remember, if eyes or joints are involved the antiseptic of choice is diluted povidone-iodine solution.)
- Dry the wound by blotting and not wiping to avoid disruption of clots.
- Apply an antimicrobial ointment if definitive assessment and treatment will be delayed. (Do not apply ointments to exposed joints.)
- Place a bandage on amenable areas to minimize further bleeding, contamination, and help stabilize the wound from further trauma.
- Vaseline or an insect repellent ointment (Swat) may be placed on the skin/hair below the wound(s) as a protective barrier against wound drainage and serum scald, and to reduce insect attack.
- For wounds of the head and face where the eye or eyelids could come in contact with the antiseptic solution and/or ointment, povidone-iodine solution and an ophthalmic antimicrobial ointment should be used.
- Animals with thick wool and fiber coats (sheep, llamas, alpacas) should have this "hair" clipped or trimmed away from the wound and the wound area to minimize contamination, decrease moisture retention, and decrease the risk of fly strike and maggot infestation. Other animals will benefit from clipping the hair from around a wound and wound edges as well, but this may be better addressed during more definitive care. Care must be taken to not allow the clipped hair to fall into the wound, and to this end packing the wound with gauze sponges and water soluble K-Y Jelly before clipping can help minimize this contamination. Some animals are not familiar with clippers and may startle at the sound and/or feel of them. It is important to remember this for safety's sake, but with patience most will accept being clipped.
- Lacerations and abrasions should be evaluated by a veterinarian as additional assessment of damage and treatment, including the possibility of primary closure (closing the wound with sutures (stitches)), and timely administration of antibiotics, nonsteroidal anti-inflammatory drugs, and tetanus vaccination booster may be indicated.

13. How should puncture wounds be managed in the first-aid setting?

There are two primary considerations in the assessment of puncture wounds.

- The first addresses immediate, life-threatening hemodynamic (cardiovascular and respiratory) issues such as bleeding, tamponade (blood accumulating in the sac around the heart), and tension pneumothorax (air escaping the lungs, but being trapped in the chest cavity).
- The second, and more common, relates to potential illness associated with bacterial infection.

If one suspects a puncture wound has penetrated into the chest cavity, abdominal cavity, pelvic canal, or jugular furrow (the groove that runs along either side of the neck where the carotid artery, jugular vein, and other vital structures run), definitive veterinary medical care should be sought immediately.

For "simple" puncture wounds that can be addressed in the field, cleanse the surface area of the wound with an antiseptic solution to decrease the contamination that could be carried into the wound. Use a syringe (without a needle attached) to deliver antiseptic solution into the wound. Antiseptic solution applied to a sterile cotton swab can also be used to probe and cleanse the wound.

If a puncture wound does not involve a joint or tendon sheath, hydrogen peroxide is a good choice for the initial irrigation and cleansing. Subsequent antiseptic flushing should be done with chlorhexidine diacetate solution or povidone-iodine solution.

If a puncture wound does, or might, involve a joint or tendon sheath, Normosol-R, 0.9% NaCl, or LRS sterile crystalloid fluids, or PSS is the irrigation agent of choice. Because of the risk of developing serious infection in these structures, definitive veterinary medical care should be obtained as soon as possible.

The goal of treating uncomplicated puncture wounds is to promote drainage, decrease the risk of developing an anaerobic environment, and encourage healing from the deep tissues outward (referred to as secondary intention healing). To this end, antimicrobial ointments should NOT be applied over the wound opening, as this forms a seal covering the opening and effectively preventing air (and therefore oxygen) from getting to the wound. Vaseline and Swat may be applied *around and below* the wound to prevent insect attack and serum scald of the skin from any wound drainage. Puncture wounds should not be bandaged, and they should not be sutured. Continued care includes gently removing surface crusts and irrigating the track with an appropriate antiseptic solution.

It is important to obtain definitive veterinary medical care for puncture wounds, as these wounds should be explored for depth and direction of track and to confirm no foreign bodies remain in the wound. In addition, systemic antibiotics, anti-inflammatory agents, and a tetanus vaccination booster are indicated.

14.   How should fractures be managed in the first-aid setting?

Fractures in large animals are devastating and frequently life-ending injuries. Aside from the prohibitive economic considerations in treating fractures in livestock, attempting treatment, regardless of the cost, in many of these animals is frequently unrewarding and doomed to failure.

In general, livestock that have sustained a fractured limb should be humanely euthanatized. Treatment may be attempted with certain types of fractures in certain types of animals. These animals tend to have a high economic or emotional value (such as horses, foundation breeding stock, insured animals, etc.); even so, the types of fracture that are amenable to repair are very limited. Any (livestock) animal with severe fractures such as spinal fractures, skull fractures with severe neurological damage, comminuted fractures (broken into many pieces), open fractures (fractures where bone ends have penetrated the skin; once called *compound fractures*), fractures resulting in nerve or vascular compromise, or multiple limb fractures should be humanely euthanatized.

An isolated limb fracture may be amenable to treatment, and first aid is directed at stabilizing the injured bone to prevent further damage. When placing a bandage or splint to support a fracture, the joint above and below the affected bone should be immobilized. Failure to do so increases the risk of creating more damage and trauma due to the fulcrum effect of the splint or bandage on the fracture site. In a first-aid setting this realistically limits the areas amenable to bandaging or splinting for fracture stabilization to the lower limbs, below the carpus ("knee") and hock.

A Robert Jones bandage uses the same bandaging principles previously discussed with *significantly more* roll cotton being used in that layer. Because a limb fracture compromises load bearing stability this bandage has to provide additional support. In addition to this abundant layer of cotton, which is the key to a successful Robert Jones bandage, rigid splint material may be incorporated to further decrease the flexibility of the bandage. The rigid splint material does not replace the necessity of a healthy cotton layer. Splint material, such as rebar, PVC half pipe, or wood strips, is placed outside of the (outer) conforming roll gauze, and an additional layer of roll gauze is used to hold the splint material in place. This is followed by the adhesive elastic wrap and Elastikon® layers. If this bandage/splint involves the carpus ("knee"), a donut hole should be cut into the bandage over the accessory carpal bone.

LAMENESS

15. What are some likely causes of lameness in livestock in a disaster?

Disasters such as tornados or earthquakes that cause tremendous damage to buildings, trees, fencing, etc. are likely to cause a significant amount of trauma to animals as well. Flying debris, individuals being picked up by wind and thrown, panicked running in fear, or having to move through ruble, downed fences, and other hazardous obstacles can all result in lameness from wounds, fractures, sprains, or blunt trauma injuries.

Disasters such as floods and hurricanes can result in animals being trapped in water or mud for extended periods of time. Prolonged exposure to water tends to macerate tissues and breaks down the skin's natural defenses. Skin infections such as deep bacterial infections (deep pyoderma), cellulitis infections (infection of soft tissues along tissue lines), and infections of the feet such as foot rot and thrush (fungi), as well as wounds sustained from debris in the water can all result in lameness.

Animals trapped in blizzards will frequently suffer frostbite of their ears, tails, and limbs. When the damage to the limbs is severe and permanent this is catastrophic for the animal.

16. How should lameness be treated by a first-aid responder?

Try to determine the cause by examining the animal for an obvious reason for the lameness. Note color changes on the skin such as bruising or blackness (seen with gangrene, frostbite, etc.). Look for trauma, note any abnormal swellings which might suggest a hematoma (blood filled swelling), abscess, or fracture; treat any wounds, lacerations, or abrasions. Pay close attention to the claws and interdigital space on cloven hoofed animals, and note any swelling, foul odor, or skin irritation (dermatitis).

For animals trapped in water there are multiple considerations. Water alone can macerate tissues and break down the skin's defenses, but in disaster situations flood waters are frequently contaminated with chemicals (gasoline, oil, household cleaners, etc.), solid waste, or other organic debris as well. With the loss of skin integrity, the risk of infection and, in severe cases, the potential for significant loss of fluids and colloids (such as occurs with plasma seepage from severely traumatized skin) is very serious.

First aid for these animals is to remove them to a dry and clean environment. For herds of animals, this may be simply moving them to higher ground that is dry and drains well. Individual animals may be confined in smaller stalls, corrals, or paddocks, but every effort should be made to assure these areas are as clean and dry as possible.

The hair and skin of these animals will need to be cleaned. If the skin is in good shape, water and shampoo, or Dawn® dishwashing liquid can be used. If the skin is significantly compromised then an isotonic fluid, such as PSS, should be used instead. When oil and other contaminates are present some sort of soap will be required to remove them from the haircoat. Mild soap products, minimal abrasive scrubbing and thorough but not copious amounts of rinsing with water or saline should be done. The skin and haircoat should be blotted dry and not wiped to prevent further damage to the skin.

Animals severely affected will require additional medical treatment, so obtaining definitive veterinary care is important.

Cloven-hoofed animals such as cattle, sheep, goats, and pigs are at risk for developing interdigital infections (infections between their claws). Interdigital infections may result from bacteria invading the skin layers or as in the case of interdigital phlegmon ("footrot"), maceration of the tissues may predispose the interdigital skin to injury which provides a portal for infection. Bacteria such as *Fusobacterium necrophorum, Dichelobacter nodosus, Escherichia coli,* and others have been identified. Most of these animals will require definitive veterinary treatment involving thorough cleansing between the claws, medicated footbaths, and/or systemic antibiotic treatment. An important consideration for an animal responder is to recognize that these animals will actively shed these organisms from the lesions in their feet, so to minimize the risk of infection to other animals, they should be isolated.

17. What is laminitis?

Laminitis is a condition seen in horses, cattle, sheep, goats, and pigs. The sensitive laminae are the vascular and nerve rich layers that lie between the outer horny hoof wall and the bone within the hoof. This layer "helps" to secure the bone to the hoof wall. While we do not completely understand all the factors involved in this disease, we recognize a variety of causes that can trigger this inflammation, including repetitive concussive forces on hard ground (such as running on asphalt or hard gravel roads), grain overloads, eating lush green grass, systemic infections, or even ingestion of a large amount of cold water in overheated horses. Animals in a disaster may develop this condition as a result of exposure to the wide variety of things that can trigger laminitis.

Clinical signs of laminitis include the appearance of "walking on eggshells," standing with the back feet farther under the body in an attempt to decrease the weight on the front feet, heat detectable over the whole hoof wall, and, in horses, bounding pulses in the medial and lateral digital arteries. This can be an extremely painful condition, so other signs of pain may also be seen such as increased respiration, muscle tremors, and anxiety.

First aid for these animals is to recognize that this condition may exist and to secure veterinary medical care as soon as possible. This is a medical emergency, and treatment is directed toward pain relief (analgesia), decreasing inflammation, and reducing the hypertensive cycle of disease in the foot.

FIRST AID FOR THE EYE

18. What is the third eyelid of animals?

Other than the "normal" dorsal (upper or superior) and ventral (lower or inferior) eyelids, domestic animals have an additional eyelid called the "nictitating membrane" or "third eyelid." This third eyelid comes up from the lower inside corner of the eye and functions to help protect the cornea (the clear surface of the eye through which light passes) among other things. Its movement is passive in that when the globe (the eyeball) retracts into the socket, it puts pressure on a fat pad behind the eye which in turn puts pressure on a gland in the third eyelid, which in turn moves the eyelid across the eye. A painful eye is frequently retracted into the socket, so sustained elevation of the third eyelid is an important sign of possible eye irritation, inflammation, or injury.

19. What are clinical signs of injury or inflammation of the eye?

In addition to obvious injury or trauma to the eye and surrounding structures, clinical signs include third eyelid elevation, squinting, excessive blinking or keeping the eyelids closed, excessive tearing, "bloodshot" eyes, swelling, or avoidance of light.

20. Describe appropriate first-aid care for eye inflammation or injuries.

When examining an animal's eyes, avoid facing him or her into direct sunlight. Move to a shaded area if possible, or provide shading to decrease the brightness and glare. Compare both eyes and note any abnormalities including injuries to the eyelids, position of the eyes and eyelids, redness of the eye(s), or injury to the surface (cornea) of the eye(s).

Irrigating the eyes can help remove particulates causing irritation and may flush a foreign body from under an eyelid. Water, PSS, or 0.09% NaCl can be used for irrigation. A 35-mL or 60-mL syringe (without a needle attached) helps significantly to irrigate an appropriate volume across the eye. Occasionally, judicious use of a moistened cotton swab or corner of a gauze sponge can help "pick up" and remove a foreign body.

If wounds are present on the eyelids or surrounding the eye, the only acceptable antiseptic solution is diluted povidone-iodine solution. As previously discussed, povidone-iodine solution 10% diluted with saline solution to a "weak tea" color (approximately 1:50 dilution) is an effective antiseptic.

All eye problems should have a definitive ophthalmic exam because a number of different eye conditions look similar, and some (corneal) injuries are very subtle and require special stains and instrumentation to detect. If veterinary care is not available (or will be significantly delayed), an ophthalmic antibiotic ointment may be placed as a precautionary measure. It is important to read the ointment label carefully and check that it is labeled for use in the eye and that it does NOT contain any corticosteroid drugs.

The easiest and safest way to apply ointment to the eye of an animal is to have clean hands, squeeze a reasonable amount of ointment onto your index finger, use your other hand to roll down the lower lid, and wipe the ointment onto the inside surface of the lower lid.

If a corneal injury is identified, obtain veterinary care immediately.

Thermal injuries from fire and explosions are particularly damaging to eyes. First-aid treatment is directed toward copious irrigation with water followed by the application of a topical antibiotic ophthalmic ointment. (Again, preparations containing corticosteroids should NOT be used.) Antibiotic ophthalmic ointments are used preferentially to antibiotic drops or solutions, as the ointment will prevent adhesions from forming between the eyelids and eyeball.

HEAT EXHAUSTION AND HEATSTROKE

21. Describe what is meant by heat exhaustion and heatstroke.

Hyperthermia is an increase in core body temperature above normal that can progress to heat exhaustion or heatstroke. These extremely high core body temperatures >105°F (40.6°C) occur when excess heat generated by body metabolism, exercise, and/or environmental conditions, exceeds the body's ability to dissipate that heat. Heat loss (transfer) occurs by convection (air currents), conduction, radiation, or evaporation. When the body's compensatory mechanisms are overwhelmed, heat exhaustion progresses to heatstroke. With heatstroke significant tissue damage occurs, which involves the brain and other organs such as liver and kidneys.

A guideline *Heat Exhaustion/Heatstroke Risk Index* for horses can be estimated by taking the summation of the air temperature and relative humidity: <130, a horse can most likely cool himself; 130 to 150, it becomes difficult for a horse to cool himself; and >180, a horse's cooling system is ineffectual—even with significant sweating, there is minimal cooling effect. This index can be used as an estimation of risk for other large animals as well. It is important to note that this index is just a guideline and common sense must prevail when assessing heat exhaustion and heatstroke risk.

Pigs rely on rolling in something cool (water or mud) to keep from overheating as they do not sweat nor can they cool down by panting. They also tend to retain heat because of their thick stout body volume relative to their surface area. Pigs are also quite susceptible to sunburn. All these factors make heat stress a high risk for these animals.

22. What are clinical signs of heat exhaustion?

Clinical signs of heat exhaustion include increased or profuse sweating (not pigs), increased heart rate, flared nostrils and increased respiratory rate. Horses CANNOT breathe through their mouths, so they will not pant like a dog. Progressively worsening signs of heatstroke include stumbling, weakness, depression, dry skin form having lost their ability to sweat, and, in horses, spasmodic jerking of the diaphragm and flanks referred to as "thumps." Poor prognostic signs of heatstroke are collapse, seizure, and coma.

23. What is the first-aid treatment for heat exhaustion and heatstroke?

First-aid treatment for hyperthermia is directed toward lowering the core body temperature. While obtaining more definitive veterinary medical treatment is vital, implementing measures to lower core body temperature should

NOT be delayed. The goal is to reduce the core body temperature to approximately 102°F (38.9°C) in 30 to 60 minutes. During the cooling process, it is important to monitor core body temperature. When the temperature drops to 103° to 104°F (39.5° to 40°C), stop active cooling measures but still monitor core body temperature as it may continue to decline and warming procedures may be indicated.

Move the animal(s) to a cooler environment that also provides good air flow, for example, into the shade of a building, tree, awning, or lean-to shed. Tarps can be rigged to provide shade and misting can be very helpful.

Apply **COOL**, 60° to 65°F (15° to 18°C) water to the legs, chest, face, head, and neck to facilitate heat loss by conduction and evaporation. A hose is ideal for this, but can also be done with a bucket of water and sponge, or using bottled water if nothing else is available. Avoid the large loin and rump muscles (especially on horses) as this relatively cold water can cause blood vessels to constrict leading to further damage in these muscles.

Do NOT use ice baths or cold, 35° to 45°F (2° to 7°C) water baths as this promotes skin vessel constriction, which impairs heat loss and induces shivering resulting in increased heat production.

In addition to the application of cool water, moving air over the animal by fanning or electric fan will help with evaporative cooling.

Cooler water can be applied to the jugular furrow (the groove on the either side of the neck) where the jugular vein and carotid artery are relatively superficial and free from large muscle groups helping to increase heat exchange of these large vessels.

Because of the potential for severe tissue damage and the sequela of tissue damage, it is imperative to obtain or transport to definitive veterinary medical care as soon as possible. While a veterinarian may implement more aggressive cooling measures that are beyond the scope of first aid such as cooled IV fluids and cool water enemas, the benefit of the rapid response of applying cool water to the body surface should not be underestimated. It is worth repeating that while obtaining more definitive veterinary medical treatment is vital, implementing measures to lower core body temperature should NOT be delayed as a consequence.

24.   What is hypothermia, and how does it differ from frostbite?

Hypothermia occurs when the core body temperature drops below normal (Table 1.19.1). "Warm-blooded" animals regulate their own body temperature, and the part of the brain responsible for this is called the *hypothalamus*. In response to changes in skin temperature and blood temperature, physiologic mechanisms are triggered, such as constricting peripheral vessels to reduce heat loss to the environment, or raising the hair (fluffing up) to trap more air against the skin and provide another layer of insulation. Other mechanisms to generate more heat include increasing muscle activity, such as shivering. Digesting food also increases metabolism and generates heat production. Animals prevented from accessing feed, as frequently happens in blizzards, are limited in their ability to generate heat and maintain body temperature.

Young animals, geriatric animals, or debilitated animals do not have the reserves to generate body heat and they do not thermoregulate as well as do healthy adult animals. Special attention should be paid to these groups as marginal environmental situations may result in hypothermia. Prolonged exposure to cold, especially cold combined with wet (rain, sleet, snow) and wind, places all animals at risk of becoming hypothermic.

Water transfers heat from the body approximately 25 to 75 times faster (standing water–fast-flowing water) than happens for the same air temperature. One can withstand being in 45°F (7.2°C) air temperature much longer than if submerged in 45°F (7.2°C) water. Animals that are trapped in water for any length of time are at risk for becoming hypothermic, even if the air temperature is warm.

When the body's mechanisms for warming are overwhelmed there is deterioration in brain function, fluids are shifted from the periphery into the core, which alters cardiovascular parameters resulting in more viscous blood, decreased output from the heart, and a drop in blood pressure. Breathing starts to decrease, and effective uptake and delivery of oxygen to cells in the body are diminished.

Hypothermia differs from frostbite in that frostbite refers to tissues actually freezing, which requires the environmental temperature to be below freezing. Hypothermia can develop in temperatures well above freezing and relates to the core body temperature dropping below normal. Certainly animals with frostbite can be hypothermic as well. Because the body attempts to preserve heat in the body core, peripheral areas such as ears, feet, and tail are at high risk for frostbite in freezing temperatures.

Many of the medical thermometers available today do not provide readings in the lower temperatures, so it may be difficult to know exactly what the core body temperature is, but they do provide enough information to confirm an animal is hypothermic and to monitor re-warming temperatures. Clinical signs may help estimate the severity of hypothermia.

25. What clinical signs are associated with hypothermia?

- Mild hypothermia: approximately 92° to 95°F (33.3° to 35°C)
  - Shivering
  - Lethargy
  - Weakness
  - Mental depression and lack of interest in surroundings
- Moderate hypothermia: approximately 82° to 92°F (27.7° to 33.3°C)
  - Muscle stiffness
  - Stumbling
  - Decreased respiratory rate and depth
  - Decreased heart rate
  - Stuporous or obtund
- Severe hypothermia: any temperature <82°F (27.7°C)
  - Difficulty breathing (very shallow, very slow)
  - Difficult to hear a heartbeat
  - Pupils are dilated and do not respond to light
  - Coma

It can be difficult to differentiate a severely hypothermic from a dead animal.

26. How should hypothermia be treated?

Hypothermic animals should be moved out of cold, wet, and/or wind environments. Smaller enclosures will warm just from the presence of "warm" bodies, but larger barns and even lean-tos with siding that provide a wind break can make a significant difference. Wet animals should be dried as much as possible. Animals that are moderately to severely affected should not be forced to move because of the risk or developing deadly heart arrhythmias; smaller animals and babies should be carried to shelter in this situation.

For mildly hypothermic animals, providing blankets or other thermal covers (e.g., straw) and feed (if not too mentally depressed) may be all that's needed. Horse blankets are ideal for the larger animals, but polar fleece vests work very well for many different animals. They are easy to come by, are easily changed and washable, and do a good job of helping to keep warmth in the body core. The vest is worn backward so it zips up the back of the animal. Groups of pigs can be protected against the cold by providing thick layers of straw that allow them to burrow in and pig pile.

A responder may be able to place a smaller sized baby animal inside their own coat, holding the animal's trunk against their body, to affect some transfer of body heat and warmth.

Heat lamps on pen enclosures and heaters may be used but ONLY if *someone is present* because of the risk of fire danger. Carefully monitored, warm water bottles can be wrapped in a towel, and nestled around the trunk of an animal that is lying down, or placed in the pockets of the polar fleece vest. Heating pads especially, but even water bottles too, can cause thermal burns to the skin (low blood pressure and decreased peripheral circulation increase this risk) and should never be placed directly against skin. In addition to being wrapped in a towel or blanket, heating pads should only be used on "Low." They should NOT be used for animals that are not mentally or physically capable of moving away from a heating element. Even with these precautions, heating pads pose a burn risk to patients, so if used, they require extra care and attention.

When rewarming hypothermic animals, it is important to apply the warmth preferentially to the trunk and core of the body and not the limbs. If the peripheral vessels dilate too soon, cold from the extremities is carried into the body core lowering core temperature further. In addition, the low blood pressure state is further compromised when these peripheral vessels dilate. Because of this, a warm water bath should only be considered for a *very mildly* hypothermic animal; otherwise this method should not be used.

Continue to monitor body temperature and be aware that the temperature may drop as you begin the rewarming because of the peripheral vessels dilating. Core body warming should be gradual at approximately 1° to 2°F (1°C) per hour.

Severely hypothermic animals will likely require more aggressive medical techniques to resuscitate them. This might include warmed IV fluids, warm water or saline gastric, peritoneal, and/or urinary bladder lavage and even warmed air delivered to the lungs via a ventilation tube. However, if this level of veterinary care is not available or not an option, it is still worth trying to save these animals by these other less costly more readily available options, as they may be able to recover.

27. How should frostbite be addressed in the first-aid setting?

As previously discussed, frostbite refers to the freezing of tissues, while hypothermia describes a decrease in core body temperature. If an animal has frostbite, he may be hypothermic as well, and the hypothermia should be addressed first for all the reasons previously discussed about warming the core before the periphery. Once the hypothermia is resolved, the current recommendation is to treat the frostbitten area with rapid rewarming. Water temperature in the range of 107° to 110°F (41.6° to 43.3°C) is recommended. Limbs may be placed in water baths or wet towels may be wrapped (and frequently changed) around ears and tails.

Frostbite of the limbs or areas of the trunk carry a guarded prognosis, and these animals may need to be humanely euthanatized.

COLIC AND BLOAT

28. What do the terms "colic" and "bloat" mean?

Colic is a term that refers to acute paroxysmal abdominal pain. Colic is a common condition of horses. In livestock, bloat is a term that refers to an accumulation of gas or froth in the first compartment of the stomach called the rumen. Bloat is a condition seen in cattle and other ruminants. Death from bloat or colic is the result of shock and cardiovascular collapse.

29. What are the clinical signs of colic?

Clinical signs of colic include the following: wanting to lie down, wanting to roll, pawing, kicking at their belly, sweating, looking back at their flanks, rapid respiration, rapid heartbeat, prolonged capillary refill time, decreased or increased bowel sound, or a change in the quality of the bowel sounds (a tympanic "pebble in a culvert" sound versus normal "distant rumbling thunder"). Horses cannot vomit, so emesis will not be a sign of colic.

30. What are clinical signs of bloat?

The rumen is a large fermenting vat on the left side of the abdomen. One can appreciate normal rumenal activity by watching the waves of contraction move down the animal's side. As the feed stuff ferments in this vat, excess gas is eructated (burped). Bloat develops when normal gastrointestinal peristalsis (movement) decreases or stops and/or when the animal is unable to burp and relieve the gas buildup. This can happen if the opening from the stomach back up the esophagus gets covered over in liquid and feed stuff such that gas cannot escape, or when certain types of feed stuff turn into froth. Froth consists of lots and lots of tiny bubbles similar to a bubble bath. These bubbles are filled with gas, but the surface tension of the bubble prevents them being burped like a gas.

Clinical signs of bloat include a decrease in the normal peristaltic wave and gut motility, a gas distended left/upper left side of the abdomen and flank, increased heart rate, increased respiratory rate, and generalized distressed appearance and look in the eye.

31.   What can an animal responder do for a horse with colic?

First aid for colic is primarily to recognize that colic may exist and to obtain veterinary medical help as soon as possible. For horses that are down, rolling, thrashing, or at risk of injuring themselves, a responder may try to walk that animal while awaiting the arrival of the veterinarian. A responder may have access to Banamine paste in certain emergency situations. If veterinary medical care will be delayed, administration of Banamine paste (flunixin meglumine paste at 1.1 mg/kg orally), can provide some pain relief and alleviate some of the effects of endotoxins.

32.   What can an animal responder do for an animal with bloat?

First aid for bloat is primarily to recognize that this condition exists and to obtain veterinary medical help as soon as possible. In an emergency where veterinary care is significantly delayed or unavailable, a responder can attempt to relieve the bloat by passing a tube. The tube should have a smooth end to avoid injuring the esophagus, and should be somewhat rigid to avoid collapsing and pinching shut. A garden hose cut to an 8-foot (2.4-m) length can work. The tube should be lubed to ease passage, and if K-Y Jelly is unavailable a light coating of liquid soap can work. Cattle have very sharp molar teeth and there is a risk that the tube may get off to the side of the mouth and the animal will bite through it. (This is very bad should an animal bite the tube in half.) Without the benefit of a Frick speculum (a metal tube inserted into the mouth to prevent the tube from being bitten), the handler should try to keep the hose centered in the mouth. There is a large bulge on the back of the tongue of bovids (cattle). When passing the hose it is important to direct the tube up and over this bump. Flexing the animal's neck (pushing the chin towards the neck) as you advance the tube will help guide it into the esophagus and not the trachea (windpipe). Allowing the animal to swallow as the tube approaches the back of the throat will also encourage the tube into the esophagus. To confirm that you are in the esophagus, suck back on the tube. The esophagus will close down around the tube and you will not be able to suck any air. If you can inhale continuously, the tube is in the trachea going to the lungs and it MUST be repositioned into the esophagus. It is fairly difficult to pass a tube into the wind pipe of cattle and generally the tube will go into the esophagus on the first pass. Gently advance the hose and when it enters the rumen there will be a release of gas, hopefully. Move the tube in short increments to find gas pockets.

Frothy bloats require additional treatment to break up the bubbles, so there may not be the gas release seen with gassy bloats. Frothy bloats are more difficult to deal with because of the surface tension of the bubbles. If a frothy bloat is suspected (minimal gas release), pouring a quart of corn, vegetable, or mineral oil down the tube via a funnel may help break up the foam.

When veterinary care is not available, animal responders passing a tube, in less than ideal conditions, with less than ideal equipment, is done as a life-saving measure in an animal that will die otherwise. Desperate times call for desperate measures.

TYING UP

33.   What is "tying up"?

Tying up is a condition seen in horses associated with excessive exercise. The exact mechanism and pathology of this exertional muscle disease are somewhat complicated, but basically these horses deplete their energy stores, are dehydrated, and have electrolyte imbalances from excessive sweating, which contribute to perfusion problems adding to the severe "cramping" of the major muscles.

34.   What are the clinical signs of tying up?

Clinical signs of tying up include muscle cramping, muscle fasciculation (twitching), a tucked-up appearance, sweating, stiff stilted gait, and a reluctance to move. The largest muscle masses are often the most severely affected, and the large rump and leg muscles may be firm and painful to the touch. A horse with colic may exhibit similar signs, but making a distinction is important to prevent a horse suffering from this condition being mistaken for a horse with colic and therapeutically walked or given Banamine before properly resuscitated with fluids. Palpating the rump and leg muscles for hardness and pain that may be seen in tying up but not colic may help in distinguishing the two conditions.

35.   What can a responder do for a horse that is tied up?

It is very important for a responder to recognize that a horse may be tied up and to seek veterinary medical care as soon as possible. These horses should NOT be moved, including walking or trailering any significant distance, as this will worsen the condition. A veterinarian may need to be transported to the horse to replace fluid and electrolyte losses, provide pain relief, and relieve anxiety.

Heat and humidity contribute to the risk of this condition. While awaiting the veterinarian, assess the animal for heat exhaustion and implement appropriate first-aid treatment as previously discussed. It is especially important to avoid hosing or cooling the large rump and leg muscles in these animals.

To avoid causing intestinal cramping and possibly cold water founder, these animals should NOT have free choice access to cold water until they are properly cooled down. Offer small amounts of tepid water while the horse cools. If the veterinarian will be delayed, the horse may drink an electrolyte water mix if available. Offer small amounts of the electrolyte water mix and small amounts of plain water.

If the horse wants to lie down provide as much soft bedding as possible. Lying on these muscles can further compromise the circulation in them so any (extra) bedding can be helpful.

Suggested Reading
Barnett KC. *Equine Ophthalmology: An Atlas and Text.* 2nd ed. Philadelphia, Elsevier Health Sciences, 2004.
Plumb DC. *Veterinary Drug Handbook,* 6th ed. Ames, IA, Blackwell Publishing, 2008.
Rose RJ, Hodgson DR. *Manual of Equine Practice.* 2nd ed. Philadelphia, WB Saunders, 1999.
Stashak TS. *Adams' Lameness in Horses.* 5th ed. Ames, IA, Blackwell Publishing, 2002.
Stashak TS. *Equine Wound Management.* Philadelphia, Lea & Febiger, 1991.

CHAPTER 1.20
EQUINE EMERGENCY SHELTERING

Rebecca S. McConnico, DVM, PhD

1. Who is the official in charge of equine sheltering in a local community during emergency or disaster situations?

The state veterinarian is in charge of animals in most states for state-declared emergencies. Animal response activities need to be coordinated both locally, regionally, statewide, and nationally using the incident command system (ICS). Establishing a network of trained people and groups with effective communication is vitally important to the overall success of any level of animal response activity.

Emergency managers in a community include officials from the parish or county Office of Emergency Preparedness (OEP) officials or local Office of Homeland Security. These officials usually employ or task a designated animal safety and control officer to be responsible for animal issues in a community. The "official" local person is usually a trained animal control officer, but it can be a public law enforcement official with some or minimal animal response training. Successful regional and community animal plan models for horses include those involved with repeated emergency responses in Florida, Southern California, Louisiana, and North Carolina.

2. Do local communities have access to state resources for local equine disaster and emergency response needs?

It is often misunderstood on the part of the public that the local community and state resources automatically come to their aid for animal rescue in disaster situations. Horse owners must work together in their respective communities and take a proactive responsibility for protecting the animals under their care. Advanced planning can help horse owners minimize the loss of animal lives and the health problems associated with disasters such as floods, tornadoes, fire, and hurricanes. Due to the vulnerability of coastal regions to hurricanes and storms and their potential to cause widespread damage due to flooding, preparedness in these most vulnerable areas is essential. It must be stressed that although help may be available from many sources following a disaster, owners themselves are ultimately responsible for the welfare of their animals and should prepare accordingly.

3. What can local equine stakeholders and owners do to plan for evacuation and response sheltering during disasters?

Local communities should have a comprehensive equine emergency plan that is part of the overall community-based animal plan that merges with regional and state animal plans. Plans should follow universal ICS structuring so that plans can dovetail with local, state, and federal emergency management systems. For equine sheltering activities, equine veterinarians, horse owners, and other equine stakeholder group members should organize a working group to determine a plan for response that includes written comprehensive (and detailed) evacuation, sheltering, and rescue plans. A critical part of any plan includes communication and ongoing public education programs. Education programs may be best coordinated through the state agriculture extension programs along with public and private universities, public and private primary and secondary education systems, and institutions of higher education.

4. What needs to be considered for determining an appropriate equine shelter for emergency response?

First, identify potential facilities to be used for equine evacuation and response sheltering. State equine councils are encouraged to take leadership roles in emergency planning in their home states and to work with local and state emergency managers. State, regional, and local community equine stakeholders should work together to identify possible sites for equine sheltering. Shelter resource options should be compiled by state animal response teams along with the state veterinarian's office and should be updated yearly.

The overall goal for equine emergency sheltering is to move (and keep) the animals away from harm's way while not putting them, or their owners and handlers, in additional risk situations (i.e., gridlock traffic in summer heat). This requires appropriate pre-storm or preevent planning and early evacuation. Typical emergencies for different areas of the country should be considered when making plans. Being prepared for the most commonly encountered emergencies before, during, or after the specific event (fire, earthquake, storm, etc.) will require some variation, but overall communication, personnel, sheltering, and other response activities will have a common template for operating. For example, sheltering that would begin after the disaster may require vehicles to be brought in to transport horses out of the area, because local transportation may be damaged or destroyed during a disaster event. Shelters need to be far enough away from harm if there is an impending disaster but in close enough proximity for practical purposes.

Shelters must provide for safe animal handling and holding areas with stalls, gates, and fences in good working condition. Shelters must have adequate and safe water sources and other utilities (electricity, trash removal). The equine shelter should have enough space so that stallions can be separated from mares and geldings. If individual stalls are not available, portable stalls, round pens, and panels can be used to separate animals as needed (Fig. 1.20.1).

Rolled plastic webbing/fencing can be used to segregate the horses if other supplies are not available. Placing two layers of fencing separated by enough space so animals cannot touch their muzzles will help keep them from fighting or pushing through this type of barrier. Many law enforcement agencies and local and state divisions of transportation use this material on a routine basis for crowd control and other safety activities and are usually willing to help with animal response activities if asked. Standard 50-foot round pens or similar-size paddocks can be used to separate horses into smaller groups if individual stalls are unavailable. Unfamiliar horses grouped together in paddocks or round pens should number no more than six to eight per 50-foot round pen or comparable-size paddock if possible to allow enough space so that pecking order activities can safely occur. In addition, shelters should be large enough to provide for a separate area for sick animals (quarantine area at least 35 feet from presumed healthy animals). Memoranda of understanding/agreement should be formed between official state or local animal response teams and shelter facility owners. Security will be discussed later. Possible locations to consider for equine shelters include the following:

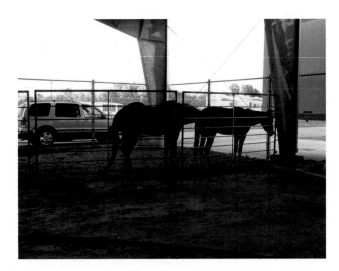

Figure 1.20.1 Portable corral panels can be used to isolate horses.

- University livestock exhibit/handling facilities
- Stockyards
- Sale barns
- Feedlots
- Private/public-owned livestock arenas/expo centers
  - Fairgrounds
  - Horse activity centers
  - Exhibition facilities
- Race tracks
- Private horse farms

5. What kinds of supplies are needed for stocking an equine shelter?

Determine the presence of retail or wholesale farm supply stores close to a community or shelter with ready supplies (as opposed to stockpiling supplies that may not be used for years). Most urgently needed supplies include water buckets, halters, and lead ropes. The Louisiana State Animal Response Team has stockpiled 100 each of these three items in three different areas of the state in the event of disaster response requiring immediate equine evacuation. Items needed for managing an equine shelter should include those shown in Table 1.20.1.

Table 1.20.1. Recommended Supplies for Equine Sheltering during a Disaster

Item	Quantity per 25 horses
Water bucket (20–26 qt)	25
Clips to hang water buckets	25
Halters of varying sizes	25
Lead ropes	10–15
Aluminum or plastic scoop shovels	3–4
Manure rakes	3–4
Manure wheelbarrows	2–3
Garden hose (75 ft)	3–4
Box fans	25
Extension cords	5–10
1–2″ PVC pipe (safety cover for extension cords)	As needed
Hay (7-day supply)	As needed
Horse feed concentrate	As needed
Bedding	As needed
Fly spray	As needed
Hoof pick	2–4
Brushes	5–10
Hand washing stations	1–2
Human first aid kit	1
Dawn® dishwashing liquid	2 gallons
Trash bags/trash cans	2 trash cans per aisle
Two-way walkie-talkie type radios	4
Laptop computer	1
Fax machine	1
Cell phones	Per volunteer
Office supplies	As needed
Animal ID tags (TabBand)	As needed

6.   What should be done to ensure that the medical needs and health maintenance of shelter horses are managed appropriately?

A veterinarian should be involved in the overall health management of an equine evacuation and/or response shelter. A licensed veterinarian should have oversight of daily nutritional management, physical condition, and medical care of all sheltered horses as well as manage shelter biosecurity. The veterinarian should work with public health officials regarding the overall human safety issues associated with taking care of shelter horses. This protects the volunteers as well as well-intentioned but curious bystanders and others.

Well in advance of a potential disaster situation, horse owners/producers should evaluate their herd health programs with their veterinarian. Horses that undergo evacuation relating to a disaster response will be stressed and are likely to commingle with other horses and livestock. Herd biosecurity will be breeched, which makes increasing herd immunity imperative. Pneumonia and abortions should be anticipated and can be minimized with proper herd nutrition and vaccination. Prior to storm seasons, horses should be vaccinated with current strains for equine herpes I and IV and equine influenza I and II, in addition to the encephalitides (Eastern and Western equine encephalitis viruses and West Nile virus) and tetanus.

All horses should be examined by a veterinarian as soon as possible (at least within 12 hours) on admission to an emergency equine shelter. Sick horses need to be separated as soon as possible (e.g., those with fever, nasal discharge, lethargy, and diarrhea) and should be kept in individual stalls in a remote area (at least 35 feet) from the rest of the sheltered animals. These animals must be handled by separate, dedicated, trained shelter personnel wearing appropriate barrier precautions (washable footwear, latex exam gloves, water-repellant barrier gowns/coveralls, etc.).

For horses sustaining injury from natural disasters such as snow storms, tornadoes, hurricanes, floods, and fires, stress is a major contributor to equine medical problems and can include colic, diarrhea, dehydration, neurologic disease, respiratory disease, laminitis, sole abscesses, skin abrasions, cellulitis, lacerations, fracture disease, smoke inhalation and burns (fire-related disasters), and corneal injuries. The innate equine flight or fight response can often accentuate even minor medical problems into sometimes life-threatening situations. If possible, injured horses should be examined by a veterinarian in the field and medically stabilized prior to transport. Animals requiring hospital level care in an equine shelter should be transported to an equipped veterinary hospital.

When large numbers of disaster affected horses arrive in large numbers at the same time to a shelter location, a plan for expedited triage should be in place so that the sickest horses may be able to receive appropriate medical treatment as soon as possible. This may require ability to call in additional volunteers at a moment's notice. A quick observation of the horse's oral mucous membranes and a skin tent evaluation will provide rapid overall physical assessment of an individual animal. The animal's temperature, pulse, and respiratory rates should be recorded. Medical records should be maintained for all shelter animals. Equine shelter workers should have prior training in equine first aid as part of their required credentialing as a shelter volunteer. More detailed information regarding equine triage is covered elsewhere in this book.

The goal of an equine emergency evacuation shelter is to keep the horses from becoming disaster victims. Basic equine husbandry practices should be followed. Some horses may require veterinary medical care (see later). Horses need to have adequate water and reasonable-quality roughage hay (grass hay) provided in a safe and secure shelter environment. Feeding concentrate feeds is not usually required and could even contribute to causing colic. It is important to minimize feed changes as much as possible. It is recommended to use local grass hay for feeding shelter horses since these horses will be less likely to colic as they would if they were fed different types of hay from various remote locations.

Rescued disaster victim horses require tetanus toxoid booster vaccination due to their increased risk for this potentially life-threatening disease. Vaccinating extremely stressed horses with respiratory and encephalitis vaccines may not be necessary and may even contribute to adverse reactions. If it is determined that the horses will remain in a shelter for a prolonged period of time, then mass vaccination for contagious equine respiratory viruses may be indicated (influenza and rhinopneumonitis).

The equine infectious anemia virus (EIAV) status of all shelter horses should be determined prior to their admission to the shelter if possible (i.e., horses admitted along with negative Coggins test). However, horses should not be turned away if their Coggins status is not available, but a plan to test these horses should be in place (see later). Louisiana is one of the only states with a mandatory permanent equine identification requirement, and it is within the state regulations that every horse must have an individual permanent identification in the form of a microchip, lip tattoo, or freeze brand. As addressed later, identification becomes a very important part of the overall planning. A specific animal identification team headed by a veterinarian is helpful with organizing EIAV testing. Animal data sheets can be created for individual horses. Information sheets should contain owner address and contact information, a description of the animal, sex, breed, permanent identification if available, the shelter arrival date, and rescue/evacuation location. Information must be stored in a secure location, away from the public to avoid animal theft, misuse of information, or misidentification. An animal release form may be used to document owner retrieval of the horse from the shelter.

7. Who pays for the equine shelter (facility rental, supplies, workforce, etc.)?

Establishment of a fund for emergency situations is critical for expediting functional equine evacuation and shelter activities. State veterinary medical foundation accounts associated with a state animal response team have been successful for emergency response and planning activities in Louisiana. State and/or federal funds may become available after a disaster event, but this is often difficult to determine at the time a disaster is imminent. It is important to note that the U.S. government requires command staff and first responders to be National Incident Management System (NIMS) compliant in order to be reimbursed for costs incurred during disaster response.

Each community, region, and state should determine funding resources available for animal care during disasters. For each state, a response operation having a nonprofit bank account/organization predetermined to act as the vehicle for accepting cash donations to assist an emergency response effort is extremely important. This became clear within the very first few hours of Hurricane Katrina's aftermath response in 2005 with the establishment of the state veterinary medical association foundation account designated for animal relief, a fund that continues to provide animal relief for the state of Louisiana. Accurate and detailed spending records must be maintained to minimize problems with reimbursements.

8. What state resources are available for emergency equine shelters?

Each state will have to determine what resources are available for their animal response activities including equine evacuation and response sheltering. States moving forward with well-functioning plans are doing so with state animal response teams. The federal veterinarian can appoint the area emergency coordinator to assist with planning. Again, the state veterinarian and associated staff are important resources to include in the planning process.

9. How do you handle horses exposed to possible contaminants?

Veterinarians should have a key role in assessment and triage of evacuated and rescued equids. Most commonly, horses require gross decontamination of mud and debris following storms so they can be examined for injuries, including lacerations, puncture wounds, and abrasions. This may require detergent bath and thorough rinsing. If animals require decontamination due to chemical, biological, or radiation exposure, then veterinarians should work with trained hazardous material personnel to determine the appropriate protocol to ensure safe handling for animals and humans. Briefly, a decontamination area should be established for animal bathing. Personnel should wear proper barrier precautions if necessary and other livestock should not be exposed to the effluent from decontaminated animals. Maintenance of appropriate and safe drainage of dirtied water and wastes from this area is critical. Dawn® dishwashing detergent or other mild shampoo can be used to bathe the horse, making sure that all skin surfaces are washed and then thoroughly rinsed. Horses can be brushed with standard equine grooming equipment.

10. How do you determine/establish a successful volunteer workforce for management and day-to-day care of the horses and supply and equipment management?

Horse owners (consider limiting the number per family) should be incorporated into the day-to-day care of their sheltered horses if possible. This will decrease the risk of human injury associated with working with unfamiliar horses. This will also limit the number of volunteers needed to run the shelter. Owners can assist with daily feeding, watering, and care of their animals as well as daily hand walking for exercise, since these horses will not be able to have pasture or paddock exercise.

It is important for disaster assistance managers and volunteers to have undergone appropriate ICS training (a minimum of ICS 100 for lay volunteers and ICS 100, 200, 700, and 800 for management positions). These courses are available free to all citizens on the FEMA website (http://training.fema.gov/IS). It is critical to understand that working outside of this system greatly hampers response efforts whether the disaster is small or the size of the Hurricane Katrina aftermath. Volunteers need to be willing to spend at least 1 week working during a disaster, perform the tasks asked of them, maintain a positive attitude, and not expect to be compensated monetarily. Volunteers should be self sufficient including daily meals and sleeping accommodations. It is critical that volunteers are physically healthy, trained, and aware of what they are volunteering to do.

Evacuation and response shelter volunteers need to be a part of local and state animal response plan. These volunteers should be preidentified so that required credentialing may be in place prior to a disaster incident. Credentialing may include criminal background check, documented ICS training, shelter training, and animal handling experience. Most communities that have a substantial number of horses already have equine interest groups in place. These groups are a natural fit for inserting into a local community animal response plan. Well-organized groups such as regional and local U.S. Pony Clubs, 4-H clubs, FFAs, breed associations, agriculture organizations, and riding clubs are often key resources for providing volunteers needed for equine shelter management and all associated tasks. National nonprofit animal and equine welfare groups are other key resources with regional volunteers in many parts of the United States. There are several experienced animal welfare groups available for assistance during disasters, often willing to carry a substantial portion of shelter management workload and associated costs. Reputable animal welfare groups are NIMS compliant, usually experienced in dealing with disaster situations, and usually well trained in animal handling. They are often willing to bear the brunt of the workload in a disaster response shelter for animals including horses. However, agreements such as a memorandum of agreement (MOA) are highly recommended so that expectations from all key players are clearly identified.

11. What can be done if the shelter response required overwhelms the resources available?

In most cases, an area command is established in emerging disaster incidents. During the first 24 to 48 hours (or longer in some situations), human lives are the primary focus, and as human response begins to stabilize, the focus will shift to the animals. Community emergency management personnel should be made aware of situations requiring animal response. Local animal response teams (a.k.a., county/parish animal response teams—SARTs, VMRCs, CARTs, or PARTs) will work with community emergency planners to ensure the existence of a functional animal response plan. Once local resources are exhausted, these local emergency managers can make requests to state-level emergency managers (usually the state veterinarian's office) as part of a specific emergency support function (ESF) specifically tasked with supporting the animal response. Disaster incidents involving human mass casualties may consume most state and federal resources; therefore, animal relief resources will need to come from well-established animal response plans within communities.

If the equine response in the local community evolves into a situation requiring equine rescue, it is extremely important for veterinarians or animal control officers to work with trained first responders such as firefighters, emergency medical technicians, or other trained law enforcement personnel to safely and effectively address the situation. Local communities should work together with first responders in their locale to identify a team appropriate for this type of response. A horse rescue situation should never preclude the safe rescue and well being of human life. However, lives of both humans and animals can be saved if there are individual and community plans in place to address these probable emergency scenarios.

12. How long should a shelter volunteer work on a shift?

Disaster response personnel (including shelter managers and workers) should work 8- to 12-hour shifts for 5 to 7 days at a time. Shift changes should overlap to allow for appropriate briefing sessions.

13. How can you keep the shelter safe and secure from theft of supplies and animals?

A secure perimeter must be set up before a shelter opens. Official law enforcement personnel may be available to provide shelter security, but often it is up to the shelter management to secure the facility. Security should be provided so that items are not stolen or vandalized (animals, supplies, drugs, fuel, feed, hay, water, and animal records) and so that personnel and animals are kept safe and secure. In addition, public health issues may become an issue as it relates to keeping the public out of animal care and holding areas.

Facility security is one of the most important parts of the animal plan and is a critical need from the start. Requests for additional shelter security support should be made to the local emergency managers early. State departments of agriculture often have their own law enforcement available to support this critical need. However, in the event of large-scale disaster situations, these officials or military police may be unavailable. Private security companies may be available, but prior agreements should be in place long before a disaster occurs.

All shelter personnel (including animal owners) must be required to check in at a single check-in location. Everyone must be able to be identified with a standardized nametag or badge system. If animal owners are taking part in the daily care of their horse, then the specific protocol must be followed and understood. Personal identification tags must be visible and required to be worn by all personnel. All animals should be able to be clearly identified by a visible ID tag or marking (see later).

Feed, equipment, veterinary drugs, other first-aid supplies, and shelter supplies should be stored in a secure location. Veterinary medical supplies are best stored in a locked veterinary ambulatory vehicle. The veterinarian(s) should be available on a 24/7 basis once the shelter opens; animal numbers and arrivals are often extremely unpredictable.

Often, during a disaster, many people truly think that these supplies are "free for all." When a local equine shelter was opened in south Louisiana during Hurricane Rita's response, a large number of bags of equine feed meant for evacuee horses were stolen from the shelter during the first couple of days.

14. How do you keep track of horses during an evacuation and sheltering situation?

Animal identification is important, and if horses are evacuated and commingled, or escape and are later captured, it is essential to be able to identify the herd of origin. Many horses look alike, so permanent brands, lip tattoos, or electronic identifications that are unique to each individual animal or farm/ranch are essential. Body condition changes with the effects of the elements or time and the horse may become more difficult to identify without permanent identification. The U.S. Horse Industry Equine Species Working Group advisors to the USDA National Animal Identification System recommends electronic microchip identification using the ISO/ANSI compatible RFID (radio frequency identification 117.84/85, 134.2 kHz) as the standard equine identification method to ensure uniformity and compatibility. A single microchip should be implanted deep in the horse's nuchal ligament halfway between the poll and the withers on the left side.

Digital photographs and/or videos of horses may also help identify them later. Owners should identify their horses two ways: (1) permanent (microchip, lip tattoo, or brand) and (2) visible tag or marking with owner name and current contact information. Livestock paint sticks, etching using electric clipper etching with a No. 40 blade, permanent marking pen, livestock stickers as used in sale barns, and bright spray paint are available household products that can be used to identify horses (Fig. 1.20.2). Copies of herd records, proof of ownership, and registration papers should be stored in a safe and secure location.

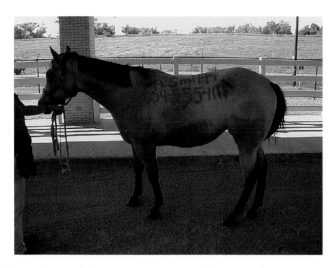

Figure 1.20.2 Predisaster body marking with horse owner's name and contact information using either a livestock paint stick or fluorescent spray paint. (Photograph by Rebecca McConnico.)

In situations such as an impending hurricane where advanced warning may be given, health papers should be provided by a veterinarian if horses are to be evacuated, particularly if there is a possibility of the horse traveling across state lines. In events where widespread evacuation is recommended, including horses, such as in the case of Category 3 or greater hurricane, state or federal veterinary officials will be the authority resource for determining travel requirements necessary for interstate transport of evacuating livestock (such as official health papers or Coggins papers).

In other situations, it may not be possible to evacuate or rescue all animals, so owners should prioritize animals so their most valuable stock will receive attention first. Due to the possibility of mass evacuation of many animals, plans should be made weeks in advance of a potential disaster. Owners should partner with other farms/ranches to provide trucking and trailering and also evacuation space so public holding areas can be used for rescued animals.

15. How is correct information disseminated during a disaster whereby an appropriate and successful sheltering response can occur?

Establishment of an area communications hub such as was done with the Horse Hurricane Helpline post Hurricanes Katrina and Rita in 2005 by the LSART–LSU Equine Health Studies partnership enabled functional lines of communication between the area command (state veterinarian's office) and field activities. The telephone number was made available to the public as early as possible, and then via appropriate command structure, the information that came into the communications center was able to be relayed to the area command. Teams were then able to be organized to move supplies and/or provide rescue teams (strike teams) for horses (and humans and other animals) in need of response.

Prestorm evacuation shelters should be identified and owners should be encouraged to leave at least 72 to 104 hours prior to hurricane force winds reaching a community. This will be at least 1 to 2 days ahead of projected evacuation of people and should allow the safe transport of livestock ahead of major traffic gridlock. Many times, there will be little warning that evacuation or rescue will require equine sheltering (such as situations involving train derailment, toxic gas release, tornadoes, etc.). Available evacuation shelters, routes, and contact information of these shelters should already be in the horse owner's personal equine emergency plan. Available shelter information should be supplied via radio, television, newspaper, Internet broadcast, etc. All communications should come through a central command system so accurate information can be ensured.

Daily situation reports (written if possible) should be communicated to emergency management personnel through the proper channels so that adequate response activities can be carried out without wasting time, effort, and ultimately human and animal lives. It is usually in the best interest of safety and public interest during disaster situations for media outlets to be allowed to make accurate reports of disaster response activities. Shelter managers should identify a specific person to handle the media on a daily basis so that accurate information may be effectively disseminated to the public. Avoid dissemination of incorrect information. Shelter volunteers may quickly set up personal websites and blogs, so correct information from the public information officer on a daily basis is important. All shelter volunteers should be required to adhere to a strict code of conduct that involves confidentiality as well as understanding the proper communication channels.

16. How long should an evacuation shelter remain open?

Evacuation shelters should be opened early, and as soon as animals arrive, exit plans should begin to be made. Shelters should stay open only for as long as it takes for the danger to pass, for damage assessments to be made, and for owners and animals to be able to return home or move on to alternate owner-organized safe locations. This is typically a matter of days (not weeks). In the case of massive devastation such as wildfire or hurricane/flood destruction of entire communities, alternative temporary or permanent plans need to be arranged. For liability and other reasons, the exit plan from the equine shelter must be the responsibility of the animal owner. With the assistance of response team members and other equine stake holders, owners, and officials in the community, alternative plans can be arranged for displaced horse owners and their animals. Remember, proof of ownership is a key to making the return of the correct horse home as seamless as possible.

17. What do you do with the leftover supplies (and animals!) once the threat has ended?

Leftover supplies may be dispersed to the community, stored for future use during emergencies, or donated to other in-state or out-of-state emergency situations. Leftover feed supplies with a short shelf-life can be readily donated and used by nonprofit equine organizations such as therapeutic riding centers or mounted law enforcement units.

Leftover and unclaimed horses can be very problematic. Each state will have specific laws that address this situation. In Louisiana, the parish of animal origin is the official "owner" of abandoned pets and livestock, including horses. Parish animal control officials should be contacted to oversee the management of these animals.

18. What workforce positions are critical for an equine response or evacuation shelter?

- Shelter manager
- Assistant shelter manager
- Shelter administrative assistant(s)
- Veterinarian (primary)
- Veterinarian (secondary)
- Veterinary technician
- Veterinary technician (back-up)
- Shelter worker crew (manure handling, bedding, feeding, watering)
- Logistics officer—supply and equipment manager (feed, hay, water, equipment)
- Logistics personnel—(available 24/7 crew since supplies may be delivered at anytime, day or night)

- Refuse service (utilities)
- Transportation (for horses)
- Transportation (for supplies/equipment)
- Personnel care team (first aid, feeding the volunteers, etc.)
- Volunteer check-in desk personnel
- Animal identification team

Suggested Reading

Heath SE, ed. *Animal Management in Disasters*. Mosby, St. Louis, 1999.

McConnico RS, French DD, Clark B, Mortensen KE, Littlefield M, Moore RM. Equine rescue and response activities in Louisiana in the aftermath of Hurricanes Katrina and Rita. *J Am Vet Med Assoc* 2007;231:384–392.

Sullivan EK. Trauma and emergency care [review]. *Vet Clin North Am Equine Pract* 2007;23(1).

CHAPTER 1.21
COMPANION ANIMAL SHELTERING

Renée A. Poirrier, DVM

1. Why should we shelter pets?

We should strive to remove all obstacles to provide shelter for people affected by a disaster, including providing shelter for their pets. Recent history has shown us that if we encourage more people to evacuate the affected area with their pets until it is safe to return, we save human lives as well (Fig. 1.21.1).

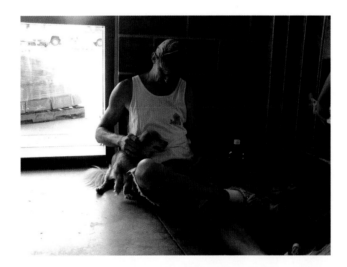

Figure 1.21.1 Allowing owners to evacuate with their pets also saved the lives of humans during Hurricane Rita.

2. Why can't the pets stay with the owners?

Some people in human shelters may be allergic and others may be fearful of pets. The overall goal of disaster response sheltering is to encourage people to evacuate in order to prevent loss of human life.

3. What is the difference between a companion animal *evacuation shelter* and a companion animal *response shelter*?

- A companion animal evacuation shelter is a companion animal shelter provided near an associated human shelter where the pets evacuated either before, during, or after the event can be housed and cared for by their owners. Evacuation shelters are most often co-located shelters where pets are housed nearby but not in the same facility as their owners. Some evacuation shelters are pet-friendly shelters where pets are housed in the same facility as their owners. Evacuation shelters are set up to encourage pet owners to evacuate.

- A companion animal response shelter is a companion animal shelter where animals rescued from the affected area are taken to be housed until identified and retrieved by their owners. The pets in a response shelter may include stray animals and may complicate identification of the rescued owned animals that were left behind. Owners are most often looking for their pets and will be an additional complication to the already stressed conditions. In smaller incidents, both types of shelters may be in the same location.

4. Who is in charge of the shelter?

During a disaster, the local emergency management organization will identify a local official responsible for companion animal issues. This official is often the local animal control official. This official, or designee, is in control of the pet shelter in their area.

5. How can veterinary personnel help?

Veterinarians are invaluable as shelter veterinarians, triaging animals as they enter and providing care for the sheltered pets. Veterinary technicians and assistants are also invaluable in assisting veterinarians (Fig. 1.21.2). Becoming involved in your local community's and state's disaster planning process gives you experience in disaster planning and will make you more knowledgeable in the issues unique to your community when faced with a disaster. Many communities need veterinary expertise to advise on the setup of a companion animal shelter, but also a workforce of shelter workers is needed to perform the actual setup.

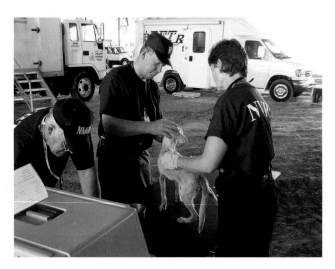

Figure 1.21.2   Veterinarians and veterinary technicians are invaluable assets to companion animal shelters during disasters such as Hurricane Rita.

6. What types of medical issues are likely to be encountered in a shelter following a disaster?

- In many cases, the medical issues in a shelter are the same as routine veterinary practice with the added stress of animal crowding.

- Chronic illnesses are exacerbated due to stress and lack of treatment. This happens when the pet is displaced from the owner or the owner did not bring medications when evacuating.
- If the shelter is not in a climate-controlled building, environmental factors will play a role in the medical cases seen.
- Depending on the type of disaster, decontamination of animals may be necessary. Animals recovered from a flood should be decontaminated by bathing. Veterinarians should work with trained hazmat personnel to determine the best method of decontamination for chemical, biological, or radiation exposure and to ensure the safety of both people and pets.

7. What were some of the companion animal medical issues documented in past disasters?

During the Katrina and Rita Hurricane response in Louisiana, Mississippi, and Texas, the most common veterinary medical issues included the following:

- Heat stress
- Heatstroke
- Dehydration
- Congestive heart failure
- Heartworm disease
- Ocular and dermal irritation
- Various dermatologic problems
- Fractures

8. Who sets the euthanasia policy during a disaster?

Both types of shelters should have a written policy in place to guide veterinarians in making the decision to euthanatize an animal.

- In a companion animal evacuation shelter, the owner and the veterinarian will discuss issues, and the owner will decide when euthanasia is appropriate, just as if the pet was in a veterinary hospital.
- In a companion animal response shelter, the accepted policy should be explained to the shelter veterinarians. For example, during Hurricane Katrina in Louisiana, two veterinarians had to agree that euthanasia was appropriate before an animal was euthanatized. The most common reasons for euthanasia included aggression (each animal with aggressive behavior was assessed by an additional behaviorist) and animals with terminal illness(es).

9. Can I show up at a shelter and offer my veterinary skills if I am not licensed in that state?

Most states currently require that a veterinarian be licensed in that state to practice veterinary medicine. In certain emergencies, a state may allow out-of-state veterinarians to come into the state to assist in the emergency response. Make sure you contact the licensing board of that state to determine if out-of-state veterinarians are allowed into the state and what information is required to allow an out-of-state veterinarian to practice in the affected state during an emergency. Each state will be different. The American Veterinary Medical Association Directory or an internet search for the veterinary licensing board will direct you to the proper contact information. There are national veterinary reserve corps (under the U.S. Department of Agriculture) and the five National Veterinary Response Teams (NVRTs) (federal teams deployed by the National Disaster Medical System of the Department of Health and Human Services) that maintain lists/teams of veterinarians who can be called on to volunteer in emergencies. In many cases, since these veterinarians and technicians have submitted their licensing information before an event and have become temporary federal employees, they can be deployed into an affected area without having to resubmit their veterinary credentials.

Veterinarians are also on several Disaster Medical Assistance Teams (DMATs) and National Disaster Medical Response Teams (NMRTs). These teams are often deployed before NVRT or veterinary reserve corps personnel.

10.   What supplies should I bring if I am asked to staff a veterinary station at a shelter?

When volunteering as a veterinarian, bring items you need to perform physical exams, such as a stethoscope, a thermometer, an otoscope, and an ophthalmoscope (Fig. 1.21.3). Some events require responders be prepared to be self-sufficient (air mattress, sleeping bags, personal items, 3–5 days of food and water, etc.). Communicate with the shelter personnel with whom you will be working to determine if the shelter needs any veterinary supplies you can bring. Be cautious with bringing controlled drugs. A personal first-aid kit will be useful. Comfortable clothes and several changes of scrubs and socks and shoes will be required. Your lab jacket with your professional name on it will give you additional credibility.

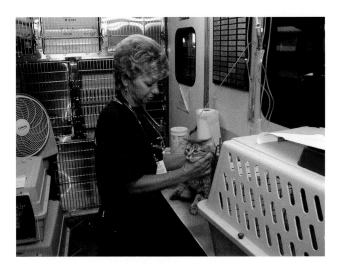

Figure 1.21.3   Basic equipment used during a physical examination will be required when responding to a disaster such as Hurricane Rita.

11.   Who pays for the medications needed for an animal in the shelter?

Each situation is different, but many times donations (of medications or money) are provided to animals affected by a disaster. In evacuation shelters, owners may be asked to pay for their animal's care. Currently, there is a federal reimbursement policy for some veterinary services for pets through FEMA and the Stafford Act. We advise planners to keep current on these frequently changing policies.

12.   Where should the shelter be located?

A companion animal evacuation shelter should be located out of harm's way as near to the human shelter as possible. This allows the animal owners to have specific time periods when the animals can be fed, watered, and walked. A companion animal response shelter should be located near the affected area to decrease the distance pets will have to be transported from their home but far enough away to be safe from the sequelae of the disaster.

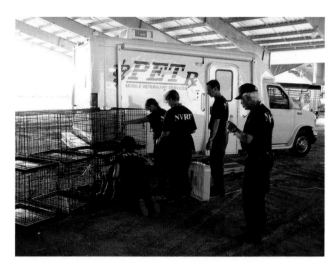

Figure 1.21.4 Animals under a fairgrounds shelter during Hurricane Rita.

13. What type of facilities may be used as companion animal shelters?

Agricultural centers, dog parks, dog training centers, existing animal shelters, fairgrounds, rodeo arenas, open fields with tents, golf courses, livestock arenas, parks, and schools all can be used as companion animal shelter facilities (Fig. 1.21.4).

14. What happens if a pet bites a human?

Each shelter should have a human bite protocol established, usually dictated by the local laws governing bites by pets. The local public health department generally has policies that dictate the requirements that need to be followed. Certainly, an animal being current on rabies vaccinations would help manage the situation more effectively. Signs warning about an aggressive dog need to be used. An area set aside for aggressive dogs, as well as an isolation ward for bite cases, needs to be created. Above all, controlling the influx of people to just the owners and limiting the visitors will also decrease the chances of bites.

15. Where do the supplies to run the shelter come from?

Many times, the supplies needed to run a shelter are donated by the local community or the neighboring areas (Fig. 1.21.5).

One of the most vital shelter supplies is caging. Every pet needs a cage in which it can be sheltered. If it is a widespread disaster, cages may be trucked in from other areas. It is very helpful to have stockpiles of cages in various areas throughout a state. After Hurricanes Katrina and Rita in 2005, the Louisiana State Animal Response Team distributed six pods across the state with supplies for a 100 animal pet shelter including 100 wire cages. Wire cages were chosen because the majority of pet shelters in Louisiana are in open agricultural facilities. Wire cages are better ventilated and therefore decrease heat stress (Fig. 1.21.6). In North Carolina, the State Animal Response Team has the supplies for a shelter including cages in a trailer that can be taken to any site in the state to set up a shelter. Often, there are humane organizations that have large numbers of cages available for use during a disaster.

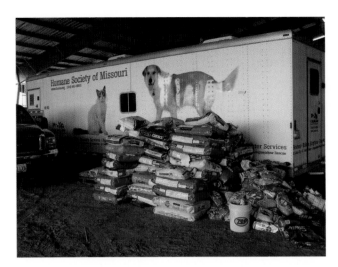

Figure 1.21.5 The generosity of surrounding communities often overwhelmed a shelter with pet foods during Hurricane Rita.

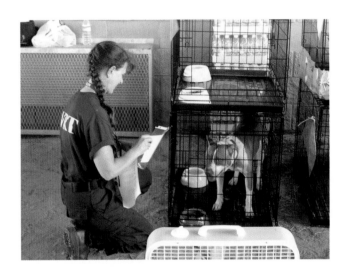

Figure 1.21.6 Wire cages with a fan helped keep animals (and veterinarians!) cooler during Hurricane Rita.

16. Is there special training required to work in a companion animal response shelter?

In most cases, veterinarians working in an affected area will be required to have taken basic incident command training that is required of all first responders. The incident command system is the system that all first responders use to manage an incident. In 2008, the required first responder courses were ICS 100, 200, 700, and 800. These courses can be taken online at the FEMA website (http://training.fema.gov/IS/).

17. How should pets be identified?

The ideal identification for an animal is a permanent identification such as a microchip. Animal neckbands may be used if microchips are not available. Clear digital or Polaroid pictures can also be used to help identify pets.

18.   How will medical records be kept?

Problem-oriented veterinary medical records should be kept on all animals examined by a veterinarian just as if the pet is in a veterinary facility.

19.   How will controlled drugs be recorded?

As with any veterinary hospital, controlled drugs need to be *very well controlled*. One or two veterinarians should be in total control of dispensing these medications. A written log will be provided for controlled drugs that keeps detailed records of the controlled drugs dispensed to patients for use at the shelter. Again, proper identification of the pet will be required in the matching of the drug output to the animals treated.

20.   What about liability insurance?

Contact your insurance carrier to ensure you are covered for liability while working in a disaster response. Most states have a Good Samaritan Law that limits the liability of volunteers during a disaster. The State Office of Emergency Preparedness will also have answers for these liability questions since a key member of the team is from the state attorney general's office.

21.   What happens to the animals after an evacuation shelter closes?

When an evacuation shelter closes, owners are responsible for picking up their pets. If an owner is not capable of retrieving and caring for his or her pet at the time the shelter closes, foster families can be identified to care for the pet until the owner is able to again house and care for the pet. In Louisiana, temporary adoption parties are planned where potential foster families and pet owners can meet at the evacuation shelter. Volunteers agree to foster a pet until an owner is capable of obtaining appropriate housing and is again able to care for the pet. These temporary adoption parties are planned if an evacuation shelter is open longer than 2 weeks. If people will be displaced longer than 1 to 2 weeks, foster families provide a more suitable environment for the pet and allow the owner to begin the process of rebuilding their lives.

22.   What happens when a companion animal response shelter closes?

Every attempt should be made to reunite pets with owners. If unclaimed pets are still present when a response shelter closes, the local official responsible for companion animals must determine the fates of the pets. The local official should be familiar with the local laws governing animal ownership and abandonment. Many of these pets can be put up for adoption and will find new homes.

CHAPTER 1.22
DISINFECTION OF AVIAN, LARGE, AND SMALL ANIMAL FACILITIES

David C. Van Metre, DVM, and Paul S. Morley, DVM, PhD

1. What is a disinfectant?

A *disinfectant* is an agent that eliminates a defined scope of pathogenic microorganisms on an inanimate object (Rutala and Weber, 2004). Disinfectants are typically chemical agents such as formaldehyde, but physical agents such as x-rays and ultraviolet light act as effective disinfectants. Efficiency and rapid activity are the implied properties of disinfectants; however, these properties are greatly influenced by the environment in which the disinfectant is applied and the types of microorganisms present. Disinfection is defined as the process of applying disinfectants for such purposes.

2. How do disinfectants relate to sterilizing agents, sanitizing agents, and antiseptics?

The relationship among these agents involves the spectrum of microorganisms eliminated, the relative efficacy of elimination of microorganisms, and the suitability for application to animate versus inanimate objects. The spectrum of microorganisms susceptible to disinfectants varies widely according to the class (type) of disinfectant used. Many disinfectants are considered relatively ineffective against bacterial spores and oocysts of certain parasites, such as *Cryptosporidium*. A *sterilizing agent* is a chemical or physical agent applied to an inanimate object that reliably eliminates *all* forms of microbial life; examples include hydrogen peroxide gas plasma and steam under pressure. Commonly used on food preparation and food handling equipment (e.g., utensils), *sanitizing agents* reduce the number of bacteria to safe levels as dictated by public health requirements. *Antiseptics* are agents applied to living tissue for the purpose of preventing or arresting the growth or activity of microorganisms. Antiseptics are frequently used to lower the risk of infection on healthy or diseased tissue.

3. Describe the role that disinfection plays in an animal care or animal housing facility.

Disinfection is a critical component of the compilation of policies that must be in place to effectively control infectious disease (ID) in an animal care facility. ID occurs as a result of interactions between the host animal, the pathogen(s), and the environment. Effective disinfection can reduce the number and/or the infectivity and viability of pathogens in the environment, thereby lowering the risk of infection to the host. Disinfection is primarily aimed at limiting or eliminating the presence of pathogenic microorganisms on objects or surfaces with which the animals or their caretakers are likely to contact, such as cages, stalls, floors, grooming equipment, and medical equipment. It is critical to understand that disinfection is only one component of a comprehensive ID control program, and if used as a sole means of managing ID, it is very likely to be ineffective. Disinfection is most effectively used as a component of a comprehensive ID control program.

4. Other than disinfection, list the components of a comprehensive ID control program for an animal care or sheltering facility.

A comprehensive ID control program consists of formal, recorded, monitored, enforced, and regularly reviewed and updated protocols related to the following:

- Sound animal husbandry practices
- Hygienic sources of food, water, and air
- Maintenance of clean, safe, and secured stores of feed and water
- Maintenance of adequate ventilation and air quality
- Maintenance of cleanable surfaces of low porosity in stalls, cages, and animal and personnel traffic areas
- Appropriately scheduled cleaning of stalls, cages, floors, tack and grooming equipment, feeding equipment, and medical equipment
- Identification of the infectious agents that pose the greatest threat to animals and personnel in the facility (both in terms of frequency and consequences)
- Identification of the most common route(s) of transmission for the targeted agents, and means by which the transmission routes can be interrupted by animal placement (location) within the facility, animal handling practices, cleaning and disinfection, traffic control, and personnel allocation
- Utilization of facility design in a manner that minimizes the risk of transmission of ID through such means as segregation of animals according to disease risk, animal proximity to animal care personnel and equipment, airflow patterns, foot and equipment traffic patterns, and risk to the general public
- Appropriate signage and access control to prevent entry of unauthorized personnel into designated areas
- Targeted, well-maintained, and lawful strategies for pest control
- Identification of animals that might be at greatest risk of acquiring or transmitting ID, with appropriate policies for segregation, isolation, feeding, medical care, and handling of such animals, including disposal of soiled bedding, waste, and cadavers
- Provision of appropriate personal protective equipment (PPE) to personnel, with appropriate ongoing training of personnel in utilization of such equipment
- Surveillance for signs of ID within the animals and personnel, with integration of surveillance data into ID control practices
- Surveillance for the presence of targeted infectious agents within the facility environment
- Diagnostic testing and treatment strategies for IDs
- Strategies for management of ID outbreaks (*Note:* Such strategies are often shaped by the disease in question and the scope of the outbreak, but a strategy to *identify* the disease in question, *measure* the scope of the outbreak, and *initiate* interventions should be preplanned.)
- Appropriate and lawful handling of infectious and hazardous waste (including animal cadavers), waste water, exit ventilation, discarded feed, and discarded equipment so as to minimize threats to public health
- Training of new personnel, and continuing education of established personnel
- Involvement of personnel of all levels in review and revision of ID control policies
- Designation of personnel as managers or directors of the infectious control program, with clear policies regarding authority/command structure
- Emergency management plans for natural and man-made disasters, including scheduled drills or exercises (*Note:* Involvement of local emergency management officials is highly recommended.)

5. When developing disinfection strategies for animal housing or care facilities, what is the most important issue that shapes the strategy?

Because disinfectants are applied to inanimate objects, the most fundamental issue to address is the nature of the surfaces within the facility that must be disinfected. More specifically, one must determine to what extent the surfaces can be *cleaned* before disinfection. *Cleaning* is defined as the removal of all visible debris, particularly organic debris such as feces, dirt, and bedding, from the area to be disinfected. Other issues that must commonly be considered are personnel safety and damage to materials (e.g., bleaching of clothing, erosion of concrete, damage to rubber and plastics, etc.).

6. Why is cleaning a necessary preliminary step to disinfection?

Because the microbiocidal activity of every disinfectant is limited to some degree by the presence of organic debris, removal of this matter by cleaning is a profoundly critical activity that *must* precede disinfection. Additionally, disinfectants cannot be expected to kill microorganisms if surfaces are encased in a protective coating of dirt and organic debris that prevents contact. Organic debris greatly increases the available colonization sites for microorganisms in the environment, provides nutrient support for bacteria, fungi, and certain stages of parasites, and shields microorganisms from both chemical and physical disinfectants. Removal of organic debris by cleaning carries the additional benefit of removing the bulk of microorganisms from the surface or object, so that fewer microorganisms remain for subsequent disinfection. Thorough cleaning and rinsing of contaminated surfaces are particularly useful in reducing persistence of disinfectant-resistant pathogens (e.g., bacterial spores) in animal environments.

7. What types of surfaces in an animal care or housing facility warrant cleaning and disinfection?

In human health care facilities, surfaces on inanimate objects are categorized as *critical*, if they come into contact with nonintact skin, deeper tissues of the body, or the mucosal surfaces of the body warrant cleaning and disinfection. Such critical materials include surgical instruments, endoscopes, thermometers, and implants. Critical surfaces, therefore, carry extremely high potential to initiate infection, and these are typically sterilized before use and either resterilized or discarded after each contact with a patient.

Noncritical surfaces are defined as those surfaces that come into contact with intact skin of patients, health care workers, or visitors of the health care facility. Of these, medical equipment (e.g., stethoscopes, blood pressure cuffs, radiographic machines) carries the highest potential to transfer pathogens among patients, and their role as fomites in nosocomial infections and health care facility–based outbreaks of ID is well documented (Rutala and Weber, 2004). Other surfaces, such as floors, telephones, computer keyboards, desks, chairs, and tables, may become contaminated by pathogenic microorganisms by contact with contaminated hands, shoes, settling of airborne microbes, and, particularly in animal housing facilities, biological fluids or animal waste.

In animal care facilities, noncritical surfaces appear to be far more likely to become heavily contaminated with pathogenic microorganisms, given that the heavy coat of hair or feathers retain contamination to a greater degree than does human skin, animals are generally bathed less frequently than people, and the elimination habits of animals in their housing environments create a far greater risk of tracking enteric pathogens onto floors by animals and caretakers. Further, if such surfaces were to be cleaned solely with a detergent, the detergent solution, mops, cloths, and sponges used for cleaning can become heavily contaminated during use and have potential to serve as fomites (Rutala and Weber, 2004). Therefore, because many noncritical surfaces in animal care and housing facilities can contribute to the spread of epidemiologically important microorganisms, cleaning and disinfection targets are numerous. These include, in order of importance:

1. Stalls, crates, and cages, particularly those occupied by ill animals and those for which the occupants frequently change
2. Floors within and leading to and from these areas
3. All surfaces of feed and water storage areas
4. Feed and water bowls, buckets, or troughs
5. Medical equipment, including equipment carried by animal care personnel (stethoscopes, penlights, clipper blades, etc.)
6. Cleaning equipment
7. Tack, blankets, toys
8. Hand contact surfaces frequently used by personnel (telephones, computer keyboards, supply shelving, door handles, etc.)
9. Other floors subject to animal traffic

It is vital to reiterate that cleaning and disinfection of the noncritical surfaces listed above represent only one component of lowering the likelihood that those surfaces could serve as a means of transmission of ID. A comprehensive ID control program is necessary to limit the extent and frequency of contamination of those surfaces with pathogens. Further, use of strategically placed hand hygiene stations and disinfectant footmats or footbaths will greatly curtail contamination of these surfaces. All personnel in the facility must be educated as to the importance of hand and footwear hygiene in ID control.

8. What types of surfaces are most easily cleaned?

The optimal surfaces for animal facilities are smooth, waterproof, resistant to corrosion, and nonporous. Examples include durable plastic and stainless steel, which are common components of small animal cages. Such cages must be inspected regularly for seams or loose fittings, into which contaminated material can become lodged. Wooden walls may be rendered less porous by the application of two coats of marine-quality epoxy or polyurethane. The depth of the small surface pockets present in concrete walls can be reduced by the application of two coats of outdoor, high-quality enamel paint. Hinges and latches that become rusted may harbor high numbers of microorganisms within their irregular surfaces, so these must be well maintained and replaced when irreparable. Other common problem areas for cleaning and disinfection include drain covers, ceiling rafters, lighting structures, vents, and fans.

9. Describe the different options for cleanable flooring.

Nonporous, smooth flooring may be used if personnel are provided with rubber footwear of adequate traction and animals are moved within cages, as in a laboratory animal facility. Sealed, well-maintained linoleum tiles are acceptable for most small animal areas. Deeply grooved or grouted tiles should be avoided because of the tendency for organic debris to be retained in grooves and cracks. Flooring in large animal facilities must offer adequate traction to animals and personnel. Although dirt flooring is inexpensive and soft and offers high traction, its very composition makes it a difficult surface to clean and nearly impossible to disinfect. When disinfection of dirt floors is necessary, the sole option is removal of the top 8 to 12 inches of dirt and replacement with fresh dirt or, optimally, a more cleanable surface, such as concrete or sealed rubber. Such floors are rendered more comfortable for large animals to stand and lay on through the application of deep bedding, consisting of sand, wooden shavings, straw, or shredded paper. Because such bedding material cannot be disinfected by most conventional means, its complete removal is required before initiation of cleaning and disinfection.

Removable, rubber floor mats are frequently placed on the floors of large animal facilities because they offer comfort and padding to animals that may have to stand or remain recumbent for long periods of time. Because tears or punctures may harbor contaminated bedding and fecal material, such mats must be inspected and repaired or replaced regularly. In addition, such mats must be regularly lifted off of the underlying floor and placed in a vertical position to allow the underside of the mat and floor to be thoroughly cleaned and disinfected. During multiple investigations of *Salmonella* outbreaks in large animal facilities, the authors have found the underside of such mats to be heavily contaminated with water and organic debris, from which *Salmonella* spp. was isolated with remarkable regularity. Cleaning of such large mats can be facilitated by integration of steel loops into one edge of the mat, which may facilitate the lifting of the mats with a forklift or block and tackle.

Although expensive, the best options for cushioning floors in large animal facilities are poured or single-piece flooring (monolayer or composite) that provide highly impermeable, comfortable surfaces, provided that the perimeter of the flooring is well sealed to the walls or underlying floor.

10. What is the optimal composition of other items, such as food bowls or tack?

Feeding containers (bowls, troughs, and buckets) should be composed of durable plastic or stainless steel, preferably with few or no exposed seams or rivets that may harbor microorganisms. These may contain oral, ocular, and nasal discharge after use, so thorough cleaning and disinfection between animals are extremely important. Heavily contaminated objects may be immersed or soaked for minutes to hours in soapy water to loosen adhered debris. Materials such as blankets, toys, combs, tack, and twitches may be composed of highly porous materials (cotton ropes, leather) and seams and buckles that make such items very difficult to clean and disinfect. After being used on an animal with a confirmed ID, disposal of such items may be the most attractive option. Failing that, meticulous cleaning by hand, followed by prolonged, complete immersion in a disinfectant may be acceptable, depending on the ID agent involved. If contaminated blankets are to be laundered, these should be stored in a clearly marked, sealed plastic container or bag and laundered separately from clothing and other cloth items (e.g., surgical drapes). Once in the laundry, use of laundry bleach and thorough, high heat drying on such items is highly recommended.

In areas with high-risk patients, such as hospital isolation units, items such as stethoscopes and other examination equipment should be designated for individual use on animals within the facility and should not be used elsewhere. These items should either be discarded after a single use, or must be cleaned and disinfected between uses. Because rectal thermometers have been incriminated as a route of transmission of pathogenic microorganisms, the safest option is to either use disposable thermometers or thermometer sleeves or to allocate a rectal thermometer to each animal in the high-risk facility. Failing these, thermometers must be cleaned and disinfected between animals.

11. Describe the steps involved in cleaning.

Before cleaning is initiated, the area to be cleaned should be inspected carefully for safety hazards, such as uncovered, nonwaterproof electrical outlets, wall or ceiling fans, electric–powered vents, and exposed wiring. Once their power supply is shut off, these may need to be cleaned and disinfected by hand, then sealed with waterproof tarps or tape while the remainder of the facility is cleaned and disinfected. Tarps and tape should be removed and the underlying electrical components checked for wetness before the power supply is restored. The anticipated path of water from the cleaned area should be determined. If animals are to remain in the facility during the cleaning process, steps should be taken to ensure that these animals are not exposed to the effluent that drains from the work area during cleaning.

Cleaning can be viewed as a four-step process. The first step in cleaning is the manual removal of soiled bedding, waste, and other debris (hair, feathers, etc.). The goal of this stage of cleaning is removal of all visible debris from the area. Typically, this step in cleaning is conducted without the application of water or other liquids; however, if these materials are particularly dusty, application of a light coat of water may be helpful in limiting the amount of dust made airborne by lifting and moving the material. Equipment such as feed buckets, food bowls, blankets, toys, and other materials should be removed from the stall or cage and either discarded or cleaned and disinfected as described later. Once disinfected, these items can be moved to a clean storage area or simply set aside in a plastic sealed container (e.g., a lidded trash can) or a sealed plastic trash bag.

The second step in cleaning is scrubbing of soiled surfaces with detergent (soap). Detergents help to loosen organic debris from surfaces by increasing the penetration of water into dirt and organic debris. Detergents also render oily substances soluble through emulsification and break-apart biofilms. Biofilms are microscopic aggregates of microbes encased in an extracellular polymeric matrix on an inanimate surface. Biofilms serve as a protective niche for microorganisms.

Objects or surfaces contaminated with dried feces may need to be wetted and soaked in a detergent for several minutes to hours to loosen the adhered debris. Surfaces should be wetted and scrubbed from the top toward the bottom, working toward the drain or exit path for water. If an entire facility is being cleaned, cleaning should progress from lightly contaminated areas toward the most contaminated area, and backtracking of equipment or personnel should be prevented. Hand-scrubbing surfaces with brushes is laborious and time consuming, but this technique minimizes splattering and aerosolization of contaminated material. This is of particular importance if other animals remain close by in the facility during the cleaning process. Power washers and pressure sprayers allow for more timely and less laborious cleaning, but these may aerosolize pathogens and push contaminated materials into previously cleaned areas or into occupied stalls or cages. The number and viability of microorganisms in splattered material may be reduced through the use of commercially available, combined detergent/disinfectant solutions during the cleaning process.

In the third step of cleaning, the detergent and mobilized debris are rinsed away with clean water. Optimally, wet surfaces should be allowed to dry (fourth step). Drying further reduces the viability and/or number of remaining pathogens and prevents dilution of disinfectants. Water that settles in puddles in low-lying areas may need to be pushed with a squeegee toward a drain or toward a faster-drying section of flooring. Applied together, these cleaning steps will optimize the efficacy of the disinfectant. Selection of detergents and disinfectants is discussed later.

12. What considerations apply when selecting and using cleaning equipment?

A critical consideration is provision of a means of *segregation* of cleaning equipment between healthy (or low-risk) and ill (or high-risk) animal housing areas. Since a well-designed facility is one in which animals are segregated by their risk of ID, it makes no sense to breach that segregation principle by using contaminated, common equipment to clean all areas. Soiled bedding and waste represent abundant sources of potentially pathogenic microorganisms; therefore, cleaning and hauling equipment becomes heavily contaminated with these pathogens during routine use. Separate cleaning equipment and disposal bins should be used to clean areas housing healthy animals and those housing ill or high-risk animals. *Under no circumstances* should cleaning implements be used to handle feed or fresh bedding, unless thoroughly cleaned and disinfected beforehand.

If maintenance of segregated cleaning equipment is not possible, the equipment itself must be cleaned and disinfected before it is moved from one segregation area to another. Such equipment should be used first in areas inhabited by healthy (low-risk) animals before being cleaned, disinfected, and moved to the high-risk animal housing areas. Cleaning and disinfection of such equipment are essential after it is used in high-risk areas.

What *type* of equipment is used is dictated in large part by whether animals are to remain in the facility or unit (i.e., the same airspace) during cleaning or if the facility is to be vacated of all animals while cleaning is being performed, such as in all-in, all-out livestock housing units. In the former case, the use of mechanized, potentially noisy equipment should be minimized or avoided altogether because of the potential stress that the remaining animals might experience; further, such equipment may volatize dust and pathogens, thereby facilitating spread to nearby animals. If a facility is to be vacated before cleaning, powered equipment (e.g., front end loaders, blowers, power washers) may be used more freely, with due consideration to protection of personnel from mechanical, heat, exhaust, or noise injury.

13. What strategies can be used for maintaining segregated cleaning equipment?

Separate mops, brooms, sponges, cloths, rakes, shovels, and pitchforks are needed for each segregated area. Ideally, multiple sets of implements should be maintained in each segregated area, thereby allowing for one set to be in use while previously soiled cleaning implements are being cleaned and disinfected before further use. Color or number coding or other clearly visible means of labeling cleaning equipment should be used to designate its dedication to a particular segregation area. Ideally, cleaning equipment should be nonporous and corrosion-resistant; implements composed of reinforced plastic and wooden handles that are sealed with polyurethane are optimal because of their limited porosity and ease of cleaning and disinfection.

14. What types of disposal equipment are needed?

In circumstances where pens, stalls, or cages are cleaned while animals remain in the facility, movable, sealed disposal bins are needed, into which soiled bedding, waste, and other debris can be placed. Bins should be sealed against leakage and covered. Again, bins should be segregated according to ID risk for a given animal or a given housing space. If material in a particular bin is destined for a specific decontamination or disinfection process (e.g., incineration or autoclaving), this should be clearly stated on the designated bin.

If the surface over which these bins are to be moved is irregular, bins with large wheels and high ground clearance are optimal. Disposal bins that traverse more smooth surfaces, such as concrete floors, can have smaller wheels with lower clearance. Bins should be large enough to allow for efficient removal of large quantities of bedding but small enough to traverse through the facility and, if necessary, to be pushed by hand. Bins that are moved outdoors should have an attached, hinged or sliding cover that can be latched in order to limit dispersion of contents by wind and access by vermin and birds. Ideally, such bins would be placed on the leeward (downwind) side of the facility, and feed and other animals should not be kept downwind from the bins.

In large animal facilities, tall bins may be of larger capacity than shorter ones, but personnel will need to lift soiled bedding and waste higher to place it into tall bins. This can result in personnel fatigue, as well as greater

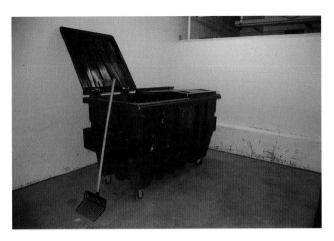

Figure 1.22.1 A well-designed disposal bin for a concrete-floored facility.

chances of dispersion of soiled materials through the air as the bedding is flung into higher bins. This can lead to dispersion of pathogenic microorganisms into the air and surrounding areas, potentially leading to cross-contamination of other stalls or cages. This problem can be limited by use of disposal bins that are shoulder height or lower for most personnel. See Figure 1.22.1 for an example of a well-designed animal waste disposal bin. This model and similar bins are available from Otto Environmental Systems North America (www.otto-usa. com).

15. How should cleaning personnel be allocated in an animal care or housing facility?

Optimally, different people should be assigned to clean the different segregated animal housing areas, with little or no cross-traffic of cleaning personnel from one area to another. In our veterinary hospital, color-coded outerwear, including waterproof footwear, is used by personnel dedicated to cleaning each unit of the hospital. If such segregation is not possible, personnel should move from cleaning low-risk areas to cleaning high-risk areas as they complete their assigned tasks. Outerwear and personal protection equipment (PPE) should be changed as personnel move from one segregation area to the next. Disposal bins for soiled clothing and PPE should be located in each segregated area.

16. Describe the most important health hazards that cleaning personnel may encounter when conducting their tasks.

The physical nature of cleaning brings personnel into aerosol and physical contact with dander, bedding, and animal waste. Contact and inhalational allergies are common ailments that may limit the ability of a particular person to conduct a particular task, although the use of appropriate PPE can limit exposure. The nature of PPE, however, renders the wearer prone to heat stress during heavy manual labor, particularly during conditions of warm ambient temperature. Physical hazards from animals also exist. Appropriate training is critical to limit the risk of injury to personnel from animal interactions, as well as to limit the chances of inappropriate animal handling or care by personnel. Cleaning equipment, detergents, and disinfectants may be hazardous as well. Use of a buddy system as cleaning tasks are conducted will limit risks as well as enable prompt reporting of an injurious event.

Zoonotic diseases represent a significant occupational health issue for cleaning personnel. For example, contact and aerosol exposure to enteric pathogens such as *Salmonella and Cryptosporidium* can occur during handling of contaminated bedding. Aerosol exposure with *Coxiella burnetti* may occur upon handling bedding or waste from livestock, particularly puerperal ruminants. Exposure to pathogenic serovars of *Leptospira* can occur when personnel are cleaning surfaces soiled by canine urine. Mucous membrane or respiratory exposure to zoonotic strains of avian influenza virus can occur if cleaning personnel in affected poultry houses are not provided appropriate PPE and the requisite training for its proper use and disposal.

Employees involved in cleaning animal housing areas should be thoroughly informed about conditions that might increase their susceptibility to zoonotic disease. Examples include immunosuppressive diseases, taking immunosuppressive medications, or physiologic states of relative immunosuppression, such as pregnancy. While privacy laws may limit the employer's ability to obtain such information from employees, at the very least, employees should be instructed on how to self-identify so that appropriate protective measures or personnel reassignment can be instituted.

Whenever possible, outerwear donned by cleaning personnel should remain on the facilities for appropriate cleaning and disinfection. If outerwear must leave the facility for cleaning, employees must understand that soiled outerwear can represent a zoonotic disease transmission threat to individuals at the employee's home. Appropriately sealed containers can be used to transport soiled outerwear, and appropriate steps for cleaning and disinfection of such clothing should be provided for employees. Ideally, outer footwear should consist of a rubber or plastic boot shoe cover that is either disposable or easily cleaned and disinfected. All outer footwear should remain on the facility grounds and not be taken home by personnel without first being thoroughly cleaned and disinfected. Showering facilities, lockers, hand washing or hand sanitization facilities, and footbaths should be available for cleaning personnel as they enter and exit the facility.

17. What items of personal protective equipment are required for effective cleaning?

It is critical to understand that the level of personal protective equipment that is adequate to protect cleaning personnel will vary according to the type of animal housing involved, the pathogens documented or suspected to be present, the type of cleaning equipment in use, and the type and means of dispersal of detergents and disinfectants to be used. The primary personal protection goals are protection of the mucous membranes, eyes, skin, and respiratory tract from microorganisms and potentially injurious chemical detergents and disinfectants. To most accurately determine the appropriate type of PPE and application equipment required for use of a particular detergent and disinfectant, the Material Safety Data Sheet (MSDS) for the disinfectant should be consulted. In addition, the anticipated method of application (e.g., hand-held sprayer or powered spray device) should be reviewed by occupational health specialists before initiation. For example, use of a gasoline-powered sprayer may create heat, fire, and exhaust hazards.

When cleaning and disinfecting high-risk areas, personnel are optimally protected by some form of waterproof barrier clothing. The characteristics of the surfaces being cleaned, the detergent and disinfectant to be used, and the application methods will determine the appropriate characteristics of the barrier clothing. As a rule, disinfectant-impervious clothing traps body heat very efficiently, and appropriate steps must be taken to ensure that employees working in such apparel are monitored for signs of heat stress and dehydration. Opportunities for personnel to rest and rehydrate are often necessary, particularly during warm weather.

Protective gloves, goggles, waterproof boots or shoe covers, and a mask or respirator are additional PPE items to be worn, the type of which is dictated by MSDS data and the facility's safety regulations. Safety regulations for PPE and related equipment may vary among private companies, public agencies, and governing bodies, because local authorities may enforce regulations that *exceed* the minimal standards set by Occupational Health and Safety Administration. Appropriate training in donning and doffing PPE, as well as storage, handling, dilution, and application of detergents and disinfectants, is critical for employee safety and efficacious cleaning and disinfection.

Selection of PPE for workers involved in decontamination of a facility in which zoonotic pathogens are known or suspected to exist involves protection against the pathogens, the detergents and disinfectants used in cleaning and disinfection, and the physical hazards that may exist in the facility (e.g., slick flooring, exhaust fumes from motorized equipment, etc.). Refer to the Suggested Readings list for Web-based resources on PPE, respiratory protection, and disinfectants approved for use in avian influenza eradication.

18. What considerations apply to selecting a detergent?

There are four general classes of detergents, based on the net charge property of the surface-active ion: anionic, nonionic, cationic, and amphoteric/zwitterionic (Meriano, 2001). This classification has relevance to the detergent's tendency to foam, the degree of detergent inactivation in hard water, and potential to interact with certain disinfectants, resulting in liberation of toxic reaction products and/or deactivation of the disinfectant. Thus, it is very important to consider the compatibility of detergents with disinfectants when making purchasing decisions. If a detergent can be reliably and thoroughly rinsed from a surface before application of the disinfectant, the potential for detergent–disinfectant interaction is greatly lessened. It is important to note that detergent solutions can become heavily contaminated with pathogens during the cleaning process. As a result, detergent solutions (e.g., mop water) and the equipment used to apply the detergents can serve as very efficient fomites. To prevent this problem, detergent solutions should be changed frequently and always discarded before moving from a segregated, high-risk area of the hospital (e.g., isolation or quarantine) to another. Certain detergents possess inherent disinfectant capacity. Certain classes of detergents and disinfectants can be mixed together to limit the potential for spreading pathogens during the cleaning process.

19. Describe the characteristics of the different classes of detergents.

- **Anionic detergents:** These include the common household soaps and laundry detergents containing alkyl sulfates (e.g., sodium lauryl sulfate) or alkyl benzene sulfonates. The anionic detergent moiety is typically compounded with sodium or potassium as the cohort ion. Water with a high dissolved calcium and magnesium content ("hard water") may partially deactivate anionic detergents, and some detergents have calcium and magnesium sequestrants (e.g., EDTA) added to limit this interaction. The deactivating properties of hard water can be limited by adding a larger dose of detergent to a given volume of hard water. Detergents are frequently mixed with phenolic disinfecants to increase the water solubility of the phenol moiety; such detergent/disinfectant combinations may be attractive for cleaning high ID risk areas. Anionic detergents may deactivate quaternary ammonium disinfectants.
- **Cationic detergents:** Most are derivatives of ammonia and characterized by the presence of a quaternary ammonium moiety. These are typically compounded as chloride or bromide salts (e.g., cetyl trimethylammonium chloride). Many compounds in this detergent class possess limited microbiocidal activity. Cationic detergents may inactivate phenolic disinfectants and hypochlorite (bleach).
- **Nonionic detergents:** These lack a net electrical charge, which makes nonionic detergents resistant to deactivation in hard water. Nonionic detergents tend to foam less than the other two types, making them useful as automated dishwasher soaps. These are particularly effective in removing greasy or fatty compounds from surfaces and can be combined with anionic detergents to reduce the overall susceptibility of the detergent mixture to hard water inactivation. The most commonly used nonionic surfactants are ethers of alcohols, such as long-chain glycols. Phenolic disinfectants are inactivated by nonionic detergents.
- **Amphoteric (Zwitterionic):** The net charge of these detergent molecules can be neutral, anionic, or cationic, depending on the pH of the solution into which they are mixed. Amphoteric detergents are commonly used in shampoos, facial soaps, and cosmetics, owing to their mild nature and tendency to foam. They are rarely used for surface cleaning, other than in carpet shampoos.

20. What is the most important criterion to consider when selecting a disinfectant?

The efficacy of a particular disinfectant against the targeted pathogen[s] in a facility is the primary consideration in selecting a disinfectant. *Limited efficacy* disinfectants are those with activity against either Gram-positive or Gram-negative bacteria. *General-purpose* or *broad-spectrum* disinfectants are effective against both of these classes of bacteria, with *Staphylococcus aureus* and *Salmonella cholerasuis* being the test organisms for these two classes. A disinfectant that has a *hospital- or medical-environment claim* is effective against Gram-positive and Gram-negative bacteria, as well as efficacy against the nosocomial pathogen, *Pseudomonas aeruginosa* (Dvorak, 2005). Disinfectant efficacy against other pathogen types, such as nonenveloped viruses (e.g., Parvovirus), bacterial spores, and Mycobacteria vary widely among disinfectant classes; efficacy claims and data for these other agents may be found on the label or in the medical literature, respectively. Table 1.22.1 provides data on the microbiocidal spectrum of the different classes of commonly used disinfectants.

Table 1.22.1 Commonly Used Disinfectants for Animal Care and Holding Facilities

Disinfectant Category	Alcohols	Aldehydes	Biguanides	Hypochlorites	Iodine Compounds	Oxidizing Agents	Phenols	Quaternary Ammonium Compounds (QACs)
Sample compounds	Ethyl alcohol, isopropyl alcohol	Formaldehyde, glutaraldehyde	Chlorhexidine	Bleach, sodium hypochlorite	Povidone iodine	Hydrogen peroxide, accelerated peroxides, peroxymonosulfates	Multiple compounds and products	Multiple compounds and products
Mechanism of action	Precipitate proteins, Denatured fats	Denatured proteins, alkylate nucleic acids	Alter membrane permeability	Denatured proteins	Denatured proteins	Denatured proteins and lipids	Denatured proteins, alter membrane permeability	Denatured proteins, bind to membranes
Advantages	Rapid action, no residue, can be used as antiseptic	Broad spectrum	Can be used as antiseptic	Broad spectrum, inexpensive, short contact time	Stable in storage, tamed compounds can be used as antiseptics	Broad spectrum, peroxymonosulfates retain activity in organic debris	Broad spectrum, retain activity in organic debris, non-corrosive, active in hard water	Effective at high pH (9–10), stable in storage, relatively non-irritating
Disadvantages	Rapid evaporation, flammable	Carcinogenic, skin / mucous membrane irritation	Only functions in pH 5–7, toxic to fish	Inactivated by sunlight, corrode metals, skin / mucous membrane irritation	Inactivated by QACs, corrode metals, stains clothing and some surfaces	Damaging to some metals and corrosive to concrete (prolonged contact), can irritate skin and mucous membranes	Skin and eye irritation	
Precautions	Flammable	Carcinogenic, personal protective equipment needed		Toxic chlorine gas can be liberated if mixed with other disinfectants	Ocular irritant (contact)		May be toxic to cats & pigs	
Vegetative bacteria	Effective	Effective	Effective	Effective	Effective	Effective	Effective	Effective vs. Gram-positive, limited efficacy vs. Gram-negative
Mycobacteria	Effective	Effective	Variable	Effective	Limited	Effective	Variable	Variable
Enveloped ciruses	Effective	Effective	Limited	Effective	Effective	Effective	Effective	Variable
Nonenveloped ciruses	Variable	Effective	Limited	Effective	Limited	Effective	Variable	Not effective
Spores	Not effective	Effective	Not effective	Variable	Limited	Variable	Not effective	Not effective
Fungi	Effective	Effective	Limited	Effective	Effective	Variable	Variable	Variable
Efficacy with organic matter	Reduced	Reduced	Reduced	Rapidly reduced	Rapidly reduced	Variable; peroxymonosulfates retain activity	Effective	Inactivated
Efficacy with hard water	?	Reduced	?	Effective	?	Check label	Effective	Inactivated
Efficacy with soap/detergents	?	Reduced	Surgical scrub solutions contain compatible detergent	Cationic detergents and ammonia-containing products will inactivate	Surgical scrub solutions contain compatible detergent	Some products contain surfactant agents with detergent activity	Cationic & non-ionic detergents will inactivate	Anionic detergents will inactivate

Adapted from and used with permission from Dvorak G, Center for Food Security and Public Health, Iowa State University, 2008; available at: www.cfsph.iastate.edu/BRM/resources/Disinfectants/CharacteristicsSelectedDisinfectants.pdf.

21. Describe the other criteria that influence selection of a disinfectant.

Precautions relative to personnel safety, chemical and fire hazards, disposal requirements, stability, storage requirements, and environmental hazards are important considerations. Certain disinfectants can be corrosive to certain types of surfaces, and others may degrade certain sealing agents, glues, and components of electrical, computer, or medical equipment. The manufacturer's guidelines for disinfection of such equipment should be consulted. Such equipment may require special cleaning and disinfection procedures such as disassembly and disinfection by hand. If sensitive equipment must remain within the facility during use of potentially harmful cleaning and disinfection compounds, the equipment can be carefully sealed within impervious tarps or plastic bags for protection. Remaining considerations include the amount of contact time necessary to achieve disinfection, the method of application of the disinfectant, the pH range within which the disinfectant remains active, and the efficacy of the disinfectant in hard water. The corrosive action of many disinfectants can be limited by rinsing or wiping away the disinfectant once adequate contact time has been allowed; use of clean water and sterile or disinfected sponges and towels is an absolute requirement. This information is provided in each product's label claims and directions for use.

The ambient temperature influences both the efficacy of certain disinfectants and the speed with which disinfectants act on target microbes. The rapidity of microbiocidal action tends to increase with increasing temperature; therefore, prolonged contact time or reapplication of disinfectant may be necessary when disinfectants are used in cold conditions. In addition, certain disinfectants may lose significant microbiocidal activity if allowed to freeze shortly after application (Dee et al, 2005). Antifreeze additives such as methanol or propylene glycol may have to be added to disinfectants to maintain activity when and where freezing is likely (Dee et al, 2005). Under conditions of dry air or high airflow, care must be taken that disinfectants do not evaporate before the required contact time for optimal disinfection. Heavy soaking and reapplication may be necessary under such conditions.

A final, but critical, consideration is the disinfectant's activity in the presence of organic debris. The critical need to clean a surface before disinfection has been emphasized previously. However, in many avian and large animal facilities, it may be impossible or impractical to remove all organic debris from certain surfaces, and as outlined in Table 1.22.1 certain disinfectants retain activity in organic debris to a greater degree than others.

22. Are there legal restrictions that apply to disinfectant use?

In the United States, disinfectants are registered and regulated by the Antimicrobial Division of the Office of Pesticides program of the Environmental Protection Agency. It is unlawful to use registered products in a manner other than what is dictated on the label.

23. What are the important considerations for using bleach as a disinfectant?

Bleach (sodium hypochlorite) is inexpensive, readily available, and broad spectrum, making it an attractive disinfectant for use as a routine disinfectant as well as for use in an emergency / disaster scenario. Commonly used dilutions for disinfection are shown below, with Chlorox® regular bleach being the reference solution (6% sodium hypochlorite):

1:64   2 ounces (1/4 cup) bleach into one gallon water
1:32   4 ounces (1/2 cup) bleach into one gallon water
1:10   24 ounces (1.5 cups) bleach into one gallon water

Several important facts should be remembered for bleach.

- It is rapidly inactivated by organic debris, so bleach is a poor choice for disinfectant footbaths.
- Bleach retains activity in hard water.
- Decolorization of clothing and corrosion of certain metals may occur.
- Vapors can cause mucous membrane irritation, particularly when concentrated solutions are used in confined spaces.
- Bleach can liberate irritating or toxic concentrations of ammonia gas when mixed with ammonia containing solutions or urine.
- Do not mix bleach with other disinfectants, as toxic chlorine gas can be liberated.
- Higher concentration solutions have a more rapid microbiocidal activity than dilute solutions.
- Cationic detergents and ammonia-containing products will inactivate bleach.
- Bleach must be protected from sunlight and heat during storage.
- Bleach solution may slowly lose efficacy during storage. Hypochlorite solutions stored at room temperature in sealed, opaque plastic containers can lose 40-50% of their available chlorine level over a period of 1 month; storage in dark brown bottles greatly limits decomposition of bleach over a similar time period (Rutala and Weber, 2004).
- Concentrated bleach solutions can etch or erode concrete surfaces over time.

24. What are the advantages and disadvantages of the phenolic disinfectants?

Phenolic disinfectants (e.g., One-Stroke Environ®, Tek-Trol®, Lysol®) have a very broad spectrum and maintain activity in organic debris. They are compatible with the widely-available household anionic detergents, and since detergents increase the water solubility and efficacy of phenolic compounds, many commercially available products are detergent/disinfectant combinations. Phenolic compounds retain activity in hard water. Certain phenolic compounds have been documented to cause systemic intoxication in cats, dermal contact lesions in swine, and occasional intoxication of other animals (Foster, 1994). Cats are hypothesized to be more sensitive to intoxication because their meticulous grooming habits might cause ingestion following cutaneous contact (Foster, 1994). To be safe, phenolic compounds should be thoroughly rinsed from surfaces with which animals might come in contact. Under conditions of routine use in equine barns, the risk of intoxication to farm cats appears to be low (Dywer, 2004).

25. Describe the pros and cons of the oxidizing agents.

Disinfectants in this class include the accelerated hydrogen peroxide products and peroxymonosulfate-based disinfectants. These are broad-spectrum disinfectants that retain activity in organic debris. They are generally regarded as efficacious against Mycobacteria and enveloped viruses, but show mixed efficacy against bacterial spores. In vitro studies indicate that the viability or infectivity of *Cryptosporidium* oocysts may be reduced with certain oxidizing agents (Ares-Mazas et al, 1997; Quiles et al, 2005). In our veterinary hospital, a peroxymonosulfate disinfectant (4% solution of Virkon® S) is used for footbaths; the efficacy of this disinfectant in reducing bacterial counts on heavily contaminated rubber boots has been documented (Morley et al, 2005). This disinfectant is also used for directed misting, by stationary motorized misters and motorized backpack misters, for decontamination of hard-to-reach surfaces (Patterson et al, 2005). These disinfectants tend to have rapid microbiocidal activity and are environmentally friendly. Although solutions of these agents are considered relatively safe for handling, powdered preparations of these products must be handled carefully, as they may irritate mucous membranes if made airborne by wind or mixing. Newer-generation products (e.g., Trifectant®) retain microbiocidal activity in hard water. Because of their oxidizing property, these products can be corrosive to a variety of materials including plain steel, iron, and concrete. However, some products in this class have claims suggesting that this is less of a concern in some newer products.

26. Describe the advantages and disadvantages of quaternary ammonium compounds.

The quaternary ammonium compounds (QACs) are relatively nonirritating and safe for handling. Their activity is greatly limited by the presence of organic debris, and they are inactivated by anionic detergents (household soaps). Nonionic detergents must be used if the detergent is to be retained on the surfaces on which the QAC is to be applied. Their limited Gram-negative spectrum is a concern when considering use in livestock housing heavily contaminated with fecal material. These compounds are ineffective for rapid disinfection of footwear when used in footbaths (Morley et al, 2005).

27. What considerations arise when using the aldehyde disinfectants?

Although aldehydes are highly effective against a variety of microbes, including spores, the primary factor that limits their use is their carcinogenic properties, which represent a hazard for both personnel and animals. Appropriate personal protective equipment, including an appropriately rated respirator, is necessary for their use. Formaldehyde is an effective fumigant, and provided that a building can be cleaned and sealed, formaldehyde fumigation is an effective means of disinfection of livestock buildings and poultry houses, particularly when an outbreak of a zoonotic or high-priority pathogen occurs. OSHA regulations regarding exposure to formaldehyde fumes also apply (See http://www.osha.gov/SLTC/formaldehyde/index.html). After fumigation with formaldehyde, a neutralizing agent, methenamine, must be applied, and the neutralization byproduct must be wiped from surfaces before use.

Glutaraldehyde is commonly used as a cold (liquid) sterilant for medical instruments that cannot be autoclaved, such as endoscopes. Because it is highly irritating to mucous membranes and the respiratory tract, it is not used as a facility disinfectant.

28. Other than formaldehyde, are there any other disinfectants that can be used as fumigants?

Vaporized hydrogen peroxide is effective against a variety of microorganisms. Once vaporized, its distribution within a facility can be irregular because it tends to condense on cool surfaces and is absorbed by celluloid materials such as paper, ceiling tiles, and cardboard. Chlorine dioxide gas is a broad-spectrum disinfectant that has been used to disinfect a large animal hospital facility contaminated by Salmonella spp. (Luftman et al, 2006). This gas was also used to decontaminate *Bacillus anthracis* spores in the Hart Senate Office Building and Brentwood postal sorting facility following the 2001 anthrax bioterrorism events.

29. What role do iodines, biguanidines, and alcohols play in a disinfection program?

Iodides (e.g., povidone iodine) and biguanidines (e.g., chlorhexidine) are frequently used as antiseptics, rather than as disinfectants, owing to their relatively high cost and tendency to be rapidly inactivated by organic debris. They are effective in reducing pathogen loads on skin and surfaces, provided that the load of organic debris on the surface has been reduced by thorough washing. Iodine-containing products can stain clothing, certain plastics, and rubber products.

Alcohols are broad-spectrum disinfectants that are rapid-acting and relatively inexpensive. Their flammability limits their use as a facility disinfectant. They are most commonly used as hand and skin disinfectants, and may be used to disinfect small, cleaned items when staining is to be avoided. Alcohol gels are highly effective for hand hygiene, although their activity is limited when hands are heavily soiled, and they possess little activity against bacterial spores.

30. Describe the relevant considerations for a disinfection program for animal facilities in an evacuation scenario.

Recently, several wildfires and floods in the United States have necessitated the evacuation of pets and livestock, along with people, to evacuation centers. Depending on the scope and nature of the disaster and the available facilities at evacuation centers, development and implementation of a cleaning and disinfection program for animal transport vehicles, holding facilities, and feed, bedding, and waste handling equipment will be critical. Pet animals may need to be held in temporary housing until reunited with their owners. Further, pet owners frequently desire contact with their pets during the evacuation process. These issues necessitate a coordinated, local and regional response plan for evacuated animals, including evacuation and relocation strategies, hazardous materials decontamination, sheltering and feed, waste management, human resource utilization, animal identification, veterinary medical care, cleaning and disinfection, and zoonotic disease control.

31. Facilities such as fairgrounds, parks, and sporting facilities have been frequently utilized as evacuation centers. What considerations apply when developing a cleaning and disinfection strategy for animal holding areas in these evacuation centers?

Of primary importance in such scenarios is the need for evaluation of evacuated animals for potential exposure to hazardous materials, including infectious materials, by hazardous materials personnel and, subsequently, by veterinary personnel before the entry of animals into the facility. Decontamination processes are dictated by the nature of the emergency and may range from no decontamination to bathing to chemical decontamination or, for animals exposed to extremely hazardous material (e.g., biological weapons or nuclear fallout), euthanasia.

Personnel assigned to disinfect stalls, crates, or equipment must be properly trained in safe use of disinfectants and must be fitted for appropriate PPE. This is of particular importance in a disaster evacuation setting, where volunteer workers may be needed for tasks such as cleaning and disinfection.

Isolation areas should be designated for animals that are ill or suspected to have been exposed to infectious agents, with appropriate signage and traffic control measures instituted to minimize contact with other animals and human evacuees. The location of such isolation facilities will be dictated by the location and available facilities, but ideal characteristics would include many of the aspects of a comprehensive ID control program listed at the beginning of this chapter. Segregation of evacuated animals by ID risk is of primary importance in evacuation center planning. Relevant considerations for high risk animals (e.g., dairy calves with signs of diarrhea) would include the following:

- Remote location with limited interaction with foot or vehicular traffic
- Fencing
- Downwind (leeward) location from other animals and people in the facility
- Drains or stand-alone, secure locations for runoff (drainage)
- Appropriate containers or storage areas for soiled bedding
- Separate feed storage and feed handling equipment. Large plastic contractor bags can serve as suitable containers for animal feeds.
- Separate feed and water containers
- Separate personnel for health care, cleaning, and husbandry
- Appropriate PPE, consisting of dedicated barrier attire (coveralls or gowns, gloves, and waterproof boots) and respiratory protection rated to the likely ID or chemical hazards

In evacuation centers, as in animal care facilities, particular emphasis should be placed on hand hygiene among caretakers. Alcohol-based hand sanitizers and/or hand washing stations equipped with disinfectant soap should be available. Disinfectant footbaths (e.g., 4% Virkon® S or Trifectant™) should be utilized at entry and exit points to areas with heavy fecal contamination, such as livestock holding pens. It may be necessary to select a detergent/ disinfectant combination product for single-step cleaning and disinfection (e.g., phenolic-detergent products), if rinse water is in limited supply. Such products are active in organic debris. Rinsing of such solutions is recommended before animal contact, particularly for equipment and housing used for cats.

When water supplies are adequate, readily available household soaps (e.g., laundry detergents) can be used for cleaning. Once these are rinsed away, inexpensive, readily available disinfectants such as bleach may then be used for disinfection. If rapid disinfection is needed for equipment or housing undergoing rapid turnaround, more concentrated solutions of bleach (e.g., 1:10) may be required. Appropriate contact time will vary according to ambient temperature, the pathogens targeted, and the nature of the surfaces being disinfected.

Suggested Reading

Ares-Mazas E, Lorenzo MJ, Casal JA, et al. Effect of a commercial disinfectant ("Virkon") on mouse experimental infection by *Cryptosporidium parvum*. *J Hosp Infect* 1997;36:141–145.

Centers for Disease Control and Prevention, Department of Health and Human Services. Interim guidance for protection of persons involved in U.S. avian influenza outbreak disease control and eradication activities. Available at http://www.cdc.gov/flu/avian/professional/protect-guid.htm.

Dee S, Deen J, Burns D, et al. An evaluation of disinfectants for the sanitation of porcine reproductive and respiratory syndrome virus-contaminated transport vehicles at low temperatures. *Can J Vet Res* 2005;69:64–70.

Dvorak G. Disinfection 101. Center for Food Safety and Public Health, Iowa State University. Available at http://www.cfsph.iastate.edu/BRM/disinfectants.htm.

Dwyer RM. Environmental disinfection to control equine infectious diseases. *Vet Clin North Am Equine Pract* 2004;20:531–542, 2004.

Foster D. Poison: Phenolics. *In Practice* 1994;330–331.

Luftman HS, Regits MA, Lorcheim P, et al. Chlorine dioxide gas decontamination of large animal hospital intensive and neonatal care units. *Appl Biosafety* 2006;11:144–154.

Merianos JJ. Surface–active agents. In Block SS, ed. *Disinfection, Sterilization, and Preservation*, 5th ed. Philadelphia, Lippincott Williams and Wilkins, 2001, pp. 283–320.

Morley PS, Morris SN, Hyatt DR, et al. Evaluation of the efficacy of disinfectant footbaths as used in veterinary hospitals. *J Am Vet Med Assoc* 2005;226:2053–2058.

National Institute for Occupational Safety and Health, Centers for Disease Control and Prevention, Department of Health and Human Services. Respirators. Available at http://www.cdc.gov/niosh/npptl/topics/respirators/.

Occupational Safety and Health Administration, US Department of Labor. Guidance for protecting employees against avian flu. Available at http://www.osha.gov/dsg/guidance/avian-flu.html.

Patterson G, Morley PS, Blehm KD, et al. Efficacy of directed misting application of a peroxygen disinfectant for environmental decontamination of a veterinary hospital. *J Am Vet Med Assoc* 2005;227:597–602.

Quilez J, Sanchez-Acedo C, Avendano C, et al. Efficacy of two peroxygen-based disinfectants for inactivation of *Cryptosporidium parvum* oocysts. *Appl Environ Microbiol* 2005;71:2479–2483.

Rutala WA, Weber DJ. Selection and use of disinfectants in health care. In Mayhall CG, ed. *Hospital Epidemiology and Infection Control*, 3rd ed. Philadelphia, Lippincott, Williams and Wilkins, 2004, pp. 1473–1522.

United States Environmental Protection Agency. Antimicrobial products to disinfect poultry and other facilities against avian (bird) flu. Available at http://www.epa.gov/pesticides/factsheets/avian.htm.

CHAPTER 1.23
PAIN MANAGEMENT IN VETERINARY DISASTER MEDICINE

Marc R. Raffe, DVM, MS

Pain management is an important component of global patient triage and management in large-scale disasters. Pain sources in disaster situations can be diverse and seemingly unrelated; however, most pain sources can be attributed to defined pain categories and managed using strategies and treatments appropriate for the pain category. The purpose of this review is to familiarize the reader with pain categories germane to disaster medicine, to globally review treatment options, and to address specific treatment for the primary cause of pain in an individual patient.

INITIAL FIELD MANAGEMENT

1. What are common causes of pain that may be seen in disaster medicine?

Pain, regardless of the cause, can be globally categorized as acute or chronic in origin. Pain associated with disasters will mainly be acute pain. Pain in disaster scenarios may be a result of musculoskeletal injury, head trauma, spinal injury, thermal injury, internal injury associated visceral pain, chemical injury, and toxic substances.

2. How does one recognize pain in small animals?

Because animals are "nonverbal" and cannot communicate pain, one must look for clues or observations that indicate pain is present. In dogs and cats, indicators can fall into five major categories: posture, temperament, vocalization, locomotion, and other. Table 1.23.1 summarizes each category for the dog and cat; Table 1.23.2 summarizes each category for the horse and cow. Small ruminants represented by sheep and goats will demonstrate signs similar to those for the cow.

3. How should one "triage" patients based on pain indicators?

Pain can be a powerful stimulus that can produce self-destructive behaviors and can lead to further injury and physiologic instability. Patients that demonstrate overt behaviors that may place the patient at risk for additional injury or physiologic decompensation should be evaluated and treated on a priority basis. These behaviors may include delirium, flailing, writhing, dragging of a torso section, and biting or striking behavior. These observed behaviors generally indicate serious injury that has produced an intense pain focus, which requires immediate attention.

Table 1.23.1   Pain Behaviors in the Dog and Cat

Appearance	Dog	Cat
Posture	Tail between legs Arched or hunched back Twisted body to protect site Drooped head Frozen sitting position Tucked abdomen Lying flat in extension	Tucked limbs Arched or hunched head, neck, or back Tucked abdomen Lying flat Slumping of body Drooping of head
Temperament	Aggressive Clawing Attacking, biting Escaping	Aggressive Biting Scratching Chewing Attacking Escaping Hiding
Vocalization	Barking Howling Moaning Whimpering	Crying Hissing Spitting Moaning Screaming Purring
Locomotion	Reluctant to move Carrying a leg Lameness Unusual gait Unable to walk	Reluctant to move Carrying one leg Lameness Unusual gait Unable to walk Inactive
Other	Unable to perform normal tasks Attacks other animals or people Chewing painful areas No interest in food, water, or play	Attacks if pain site is touched Failure to groom Dilated pupils No interest in food or play

Adapted from Pfizer Animal Health Pain Management Toolkit, 2007.

4. What initial steps should be taken by disaster workers to manage pain in these patients as they reach the medical triage area?

As with other disaster patients, primary survey and assurance of A-B-C stability are the highest priorities. Once stability is confirmed, "first-aid" practices to manage pain and improve patient comfort/cooperation are initiated. First actions may include gaining patient control by physical or chemical restraint, immobilizing limb fractures with splint or bulk bandage techniques, immobilizing spinal injury with a "back board" device, beginning burn management, and initiating chemical or toxic substance decontamination measures.

5. What additional options for pain management can be used following initial evaluation?

As noted, pain medications can be initiated once initial evaluations suggest patient stability. In most cases, pain will be initially managed with systemic opioid administration in conjunction with local anesthetic injection at the

Table 1.23.2 Pain Behaviors in the Horse and Cow

Appearance	Horse	Cow
Posture	Tail between legs Arched or hunched back Twisted body to protect site Drooped head Tucked abdomen Lying flat on side with legs in extension	Arched or hunched head, neck, or back Tucked abdomen Lying flat Drooping of head
Temperament	Attacking Biting Striking Escaping	Attacking Escaping
Vocalization	Loud whinny Groaning	Soft or loud "grunts" Bellowing
Locomotion	Reluctant to move Carrying a leg Lameness Unusual gait Unable to walk Thrashing while lying on side	Reluctant to move Carrying one leg Lameness Unusual gait Unable to walk Sternal or lateral posture Inactive
Other	Rapid breathing Dilated pupils Grinding of teeth No interest in food, water, or play	Attacks if pain site is touched Dilated pupils Grinding of teeth No interest in food or play

Adapted from Pfizer Animal Health Pain Management Toolkit, 2007.

primary pain focus where indicated. The rationale for this treatment strategy is that opioid and local anesthetic class drugs have the highest safety margin and the greatest range of efficacy in unstable or potentially unstable pain patients.

6. What is recommended for transport of high-grade pain patients to the primary casualty center?

All pain patients should be handled as "high risk." Measures to ensure safety of both the patient and rescue worker are important during the transport process. Physical restraint measures appropriate to the situation including use of muzzles may be necessary to ensure patient cooperation. As noted, support devices such as stretchers or rigid back boards fashioned from wood or metal are encouraged for patients that have unstable musculoskeletal or spinal injury. Use of blankets or other soft material to fashion a "stretcher" or a whole body wrap to help restraint during transport may be used. Finally, the patient may need to be "suspended" by use of blanket or material stretcher in the rescue vehicle in order to provide a "cushion" from irregular road surface motion and shock impact, which may further exacerbate the injury.

PRIMARY ASSESSMENT AND TREATMENT AT THE MEDICAL TRIAGE AREA

7. How can pain be "triaged" at a medical triage area?

All pain patients are assessed and initially prioritized based on the clinical impact that pain may have. Patients that demonstrate overt behavior characterized by delirium, flailing, writhing, dragging of a torso section, and biting or striking behavior should be considered high priority for evaluation and early management.

8. What are initial "steps" that nonmedical workers can implement to help address pain?

Good nursing care is an important first step in providing good pain management to injured patients. Wound management is a primary consideration in these patients. Techniques for wound care and management are described in the chapters on large and small animal first aid. Fracture stabilization using splints, bulk bandages, or immobilizing boards should be performed unless poor patient cooperation requires the use of analgesia and/or anesthesia to accomplish the goal. Use of soft bedding materials for housing these patients will increase comfort level.

9. What initial "steps" should medical workers implement to address pain?

Identification of the primary pain focus is the first step. Once the pain source is identified, decisions regarding treatment strategy should be quickly formulated. Options will include use of local/regional nerve blocks or systemic analgesic administration.

10. What drugs can be used for local/regional pain control?

Drugs of the local anesthetic class are generally selected for local/regional pain control. Common members of this drug class include 2% lidocaine, 1% mepivacaine (Carbocaine), and 0.5% bupivacaine (Marcaine). Any of these class members can be effectively used for pain control. The major differences between class members include the time from administration to onset (lidocaine < mepivacaine < bupivacaine) and duration of effect (lidocaine < mepivacaine < bupivacaine).

Drugs of the opioid class (morphine, hydromorphone, buprenorphine) can be mixed with local anesthetic drugs prior to administration for joint or epidural administration. Other drugs reported to enhance regional/local analgesia include xylazine, metdetomidine, ephedrine, and epinephrine.

11. Are there "safety" issues with these drugs?

Local anesthetic drugs are considered a safe drug class for many applications. The main consideration is to make sure that dose guidelines are not exceeded to prevent toxic side effects. The guidelines for the dog are a MAXIMUM of 2 mL/10 lb local anesthesia in any patient regardless of the administration site. In cats, a maximum of 1.25 to 1.5 mL/10 lb should be used. Opioids have a very high safety margin and can be used in pain patients without fear of toxicity. Xylazine and metdetomidine should be used in low doses as "adjunctive" drugs along with opioids.

12. How can these drugs be used to control pain?

Local anesthetic drugs play an important role in pain control. Local anesthetic drugs can used in irrigation solutions for wound decontamination; can be discretely injected into injury sites, joints, or around individual peripheral nerves; can be locally infiltrated in a specific tissue site or region; or can be regionally administered (epidural, brachial plexus) to desensitize specific regions to effect pain control. Lidocaine can also be incorporated into intravenous solutions that are parenterally administered to manage visceral pain.

As noted, opioids can be coadministered with local anesthetic drugs to enhance pain control in joints for regional pain control via epidural or brachial plexus blockade.

13. What are specific techniques in which local anesthetic drugs can be used?

There are many sites and techniques that have been described for local or regional analgesia. Simple techniques include a quadrant block performed by local tissue infiltration. Anatomic sites into which local anesthetic drugs can be injected include joints, bone fracture site, and specific nerves or groups of nerves to create regional desensitization. Single nerve injection techniques include dental blockade of the infraorbital and mandibular nerves, sciatic nerve block, and intercostal nerve block. Regional techniques include brachial plexus block and epidural injection. Intrathoracic analgesia can be created by injection of local anesthetic agents into the interpleural space in addition to intercostal nerve block to desensitize the thoracic wall.

14. What precautions should one be aware of when performing local/regional techniques?

In the awake or mildly sedated patient, local anesthetic drug injection will induce discomfort and reaction due to the acidic pH of all local anesthetic drugs. Warming local anesthetic agents to 40° C prior to use has been shown to reduce injection associated pain. Mixing the local anesthetic drug with sodium bicarbonate just before administration also reduces this reaction by buffering the drug pH. One part of sodium bicarbonate is mixed with five parts of local anesthetic drug to reduce injection related irritation.

Anatomically, nerves generally are "bundled" with blood vessels. Following needle placement, aspiration should be done prior to injection to confirm that the needletip has not been accidentally placed into a blood vessel.

DEFINITIVE PAIN MANAGEMENT

15. What pain management control strategies can be considered for extended care?

Once initial triage and stabilization have occurred, additional pain control measures can be considered. Drug delivery routes for extended pain management include wound infiltration and irrigation, intramuscular, subcutaneous, intravenous, regional administration, transdermal, and oral. In disaster scenarios, periodic intramuscular or subcutaneous administration, transdermal, and oral techniques require the least personnel involvement. Regional administration requires intermediate personnel involvement, and continuous intravenous infusion requires the most personnel involvement.

16. What drugs can be used for parenteral administration?

Drug classes used systemically include opioids, nonsteroidal anti-inflammatory (NSAID), α_2 drugs, and local anesthetics. Opioids and nonsteroidal anti-inflammatory drugs (NSAIDs) are the most commonly used. Opioids have excellent pain control properties following parenteral administration. Selection of parenteral administration route (subcutaneous, intramuscular, and intravenous) is based on desired response speed and duration of effect. In general, opioids that have an extended duration of effect (morphine, hydromorphone, buprenorphine) are selected for subcutaneous or intramuscular injection. Opioids that have a short life span (fentanyl) will require continuous intravenous administration.

NSAIDs can be an effective choice for soft tissue based pain in patients that are NOT in shock or have evidence of renal or gastrointestinal disease. In general, oral NSAIDs are administered once a day to accomplish pain control. If quicker response is needed, the first NSAID dose may be given by injection if the selected product has that formulation option.

α_2-Agonist drugs (xylazine, metdetomidine, dexmetdetomidine) are excellent analgesics and produce dose-dependent calming or sedation. They can be used in cardiovascular stable patients as a primary or adjunctive pain control. One of their strong values is sedation that can calm a dysphoric or agitated patient.

17. What is CRI, and how is it used?

Continuous rate infusion (CRI) is a method that is used to constantly deliver medications by intravenous infusion. It is used when drugs have short duration of effect following a single dose administration or when a "steady state" drug level across time is desirable. CRI delivery is used in pain management to reduce the "peak and valley" effect associated with periodic administration of analgesic drugs. It has been shown that "breakthrough" pain associated with subtherapeutic drug level requires higher pain medication doses to "capture" and regain patient comfort. Using a CRI avoids the "peak and valley" blood level of single drug dose administration and provides a consistent clinical response to treatment.

18. What drugs can be given by CRI?

In theory, all drugs that can be intravenously administered can be delivered by CRI technique. Pain medications that have been delivered by CRI in veterinary medicine include opioids (morphine, oxymorphone, hydromorphone, and fentanyl), local anesthetics (lidocaine), ketamine, and α_2-agonists (metdetomidine, dexmetdetomidine, xylazine).

19. How does one formulate a CRI?

The key factor in formulation is to know how much drug to give over a specific time period. There are standard tables that contain precalculated information based on dose, body weight, and fluid administration rate. These are the key variables that must be known in order to calculate a CRI.

Let's use an example to illustrate how to calculate a CRI formula. Lidocaine CRI can be very effective for visceral pain control. Lidocaine 2% (without epinephrine) is added to an intravenous fluid unit (lactated Ringer's, Normosol-R, or 5% dextrose solution) to create a lidocaine infusion. The final concentration of lidocaine in the fluid unit is set at 1 mg/mL. In order to achieve the desired lidocaine concentration in a 1-L fluid bag, add 50 mL of 2% (20 mg/mL) lidocaine. This works out to the target concentration of 1 mg (1000 µg) per mL. If a smaller fluid unit (100 mL, 250 mL, and 500 mL) is used, proportionately less lidocaine is added to the fluid unit.

Prior to starting the lidocaine infusion, an initial intravenous "bolus" of 1 to 2 mg/kg lidocaine is SLOWLY given to build therapeutic blood lidocaine concentration. Following the initial bolus, the lidocaine-containing fluid is dosed at 25 to 50 µg/kg/min until clinical effect is noted. This is the published dose range for CRI lidocaine to produce pain control in dogs and horses. Administering lidocaine at this targeted dose rate translates into an infusion rate of ½ to 1 × maintenance fluid rate (3 mL/kg/hr) to achieve the targeted drug concentration in the patient.

20. What pain medications can be delivered by CRI?

All opioid class drugs (morphine, hydromorphone, fentanyl, oxymorphone, butorphanol) have published CRI dose rates. As noted, lidocaine can be administered as a CRI for visceral pain control. The α_2 drugs (metdetomidine, dexmetdetomidine) can also be delivered by CRI technique.

CRI dosages have been extensively published for dogs and cats. Less information is available for horses and cattle. One exception is lidocaine in horses, studied due to its favorable effects on gastrointestinal motility. As noted, the CRI lidocaine dose is similar to that in dogs.

21. How can local anesthetic drugs be regionally delivered for extended pain control?

Multifenestrated pain catheters can be percutaneously or surgically implanted proximate to a primary pain focus including wounds, regional nerves, or nerve groups to provide continuous pain control. Following catheter placement, a reservoir of local anesthetic (lidocaine, bupivacaine) is attached to the catheter hub adapter to provide continuous infusion. Commercial elastomeric reservoirs ("pain buster" bulb or pump) have a mechanism to provide continuous local anesthetic delivery at a controlled rate (generally 1 to 3 mL/hr). This technique may be used to provide sustained pain control over a 12- to 24-hour period. The reservoir can be refilled to extend the duration of pain control if needed.

GENERAL POINTS IN PAIN MANAGEMENT

22. Can pain management be included in wound care?

Yes. Initial wound cleaning and irrigation can use lidocaine-containing flush solutions compounded as noted for CRI formulation. Including lidocaine in the flush provides desensitization of the wound site at a low risk level for toxicity. Lidocaine flush solution can also be used to moisten bandages used in "wet-to-dry" bandage technique. Incorporation of lidocaine facilitates dressing change and desensitizes the area immediately following bandage change. Studies of local anesthetic use in wounds do not support delayed healing due to use of local anesthetic drugs directly in wounds.

23. Can "patch" delivery systems be used for pain control?

Fentanyl and lidocaine are commercially available in a slow-release dermal patch formulation. Fentanyl patches can be used for extended duration (3- to 4-day) pain control; however, they may require 12 hours (cat) to 18 hours (dog) to become clinically effective. As such, supplemental analgesia with another opioid class drug is required until the patch becomes effective. Also, the release fentanyl is "fixed" at a specific dose (about 1 to 2 μg/kg/hr) and may not be adequate for pain control in a specific patient.

Lidocaine patches are effective for superficial pain control; their efficacy for deep tissue and visceral pain control is unknown at this time.

24. What strategy is better, unimodal or multimodal pain control?

Multimodal pain control is preferred in almost all pain classes. The rationale for the superiority of multimodal control is that it inhibits pain transmission at multiple sites in pain pathways, thus providing improved quality of pain control with lower doses of individual drugs.

25. How long should pain management be provided?

Pain has two major components: direct tissue damage and inflammation. In acute pain, the first component is dominant for up to 48 hours; inflammation may persist for 4 to 7 days. As such, good pain management requires treatment for a minimum of 4 to 7 days' duration or until the pain source is stabilized and healing begins.

26. When should pain management be withheld?

The only relative indication for delayed pain management is acute head trauma. Until loss of consciousness is determined to be stabilized, central nervous system depressants such as opioids and α_2 drugs should be judiciously used so that stable loss of consciousness can be confirmed. In all other settings, pain control should be initiated as a primary step in triage and stabilization.

Suggested Reading

Gaynor J, Muir WW: Handbook of Veterinary Pain Management, 2nd ed. New York, Elsevier, 2008.

International Veterinary Academy of Pain Management. Available at www.ivapm.org.

Pfizer Animal Health. *Anesthesia/Pain Management Techniques for Veterinary Professionals.*

Pfizer Animal Health. *Pain Management Toolkit for Companion Animals.*

Tranquilli WJ, Grimm KA, Lamont LA. *Pain Management for the Small Animal Practitioner,* 2nd ed. Teton, New Media, 2004.

CHAPTER 1.24
HUMANE EUTHANASIA OF ANIMALS

Wayne E. Wingfield, MS, DVM

1. What is euthanasia?

In the context of this learning module, euthanasia is the act of inducing humane death in an animal.

2. Where was the term "euthanasia" derived?

Euthanasia is derived from the Greek terms *eu* meaning "good" and *thanatos* meaning "death." A good death is one that occurs with minimal pain and distress.

3. Why is euthanasia important in a disaster setting?

As veterinary disaster workers, it is our responsibility to ensure that if an animal's life is to be taken, it is done with the highest degree of respect and with an emphasis on making the death as painless and free of distress as possible.

4. What are the goals of euthanasia techniques?

Euthanasia techniques should result in rapid loss of consciousness, followed by respiratory and cardiac arrest, and the ultimate loss of brain function. In addition, the technique should minimize distress and anxiety experienced by the animal prior to loss of consciousness.

5. Can we always ensure that alleviation of pain and distress is achieved?

No, but in every case, pain and distress should be minimized. If in doubt, you should always seek a veterinarian with training and expertise for that species to ensure proper procedures are followed.

6. What is pain?

Pain is the sensation (perception) that results from nerve impulses reaching the cerebral cortex via ascending neural pathways. For pain to be experienced, the cerebral cortex and subcortical structures must be functional.

7. Why do we discuss pain in the topic of euthanasia?

If the cerebral cortex is nonfunctional because of hypoxia (decreased blood oxygen levels), depression by drugs, electric shock, or concussion, pain is not experienced. Therefore, the choice of the euthanasia agent or method is less critical if it is to be used on an animal that is already unconscious, provided the animal does not regain consciousness prior to death.

8. How is pain identified in animals?

This is one of the most difficult questions to answer. Some of the following may help define the animal that is painful.

- Vocalization may indicate pain; however, it is an insensitive and nonspecific indicator of pain.
- Pain is frequently associated with abnormal activity, which may appear as either an increase or a decrease in activity.
- Some animals may appear restless, agitated, or even delirious. At the other end of the spectrum, other animals may be lethargic, withdrawn, dull, or depressed. These animals may not pay attention to environmental stimuli.
- Animals may bite, lick, chew, or shake painful areas.
- Painful animals may adopt abnormal body postures in an attempt to relieve or cope with pain in a given area. For example, dogs with abdominal pain may assume a posture with a rigid torso and arched back. Animals with thoracic pain may be reluctant to lie down despite obvious exhaustion. Disuse or guarding of a painful area is a fairly reliable indicator of pain. The animal's gait may be abnormal or may appear much more rigid than normal.
- Interactive behaviors are frequently changed in the painful animal. Some animals may become more aggressive and resist handling or palpation. In contrast, they may become more timid than usual and seek increased contact with caregivers. Although most animals do not have the same degree of motor control over their facial muscles as do primates, changes in facial expression can be used in some to detect pain. Animals may hold their ears back or in a down position. The eyes may be wide open with dilated pupils, or partially closed with a dull appearance. Many animals will display a "fixed stare" into space, apparently oblivious to their surroundings. Some may display a type of grimace uncharacteristic when not painful.

9. Are the outwardly recognizable clinical signs of pain ever masked by the underlying cause of the pain?

Yes, trauma and other causes may blunt an animal's behavioral response to pain. Lack of overt signs of pain (vocalizing, thrashing, etc.) does not confirm the animal is not painful.

10. Identify one common rule of thumb for recognizing the importance of pain in animals.

The greater the amount of trauma, the more intense is the pain.

11. What are some of the physiologic signs of pain in animals?

Tachypnea, tachycardia, hypertension, dilated pupils, and salivation are physiologic signs suggestive of pain.

12. What is stress?

Stress is defined as the effect of physical, physiologic, or emotional factors (stressors) that induce an alteration in an animal's homeostasis or adaptive state. The response of an animal to stress represents the adaptive process that is necessary to restore the baseline mental and physiologic state.

13. What determines an animal's response to stress?

An animal's response to stress varies according to its experience, age, species, breed, and current physiologic and psychological state.

14. What are the three phases of stress in an animal?

- *Eustress* results when harmless stimuli initiate adaptive responses that are beneficial to the animal.
- *Neutral stress* results when the animal's response to stimuli causes neither harmful nor beneficial effects to the animal.
- *Distress* results when an animal's response to stimuli interferes with its well-being and comfort.

15. Is it important to understand animal handling in euthanasia?

Yes! Proper handling is vital to minimize pain and distress in animals, to ensure safety of the person performing euthanasia, and, often, to protect other people and animals. Some methods of euthanasia require physical handling of the animal. The amount and kind of restraint will be determined by the animal's species, breed, size, state of domestication, degree of taming, presence of painful injury or disease, degree of excitement, and method of euthanasia.

16. Describe means of handling domestic animals that are NOT appropriate prior to euthanasia.

- Electric prods or whips should not be used to encourage movement of animals. Instead, properly designed chutes and ramps should be used.
- Placing the animal in a painful position should NOT be allowed.
- Inducing undue stress on the animal is not condoned.

17. When preparing to euthanatize an animal, list several animal behavioral considerations that should be followed.

- Gentle restraint, careful handling, and talking during euthanasia often have a calming effect on animals that are used to being handled.
- Sedation and/or anesthesia may assist in achieving the best conditions for euthanasia.
- Observers of the euthanasia should be aware of what is to take place.
- Show compassion toward the animal, the animal owner, and professionals involved with the euthanasia.

18. How does euthanasia of animals that are wild, feral, injured, or already distressed from disease differ from euthanasia of healthy, unwanted pets?

These animals are already distressed and methods of preeuthanasia handling may not be effective. Because handling may stress animals unaccustomed to human contact, the degree of restraint required to perform euthanasia should be evaluated prior to the procedure. When handling these animals, calming may be accomplished by minimizing visual, auditory, and tactile stimulation.

19. What techniques may be required prior to euthanasia of wild, feral, injured, or already distressed animals?

Because struggling during capture or restraint may cause pain, injury, or anxiety to the animal, or danger to the rescuer, the use of tranquilizers, analgesics, and/or anesthetics may be necessary.

20. What is the most common human psychological response to euthanasia of animals?

The most common human psychological response is *grief at the loss of life*.

21. What are the three main methods in which euthanatizing agents cause death?

• Hypoxia, direct and indirect
• Direct depression of neurons necessary for life function
• Physical disruption of brain activity and destruction of neurons necessary for life

22. What physical state must exist to ensure death is painless and distress free?

Loss of consciousness should precede loss of motor activity (muscle movement).

23. Does the loss of motor activity equate with the loss of consciousness and the absence of distress?

No! There are agents that induce muscle paralysis without the loss of consciousness and these agents should NOT be used as sole agents for euthanasia. Examples of these unacceptable euthanasia drugs include depolarizing and nondepolarizing muscle relaxants, strychnine, nicotine, and magnesium or potassium salts.

24. How does the physical destruction of brain activity result in the death of an animal?

Physical destruction of brain activity, caused by concussion, direct destruction of the brain, or electrical depolarization of neurons, induces rapid loss of consciousness. Death occurs because of destruction of midbrain centers controlling cardiac and respiratory activity or as a result of adjunctive methods (e.g., exsanguination) used to kill the animal.

25. List the physical methods of euthanasia.

- Captive bolt
- Gunshot
- Cervical dislocation
- Decapitation
- Electrocution
- Kill traps
- Thoracic compression
- Exsanguination
- Stunning
- Pithing

26. From the list above (question No. 25), which physical methods of euthanasia are NOT recommended as a sole means of euthanasia?

- Exsanguination
- Stunning
- Pithing

27. What are some of the concerns that should be considered when using the physical means of euthanasia?

Since most physical means of euthanasia involve trauma, there is inherent risk for animals and humans. Extreme care and caution must be practiced. Skill and experience of personnel are essential. If the method is not correctly performed, animals and personnel may be injured.

28. Describe euthanasia induced by a blow to the head.

Euthanasia by a blow to the head must be evaluated in terms of anatomic features of the species on which it is to be performed. A blow to the head can be a humane method of euthanasia for neonatal animals with a thin cranium. The blow to the head of all animals must be delivered with sufficient force to the central skull bones to produce immediate depression of the central nervous system and destruction of brain tissue.

29. Is a physical blow to the head an acceptable means to euthanatize neonatal calves?

No, the anatomical features of neonatal calves make this method of euthanasia unacceptable.

30. Describe some of the concerns in using a gunshot to euthanatize an animal (Appendix 1.24.1).

A properly placed gunshot can cause immediate insensibility and humane death. In some cases, gunshot may be the only practical method of euthanasia. Shooting should be performed only by highly skilled personnel trained using appropriate caliber firearms. Personnel, public, and nearby animal safety should be of paramount importance. The procedure should only be performed outdoors and away from public access.

31. Approximately how long does brain activity persist following cervical dislocation or decapitation?

Electrical activity persists for 13 to 14 seconds following cervical dislocation or decapitation.

32. Describe electrocution as a means of euthanasia in animals.

Electrocution, using alternating current, induces death by ventricular fibrillation, which causes cerebral hypoxia. However, animals do not lose consciousness for 10 to 30 seconds after the onset of ventricular fibrillation. It is imperative that animals be unconscious before being electrocuted.

33. When choosing thoracic (cardiopulmonary, cardiac) compression as a means of euthanasia, which animals is this most commonly used upon?

Thoracic compression is used to euthanatize small to medium-sized free-ranging birds when alternate techniques are not immediately available.

34. Describe some of the special concerns when euthanatizing amphibians, fish, and reptiles.

Euthanasia of ectothermic animals must take into account differences in their metabolism, respiration, and tolerance to cerebral hypoxia. In addition, it is more difficult to ascertain when an animal is dead. Many reptiles and amphibians are capable of holding their breath and converting to anaerobic metabolism. Thus, they can survive long periods of hypoxia (up to 27 hours in some species!).

35. Describe mass euthanasia techniques used in disease eradication and natural disasters.

Undoubtedly, euthanasia options are limited in these circumstances. The most appropriate technique minimizes human and animal health concerns. These options include, but are not limited to, CO_2 and physical methods such as gunshot, penetrating captive bolt, and cervical dislocation.

36. List the agents and methods of euthanasia by species (Table 1.24.1). (Refer to Question No. 39 for unacceptable agents and methods.)

Table 1.24.1 Agents and Methods of Euthanasia by Species

Species	Acceptable* (refer to Table 1.24.2 for details)	Conditionally Acceptable† (refer to Question 38 for details)
Amphibians	Barbiturates, inhalant anesthetics (in appropriate species), CO_2, CO, tricaine methane sulfonate (TMS, MS 222), benzocaine hydrochloride, double pithing	Penetrating captive bolt, gunshot, stunning and decapitation, decapitation and pithing
Birds	Barbiturates, inhalant anesthetics, CO_2, CO, gunshot (free-ranging only)	N_2, Ar, cervical dislocation, decapitation, thoracic compression (small, free-ranging only), maceration (chicks, poults, and pipped eggs only)
Cats	Barbiturates, inhalant anesthetics, CO_2, CO, potassium chloride in conjunction with general anesthesia	N_2, Ar
Dogs	Barbiturates, inhalant anesthetics, CO_2, CO, potassium chloride in conjunction with general anesthesia	N_2, Ar, penetrating captive bolt, electrocution
Fish	Barbiturates, inhalant anesthetics, CO_2, tricaine methane sulfonate (TMS, MS 222), benzocaine hydrochloride, 2-phenoxyethanol	Decapitation and pithing, stunning and decapitation/pithing
Horses	Barbiturates, potassium chloride in conjunction with general anesthesia, penetrating captive bolt	Chloral hydrate (IV, after sedation), gunshot, electrocution
Marine mammals	Barbiturates, etorphine hydrochloride	Gunshot (cetaceans <4 m long)
Mink, fox, and other mammals produced for fur	Barbiturates, inhalant anesthetics, CO_2 (mink require high concentrations for euthanasia without supplemental agents), CO, potassium chloride in conjunction with general anesthesia	$N_2$2, Ar, electrocution followed by cervical dislocation
Nonhuman primates	Barbiturates	Inhalant anesthetics, CO_2, CO, N_2, Ar
Rabbits	Barbiturates, inhalant anesthetics, CO_2, CO, potassium chloride in conjunction with general anesthesia	N_2, Ar, cervical dislocation (<1 kg), decapitation, penetrating captive bolt
Reptiles	Barbiturates, inhalant anesthetics (in appropriate species), CO_2 (in appropriate species)	Penetrating captive bolt, gunshot, decapitation and pithing, stunning and decapitation

*Acceptable methods are those that consistently produce a humane death when used as the sole means of euthanasia.
†Conditionally acceptable methods are those that by the nature of the technique or because of greater potential for operator error or safety hazards might not consistently produce humane death or are methods not well documented in the scientific literature.
[a]http://www.avma.org/issues/animal_welfare/euthanasia.pdf (2007).

37. Describe the acceptable agents and methods of euthanasia.

Refer to Table 1.24.2 for acceptable agents and methods of euthanasia.

38. Describe the conditionally acceptable agents and methods of euthanasia.

Refer to Table 1.24.3 for conditionally acceptable agents and methods of euthanasia.

Table 1.24.2 Acceptable Agents and Methods of Euthanasia

Agent	Classification	Mode of Action	Rapidity	Ease of Performance	Safety for Personnel	Species Suitability	Efficacy and Comments
Barbiturates	Hypoxia attributable to depression of vital centers	Direct depression of cerebral cortex, subcortical structures, and vital centers; direct depression of heart muscle	Rapid onset of anesthesia	Animal must be restrained; personnel must be skilled to perform IV injection	Safe except human abuse potential; DEA-controlled substance	Most species	Highly effective when appropriately administered; acceptable IP in small animals and IV
Benzocaine hydrochloride	Hypoxia attributable to depression of vital centers	Depression of CNS	Very rapid, depending on dose	Easily used	Safe	Fish, amphibians	Effective but expensive
Carbon dioxide (bottled gas only)	Hypoxia attributable to depression of vital centers	Direct depression of cerebral cortex, subcortical structures, and vital centers; direct depression of heart muscle	Moderately rapid	Used in closed container	Minimal hazard	Small laboratory animals, birds, cats, small dogs, rabbits, mink (high concentrations required), zoo animals, amphibians, fish, some reptiles, swine	Effective, but time required may be prolonged in immature and neonatal animals
Carbon monoxide (bottled gas only)	Hypoxia	Combines with hemoglobin, preventing its combination with oxygen	Moderate onset time, but insidious so animal is unaware of onset	Requires appropriately maintained equipment	Extremely hazardous, toxic, and difficult to detect	Most small species including dogs, cats, rodents, mink, chinchillas, birds, reptiles, amphibians, zoo animals, rabbits	Effective; acceptable only when equipment is properly designed and operated
Inhalant anesthetics	Hypoxia attributable to depression of vital centers	Direct depression of cerebral cortex, subcortical structures, and vital centers	Moderately rapid onset of anesthesia, excitation may develop during induction	Easily performed with closed container; can be administered to large animals by means of a mask	Must be properly scavenged or vented to minimize exposure to personnel	Some amphibians, birds, cats, dogs, furbearing animals, rabbits, some reptiles, rodents and other small mammals, zoo animals, fish, free-ranging wildlife	Highly effective provided that subject is sufficiently exposed; either is conditionally acceptable

374

Table 1.24.2 (Continued)

Agent	Classification	Mode of Action	Rapidity	Ease of Performance	Safety for Personnel	Species Suitability	Efficacy and Comments
Microwave irradiation	Brain enzyme inactivation	Direct inactivation of brain enzymes by rapid heating of brain	Very rapid	Requires training and highly specialized equipment	Safe	Mice, rats	Highly effective for special needs
Penetrating captive bolt	Physical damage to brain	Direct concussion of brain tissue	Rapid	Requires skill, adequate restraint, and proper placement of captive bolt	Safe	Horses, ruminants, swine	Instant loss of consciousness, but motor activity may continue
2-Phenoxyethanol	Hypoxia attributable to depression of vital centers	Depression of CNS	Very rapid, depending on dose	Easily used	Safe	Fish	Effective but expensive
Potassium chloride (intracardially or intravenously in conjunction with general anesthesia only)	Hypoxia	Direct depression of cerebral cortex, subcortical structures, and vital centers secondary to cardiac arrest.	Rapid	Requires training and specialized equipment for remote injection anesthesia, and ability to give IV injection of potassium chloride	Anesthetics may be hazardous with accidental human exposure	Most species	Highly effective, some clonic muscle spasms may be observed
Tricaine methane sulfonate (TMS, MS 222)	Hypoxia attributable to depression of vital centers	Depression of CNS	Very rapid, depending on dose	Easily used	Safe	Fish, amphibians	Effective but expensive

http://www.avma.org/issues/animal_welfare/euthanasia.pdf (2007).

Table 1.24.3 Conditionally Acceptable Agents and Methods of Euthanasia

Agent	Classification	Mode of Action	Rapidity	Ease of Performance	Safety for Personnel	Species Suitability	Efficacy and Comments
Blow to the head	Physical damage to brain	Direct concussion of brain tissue	Rapid	Requires skill, adequate restraint, and appropriate force	Safe	Young pigs <3 weeks old	Must be properly applied to be humane and effective
Carbon dioxide (bottled gas only)	Hypoxia due to depression of vital centers	Direct depression of cerebral cortex, subcortical structures and vital centers; direct depression of heart muscle	Moderately rapid	Used in closed container	Minimal hazard	Nonhuman primates, free-ranging wildlife	Effective, but time required may be prolonged in immature and neonatal animals
Carbon monoxide (bottled gas only)	Hypoxia	Combines with hemoglobin, preventing its combination with oxygen	Moderate onset time, but insidious so animal is unaware of onset	Requires appropriately maintained equipment	Extremely hazardous, toxic, and difficult to detect	Nonhuman primates, free-ranging wildlife	Effective; acceptable only when equipment is properly designed and operated
Cervical dislocation	Hypoxia due to disruption of vital centers	Direct depression of brain	Moderately rapid	Requires training and skill	Safe	Poultry, birds, laboratory mice, rats (<200 g), rabbits (<1 kg)	Irreversible; violent muscle contractions can occur after cervical dislocation
Chloral hydrate	Hypoxia from depression of respiratory center	Direct depression of brain	Rapid	Personnel must be skilled to perform IV injection	Safe	Horses, ruminants, swine	Animals should be sedated prior to administration
Agent	Classification	Mode of action	Rapidity	Ease of performance	Safety for personnel	Species suitability	Efficacy and comments
Decapitation	Hypoxia due to disruption of vital centers	Direct depression of brain	Rapid	Requires training and skill	Guillotine poses potential employee injury hazard	Laboratory rodents; small rabbits; birds; some fish, amphibians, and reptiles (latter 3 with pithing)	Irreversible; violent muscle contraction can occur after decapitation
Electrocution	Hypoxia	Direct depression of brain and cardiac fibrillation	Can be rapid	Not easily performed in all instances	Hazardous to personnel	Used primarily in sheep, swine, foxes, mink (with cervical dislocation), ruminants, animals >5 kg	Violent muscle contractions occur at same time as loss of consciousness
Gunshot	Hypoxia due to disruption of vital centers	Direct concussion of brain tissue	Rapid	Requires skill and appropriate firearm	May be dangerous	Large domestic and zoo animals, reptiles, amphibians, wildlife, cetaceans (<4 meters long)	Instant loss of consciousness, but motor activity may continue

Table 1.24.3 (Continued)

Agent	Classification	Mode of Action	Rapidity	Ease of Performance	Safety for Personnel	Species Suitability	Efficacy and Comments
Inhalant anesthetics	Hypoxia due to disruption of vital centers	Direct depression of cerebral cortex, subcortical structures, and vital centers	Moderately rapid onset of anesthesia; excitation may develop during induction	Easily performed with closed container; can be administered to large animals by means of a mask	Must be properly scavenged or vented to minimize exposure to personnel; ether has explosive potential and exposure to ether may be stressful	Nonhuman primates, swine; ether is conditionally acceptable for rodents and small mammals; methoxyflurane is conditionally acceptable for rodents and small mammals	Highly effective provided that subject is sufficiently exposed
Agent	Classification	Mode of action	Rapidity	Ease of performance	Safety for personnel	Species suitability	Efficacy and comments
Nitrogen, argon	Hypoxia	Reduces partial pressure of oxygen available to blood	Rapid	Used in closed chamber with rapid filling	Safe if used with ventilation	Cats, small dogs, birds, rodents, rabbits, other small species, mink, zoo animals, nonhuman primates, free-ranging wildlife	Effective except in young and neonates; an effective agent, but other methods are preferable
Penetrating captive bolt	Physical damage to brain	Direct concussion of brain tissue	Rapid	Requires skill, adequate restraint and proper placement of captive bolt	Safe	Dogs, rabbits, zoo animals, reptiles, amphibians, free-ranging wildlife	Instant loss of consciousness but motor activity may continue
Pithing	Hypoxia due to disruption of vital centers, physical damage to brain	Trauma of brain and spinal cord tissue	Rapid	Easily performed but requires skill	Safe	Some ectotherms	Effective, but death not immediate unless brain and spinal cord are pithed
Thoracic compression	Hypoxia and cardiac arrest	Physical interference with cardiac and respiratory function	Moderately rapid	Requires training	Safe	Small-to medium-sized free-ranging birds	Apparently effective
Maceration	Physical damage to brain	Direct concussion of brain tissue	Rapid	Easily performed with properly designed, commercially available equipment	Safe	Newly hatched chicks and poults, and pipped eggs only	Effective when equipment is properly designed and operated

http://www.avma.org/issues/animal_welfare/euthanasia.pdf (2007).

39. List some unacceptable agents and methods of euthanasia (Table 1.24.4).

Table 1.24.4 Unacceptable agents and methods of euthanasia

Agent or method	Comments
Air embolism	Air embolism may be accompanied by convulsions, opisthotonos, and vocalization. If used, it should be done only in anesthetized animals.
Blow to the head	Unacceptable for most species.
Burning	Chemical or thermal burning of an animal is not an acceptable method of euthanasia.
Chloral hydrate	Unacceptable in dogs, cats, and small mammals.
Chloroform	Chloroform is a known hepatotoxin and suspected carcinogen and, therefore, is extremely hazardous to personnel.
Cyanide	Cyanide poses an extreme danger to personnel and the manner of death is aesthetically objectionable.
Decompression	Decompression is unacceptable for euthanasia because of numerous disadvantages. (1) Many chambers are designed to produce decompression at a rate 15 to 60 times faster than that recommended as optimum for animals, resulting in pain and distress attributable to expanding gases trapped in body cavities. (2) Immature animals are tolerant of hypoxia, and longer periods of decompression are required before respiration ceases. (3) Accidental recompression, with recovery of injured animals, can occur. (4) Bleeding, vomiting, convulsions, urination, and defecation, which are aesthetically unpleasant, may develop in unconscious animals.
Drowning	Drowning is not a means of euthanasia and is inhumane.
Exsanguination	Because of the anxiety associated with extreme hypovolemia, exsanguination should be done only in sedated, stunned, or anesthetized animals.
Formalin	Direct immersion of an animal into formalin, as a means of euthanasia, is inhumane.
Household products and solvents	Acetone, quaternary compounds (including CCl_4), laxatives, clove oil, dimethylketone, quaternary ammonium products*, antacids, and other commercial and household products or solvents are not acceptable agents for euthanasia.
Hypothermia	Hypothermia is not an appropriate method of euthanasia.
Neuromuscular blocking agents (nicotine, magnesium sulfate, potassium chloride, all curariform agents)	When used alone, these drugs all cause respiratory arrest before loss of consciousness, so the animal may perceive pain and distress after it is immobilized.
Rapid freezing	Rapid freezing as a sole means of euthanasia is not considered to be humane. If used, animals should be anesthetized prior to freezing.
Smothering	Smothering of chicks or poults in bags or containers is not acceptable.
Strychnine	Strychnine causes violent convulsions and painful muscle contractions.
Stunning	Stunning may render an animal unconscious, but it is not a method of euthanasia (except for neonatal animals with thin craniums). If used, it must be immediately followed by a method that ensures death.
Tricaine methane sulfonate (TMS, MS 222)	Should not be used for euthanasia of animals intended as food.

*Roccal D Plus, Pharmacia & Upjohn, Kalamazoo, Michigan.
http://www.avma.org/issues/animal_welfare/euthanasia.pdf (2007).

Suggested Reading

Animal Welfare Committee of the American Association of Bovine Practitioners. Practical euthanasia of cattle. Available at http://www.aabp.org/euth.pdf.

AVMA panel on euthanasia. 2007. Available at http://www.avma.org/issues/animal_welfare/euthanasia.pdf.

Blackmore DK. Energy requirements for the penetration of heads of domestic stock and the development of a multiple projectile. *Vet Rec* 1985;116:36–40.

Blackmore DK, Bowling MC, Madie, P, et al. The use of a shotgun for emergency slaughter or euthanasia of large mature pigs. *N Z Vet J* 1995;43:134–137.

Daly CC, Whittington PE. Investigation into the principal determinants of effective captive bolt stunning of sheep. *Res Vet Sci* 1989;46:406–408.

Denicola AJ. Non-traditional techniques for management of overabundant deer populations. *Wildl Soc Bull* 1997;25:496–499.

Dennis MB, Dong WK, Weisbrod KA, et al. Use of captive bolt as a method of euthanasia in larger laboratory animal species. *Lab Anim Sci* 1988;38:459–462.

Fowler ME, Miller RE, eds. *Zoo and Wild Animal Medicine: Current Therapy*, 4th ed. Philadelphia, WB Saunders, 1999, pp. 1–747.

Hughes HC. Euthanasia of laboratory animals. In Melby EC, Altman NH, eds. *Handbook of Laboratory Animal Science*. Vol 3. Cleveland, CRC Press, 1976, pp. 553–559.

Longair JA, Finley GG, Laniel M-A, et al. Guidelines for euthanasia of domestic animals by firearms. *Can Vet J* 1991;32:724–726.

Not between the eyes! Humane euthanasia procedures for sick, injured, and/or debilitated livestock. University of Florida College of Veterinary Medicine and University of Florida Institute of Food and Agricultural Sciences. Available at http://www.vetmed.ufl.edu/lacs/HumaneEuthanasia/acrobat/wallchart.pdf.

On-Farm Euthanasia of Swine: Options for the Producer. Perry, IA, American Association of Swine Practitioners/Des Moines, IA, National Pork Producers, 1997.

Operational Guidelines. Euthanasia. National Animal Health Emergency Management, Systems Guidelines, USDA, January 2004.

Practical Euthanasia of Cattle: Considerations for the Producer, Livestock Market Operator, Livestock Transporter, and Veterinarian. Rome, GA, American Association of Bovine Practitioners, 1999.

Rietveld G. On-farm euthanasia of cattle and calves. October 2003. Available at http://www.gov.on.ca/OMAFRA/english/livestock/animalcare/facts/info_euthanasia_cc.html.

Shearer JK, Nicoletti P. Procedures for humane euthanasia for sick, injured or debilitated livestock. University of Florida College of Veterinary Medicine. Available at http://www.vetmed.ufl.edu/lacs/HumaneEuthanasia/acrobat/brochureEng.pdf.

The Center for Animal Welfare. College of Agriculture and Environmental Sciences. Euthanasia of poultry. University of California, Davis. Available at http://animalwelfare.ucdavis.edu/publication/poultryeuth.html.

The Emergency Euthanasia of Horses. Sacramento, California Department of Food and Agriculture/Davis, CA, University of California's Veterinary Medical Extension, 1999.

The Emergency Euthanasia of Sheep and Goats. Sacramento, California Department of Food and Agriculture/Davis, CA, University of California's Veterinary Medical Extension, 1999.

The use of cervical dislocation as a method of euthanasia of poultry. office of research protections. Pennsylvania State University, IACUC Guideline. Available at http://www.research.psu.edu/orp/ANI/GUIDE/XV.pdf.

APPENDIX 1.24.1
EUTHANASIA IN A VARIETY OF VETERINARY SPECIES

1. Euthanasia using either a captive bolt or gunshot[a,b]

1.1. Aesthetic concerns

1.1.1. Both gunshot and penetrating captive bolt are aesthetically displeasing procedures. Euthanasia by either technique results in involuntary movements, and occasionally vocalization, that may be inaccurately interpreted as painful to an inexperienced person. Therefore, when and where possible, it is recommended that such procedures be performed in areas out of the public view.

1.2. Anatomical landmarks

1.2.1. Cattle

I. **Proper positioning** of the firearm or penetrating captive bolt is necessary to achieve the desired results. When euthanasia is performed by gunshot, the firearm should be held within a few inches of the intended target. Ricochet may be prevented if the barrel of the firearm is positioned perpendicular to the skull as shown in the diagram. In cattle, the point of entry of the projectile should be at the intersection of two imaginary lines, each drawn from the inside corner of the eye to the base of the opposite horn (or to a point slightly above the opposite ear in a cow without horns). As seen in Figures 1.24.1 and 1.24.2, this places the recommended point of entry in the center of the forehead somewhat above a line drawn between the eyes.

II. **Special considerations for euthanasia of bulls**

A. Bulls present particular challenges because of the size, attitude, and physical thickness of their skulls. Specialized heavy-duty penetrating captive bolt guns or higher-caliber firearms (9 mm or .357) are required for euthanasia of bulls. As described previously, safety is of paramount importance. Since ideal positioning of either device requires close contact with the animal, restraint is usually necessary. Operators should recognize that restraint alone causes significant distress. By preparing the euthanasia device for use prior to restraining the animal, one can limit the restraint-related stress period.

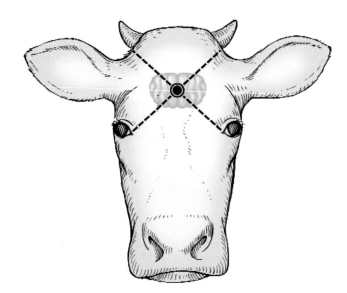

Figure 1.24.1. When using either a captive bolt or gunshot for euthanasia in cows, **do NOT aim between the eyes**, but rather above eyes, as illustrated.

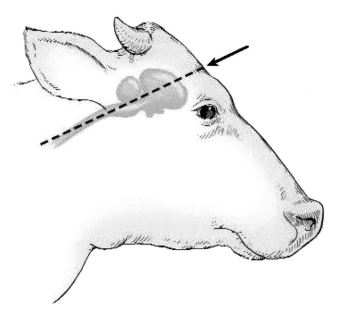

Figure 1.24.2. Direct the captive bolt/gunshot down in the direction of the vertebral column in cattle.

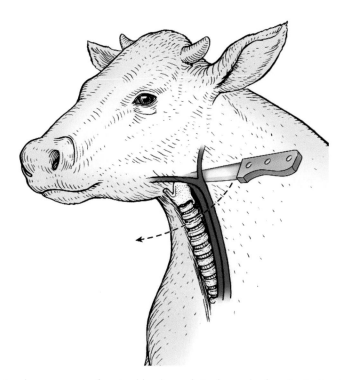

Figure 1.24.3. Exsanguination by severance of major blood vessels in the neck of cattle. 1, Jugular vein (blue); 2, carotid artery (red); 3, trachea or windpipe (white).

III. Penetrating captive bolt or gunshot followed by immediate **exsanguination** is preferred in cattle.

A. Once the animal has been rendered unconscious, exsanguination procedures should be initiated to ensure death using a pointed, very sharp knife with a rigid blade at least 6 inches in length. As indicated previously, exsanguination procedures are required with the use of penetrating captive bolt. The knife should be fully inserted through the skin just behind the point of the jaw and below the neck bones (Fig. 1.24.3). From this position, the knife is drawn forward, severing the jugular vein, carotid artery, and windpipe. When the procedure is properly performed, blood should flow freely with death occurring within a few minutes.

1.2.2. Sheep, Goats, and Llamas

I. Penetrating captive bolt or gunshot followed by immediate exsanguination is the preferred method of euthanasia in sheep.

A. For hornless sheep, goats, and rams, the recommended sites for placement of the gun or penetrating captive bolt include the top of the head or slightly behind the poll.

1. In horned sheep and rams, the top of the head is not a recommended site because of the thickness of the skull in this region. Instead, the preferred position and orientation of penetrating captive bolt or gunshot are on a line starting from behind the poll and aimed in the direction of the animal's muzzle as shown in the figure. An alternative position for placement of the stunning device is the front of the skull as shown in Figures 1.24.4 through 1.24.6. One must be careful to avoid ricochet by placing the firearm within inches of the intended target.

II. Site in **llamas** is on theforehead as shown in Figure 1.24.7.

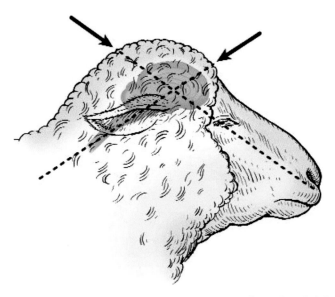

Figure 1.24.4. In nonhorned sheep, again, **do not aim between the eyes**, but rather slightly behind the poll or on the top of the head.

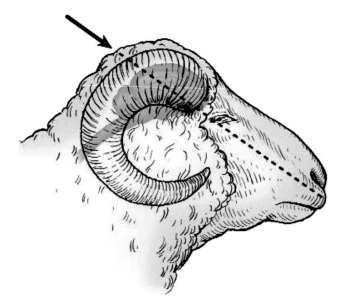

Figure 1.24.5. Proper site for gunshot or captive bolt in horned sheep is behind the poll as shown.

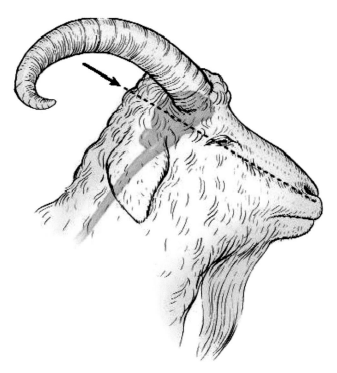

Figure 1.24.6.   In goats, direct the captive bolt or gunshot from the animal's poll toward the midline of the face.

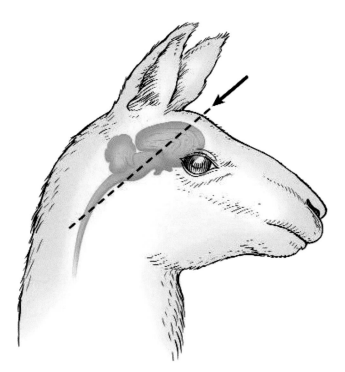

Figure 1.24.7.   Site in llamas is on the forehead as shown.

III. Sheep should be exsanguinated within 10 seconds after stunning by penetrating captive bolt or they may regain consciousness. Exsanguination of sheep should be performed as shown in Figures 1.24.8 and 1.24.9.
A. One may sever the brachial vasculature by lifting a front leg and inserting the knife deeply into the axillary area at the point of the elbow and cutting the skin, blood vessels, and surrounding tissue until the limb can be

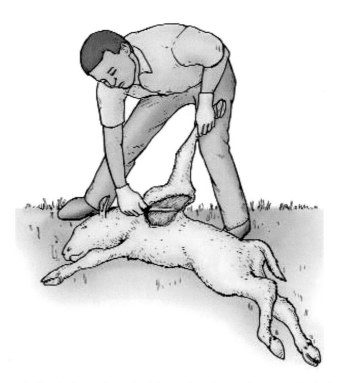

Figure 1.24.8. One may sever the brachial vasculature by lifting a front leg and inserting the knife deeply into the axillary area at the point of the elbow and cutting the skin, blood vessels, and surrounding tissue until the limb can be laid back away from the thorax of the stunned or gunshot animal.

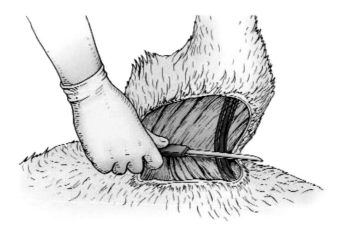

Figure 1.24.9. Sever the brachial vasculature by lifting a front leg and inserting the knife deeply into the axillary area in the stunned or gunshot animal.

laid back away from the thorax of the animal (Fig. 1.24.9). Regardless of the method used, great care should be exercised in performing exsanguination procedures. Although unconscious, animals in this state are capable of violent involuntary movement that may cause personal injury.

1.2.3. Swine

I. There are two options for captive bolt or gunshot:

A. A frontal site (Fig. 1.24.10).

B. A temporal site (Fig. 1.24.11).

II. Recommended placement of the penetrating captive bolt or gunshot for use of the frontal site is in the center of the forehead slightly above a line drawn between the eyes (Fig. 1.24.10).

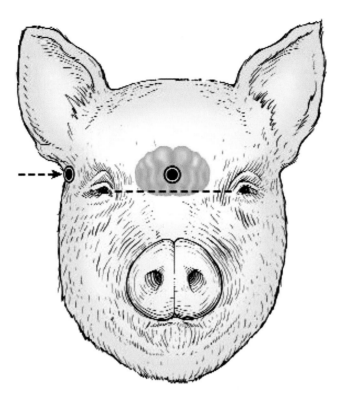

Figure 1.24.10. Recommended placement of the penetrating captive bolt or gunshot for use of the frontal site in swine is in the center of the forehead slightly above a line drawn between the eyes. The temporal site (for gunshot only!) is located on the left side of the figure (*arrow*).

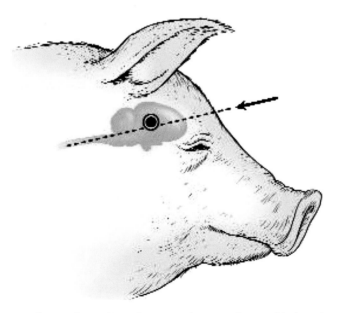

Figure 1.24.11. An alternative site for gunshot (only) is the temporal region of swine (black circle just in front of the ear).

A. Proper placement or aim of the euthanasia device is particularly important since the brain is relatively small and well protected by sinuses.

B. An alternative site for gunshot (only) is the temporal region (Fig. 1.24.11).

1.2.4. Horses may be euthanized by gunshot or penetrating captive bolt.

I. As described previously, use of the captive bolt requires good restraint so that the device may be held in close contact with the skull when fired.

II. The site for entry of the projectile is described as a point slightly above the intersection of two diagonal lines each running from the inside corner of the eye to the base of the opposite ear (Figs. 1.24.12 and 1.24.13). Note that *contrary to that described for cattle,* the optimum site in the horse is slightly above the intersection of these two lines.

1.2.5. Deer

I. The methods described for emergency euthanasia of deer are similar to those described previously for cattle and small ruminants. Recommended positions and direction for firing of a penetrating captive bolt or gunshot in deer are as shown in Figures 1.24.14 and 1.24.15.

II. Since deer requiring euthanasia may be encountered on farm or roadside, it is important to consider the natural instincts of fear and anxiety of farm-raised versus a wild animal.

III. Approaching an injured wild deer will likely increase its distress, causing it to attempt to flee, which may only compound its misery.

IV. In general, whenever wildlife is involved in highway accidents, the best advice is to contact the appropriate state authorities (e.g., Fish and Wildlife Conservation Officers). Their personnel are properly trained to handle these emergencies.

1.3. Confirmation of Death.

1.3.1. Regardless of the method of euthanasia used, death must be confirmed before disposal of the animal. The following should be used to evaluate consciousness or confirm death:

I. **Absence of a heartbeat**

A. The presence of a heartbeat can best be determined with a stethoscope placed under the left elbow. Please note that a pulse is usually not palpable under such circumstances and palpation should not be used to confirm death.

II. **Absence of respiration**

A. Movement of the chest indicates respiration; however, respiration rates may be very erratic and slow in unconscious animals. Therefore, one must be cautious in the interpretation of respiration for confirmation of death.

III. **Absence of a corneal reflex**

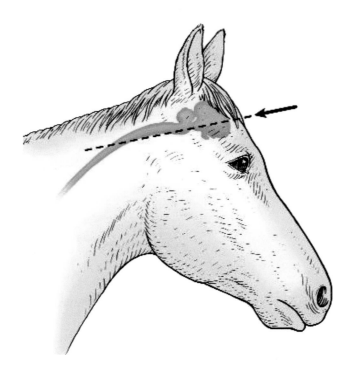

Figure 1.24.12. The site for entry of the projectile is described as a point slightly above the intersection of two diagonal lines each running from the inside corner of the eye to the base of the opposite ear. Note that *contrary to that described for cattle,* the optimum site in the horse is slightly above the intersection of these two lines.

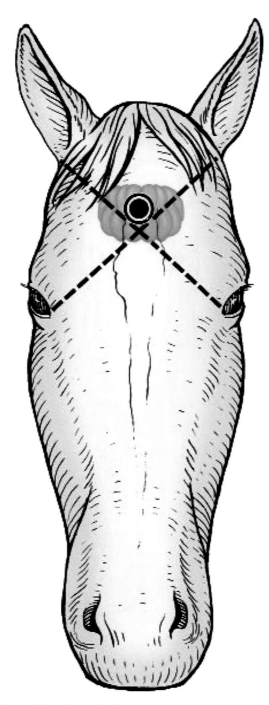

Figure 1.24.13. Direct the projectile parallel to the neck of a horse during euthanasia.

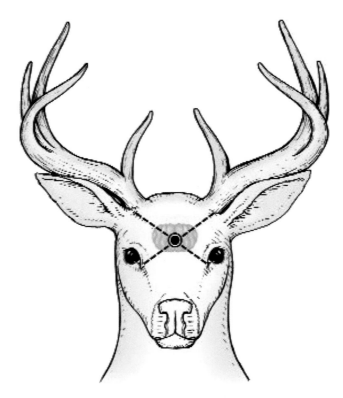

Figure 1.24.14. Proper site for euthanasia in deer is similar to that in cattle.

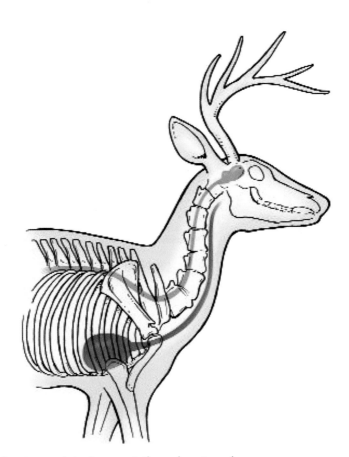

Figure 1.24.15. Brain and major vessels in deer are similar to those in cattle.

A. One may test for evidence of a corneal reflex by touching the surface of the eyeball. Normal or conscious animals will blink when the eyeball is touched. Absence of a corneal reflex, failure to detect respiration, and absence of a heartbeat for a period of more than 5 minutes should be used to confirm death.

1.3.2. An alternative is to observe the animal over a period of several hours. Lack of movement and absence of a heartbeat, respiration, or corneal reflex over an extended period of time provides further confirmation of death.

[a]This document is modified from VM152, one of a series from the Veterinary Medicine-Large Animal Clinical Sciences Department, Florida Cooperative Extension Service, Institute of Food and Agricultural Sciences, University of Florida. Original publication date April 2007. Visit the EDIS Website at http://edis.ifas.ufl.edu.

[b]Jan K. Shearer, DVM, Professor, and Paul Nicoletti, DVM, Professor, College of Veterinary Medicine–Large Animal Clinical Sciences, Cooperative Extension Service, University of Florida, Gainesville, FL 32611.

CHAPTER 1.25
CARCASS DISPOSAL FOLLOWING
A VETERINARY DISASTER

Ryan Gordon Leon Murphy, MS, and Anthony P. Knight, BVSc, MS

DISCUSSION OF ANIMAL CARCASS DISPOSAL

1. What sort of hazards do improperly disposed animal carcasses pose to people, animals, and the environment?

Decomposing carcasses can maintain and transfer diseases to humans, livestock, wildlife, and pets. Furthermore, these hazards are not limited to the diseases or ailments that may have led to the animals' deaths but also can include organisms naturally present in the animal that could contaminate surface and ground water systems.

2. Name a few organisms that occur naturally in animals and can pose a hazard to people handling animal carcasses.

- *Clostridia* spp.
- *Cryptosporidium* spp.
- *Escherichia coli* O157:H7
- *Giardia* spp.
- *Listeria* spp.
- *Salmonella* spp.

3. What is a "zoonotic" disease?

Zoonotic diseases are diseases caused by infectious agents that can be transmitted (or shared) between animals and humans.

4. Approximately how many diseases of humans with known etiologies are zoonotic diseases?

Woolhouse and Gowtage-Sequeria (2005) reported that of the 1407 human diseases of known etiology, 816 (58%) are zoonotic.

5. List some examples of important zoonotic disease agents.

- Anthrax
- Avian influenza
- Brucellosis

- Hantavirus
- Plague
- Rabies
- Tuberculosis
- Tularemia
- West Nile virus

6. Are there laws that govern disposal of animal carcasses?

Many states require that dead animals be disposed of within 48 to 72 hours of death; however, acceptable disposal methods are not always clearly identified. Contact the local and/or state government to determine which disposal methods are acceptable and which methods are strongly discouraged or prohibited. Ideally, this should be done in advance of any disaster and is part of the planning process that should take place on all livestock premises.

7. What are the most common methods of animal carcass disposal?

- Burial
- Incineration
- Composting
- Rendering
- Alkaline hydrolysis

METHODS OF ANIMAL CARCASS DISPOSAL

BURIAL

8. What kind of burial methods are most commonly used for carcass disposal?

- Landfill disposal
- Mass burial

9. Can I take animal carcasses to the landfill for disposal?

Many landfills are operated by private companies and are free to decide which materials they will or will not accept. It is necessary to check ahead of time with regard to the acceptability of animal carcasses.

10. What are some of the issues related to landfill disposal that need to be addressed before an animal emergency?

- Number of carcasses allowed at one time or in total
- Under what conditions will restrictions on animal carcasses be waived (i.e., natural disaster, disease outbreak, etc.)?

- Will cause of death (i.e., transmissible or zoonotic disease agents) affect acceptance of carcasses?
- Carcass disposal fees (i.e., flat fee per head or based on weight)

11. What is mass burial?

Carcasses are buried in large earthen pits that are specially designed to control the byproducts of decomposition. Complete decomposition of a carcass may take 5 to 10 years after burial, but leachate may be released for 20 years or longer. Leachate collection systems are used to direct the leachate to collection sumps so that it can be removed from the burial pit for proper treatment and disposal.

12. Are there serious risks from leachate that is produced as a byproduct of mass burial?

Buried animal carcasses produce tremendous amounts of leachate. The United Kingdom Environment Agency (2001) estimated that in the first 2 months of burial, an adult sheep would produce 16 L (4 gal) of leachate and an adult cow would produce 170 L (45 gal) of leachate. For example, the Throckmorton disposal site in the United Kingdom buried over 133,000 carcasses during the 2001 foot and mouth disease outbreak. Within the first few months of burial, 74 million L (19.5 million gal) of leachate was produced. The leachate was collected daily and transported off-site for treatment at a waste treatment facility before release into the sanitary sewer system. As a consequence of the tremendous volume of leachate produced at these burial sites, the British government developed a 20-year monitoring program to test for ground water contamination (United Kingdom Environment Agency, 2001).

13. How deep do I have to bury animal carcasses?

The depth to which animal carcasses must be buried varies widely among states but generally ranges from 0.6 to 1.8 m (2 to 6 ft). For example, according to the National Biosecurity and Resource Center (undated), the Minnesota Board of Animal Health requires that animal carcasses be buried 1.5 m (5 ft) above the high water level and covered with 0.9 m (3 ft) of soil. However, it is imperative to check the acceptability of burial with local governments before pursuing as a potential disposal method. Where dogs or wildlife may expose carcasses, the carcasses should be buried at least 1.8 m (6 ft).

14. What factors must be considered when considering burial as a means of disposal?

- Topography
- Soil type
- Slope
- Hundred-year flood plains
- Disease agent (infectivity, as well as persistence in environment)
- Number of carcasses
- Depth to water table
- Proximity to bodies of water (e.g., lakes, rivers, and streams)
- Proximity to drinking wells
- Property lines and residences

15. Is it legal to bury animal carcasses within city limits?

Burial is not a legal method of disposal within city limits. Regulations may vary by city, but within the limits of many cities, it is illegal to bury animal carcasses, including family pets, on one's property.

INCINERATION

16. What methods of incineration are available?

- Open-air burning
- Air-curtain incineration
- Fixed-facility incineration (crematorium)

17. What is open-air burning?

- A state permit is required for open-air burning; however, not all states allow open-air burning.
- It was used extensively in the United Kingdom during the 2001 foot and mouth disease outbreak and in North America for small-scale outbreaks of anthrax.
- A shallow pit should be dug to ensure a steady supply of fresh air, which will promote hotter and cleaner combustion.
- It requires large volumes of combustible materials (e.g., straw, hay, untreated timber or lumber, kindling wood, diesel fuel, etc.).
- It poses a significant fire hazard under dry and/or windy conditions.

18. How does air-curtain incineration compare to open-air burning (Fig. 1.25.1)?

- Curtain of high-velocity air traps unburned particles and overoxygenates the air to increase combustion.
- Temperatures can reach 600° to 700° C, even as high as 1000° C, compared with open-air burning, which produces lower peak temperatures with greater variability.
- Burns it up to 6 times faster than for open-air burning and ensures more complete combustion.
- *Rule of thumb:* Require 0.45 kg (1 lb) of fuel per 0.45 kg (1 lb) of carcass.
- It is used successfully in Colorado and Montana for disposal of depopulated chronic wasting disease–positive herds.

19. What are the principles of air-curtain incineration (Fig. 1.25.2)?

- Manifold directs high-velocity airflow into fire box or trench.
- Refractory lined wall or earthen wall
- Material to be burned
- Initial airflow forms high-velocity "curtain" over fire.
- Continued airflow overoxygenates fire, keeping temperatures high.

20. How much fuel (i.e., combustible materials) is needed to incinerate a carcass?

The amount of fuel required is highly dependent on the materials being incinerated, as well as the incineration method being used (Table 1.25.1). For example, air-curtain incinerators require wood for combustion at a 1:1

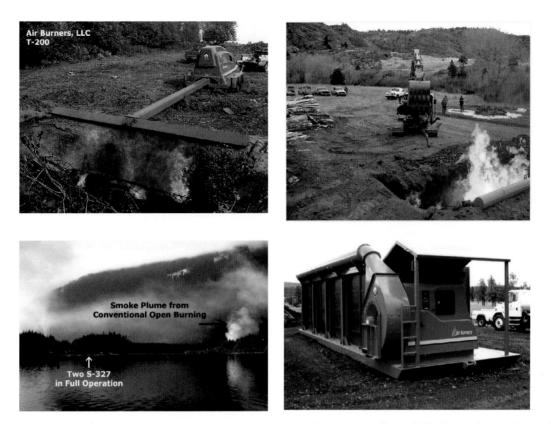

Figure 1.25.1 Pictures of air-curtain incinerators in operation. *Bottom right,* commercially available firebox that can be used in place of an earthen trench. (Used with permission © 1996–2007, Air Burners, LLC.)

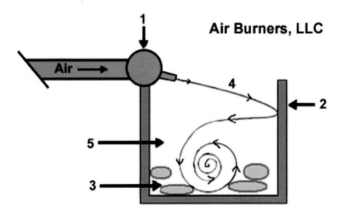

Figure 1.25.2 The wood waste is the fuel. (Used with permission © 1996–2007, Air Burners, LLC.)

Table 1.25.1 Comparison of Different Incineration Methods

	Advantages	**Disadvantages**
Open-air	• Inexpensive	• Not suitable for TSE prions • Poor public perception • Dependent on weather and availability of materials
Air-curtain	• Mobile • Environmentally sound • Suitable for TSEs	• Fuel intensive • Logistically challenging • Dependent on weather and availability of materials
Fixed-facility	• Suitable for TSE-prions	• Expensive • Difficult to operate and manage • Stationary • Permitting

Adapted from Kastner and Phebus (2004).

or 2:1 wood-to-carcass ratio, as well as diesel fuel to power the engines that drive the fans. Open-air burning is more variable than air-curtain incineration but can be expected to require, at a minimum, an equal amount of "dry" wood.

COMPOSTING

21. What are the basic elements needed for successful composting (Byers, undated; Mukhtar et al., 2004)?

1. Carbon source
   • Carbon is the energy that drives decomposition.
   • A proper carbon-to-nitrogen (C:N) ratio will ensure complete decomposition of carcasses and will minimize odors.
   • C:N ratio should be in the range of 25:1 to 40:1.
   • Materials that can be used as a carbon source include sawdust, cornstalks, straw, hay, poultry litter, etc.
2. Bulking agents
   • These agents have larger particle sizes than carbon source materials to maintain adequate air spaces and prevent packing.
   • They provide at least 0.03 m³ (1 ft³) of bulking material per 4.5 kg (10 lb) of expected mortality.
   • Materials can include coarse wood chips, and cornstalks, straw.
3. Moisture
   • Ideal range of moisture is 40% to 60%.
   • Process will not operate effectively if material is too dry or too wet.
4. Temperature
   • Under optimal conditions, thermophilic aerobic bacteria will raise the temperature of the composting pile to 57° to 63° C (135° to 145° F).

22. What are the two phases of composting (Mukhtar et al., 2004)?

First Phase:

• Temperature of compost pile should rise to at least 55° to 60° C (130° to 140° F) within 10 days and remain within this range for several weeks.
• Organic materials break down, soft tissue decomposes, and bones partially soften.
• Core of compost pile should reach 65° C (149° F) for 1 to 2 days to inactivate pathogenic bacteria and destroy weed seed germination.

Second Phase

- Compost pile is cultivated or reworked.
- Water is added (if needed) to reheat composting materials.
- Remaining materials (mainly bones) break down.
- Second phase is completed when core temperature reaches 25° to 30° C (77° to 86° F).
- Compost turns to a dark brown to black soil.

23. How does one construct a compost pile for animal carcasses (Figs. 1.25.3 and 1.25.4, Table 1.25.2)?

- A base layer of dry material should be placed at least 0.3 m (1 ft) deep under the animal.
- The base layer will insulate the composting material from the outside environment, provide carbon to fuel the composting process, provide sufficient space between organic particles to allow gas exchange, and soak up leachate that is released from the carcass.
- The bigger the animal, the deeper is the base layer.
- The base layer should extend at least 0.6 m (2 ft) beyond all sides of the animal.
- The animal should be covered with compost ingredient material to form a peaked pile such that a minimum of one foot of cover exists all around the animal.

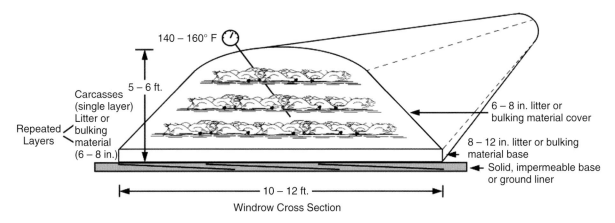

Figure 1.25.3 Schematic of a mortality compost windrow. (From Ritz, 2005.)

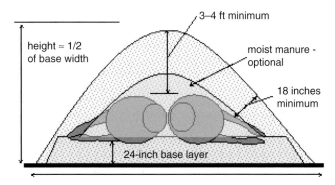

Figure 1.25.4 Recommended cross section for composting full-sized cattle carcasses. (From Iowa State University, 2002; http://www3.abe.iastate.edu/cattlecomposting/guidelines/draft_guidelines.asp.)

Table 1.25.2 Dimensions of Compost Windrows Based on Size of Animal Carcasses

Carcass Size	Bottom Width	Top Width	Height
Small	3.6 m (12 ft)	1.5 m (5 ft)	1.8 m (6 ft)
Medium	3.9 m (13 ft)	0.3 m (1 ft)	1.8 m (6 ft)
Large and very large	4.5 m (15 ft)	0.3 m (1 ft)	2.1 m (7 ft)

Adapted from Mukhtar et al. (2004).

24. Is it necessary to quarter large carcasses before composting?

It is not necessary to quarter, cut up, or puncture the stomach of large carcasses before composting. However, performing these steps will increase the surface area of carcass that is available to microbial decomposition, which can significantly speed up the composting process.

25. What additional materials are needed for composting?

- Thermometer with a 0.9 m (36 in) stem to monitor temperatures
- Method to get water to compost pile
- Heavy equipment for moving carcasses to the composting site, for "turning" the compost after the first phase, and for loading out finished compost

26. What are the advantages of composting?

- On-site disposal
- Inexpensive
- Environmentally sound
- Produces valuable soil fertilizer

27. What are the disadvantages associated with composting mortalities?

- Labor intensive
- Spore-formers such as *Bacillus anthracis* (anthrax) and other pathogens such as *Mycobacterium tuberculosis* and TSE prions can survive.
- Not a quick method for destroying infected carcasses
- Potential for scavengers (e.g., rodents, coyotes, birds) and insects to spread disease

28. Is composting poultry carcasses in-house (i.e., inside the poultry barn) an effective method for disposal?

In-house composting is very effective and is becoming the preferred method for managing flocks that were depopulated for disease control and eradication purposes. For example, in 2004 the Canadian Food Inspection Agency used in-house composting in British Columbia to successfully destroy poultry carcasses infected with the highly pathogenic avian influenza subtype H7N3.

29. What are the advantages of composting poultry carcasses in-house?

- Reduce potential for inadvertent disease transmission
- Protect against disease transmission to native birds and waterfowl
- Controlled environmental conditions
- Carcasses do not have to be moved outside or off-site.
- Inactivate disease agent in poultry manure
- Poultry manure can be used as carbon and nitrogen source.
- Possible to contain outbreak to a single infected barn or property

30. Are there disadvantages to composting poultry carcasses in-house?

- Composting can extend as long as 3 months.
- Must remove and dispose of composted material before restocking

RENDERING

31. Is rendering an acceptable means of carcass disposal?

This is one of the most efficient and safest methods of disposal, but it is often limited by the capacity of the facilities and is not appropriate for handling highly contagious infectious and zoonotic diseases such as anthrax and foot and mouth disease.

32. Explain the commercial rendering process.

Rendering recycles perishable animal byproducts (e.g., slaughter plant waste, restaurant grease, expired meat from grocery stores, animal carcasses, etc.) into valuable ingredients that are used in industrial processes and in the animal feed industry.

33. Are there advantages of rendering?

- Highly regulated industry (permitted and licensed by state agencies; inspected by FDA and Animal and Plant Inspection Service [APHIS])
- Generates usable end product
- Can be performed year-round

34. What are some disadvantages of rendering?

- Fixed facilities (Fig. 1.25.5)
- High biosecurity risk from transporting carcasses
- Cannot destroy Transmissible Spongiform Encephalopathy (TSE) prions; therefore, sheep and goat carcasses, as well as deer and elk carcasses, are prohibited
- Cannot render companion animals (i.e., cats and dogs)
- Local and regional availability

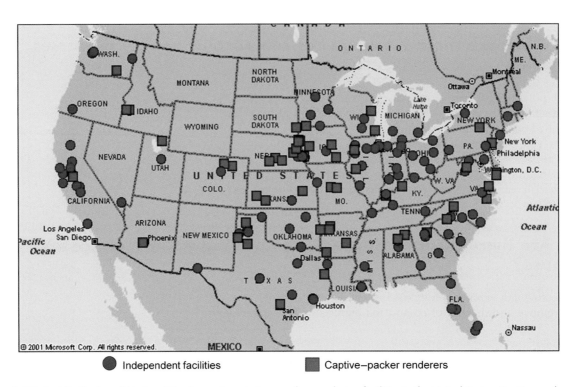

● Independent facilities   ■ Captive–packer renderers

Figure 1.25.5 Distribution of National Renderers Association member rendering facilities in the United States. Captive-packer renderers are rendering facilities that are attached to packing plants. These facilities typically do not accept outside materials (i.e., animal carcasses) for rendering. (Source: D. Meeker, Vice President, Scientific Affairs, National Renderers Association, Inc., 801 North Fairfax Street, Suite 205, Alexandria, VA 22314; undated.)

ALKALINE HYDROLYSIS

35. What is alkaline hydrolysis?

This process uses heat, pressure, time, and an alkali catalyst (i.e., sodium or potassium hydroxide) to hydrolyze biological materials into small peptides, proteins, sugars, and soaps. The end product, or "effluent," is sterilized during the hydrolysis process.

36. Are there advantages to alkaline hydrolysis?

- Environmentally friendly nonburn carcass disposal technology
- Sterilization and digestion in one operation
- Complete destruction of pathogens, including TSE prions
- Generates reusable end product that could be used as a valuable carbon source for composting or anaerobic digestion

37. What are the disadvantages to alkaline hydrolysis?

- Limited capacity for large volumes of carcasses
- Large initial investment
- Expensive disposal method on a per-carcass basis in comparison to other methods

38. Are there other applications for alkaline hydrolysis besides carcass disposal?

Large carbohydrates (e.g., cellulose) are resistant to alkaline hydrolysis. Although items such as wood shavings, undigested plant material, and soil will not be digested, these materials can still be sterilized by the process. Alkaline hydrolysis could be useful for inactivating infectious disease agents in contaminated soil, as well as in other materials when incineration is not an option (Thacker, 2004).

MORTALITY MANAGEMENT IN THE EVENT OF A DISASTER

39. In a dairy with over 2,000 cows that have to be depopulated, is it appropriate to bury the animals on the farm?

Burying large numbers of animals requires some special considerations. It is important to know the depth of the water table for the proposed burial site to avoid contaminating ground water. To determine this depth, as well as to determine the feasibility of using burial as a means of carcass disposal, the local water authorities and EPA should be contacted.

40. Are there regulations that prohibit the disposal of animal carcasses on public lands?

Restrictions may exist and will depend on the public land's local, state, or federal statutes. For example, cattle lost during the 2007 High Plains Winter Storm in Colorado could not be buried on public lands. Cattlemen were required to move the carcasses off of public land for disposal.

41. What methods of disposal are appropriate in the event of a devastating blizzard such as the 2007 High Plains Winter Storm?

Rendering was the favored method of disposal for animals lost to the blizzard. Rendering companies increased collection in affected areas to facilitate proper and responsible disposal. One advantage of the blizzard was that carcasses were frozen, which made rendering more feasible. However, in some situations, carcasses were not discovered until spring, which resulted in many being too badly decomposed to be acceptable for rendering. As a consequence, it was necessary to seek alternative methods such as burial or composting.

SPECIAL CONSIDERATIONS

CONTAGIOUS DISEASES

42. How do I dispose of carcasses infected or contaminated with anthrax?

- Any method of incineration should destroy anthrax spores.
- Open-air burning is commonly used in small-scale anthrax outbreaks in North America.
- Rendering and alkaline hydrolysis also can inactivate anthrax spores but pose significant hazards to those workers who handle and transport the carcasses.
- There is always the risk of inadvertently distributing spores during transport.

43. How should animal carcasses infected with foot and mouth disease virus be disposed?

- Burial and open-air burning were both used extensively during the 2001 foot and mouth disease outbreak in the United Kingdom.
- Composting could work, but there is a significant risk of spreading the disease as it takes time for the virus to be inactivated.
- Any disposal method used for foot and mouth disease–positive carcasses must meet federal and state regulations.

PENTOBARBITAL

44. Are there any restrictions on disposal methods for animals that have been euthanized with pentobarbital?

Most rendering companies will not accept animal carcasses euthanized with pentobarbital. However, some companies may accept such carcasses but then take great efforts to dilute that material over an extended period of production. It is critical to check with local rendering companies before euthanizing animals that are to be disposed of through a rendering company.

45. What could be the consequences of not disclosing to a rendering company that the animals were euthanized with pentobarbital?

It is possible charges could be filed against parties that knowingly submitted animal carcasses containing pentobarbital for rendering. In addition, the guilty party could be responsible for the cost of diluting a batch of contaminated feed or, worse, be responsible for paying the costs associated with a recall of contaminated feed.

46. Are there any risks to wildlife from animal carcasses that were euthanized with pentobarbital?

There are many verified reports of accidental poisonings of scavenger animals (e.g., coyotes, foxes, etc.) and birds of prey (e.g., Bald Eagles, Golden Eagles, etc.) from feeding on animal carcasses containing pentobarbital. For example, in 1999, a Colorado veterinarian euthanized two mules on a ranch and left without instructing the owner on how to properly dispose of the carcasses. Five Golden Eagles and two Bald Eagles died after feeding on the carcasses. As a result of their negligence, the veterinarian, as well as the rancher, were given considerable monetary fines for violations of the federal Endangered Species Act.

47. Describe a checklist that can be used for making animal carcass disposal decisions.

✓ Can all animal carcasses be disposed of in a similar manner?
- Commercial livestock
- Companion animals (e.g., cats, dogs, and horses)

✓ **Does the cause of death matter when deciding on how to dispose of the carcasses?**
  - Is this an isolated incident or a widespread disease outbreak or disaster?
  - Bacterial—anthrax, brucellosis, tuberculosis
  - Viral—foot and mouth disease, pseudorabies, rabies, vesicular stomatitis
  - Prions—Bovine Spongiform Encephalopathy (BSE), Chronic Wasting Disease (CWD), scrapie
  - Chemical—pentobarbital, Compound 1080 (sodium fluoroacetate), strychnine, pesticides, etc.

✓ **Are there special considerations that must be taken into account when disposing of carcasses that have died from a zoonotic disease?**
  - What is the potential for the transfer and maintenance of disease in humans, livestock, wildlife, and pets?
  - Examples: anthrax, tuberculosis, plague

✓ **Can the method of carcass disposal contribute to the potential spread of the disease?**
  - Can the disease agent be spread via airborne transmission, direct contact, vectors, fomites, etc.?
  - How long can the disease agent persist in the environment?

✓ **Where are the carcasses located?**
  - What is the proximity of the carcasses to intensified feeding operations and other livestock, as well as densely populated areas?

✓ **Are there environmental concerns that need to be considered when disposing of carcasses?**
  - Contamination of surface and ground water, as well as soil
  - Odor control
  - Fly control

✓ **What is the availability of equipment, transportation, fuel, manpower, etc.?**
  - Is timber or similar fuel source available for incineration? How much?
  - Does the availability of the fuel source vary by season?
  - How many trucks with watertight and, potentially, sealable trailers would be available to haul carcasses off-site for disposal?
  - In the event of a natural disaster, would resources be directed to cleanup and other public needs before carcass disposal?

✓ **Has informed public consent been obtained?**
  - Were local, city, and county officials involved in response plan development?
  - Do written agreements exist that stipulate which carcass disposal methods are acceptable, and under what circumstances?

Suggested Reading and Sources

Air Burners, LLC. Photo gallery. Available at http://www.airburners.com/ab-photogal.htm.

Air Burners, LLC. The principle of air-curtain incineration. Available at http://www.airburners.com/ab-principle.htm.

Byers M. Carcass disposal options. National Biosecurity and Resource Center (for Animal Health Emergencies), Purdue Homeland Security Institute. Undated. Available at http://www.biosecuritycenter.org/article/carcass Disposal.

Ellis DB. Carcass disposal issues in recent disasters, accepted methods, and suggested plan to mitigate future events [thesis]. Public Administration, Political Science Department, Texas State University-San Marcos, 2001 Available at http://ecommons.txstate.edu/cgi/viewcontent.cgi?article=1068&context=arp.

Iowa State University. Draft guidelines for emergency composting of cattle mortalities. Department of Agricultural and Biosystems Engineering, College of Engineering, Iowa State University, 2002. Available at http://www3.abe.iastate.edu/cattlecomposting/guidelines/draft_guidelines.asp.

Kastner J, Phebus R. Incineration. Carcass disposal: A comprehensive review. National Agricultural Biosecurity Center, Kansas State University, 2004. Available at http://fss.k-state.edu/FeaturedContent/CarcassDisposal/PDF%20Files/CH%202%20-%20Incineration.pdf.

Larson J. Disposal of dead production animals 1988–2006. Animal Welfare Information Center, National Agricultural Library, Agricultural Research Service, US Department of Agriculture, 2006. Available at http://www.nal.usda.gov/awic/pubs/carcass.htm.

Mukhtar S, Kalbasi A, Ahmed A. Composting. Carcass disposal: A comprehensive review. National Agricultural Biosecurity Center, Kansas State University, 2004. Available at http://fss.k-state.edu/FeaturedContent/CarcassDisposal/PDF%20Files/CH%203%20-%20Composting.pdf.

National Biosecurity and Resource Center (for Animal Health Emergencies). Carcass disposal options. Hosted by: Purdue Homeland Security Institute. Available at http://www.biosecuritycenter.org/article/carcassDisposael.

Ritz CW. Composting mass poultry mortalities. University of Georgia, College of Agricultural and Environmental Sciences, Department of Poultry Science, 2005. Available at http://www.thepoultrysite.com/articles/403/composting-mass-poultry-mortalities.

Thacker HL. Alkaline hydrolysis. Carcass disposal: A comprehensive review. National Agricultural Biosecurity Center, Kansas State University, 2004. Available at http://fss.k-state.edu/FeaturedContent/CarcassDisposal/PDF%20Files/CH%206%20-%20Alkaline%20Hydrolysis.pdf.

United Kingdom Environment Agency. The environmental impact of the foot and mouth disease outbreak: An interim assessment, 2001. Available at http://www.environment-agency.gov.uk/commondata/acrobat/fmd_report.pdf.

Woolhouse MEJ, Gowtage-Sequeria S. Host range and emerging and reemerging pathogens. *J Emerg Infect Dis* 2005;11:1842–1847.

SECTION 2
PLANNING

CHAPTER 2.1
ELEMENTS OF A DISASTER PLAN FOR ANIMALS

Anthony P. Knight, BVSc, MS

In preparing for battle I have always found plans are useless, but planning is indispensable.
Dwight D. Eisenhower

1. Why is there a need for a disaster plan for animals?

Significant health and safety risks in a disaster area are exacerbated by abandoned pets and livestock. A well-organized and rehearsed disaster plan for animals is essential if all types of animals are to be safely protected, evacuated, or rescued from hazardous situations.

Disaster plans must start locally with people being prepared to take care of themselves, their families, and their pets and livestock for a minimum of 72 hours. This may include sheltering in place or evacuating themselves and their animals safely and efficiently. In addition, neighbors may need assistance with their animals, especially those who are elderly or disabled.

2. Is there a national, state, and/or county disaster plan for animals?

The Pets Evacuation and Transportation Standards Act of 2006, which amends the Robert T. Stafford Disaster Relief and Emergency Assistance Act, requires that state and local emergency preparedness operational plans address the needs of individuals with household pets and service animals following a major disaster or emergency.

In addition, the Department of Homeland Security National Response Framework has identified 15 Emergency Support Functions (ESF) that deal with the overall disaster plans for the country (http://www.fema.gov/pdf/emergency/nrf/).

The means by which animals are to be handled in a disaster situation are defined in ESF #6, #8, #9, #11, and #14. There is therefore legislation in place that requires states and counties to develop and implement disaster plans, especially if they wish to obtain federal funding to assist with a disaster response.

A useful resource for veterinarians, animal owners, and others involved in planning for disasters involving animals is the American Veterinary Medical Association's disaster preparedness website (http://www.avma.org/disaster/default.asp) (Fig. 2.1.1).

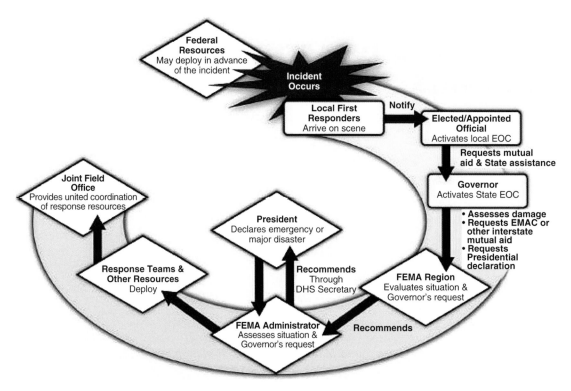

Figure 2.1.1 Overview of the Stafford Act support to states January 2008. (Available from public domain: http://www.fema.gov/pdf/emergency/nrf/nrf-overview.pdf.)

3. What is included in the emergency support functions (ESF) that is relevant for animals?

- Animal evacuation
- Transportation of animals and animal support materials
- Animal sheltering
- Animal feeding and water
- Animal search and rescue
- Animal control/capture
- Veterinary medical care
- Animal decontamination
- Animal disease management
- Zoonotic disease management
- Animal mortality management
- Animal/owner reunion

4. What are the elements of a disaster plan?

Basic elements to be considered in a disaster plan are as follows:

- Planning for disaster mitigation
- Response to a disaster
- Recovery from a disaster

5. Are there specific components to planning for disaster mitigation?

There are four basic steps in disaster planning in a veterinary setting that require forming a planning team or committee with goals and timelines.

1. Identify the most probable disasters for your area and the effects on your facility and practice.
2. Take a census of animals in your area that would impact your practice in the event of a disaster.
   - Develop a list of facilities that can shelter or house animals.
   - Define a plan for handling injured or sick animals.
   - Have a plan for:
     - Handling stray or abandoned animals disasters that requires maintaining animals on the premises.
     - When an animal evacuation is necessary
     - Disposing of dead animals
3. Make a written plan and distribute it to all members of the team.
4. Periodically update and practice the plan.

6. What kinds of disaster should be planned for?

Ideally a disaster plan should cover the possibility of any hazard or disaster. However, it is not realistic to plan for every conceivable kind of disaster, but by determining what the most probable risks are in your area, the most important elements of a plan can be developed. For example, it is unlikely that a hurricane will directly affect Colorado, but snowstorms, forest fires, floods, and man-made disasters such as a chemical spill are likely! It is especially important to identify animal facilities such as veterinary hospitals, animal shelters, and fairgrounds that could be affected by a disaster. For example, is the county animal shelter built in a flood plain? Is the veterinary hospital situated close to an oil refinery or chemical plant?

7. Who should participate in a disaster plan involving animals?

Veterinarians, veterinary technicians, veterinary practice managers, animal extension specialists, animal shelter personnel, brand inspectors, animal control officers, animal rescue units, the fire department, and law enforcement are some of the critical participants involved with developing an animal disaster plan. Coordination of this diverse group in the event of a disaster is handled through the Incident Command System (ICS) (see Chapter 1.1 on ICS training).

8. How does one estimate the number of animals to accommodate in disaster planning?

An animal census of animal shelters, rescue groups, veterinary hospitals, pet stores, boarding stables, and livestock operations and their locations will facilitate the planning process. To estimate the number of pets in your area, use the American Veterinary Medical Association's statistics that 59.5% of American households have pets, and multiply by the number of households in your county, town, etc. (*U.S. Pet Ownership and Demographics Sourcebook*, 2007 edition). For example, if you have a city with 20,000 homes, the number of pets would be $20,000 \times 0.595 = 11,900$. Using the same source of statistical information, the number of dogs, cats, birds, and horses can also be calculated. Estimates of wildlife and feral animals in the area may be available through the state agencies involved with wildlife.

9. What facilities can be used to shelter or house animals in a disaster?

Veterinary hospitals, animal shelters, pet stores, etc. need to determine what options are available for housing their animals should it be necessary to evacuate them from the disaster zone. An inventory of facilities and the number and species of animals that can be accommodated at safe facilities such as neighboring county animal shelters, fairgrounds, vacant warehouses, business parking lots, and veterinary hospitals is invaluable in the planning process. Where livestock and horses are involved, different facilities capable of handling and feeding large animals will need to be identified such as county fairgrounds, sale barns, and feedlots.

An inventory of local motels and hotels that would allow people and their household pets to stay in the same facility in the event of an emergency evacuation can be valuable information to have to pass out to people being evacuated.

10. How should injured or sick animals be handled?

In a disaster zone, a plan needs to be in place to have a veterinarian triage patients as they are rescued. The injured or sick animals that have a reasonably good prognosis and need immediate lifesaving treatment can be treated by the emergency/critical care veterinary staff, while less severe cases will be designated for transport to a veterinary facility that has agreed to accept animals in the event of a disaster.

11. What forms of animal identification are acceptable in a disaster?

Appropriate animal identification and ownership become a critical issue in a disaster and especially in the recovery phase when animals need to be reunited with their owners.

In the case of pet animals, veterinarians and animal shelters should strongly encourage pet owners to have their animals microchipped with a chip that is readable by a universal scanner. Identifiable tattoos may also work well. Livestock may be identified through a variety of methods including brands, ear tags, microchips, and radiofrequency identification tags.

Should your veterinary practice or animal shelter be designated as a holding area for animals in a disaster, plan on what method of identification will be used for animals that have no identification. This will help ensure animals recovered in a disaster are reunited with their appropriate owners during the recovery phase.

12. What if an animal is rescued or abandoned and has no owner?

A system to record pertinent information about the animal and where it was found is essential and must be established ahead of time. Digital photographs of each animal can be valuable in reuniting people with their pets. Collars with numbers should be available to provide a means of identification for animals in a designated collection area. Spray painting identification on the sides of large animals can be effective in the short term.

13. Should veterinary hospitals, animal shelters, livestock enterprises, etc. have a disaster plan?

Successful management and outcomes of a disaster depend on a plan to ensure the safety of one's person and family first. Employees must be informed and have rehearsed the disaster plan for the premises. Written plans in English and Spanish should be reviewed and rehearsed with employees regularly. Pets and livestock must be included in the plan.

Items that need to be considered in a disaster plan should include:

- Escape routes, meeting points, family contacts outside the area.
- Gas, electricity, and water shutoff
- Important records; make backup copies of computer hard drives and store elsewhere.
- Photographic inventory of the facilities
- Special provisions for disabled people

14. What are the elements of a disaster plan if animals do not need to be moved?

Assuming that utilities will be disrupted for several days at a minimum (electricity, water, sewage), plans must include means to provide light, food, water, warmth, and garbage and sewage disposal if the premises are not to be evacuated. There are many resources that provide information on planning for a disaster (CDC Emergency Preparedness for Businesses, http://www.cdc.gov/niosh/topics/prepared/; Federal Emergency Management Agency, http://www.fema.gov/plan/index.shtm). At a minimum, a disaster plan should include:

- Potable water sources
- Flashlights/lantern, extra batteries
- Nonperishable food reserves (1 week)
- Prescription medications for people and pets (1 week minimum)
- Pet food (minimum 1 week supply)
- For aquariums (battery operated air pump with extra batteries)
- Alternative heating sources (propane, kerosene heaters)
- Cars/trucks at least 50% full of gas whenever possible; ensure gas tanks are full before major storms.
- Snow shovel, snow shoes, cold weather gear where appropriate
- Means to transport pets and livestock should an evacuation be necessary

15. What are the elements of a disaster plan for a small animal practice?

A small animal practice needs to develop plans for different circumstances: an evacuation plan, a "stay in place" plan, and a "shelter" plan for animals rescued from the disaster area. Veterinary practices may become a "shelter" for animals if they are not in the immediate disaster zone. What is planned for handling additional animals? How many animals can be sheltered in an emergency?

16. Are there additional considerations for a livestock disaster plan?

- Disaster plans for horses and livestock will entail some different considerations. This was well exemplified by the equine rescue activities associated with the hurricanes in Louisiana in 2005 (McConnico, 2007).
- Location of hay and water sources must remain accessible during a disaster.
- Maintain at least a 2-week supply of hay and water that is accessible if there is no electricity for pumps, fans, lights, etc.
- Transportation options for large animals
- Evacuation routes/destinations
- Holding areas, pens, etc.
- Carcass disposal

17. What special considerations are necessary in a large animal disaster plan?

Proper identification of animals helps avoid disputes over ownership and greatly assists in reunification of animals with their owners, especially if the identification system used is linked to registered premise identification.

Dairy farms will need backup generators to provide the electricity to run milking machines. Similarly, ventilation systems in poultry and swine houses will need adequate backup electrical generators.

18. How should dead animals be handled in a disaster?

This is a complex issue in a disaster as normal means of carcass disposal may be disrupted or overwhelmed by the numbers of animals involved. Each county and municipality must develop a plan to handle carcass disposal that is not a threat to public health, and meets with state and federal requirements. Landfills may be unable to accommodate mass burials or may be inaccessible because of the disaster. Alternative burial sites that do not run the risk of contaminating water sources need to be identified ahead of time.

Livestock enterprises also need to develop plans for burial sites on the farm that do not pose a risk to human and animal health. If burial is not possible in a given area, alternative means of carcass disposal need to be established such as incineration, and composting. (See chapter 1.25.)

19. Are there any states with disaster animal response plans for animals that could serve as a template from which to develop a disaster or emergency response plan?

Several states have developed plans that can serve as a model for developing a state, county, or local animal disaster plans: http://www.vetmed.ucdavis.edu/vetext/DANR/DANRGuide2.pdf and http://www.dola.state.co.us/dem/operations/seop2007/base_plan.pdf.

Suggested Reading
American Veterinary Medical Association. Disaster preparedness. Available at http://www.avma.org/disaster/default.asp, 2007.
Centers for Disease Control and Prevention, Emergency Preparedness for Businesses. Available at http://www.cdc.gov/niosh/topics/prepared/, 2008.
FAO Biosecurity Toolkit 2007. Available at http://www.fao.org/docrep/010/a1140e/a1140e00.htm.
Federal Emergency Management Agency. Available at http://www.fema.gov/plan/index.shtm, 2007.
LSU Emergency Animal Shelter Disaster Response Manual, 2006. Available at http://www.lsuemergencyanimalshelter.org/operat4.htm.
McConnico RS, et al. Equine rescue and response activities in Louisiana in the aftermath of Hurricanes Katrina and Rita. J Am Vet Med Assoc 2007;231:384–392.
National Response Framework. Available at http://www.fema.gov/pdf/emergency/nrf/nrf-overview.pdf, 2008.
Pets Evacuation and Transportation Standards Act of 2006. Available at http://sema.dps.mo.gov/Planning/Pets%20Law.pdf, 2006.
Robert T. Stafford Disaster Relief and Emergency Assistance Act (Pub. L. 106–390, § 301, October 30, 2000). Available at www.hidlnr.org/eng/nfip/pdf/leg/staffordAct.pdf, 2007.
U.S. Pet Ownership & Demographics Sourcebook. Available at http://www.avma.org/reference/marketstats/ownership.asp, 2007.

CHAPTER 2.2
DISASTER PLANNING FOR PRIVATE PRACTICE

Dirk B. Yelinek, DVM

1. Why should a private veterinary practice concern itself with disaster preparedness?

- Animal concerns parallel the human counterpart and may increase as a direct effect of the disaster or by the need to evacuate.
- Historically, in the event of a disaster, many animals are left behind to fend for themselves
- The veterinarian typically has the respect in the community as a health care professional and leader and will be important in the response and recovery phases with proper planning and preparation.
- The veterinarian is in the forefront of knowledge on recognizing emerging zoonotic diseases that can be potential bioterrorist agents.

2. Is it important to have a written disaster plan for each practice?

- Every practice should have a written plan that is practiced at least once a year by all employees and reviewed with any new employee as part of the orientation program.
- The purposes of the plan are to prevent accidents and to have a safe and controlled response should an event occur.
- When this becomes requisite for continued employment the participants will also be better prepared in their own personal home response.
- The plan can be administered and shared by area veterinary practices for a more calculated, uniform, and cooperative response.
- Assign a staff member to develop, update and explain the plan. Communicate regularly before, during, and after an incident. Evaluate and make revisions of the plan based on experiences and keep training records.

3. What are the six essentials of a written disaster plan for private veterinary practice?

- Life safety
  - First, for your staff and clients
  - Second, for the animals
- Animal relocation and transport
  - When?
  - Where?
  - How?
  - Who?
- Property and intellectual preservation of important documents
  - Computer backup and conservation of medical records
  - Know how to protect and access vital business records.

- Continuity of operations
  - Same location?
  - Temporary location?
- Security and incident stabilization—How can you protect the facility and equipment from further damage?
- Insurance and legal issues—Do you have adequate coverage for damage and losses due to natural or man-made disasters?

4. If my employees are not yet at work and have sustained damages and losses at the home, what are my expectations for being able to open for business?

- Those with immediate family should think family first—the welfare of the children and family unit overrides any thoughts to breaking the circle to come to work at that critical time.
- Among others, there is acceptance of the situation and some solace in coming to work to help others in need and to try to keep schedules as normal as possible.
- Employees, if able to leave the home and travel safely, will continue to work as they need to make a living wage.
- Others may enlist the family to come to the practice to work for the common cause of helping the injured animals, support the community practice, assist in clean up, and by doing so, be together. In this way they can experience and work through the initial stages of stress and/or grief together.

Our employees and co-workers are our practice's most important and valuable asset and so it goes for their families. Nothing is more important in that critical moment than taking care of ourselves and each other, so that we may be able to take care of others.

5. What communications are needed internally for the purposes of planning?

- Know what natural and man-made disasters could potentially affect the business.
- Identify operations critical to survival and recovery. Prioritize a list of daily operations, staffing, equipment, and procedures needed to recover from the disaster.
- Establish procedures for succession of management including at least one person who is not at this location.
- Know the other area practices (and other nonrelated businesses) that will be participating in the emergency planning team and coordinate and practice drills with them.
- Determine in advance how all communications are to be performed by situation or preference (e.g., direct via cell telephone call tree, relay via out-of state contact, an email alert, message machine, etc.). You may choose to sort your employee call list alphabetically or by call-down priority order.
- If there are employees with disabilities ask them what assistance, if any, they require.
- Establish a warning system including plans to communicate with people who are hearing impaired or that do not speak English.

6. Provide a plan for integrating the incident command system (ICS) into a private practice disaster plan (Fig 2.2.1). (For a review of ICS, see Chapter 1.1.)

Create a chain of command so that others are authorized to act in case your designated person is not available.

- Determine in advance who is responsible for all aspects of transportation including fuel and maintenance.
- Determine who will be responsible for the safety of the animals.

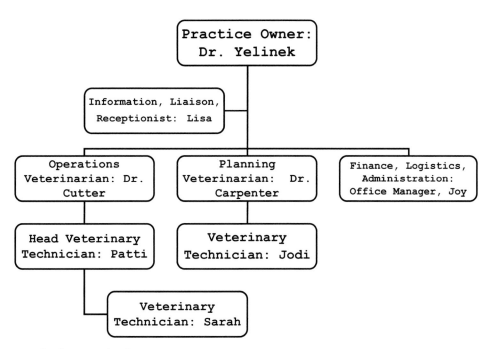

Figure 2.2.1 Example of an ICS plan for a private practice.

- Know who will be in charge of security.
- Know who will lead the charge to evacuate versus make the decision to maintain operations and work with the planning group of the hospital (assembly site manager and alternate, shutdown manager and alternates)
- Know who will perform the interhospital/agency communications and keep the practice team advised of updates and changes in the disaster scene (primary crisis manager and alternate).
- If the disaster event renders operations to cease, and there is clearly no option for evacuation, know who decides that it would be best for all to shelter in place.
- Who is responsible for issuing an "all clear" or return-to-work notification?

The ICS system is a standardized, efficient, on-site management tool used to organize both short- and long-term operations among all levels of organizations and agencies.

7. If risk assessment indicates the need to perform a safe and effective evacuation from the business, what initial concerns should be planned in advance for personal safety?

- Are all present and accounted for?
  - This must be determined on safe exit to the outside if not before.
- Where are the exits?
  - Have a floor plan complete with a minimum of two exits clearly marked and posted on the inside rear door of the facility and by the front entrance. Exits must be left unobstructed.
- Where should an off-site meeting place be located for regrouping?
  - The team must designate a meeting place in advance of any destructive disaster. One site can be within a few blocks of the actual facility but a backup plan with a meeting site several miles away may be needed for safety reasons. A nearby open lot can serve as the initial site to gather and consider options available following a well-planned and practiced evacuation plan.

8. What are some other potential post-evacuation meeting sites?

- Livestock show grounds or fairgrounds
- Church
- Community college
- Mall parking lot
- Grocery store parking lot

9. What is the system of checks and balances? How do we account for everyone?

- Formal check-in and check-out procedures are required.
- Maintain standard operating procedures for the hospital that include rules for the staff reporting to work and for ending their shift. Provide employees information on when, if, and how to report to work following an emergency.
- Keep updated emergency contact information on all of the employees as well as an out-of-state number for each employee.
- Be able to discharge employees to safe surroundings and inform those planning to cover any shifts of any change of events.
- Have a "buddy system" in place.
- Institute the use of an operational format such as the incident command system (ICS) to ensure accountability.

10. If we are able to remain on the premises at least until help arrives, determine what necessary items will be supplied in preparation of taking care of employees and clients for at least the short term.

- NOAA weather alert radio
- Battery-powered AM/FM radio
- Emergency contact list
- Working smoke detectors and fire extinguishers
- Flashlights and light-sticks
- First-aid kit
- Bottled water
- Nonperishable foods
- Can opener, utensils, and any tools
- Heat source and blankets
- Camera
- Cash/ATM and credit card
- Extra batteries of required sizes

11. What contacts should be made at the outset of a *major disaster*?

- Avoid calling 911 or emergency services unless there is an obvious life-threatening situation or physical injuries that require immediate attention.
- Listen to your battery-operated radio (or local TV station) to determine what the effect has been and where you might seek assistance. In the event that help is not immediately available have everyone trained in turning off the gas, water, and electricity.

- Ask someone outside the area to be an information clearing house for you and your family (practice). Since it will probably be easier to call out of the disaster area, let that person know how and where you are, so they can let your friends and relatives know. If you need to make an emergency call and do not hear a dial tone right away, stay on the line as the tone could be delayed a minute or more. If there is damage to your facility, wiring, or the equipment of the telephone company, you may not be able to make a call. If possible, first make contact with your out-of-state contact to let them know the status of the practice and if you are able to continue to function or not.
- Communicate to local, state, and federal authorities what emergency assistance is needed for you to continue essential business activity.
- Have emergency numbers posted in your hospital (Table 2.2.1). Keep one copy by the main reception area telephone, another posted in the treatment area, and one with the evacuation supply kit.

12. What two radio sources will provide the information I need?

- The Emergency Alert System (EAS) provided by local radio stations
- National Oceanic and Atmospheric Administration (NOAA) Weather Radio (NWR) with Specific Area Message Encoding (S.A.M.E.)
  - This radio remains silent until an alert is broadcast giving specific information and instructions as to how best to avoid danger.

13. What preparation and planning is needed for the safe and efficient emergency relocation of animals? What do I do with the animals? Can I shelter them elsewhere?

- Secure the building and contents, if possible, and exit safely.
- Have a planned evacuation list for boarded and hospitalized animals.
- Be ready to transport. Keep vehicles fueled and practice good maintenance. If at all possible, it is best to load the animals, in confinement cages, into vehicles for transport to a safer area or facility. Portable cages (i.e., airline carriers), vans, and horse trailers are best suited for this purpose.
- Know published evacuation routes from your local Emergency Operations Center. Having a local and regional map and a battery-operated radio will facilitate a more rapid egress. If versed in the use of GPS, log the positions of your base hospital, as well as animal clinics, shelters, emergency clinics, boarding and grooming facilities, equine stables, and mobile clinic home bases so you will be able to locate them in the event of road closures or detours. Do not take shortcuts as they will likely be blocked.
- It is important to coordinate and practice with other local tenants and/or businesses to avoid confusion and potential gridlock.

14. How do I identify the animals that are under my care at the time of the disaster?

- Identify animals with secure and weather resistant methods. This may be a tag attached to the collar or a neckband (or brand) in the emergency exit situation (see Chapters 1.5 and 1.9).
- For large animals the same applies, or one may use a mane clip, luggage tag braided into tail or mane, or shave information in the animals' hair. A nontoxic marking crayon, non–water-soluble spray paint, or non–water-soluble markers can be used to write on the animals' side or a permanent marker can be used on the hooves of livestock.
- Designate an employee to take digital photographs of the animals as they are systematically evacuated.
- Clearly label each carrier with your identification and contact information. Bird cages may be needed and reptiles/amphibians can be placed separately in plastic food containers with adequate ventilation holes.

Table 2.2.1 Example of a Hospital Contact List

Hospital Contact List	Title	Home Telephone	Cell Phone
Dr. Dirk Yelinek	Owner/Veterinarian	310-555-1234	310-555-8970
Dr. Sam Carpenter	Veterinarian	310-555-5678	310-555-6843
Dr. Sky Cutter	Veterinarian	310-555-9012	310-555-9812
Lisa Talker	Receptionist	310-555-3456	310-555-9485
Joy Banker	Hospital Administrator	310-555-7890	310-555-2085
Beth Busy	Office Assistant	310-555-0987	310-555-9034
Patti Quick	Head Veterinary Technician	310-555-6543	310-555-9008
Jodi Washer	Veterinary Technician	310-555-2109	310-555-9192
Sarah Finish	Veterinary Technician	310-555-8765	310-555-4923
Mary and Bob Breaker	Hospital Tenants	310-555-1357	310-555-0089

Building Emergency Contact	Name	Telephone Number	Cell Phone
Building Manager	Ralph Gotcha	310-555-6195	310-555-1029
Insurance Agent	Bob Protection	310-555-2908	310-555-1592
Electric Company	Edison Electric	310-555-3691	
Gas Company	Light-M-Up	310-555-5937	
Plumber	Parks Plumbing	310-555-9600	
Security Company	All Alarms	310-555-5523	
Water Company	Always Irrigation	310-555-5902	
Telephone Company			
Snow Removal			
Electrician			
Plumber			
Contractor			

Emergency Contact	Name	Telephone Number	Contacted By
Police Department		310-555-0911	
Harbor Patrol		310-555-3582	
Fire Department		310-555-3579	
Out-of-State Contact		310-555-4600	
Hospital		310-555-4321	
Children's Hospital		310-555-0909	
Pharmacy		310-555-8653	
Health Department		310-555-4123	
Evacuation Hospital Site		310-555-5151	
Poison Control		310-555-5640	
Animal Control		310-555-4952	
Ambulance		310-555-7893	
EMS Animal Coordinator		310-555-6321	
State Veterinarian		612-555-9090	
Animal Rescue Coordinator		310-555-9999	
Red Cross Coordinator		310-555-6644	
American Humane Society		310-555-6378	
Local News Media		310-555-7776	
Vendor A			
Vendor B			
Payroll			
Bank			
Accountant			
Attorney			
Taxi			

15. What if I cannot take the animals from the facility yet? How can I provide for them assuming I can gain access?

- Separate dogs from the cats. Leave enough food and water to last at least 48 hours. Leave only dry foods and fresh water in nonspill containers. Do not tie or confine them to anything other than a room or rooms with adequate ventilation in areas that can be easily cleaned. Fill sinks and bathing tubs half full with water.
- Post notices on the doors to your hospital that advises there are animals inside and leave concise information on where you are evacuating to as well as your contact telephone numbers.
- If evacuation of any livestock seems impossible do your best to relocate them out of harm's way based on the type of imminent disaster present and your environment. Move these animals to higher ground to avoid flood levels. Provide food and water and do not rely on automatic watering systems. If time permits, secure or remove all outdoor objects that may become dangerous if they become airborne (see Chapter 3.3).

16. What arrangements can I make in advance to have a cooperative response with other area veterinary practices?

- Establish cooperative agreements with neighboring veterinary hospital/clinics that will allow you to move your animals to their facility or theirs to yours should disruption of services occur.
  - A list of such participants can be generated at local veterinary association meetings focused for the purpose of disaster planning and preparedness.
  - Have number one and two choices clearly identified and listed on the emergency contact list complete with address and telephone number. These lists should be updated at least biannually.
  - Training staff response and evacuation with a practice in a distant community helps to provide reciprocal care in the event that one is affected and the other can receive patients.
  - Prepare to receive patients and prepare to send patients so you are ready for both scenarios.
  - Discuss this in preparation for servicing the needs of the veterinary community. It may be best to agree to be available in "shifts" so that one facility can back another.
- Know in advance which other hospitals, clinics, kennels, stables, and grooming facilities in the area have volunteered to take on patients if you cannot adequately handle the load at your site.
- Prepare personalized individual employee business cards/badges so that employees may gain access to an otherwise restricted area.
- As a safeguard it would be wise to find out ahead of time which motels and hotels in your area allow pets so this information can be conveyed to callers if you cannot accommodate them. Red Cross shelters do not allow pets for human health reasons but your pet can be sheltered nearby thanks to the new congressional PETS Act.

17. How can I prepare my clients to be "pet-ready" in the event of disaster?

Provide a checklist that may include the following for them to have in their water-proof animal first-aid and evacuation kit (see Chapters 1.18 and 4.2). For proof of ownership have pet owners keep a duplicate ID tag on their key chain with current telephone information in addition to having a photograph of themselves with their pet.

---

18. How do I know who and where to contact clients for whom I have their pet animals following a major disaster? What minimum record-keeping practices would help me to maintain identification and facilitate reuniting the pets with their owners? (Also see Chapter 1.5.)

- It is helpful to have an in-hospital census of patients and boarding animals complete with the animal's name, description, owners name, and best contact number. Ask your computer software technical services department to show you how to do this daily or during the course of the day at any moment's notice.
- Encourage all clients to "microchip" their animals in the event that they escape or must be turned loose for their own safety's sake.
- Leave a message on your business answering machine as well as your cell telephone of the contact number(s) so that clients know the status of the practice and where their pets might be located.
- For any lost pets, contact or visit area shelters, humane societies, shelters, and stables at least once every other day. Listen to the EBS for groups that broadcast lost animals.

19. How do I preserve computer, intellectual backup, medical records, and important documents?

- Maintain a laptop computer with the same programs and a portable printer if possible.
- Have an exit list of the most valuable items to evacuate after staff and animals. Be sure to try to grab and run with the backup if it is safe to do so.
- Keep daily, weekly, and monthly backup copies off-site.
- Use antivirus software and firewalls. Keep them up to date.
- Do not open email from unknown sources, and use hard-to-guess passwords.
- If possible have the ability to transport important business documents in a secure carrying case related to banking, leases, real estate, equipment purchases, trusts, and wills if you suspect they may be safer if removed from the premises. Include copies of tax records and insurance policies.
- Elevate any records that are maintained at floor level. Always have available an extra set of keys for business, automobiles, and home.

20. What factors need to be considered in securing the building and insuring the safety of our staff personnel?

- Consider whether shutting off the gas, water, and electricity sources is advisable.
- Be aware of fire hazards and know where the extinguishers are and how to use them. Make sure they are inspected annually. In larger facilities, with more than one level, adequate fire protection in the way of built in sprinklers and accessible extinguishers should be supplied.
- Do not use open flames as a light source as there may be unknown flammable gases.
- Review OSHA guidelines for safely storing items on shelves, etc.
- Have the oxygen stored in an outside regulated area if possible.
- Stay away from downed power lines and avoid standing in water if the electricity is still on.
- If you have horses or livestock, practice good barn and field maintenance to reduce danger.
- Minimize debris and dead trees and assess the stability of structures.

21. What hazards are unique to my situation? Which do I need to be concerned about in my practice area?

- Tornadoes
- Hurricanes

- Earthquakes
- Floods
- Landslides
- Fires
- Extremes of weather causing excess wind, heat, cold, or lightning
- Accidental or intentional release of hazardous materials that are flammable or combustible, explosive, toxic, noxious, corrosive, chemical, nuclear, or radioactive
- Intentional release of biological or zoonotic emerging diseases
- Riots/robbery
- Potential terrorist targets in the area
- Economic depression

Risk factors may make one or more hazards more likely than others based on geographic region (floods, fires, earthquakes, hurricanes), seasonality (floods, fires, hurricanes), and regional risk occupancy (hazards spills, terrorism).

22.   How do we protect ourselves from the various disaster elements as they are occurring?

- **Tornadoes:** Stay away from windows, seek a basement. Otherwise hole up in an interior closet or bathtub. Shield from falling and flying debris. Stay away from corners because they attract debris.
- **Hurricanes:** Same as tornadoes.
- **Earthquakes:** Get out from under areas where things can fall on you; drop, cover and hold, and avoid driving.
- **Floods:** Use the roof level if necessary but avoid being trapped inside when there are rising water levels.
- **Landslides:** Avoid landslide areas.
- **Fires:** Evacuate! If the building is on fire let the animals loose and crawl low to the floor to the nearest exit. If you see smoke flowing beneath a door, do not open it.
- **Extremes of weather causing excess wind, heat, cold, or lightening:** Prepare in advance by listening to appropriate weather stations
- **Hazardous materials release:** Take advice from your local EMS on evacuation or limiting travel. Make sure the building's HVAC system is working properly and well maintained to secure outdoor air intakes and increase filter efficiency. May need to shut down systems because of outdoor air intake.
- **Terrorism:** Take advice from your local EMS on evacuation, limiting travel, and self protection. Make sure the building's HVAC system is working properly and well maintained to secure outdoor air intakes and increase filter efficiency. May need to shut down systems because of outdoor air intake.
- **Riots/robbery:** Secure the building and yourself from potential harm. Stay away from windows. Be able to manually activate your security system with a remote switch panic button carried by the acting front office coordinator. This will contact the police department directly.
- **Economic depression:** Have an intact business plan with a breakeven analysis, cash flow projections, and proforma income statements so you know what you must achieve to survive any downturns.

23.   If I am to remain open and operable how can we prepare ourselves to assist the community?

- This is part of the local veterinary disaster plan as well as the community plan. Share your ability to provide services with or to the other area facilities by calling into an out of state number that you know will be operational and have a person that can actively relay the information to others as they call and keep the information current.
- Have an adequate supply of food and water
- A minimum of 3 days of food and water is needed for the immediate response for the animals as well as personnel but planning for 7 days is better. Store canned or bottled water, fruit juices, and canned and dried foods in

airtight, water-proof protective containers, and date them with a label. Store at least 1 gallon of water per person per day. Under no circumstances should a person drink less than 1 quart of water per day. Add eight drops of unscented bleach per gallon of water and let stand for 30 minutes to disinfect. Water can also be boiled for 5 minutes (add another minute per 1000 ft above sea level). Food can be rationed. Twenty-five pounds of dry ice will keep a 10 cubic foot freezer below freezing for 3 to 4 days. Rotate stored water and foods at least every 6 months.
- Have a flashlight, first-aid kit, basic tool kit, portable radio, and an adequate supply of batteries.
- Provisions must also be made for waste management, both human and animal. Large plastic waste cans filled to half of their capacity and lined with plastic may be all that you can make available for disposal in the short term. Add bleach as a disinfectant. Drains may or may not be useable for liquid excrement.
- Consider a backup generator as a source of power and know how to use it. Is it gasoline powered or diesel? Does it have an automatic start that needs to be hooked up in advance by an electrician? Which devices will you need or require making your hospital/clinic operable? Lights? Refrigeration? Ventilators? Infusion pumps? Have the staff practice operating the generator and communication devices. Be sure you have adequate back-up fuels for the generator.
- Consider that vendors may not be able to get to you and supplies may be limited. Have a back-up supplier listed in case that vendor has been affected by the incident.

24. Do I have the proper insurance coverage? What type of insurance coverage would be relative to a catastrophic event?

Ask your insurance agent. Review and update your policy at least every 2 years or when dramatic changes in the business have occurred, for better or for worse. Property and casualty coverage that veterinarians should consider when insuring their practice to protect against disasters include property liability, general liability, professional liability, and umbrella liability. Major medical, disability, and life insurance also should be considered because of the risk of disasters causing bodily harm to veterinarians or staff. Ask about deductibles.

A Business Owner's Policy (BOP) package is an insurance contract that includes property and general liability coverage. The following considerations must be addressed:

- Contents (at replacement cost). Inventory, equipment, furniture, and fixtures—take digital photographs or, better yet, video and keep it updated at least annually.
- Buildings and property (at replacement cost)
- Accounts receivable
- Business interruption
- Loss of income
- Water damage
- Fire damage
- Automatic inflation
- Valuable papers
- Coverage of leased equipment
- Theft or destruction of money
- Employee dishonesty
- Debrief removal/cleanup
- Property away from your premises and in transit
- Professional extension—injury, loss, death of animals, or accidental loss by fleeing
- Workers' compensation coverage
- Auto, disability, and life insurance

There is no standard package policy that exists in the insurance industry. All of the coverage mentioned is subject to extensions, limitations, and exclusions that vary by insurer. Some policies, therefore, are broader than others, which is why it is important for veterinarians to base their selection of an insurer on more than price.

Beyond the basic coverage described, practice owners should be aware of coverage available for damage to outdoor signs, computers, and software; losses resulting from off-premises power interruption, breakdown of heating and air conditioning equipment, and problems with the sewer system.

As a recommendation, building plans and construction records can be examined by an engineer to determine whether structures were built to code. Changes in construction and operations may be considered. Doors should be examined and changed if necessary to help guarantee easy exit or be upgraded to fire retardant. Roofs may be repaired or improved, walls may be reinforced, and window protection may be considered. By taking into account necessary structural changes for the purpose of safety and prevention one has taken a proactive position in disaster response. Keep a diary once the event has occurred and take pictures or video the damages to assist in your reporting losses to your insurance company.

25. What are three benefits of performing disaster exercises with your practice team?

- Planning and preparation reduce morbidity and mortality. The likelihood of surviving any future disaster depends largely on emergency planning today and practicing that plan.
- Damage can be mitigated to the extent that factors are identified and stop losses are effectively put into place.
- Preparation makes you feel better; experience begets reassurance and piece of mind. Learn, train, identify your needs, practice, and establish a rapport with the local office of emergency services (OES) personnel and the county animal control/animal coordinator in advance of any future needs as one never knows what the future may bring.

26. What are postdisaster business concerns that I should think about in advance for planning?

- Recovery location: What if I am forced to relocate temporarily after a disaster?
  - Can I share space with another clinic and how/what do I pay them for use of the facility and resources?
  - Can I temporarily set up in a trailer, mobile veterinary clinic, or other space and what would be minimally inexpensive to equip it?
  - Will I have to rebuild or relocate?
- How many employees can I maintain on the payroll and what will their functions be at various stages of the recovery?
- How will I pay creditors? Risk management involves sound business planning.
- Before reentering the facility after the incident what do I need to take into consideration for reasons of safety?
  - Survey the outside for sharp objects, dangerous material or gases, dangerous wildlife, downed power lines, and structural integrity.
- How do I recover lost animals?
  - Familiar scents and landmarks may be altered causing confusion and abnormal behavior for animals trying to find their ways home.
  - If animals have been lost, post waterproof notices and notify local officials, neighboring veterinary hospitals, and animal shelters. Check shelters at least every other day, if possible.
- What provisions must be in place for the disposal of dead animals?
- How will we handle post-traumatic stress among our team?
  - How the practice responds to the medical needs of the injured and the emotional care of others is an important part of disaster preparedness.
  - Severe injuries, or even a death, may lead to panic, stress, rumors, and confusion.
  - Encourage adequate food, rest, and recreation.
  - Have an open door policy that includes seeking care when needed.
  - Offer professional counselling to address anxiety and fears.

Suggested Reading

http://www.avma.org/disaster/responseguide/responseguide_toc.asp.
http://www.cdfa.ca.gov/ahfss/Animal_Health/Disaster_Preparedness.html.
http://www.cvma.net/images/cvmapdf/DisasterPlan.pdf.
http://www.fema.gov/pdf/areyouready/basic_preparedness.pdf.
http://www.fema.gov/pdf/business/guide/bizindst.pdf, Emergency Management Guide for Business and Industry.
www.areyouprepared.com.
www.hsus.org/disaster.
www.ibhs.org/business_protection.
www.osha.gov.
www.ready.gov.
www.readypets.com.
www.redcross.org.
www.sba.gov.
www.us-cert.gov.

CHAPTER 2.3
COMMUNITY ANIMAL EMERGENCY PLANNING

Kevin M. Dennison, DVM

1. Why should each community have an animal emergency plan within their local emergency operations plan?

Animal emergency issues impact public health and safety, animal health and safety, our agricultural system, and our environment. People will risk their lives to protect their animals, including both pets and livestock. Animal health and public health are interwoven issues that must be addressed during disasters. Livestock serve in a multitude of roles, including commercial food and fiber production, transportation, recreation, education (e.g., 4-H programs), and even companionship. Communities may contain animal facilities such as biomedical research facilities, zoos, wildlife sanctuaries, kennels, veterinary hospitals, and other facilities that may contain large numbers of animals and present special challenges. Finally, wildlife populations and habitat may be impacted by disasters. Over 95% of disasters are managed locally from start to finish. To protect people, animals and agriculture, local communities must be able to rapidly mobilize their resources to this task. Even if the community needs to seek additional outside resources, those responsible for the local animal emergency plan must be able to manage those incoming animal resources within the framework of the local plan.

2. What is the PETS Act?

In October of 2006, the Pet Evacuation and Transportation Standards Act (PETS Act) was signed into law. This bill is an amendment to the Stafford Act, a law that provides a cost-sharing mechanism between the federal government and state or local governments during response to and recovery from major disasters. The act also provides a mandate for states and local communities to take into account people with household pets and service animals within their local emergency plans. In addition, the PETS Act provides that expenses related to services for people with household pets and service animals (and for the care of those animals) qualify for cost sharing under the Stafford Act. The law also allows the FEMA administrator to support such state and local planning processes with grants. While there is no specific funding appropriated within the PETS Act, this clearly qualifies PETS-Act related efforts for inclusion under existing Emergency Management Performance Grants (EMPG) and State Homeland Security Grants (SHSG). While a case could already be made for the incorporation of animal issues into state and local emergency operations plans, the PETS Act created a specific federal mandate for inclusion of at least the household pets and service animal portions of an all-hazards, all-species animal emergency management plan.

3. What is the Post Katrina Emergency Management Reform Act?

The Post-Katrina Emergency Management Reform Act (PKEMRA) also became law in 2006. The statute provided some broad reforms for the Department of Homeland Security (including FEMA) and the broader emergency management community. Within the PKEMRA, is a provision that "Authorizes the provision of rescue, care, shelter, and essential needs to individuals with household pets and service animals and to such animals." The bill also "Directs the Administrator: (1) in approving standards for state and local emergency preparedness plans, to ensure that such plans take into account the needs of individuals with special needs and individuals with pets; (2) to ensure that each state, in its Homeland Security Strategy or other homeland security plan, provides comprehensive pre-disaster and post-disaster plans for individuals with special needs and their care givers and that such plans address the evacuation planning needs of those unable to evacuate themselves; and (3) to ensure that state and local emergency preparedness, evacuation, and sheltering plans take into account the needs of individuals with household pets prior to, during, and following a major disaster or emergency." Essentially, the PETS Act provides a mandate for state and local actions and the PKEMRA provides the federal government with a mandate to support such state and local plans and to provide federal support for such responses when needed.

4. Does FEMA set standards for state and local animal emergency plans that support people with household pets and service animals?

Since the PETS Act and the PKEMRA passage in 2006, the federal government has provided a number of policy or guidance documents for state, territorial, tribal, and local planners. These documents have included:

- Interim guidance issued to federal agencies and states in late 2006, based on a set of recommendations developed by the U.S. Animal Health Association (USAHA) Committee on Animal Emergency Management.
- *FEMA Disaster Assistance Policy DAP9523, Eligible Costs Related to Pet Evacuations and Sheltering*: This guidance defines household pets by animal types and lists the services and parties eligible for Stafford Act cost sharing.
- *Best Practice Shelter Operations: Pet-Friendly Shelters*: published in 2007 on the Lessons Learned Information Shared site www.LLIS.gov.
- *National Response Framework*: Released in early 2008, this document provides key changes in how companion animals are addressed in emergency management systems. Emergency Support Function (ESF) #11 (Agriculture and Natural Resources), led by the U.S. Department of Agriculture provides overall coordination for the safety and welfare of pets. In addition, ESF #6 (Mass Care and Human Services), ESF #8 (Public Health and Medical), ESF #9 (Search and Rescue), and ESF #14 (Long-Term Recovery) all now have responsibilities to address specific issues related to pets and service animals.
- In 2008, FEMA will also release a comprehensive guidance document on standards and best practices for state, territorial, tribal, and local plans that take into account people with household pets and service animals.

5. Who is responsible for creating the community animal emergency plan?

The community emergency manager is responsible for overall development of the local emergency operations plan. The emergency manager, however, is more like a conductor of an orchestra, with each community sector providing the bulk of planning for their specific area of expertise. While the elected officials and the local emergency manager are ultimately responsible for creating the animal plan, the local agencies and organizations within the community animal and agricultural sector must provide the bulk of the expertise and the actual work behind the plan.

6. Who should write the community animal emergency plan?

The community animal emergency plan should be written by a drafting group that includes the county emergency manager and a handful of community animal or agricultural experts. This core group of essential stakeholders and experts can get the first draft ready for discussion by a broader group of agencies, organizations, and individuals. Based on input from the stakeholders, the drafting group then develops additional draft versions until the plan is ready for final approval by elected officials.

7. How do you organize the essential stakeholders to develop the community animal emergency plan?

Identification of the essential stakeholders should be done early in the planning process. Agencies, organizations, and individuals that should be engaged in the planning process may include:

- Local emergency management
- Animal control agencies
- Law enforcement
- Public health agencies
- Veterinary professionals
- Cooperative Extension
- Animal shelters
- Fairgrounds
- Livestock associations
- Brand inspectors (mostly in western states)
- Livestock producers
- Pet rescue organizations
- Kennels and pet service providers
- Fire and EMS responders
- County mapping
- Wildlife agencies
- Significant at-risk facilities (zoos, wildlife sanctuaries, biomedical research facilities, etc.)
- Local chapters of Voluntary Organizations Active in Disaster (VOAD) and community voluntary organizations such as the American Red Cross, Salvation Army, United Way, 211, food banks, Amateur Radio Emergency Service (ARES), Adventist Community Services, and many more
- Concerned citizens/volunteers
- Community foundations/philanthropy organizations
- Jurisdictional legal staff (to address volunteer liability and workers compensation issues)

8. What is a community animal response team (CART)?

The term county or community animal response team (CART) is one of the more common nomenclatures for local animal emergency planning, preparedness, and response networks. In some communities, the CART program is a network of agencies and nongovernment organizations with volunteer participation routed through existing community organizations. Other communities, particularly ones with fewer preexisting community organizations that use volunteers, may establish a voluntary program in which volunteers are affiliated directly with local government. While the exact format and nomenclature varies greatly among local programs, they share some basic commonalities, including:

- Creates a unified network of community animal response resources in a system connected to local emergency management which collectively develops and executes the community animal emergency plan
- Helps communicate lead and supporting roles for various mission tasks to the network of stakeholders. This is particularly important since there is often high turnover in personnel over time within government, nongovernment organizations, private sector businesses, and community volunteers.
- Creates a pathway for volunteer involvement and provides a mechanism to address volunteer liability and accident issues
- Serves to facilitate training and exercises
- Supports community preparedness outreach

9. What are the components of a community animal emergency plan?

While the exact format and content of community animal emergency plan may vary significantly, one typical format for local emergency plans is as follows:

- Purpose and scope
- Authority
- Lead and support agencies
- Planning assumptions
- Activation
- Concept of operations
- Organizational summaries and planning matrix
- Attachments or appendices
  - Contact list
  - Resource list
  - Agreements
  - Operational guidelines or standard operating procedures

10. What is the Purpose and Scope section?

The Purpose and Scope section summarizes why the community needs the plan and discusses the span of the issues covered in the plan, for instance whether the plan covers companion animals, livestock, wildlife, zoological facilities, biomedical facilities, etc.

11. What is the Authority section?

The Authority section references the local, state or federal statutes or regulations that either provide local agencies with authority to enact the plan or create a mandate for such planning. The PETS Act and National Response Framework would be examples of federal mandates for community animal plan development. Emergency managers and community legal advisors can generally provide this information.

12. What is the Lead and Support Agencies section?

The Lead and Support Agencies section lists the local agency that has primary responsibility for implementation of the community animal emergency plan. Animal Control is most commonly the lead agency in urban communities. In smaller or more rural communities, Cooperative Extension is commonly the lead agency. In some cases, a nongovernment organization may be the lead agency (such as a humane organization) or local emergency management may provide that role directly. In a few cases, the CART program may be incorporated as a not-for-profit organization and serve as the lead agency. Supporting agencies and organizations are typically listed in this section, but their precise role is listed later in the plan. State agencies and organizations can be listed as supporting agencies, but the local community cannot assign state or federal agencies to perform specific functions. Local communities can list these higher levels of government as sources from which to request assistance. State or national nongovernment organizations may be listed as support agencies but should not be counted on for core elements of the plan since there is no guarantee that those resources will not be deployed elsewhere during a major disaster.

13. What are Planning Assumptions?

Planning Assumptions are key concepts that are used in development of the local animal emergency plan. Planning assumptions might include the following examples:

- Inability to evacuate animals is a leading cause for failure of people to evacuate during disasters.
- Failure by citizens to evacuate may both endanger those citizens and the emergency responders who attempt to protect them.
- The Americans with Disabilities Act mandates that service animals must be treated as an extension of a disabled person and must receive necessary services as such.
- While most owners of pets and livestock will take reasonable steps to evacuate, shelter and provide for their animals, others cannot or will not take adequate actions for the protection of their animals due to, for example, special needs, senior citizen issues, limited mobility, large numbers of animals in their possession, and language or cultural barriers.
- Animal agriculture is a critical element of our economy and national food supply.

14. What is the Activation section?

The Activation section describes the mechanisms and protocols for mobilizing and tasking community resources during an emergency incident. The plan should describe how local emergency management or incident command personnel will contact the lead agency and how the lead agency will begin mobilizing community animal resources. Activation should include mechanisms for both placing resources on standby and actually mobilizing them into the incident. The plan may contain a precaution against volunteer self-mobilization.

15. What is the Concept of Operations section?

The Concept of Operations section contains a description of the anticipated animal-related mission tasks and how these tasks will be addressed under the plan. For each mission area, there should be a short discussion of the lead entity (which may be a shared lead between two or more entities) and the support entities for each mission area. Some key operational policies may be included, but *detailed operational procedures should not be included in this section* since the community animal emergency plan will become part of policy of the elected officials. Adding too much detail to this section of the plan can hinder flexibility and perhaps even create liability if the policies set forth in the plan are not followed precisely. Too much information in this section also makes the plan difficult to understand.

16. What are the animal mission tasks that should be covered in the Concept of Operations?

Anticipated animal-related mission areas will vary somewhat among communities, but the following list should help planners determine what should be included in their community plan.

- **Rapid needs assessment:** Initial steps taken to size up responder safety, community needs, and create initial mission assignments under the community animal emergency plan.
- **Animal sheltering:** Companion animals, backyard livestock, commercial livestock, service animals, and animal facilities such as zoos, veterinary hospitals, kennels, etc. Sheltering may be collocated in close proximity to citizen emergency shelters, allowing people to help take care of their animals.
- **Animal evacuation and transportation**
- **Animal control and stray management**
- **Owner-pet reunion efforts:** To reunite owners and pets that might be separated during the incident.

- **Animal search and rescue:** including removal of animals stranded in evacuated areas, searching for trapped animals, and technical animal rescue (rope rescue, trailer extraction, ice, flood water, etc.)
- **Sheltering in place support:** Providing food, water, essential services for people sheltering in place with pets or livestock, and for animal facilities.
- **Support of commercial agricultural operations,** including maintenance of power, critical support services, feed, water, and movement of product to market (dairy, eggs, etc.)
- **Veterinary medical care and veterinary support for animal facilities,** including veterinary triage, veterinary medical services, infectious disease control, and veterinary support of public health needs.
- **Animal decontamination** for animal exposure to hazardous substances, including flood waters.
- **Wildlife management:** Typically this mission will be coordinated by state wildlife agencies but may include animal control, veterinary medical professionals and wildlife rehabilitation facilities.
- **Animal mortality management:** Dealing with dead animal carcasses or euthanasia of animals for disease control, public safety, or humane reasons.
- **Animal disease emergency support,** which includes the anticipated role of the community in supporting the response to a significant animal disease outbreak, such as highly pathogenic avian influenza, foot and mouth disease, or other foreign animal diseases.

17. What is the role of the community in supporting an animal disease emergency response?

Animal disease emergency response is generally led by state and federal agencies, but many community resources will be needed in large scale animal disease incidents. Mission tasks during animal disease emergency events may include:

- Clinical diagnosis and laboratory confirmation
- Quarantine management and enforcement
- Surveillance for disease
- Epidemiology (tracing back and forward)
- Appraisal and government indemnity payments
- Euthanasia and mortality management
- Decontamination and disinfection
- Movement permits & biosecurity compliance agreements (to keep healthy animals and product moving in the system)
- Mental health support for citizens impacted emotionally and economically
- Public information outreach
- Repopulation and recovery

Community resources that may be directly involved in supporting these mission tasks include:

- Local emergency management
- Law enforcement, brand inspectors, and animal control
- Cooperative Extension (an absolute key resource)
- Veterinary professionals
- Public health and mental health professionals
- Public works (heavy equipment)
- Fire and HAZMAT resources (decontamination)
- County mapping
- Livestock associations
- Local Voluntary Organizations Active in Disaster (VOAD)

18. What are Organizational Summaries?

Organizational Summaries list the lead and support entities individually and summarize the entity's responsibilities under the plan. Every organization listed in the lead and support entities should have an organizational summary, even if it is a brief description in bullet points about their responsibilities.

19. What is a Planning Matrix?

A Planning Matrix is a chart of the participating lead and support entities on one axis and the anticipated mission tasks on the opposite axis. This matrix creates a one-page summary of the entire plan in an easily understood visual representation. Lead and support agencies may be listed as a primary/lead entity, a shared/unified lead entity, a support entity, or not involved for each mission task. A sample of a simple planning matrix is included as Table 2.3.1.

Table 2.3.1 A Simple Community Animal Planning Matrix

Community agencies and organizations	Needs assessment	Sheltering companion animals	Sheltering livestock	Evacuation companion animals	Evacuation livestock	Animal control—stray management	Owner-animal reunion	Animal search and rescue	Veterinary medical response	Animal decontamination	Wildlife management
Emergency management	P	S	S	S	S	S	S	S	S	S	S
Animal control	S	S	S	P	S	P	S	P	S	S	S
Animal shelter		P					U		S	S	S
Brand inspector (state)	S		S		S		U	S		S	
Cooperative Extension	S		S	S	P		S			S	
Fairgrounds			P		S		S			S	
Fire department	S							S		S	
Law enforcement	S			S	S	S		S		S	S
Livestock associations			S		S		S			S	
Public health	S	S	S			S			S	S	S
Search and rescue organization	S			S	S			S		S	
Veterinary community	S	S	S	S	S		S	S	P	P	S
Wildlife agency (state)	S							S		S	P

P, primary responsibility for mission task; S, support responsibility for mission task; U, unified or shared primary responsibility for mission task.

20. What other components could be included in the community animal emergency plan?

Communities may want to add additional components to their animal emergency plan, including:

- **Preparedness outreach plan** to communicate essential preparedness information to animal service businesses, agribusinesses, and citizens.
- **Mitigation plan**—strategies to prevent or reduce the impact of hazards on community animal populations or agricultural operations.
- **Recovery plan**—listing the tasks and responsibilities for short-term and long-term recovery issues related to animal populations. After many disasters, a long-term recovery committee is formed to help address unmet needs and long-term issues. Community animal and agricultural stakeholders should participate in this committee.

21. What attachments should be developed for the community animal emergency plan?

Attachments or appendices to the community animal plan are documents that do not require the approval of elected officials. For that reason, most of the tactical elements of the plan should be invested in these documents. The more concise document will make the strategic elements of the plan more easily understood. Attachments commonly added to emergency plans include:

- Contact list
- Resource list
- Agreements
- Operational guidelines and forms

22. What is a contact list?

A contact list is a list of the lead and support entities and specific (preferably 24-hour) contact information for the individuals that represent those entities. A list of key volunteers along with their contact information could be included as well, although in many instances, volunteer contact information will be kept by the organization with which they are affiliated. In addition, the contact list should include state and federal entities that may be able to provide resource and technical support, such as:

- State veterinarian and/or state agriculture agency
- State animal response team or similar program
- State veterinary medical reserve corps or similar program
- State emergency management agency
- State wildlife agency
- State public health agency
- State land-grant university/Cooperative Extension
- State veterinary medical association
- State animal control and/or animal welfare association
- State voluntary organizations active in disaster
- Federal Emergency Management Agency (FEMA)
- U.S. Department of Agriculture (USDA)
- U.S. Department of Health and Human Services (DHHS)
- State or national animal welfare organizations with which the community has a working relationship

23. What is a resource list?

A resource list would be the list of the location and point of contact for equipment, facilities, specialized services, and supplies that can be accessed to support the community animal emergency plan. Examples of such resources include:

- Facilities that could be used for animal sheltering or warehousing animal or agricultural supplies
- Animal control and animal handling equipment
- Animal transportation equipment
- Veterinary facilities and mobile veterinary units
- Agricultural equipment, such as portable corral panels, portable chutes, pressure sprayers, and much more
- Wildlife rehabilitation facilities and chemical capture teams
- Teams that are "typed" as to their kind of service and level of capability (animal sheltering, animal search and rescue, veterinary teams, etc.)
- Any community resource that would be potentially useful in supporting the community animal emergency plan

24. What agreements should be listed or attached?

The Agreements section can include copies of contracts or agreements that are created in support of the local animal emergency plan, including:

- Agreements with facilities to be used for emergency animal sheltering
- Agreements with various local, state, or national organizations that could be requested to perform specific missions during an emergency incident
- Agreements between key stakeholders, such as a memorandum of agreement between the local animal shelter and the local chapter of the American Red Cross
- Contracts or agreements with private sector companies, such as heavy equipment contractors, vendors, private kennels or stables, veterinary hospitals, or any other private business

25. What are operational guidelines?

Operational guidelines are the anticipated tactical details of the community animal emergency plan. The core plan addresses what needs to be done and who will do it. Operational guidelines frame out how it will be done. The purpose of the guidelines is to be both conceptual and educational. There is no end to the amount of information that *could* be put into these supporting guidelines, but planners may need to limit this section to those elements necessary to ensure safety, mission success, and tactical coordination among the participating entities. Each participating entity may also develop internal policies and guidelines, but these do not necessarily have to be attached to the community animal emergency plan.

26. Where can a person find model community animal emergency plans?

There are numerous community animal emergency plans available on the Internet and links to a few of these are included at the end of this chapter. These plans are highly variable and should be evaluated carefully as to format and content. No single plan is suitable for every community! While these plans are helpful references, communities should be cautioned that your plan will only be effective because the stakeholders worked to create the plan. *Simply adapting even a well-written model plan to your community has little value unless your community's stakeholders become actively engaged in the planning process!*

27. How are community animal emergency plans approved?

In most communities, elected officials, such as a mayor, city council or county commissioners must approve emergency plans that are submitted to them through local emergency management agencies. For this reason, it is critical for local CART/planning networks to ensure that the planning process is guided by local emergency management. This process also reflects the need to keep the main part of the plan focused on strategic responsibilities and allow the tactical elements to fall to attachments. In this way, approval will not be needed from elected officials each time a tactical change is made.

28. Who needs to know about the community animal emergency plan?

A community animal emergency plan is only optimally effective if understood by all the relevant stakeholders. The lead and support agencies in the plan must make an ongoing effort to educate the community on the plan. Outreach should include the following:

- Local elected officials
- Emergency management and the lead and support agencies listed in the plan (as the leadership of these entities will change periodically)
- Community animal service businesses and agribusinesses
- Local media
- Community citizens

29. How does a community keep their plan functional?

Emergency plans will become outdated due to changing circumstances and normal leadership turnover in the lead and support agencies that will breed unfamiliarity with the plan. In order to maintain a functional plan, communities must adopt the following maintenance cycle after the initial development of the plan:

1. Educate the stakeholders on the plan
2. Periodically exercise the plan at least once yearly (or an element of the plan, as it may be very difficult to exercise the *entire* plan)
3. Review and revise the plan based on the outcome of the exercise.
4. Start over with No. 1.

30. What is the most important factor in the success of a community animal emergency plan?

Communities invest in animal and agricultural resources typically at the amount they can afford in order to address daily challenges. There is no community that will ever possess all the government and organizational resources they need to care for every animal and every related need during a major disaster. In order to achieve success, any plan must be supported by family preparedness plans that incorporate pets and livestock into the owner's plan and by business contingency plans for animal service businesses and agribusinesses. If 95% of the impacted families and businesses can take care of their own animals, the community animal emergency plan can focus on the 5% that have special needs or are so severely impacted that their personal or business plans were not enough. The most important element of the community animal emergency plan, therefore, is the personal and business preparedness plans of the citizens of that community!

Suggested Reading

American Veterinary Medical Association. Disaster resources page including links to state resources, 2008. Available at http://www.avma.org/disaster/default.asp.
Colorado Division of Emergency Management, model community animal emergency plan. Available at http://www.dola.state.co.us/dem/plans/plans.htm, 2007.
Colorado State Animal Response Team site. Available at http://www.cosart.org, 2008.
Department of Homeland Security. Lessons Learned and Information Shared site—Registration and password needed to access. Available at http://LLIS.gov, 2008.
Extension Disaster Education Network site. Available at http://www.eden.lsu.edu/, 2008.
Florida State Agricultural Response Team site. Available at http://flsart.org/, 2008.
Hillsborough County, Florida: County Animal and Agricultural Response Team site. Available at http://chaart.org/, 2008.
Minnesota local animal emergency plan template. Available at http://www.hsem.state.mn.us/uploadedfile/state_animal_eog.pdf, 2005.
National Alliance of State Animal and Agricultural Emergency Programs. Available at http://www.nasaaep.org (under development 5/2008).
North Carolina State Animal Response Team site. Available at http://ncsart.org, 2008.
Texas State Animal Resource Team site. Available at http://txsart.org, 2008.

CHAPTER 2.4
STATE RESPONSE TO VETERINARY DISASTERS

Terry K. Paik, DVM

1. What constitutes an emergency?

An emergency is a critical event that threatens lives, property, or resources. Emergencies can usually be handled by a local practitioner, rescue group, humane association, etc.

2. What constitutes a disaster?

A disaster is a critical event that threatens lives, property, or resources *and overwhelms* the local ability to manage the situation. Disasters require a coordinated effort to respond and aid in recovery effectively and efficiently.

3. What are the stages in planning for disaster?

Disaster planning is not something you can do once, put it on a shelf, and expect it to work when the next "big one" occurs. It is an ongoing, growing, ever-changing, evolving process. After every exercise, training, or event there are lessons to be learned—what went well and what did not? How can we improve and be more prepared and more responsive next time? Create your after-action reports and read them; share them with your cohorts as well as up and down the chain of command.

The following are the components in disaster planning. Note that they do not create a static list, but a cycle for knowledge, learning, and improvement (Fig. 2.4.1).

- **Awareness:** becoming knowledgeable and cognizant of populations, hazards, risks, and vulnerabilities. Hazard analysis is a process used to assess risk and increase awareness.
- **Preparedness:** a continuous process involving efforts at all levels of government and between government and private sector and nongovernmental organizations to identify threats, determine vulnerabilities, and identify required resources.
- **Mitigation:** activities designed to reduce or eliminate risks to persons or property or to lessen the actual or potential effects or consequences of an incident and may include actions taken to avoid an incident or to intervene to stop an incident from occurring. This includes applying intelligence and other information to a range of activities that may include such countermeasures as deterrence operations; security operations; investigations to determine the full nature and source of the threat; public health and agricultural surveillance and testing; and law enforcement operations aimed at deterring, preempting, interdicting, or disrupting illegal activity and apprehending perpetrators. Mitigation measures are often developed in accordance with lessons learned from prior incidents.
- **Detection:** the finding out or being found out, especially of what tends to elude notice. The sooner we know an event has occurred, the sooner we can respond and minimize losses. This can be especially critical in a foreign animal disease outbreak, e.g., foot and mouth disease.
- **Response:** activities that address the short-term, direct effects of an incident. These activities include immediate actions to preserve life, property, and the environment; meet basic human needs; and maintain the social,

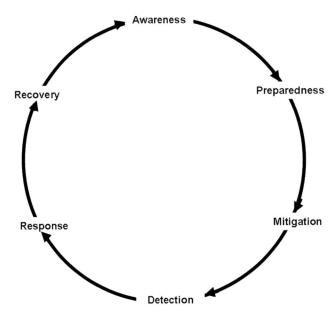

Figure 2.4.1 Stages of planning for a disaster.

economic, and political structure of the affected community. Response also includes the execution of emergency operations plans designed to limit loss of life, and property.

- **Recovery:** actions and the implementation of programs necessary to help individuals, communities, and the environment directly impacted by an incident return to normal. These actions assist victims and their families, restore institutions to regain economic stability and confidence, rebuild or replace destroyed property, address environmental contamination, and reconstitute government operations and services.

4. What is the role of the state during an animal disaster?

Every state has a written disaster plan. This plan will be with the Department of Homeland Security, Office of Emergency Services, or your state's equivalent.

Here are some examples:

- California—The Governor's Office of Emergency Services (www.oes.ca.gov/)
- Colorado—Colorado Department of Local Affairs (http://www.dola.state.co.us/dem/plans/plans.htm)
- Florida—Division of Emergency Management (http://www.floridadisaster.org/index.asp)
- Texas—The Governor's Division of Emergency Management (GDEM) (http://www.txdps.state.tx.us/dem/pages/index.htm)
- New York—New York State Emergency Management Office (http://www.semo.state.ny.us/)

The governor, as the executive head of state, has the responsibility and the authority to commit state and local resources (personnel, equipment, and financial) to meet the dangers presented by disasters.

The governor's Office of Emergency Services (OES) is the state agency charged as the lead organization in disasters. The OES is responsible for the coordination and leadership of all state agencies during declared emergencies.

The State Operations Center (SOC) will be activated at the governor's proclamation of a state of emergency. In California, the SOC will also be activated when a Regional Level Emergency Operations Center (REOC) is activated or after the governor's proclamation of an earthquake or volcanic prediction.

During a declared local emergency, an Emergency Operations Center (EOC) is activated to provide resources from the non-impacted areas to the impacted areas within the Operational Area.

5.   What is a hazard analysis?

A hazard analysis is a process used to assess risk. The goal of a hazard analysis is the identification of unacceptable risks and the selection of means of controlling or eliminating them to reduce the vulnerability of people and property to the effects of emergencies and disasters.

It will include a synopsis of the state's at-risk populations and the major hazards to which the state is vulnerable.

The Emergency Response Plan should determine the types of disasters likely to affect the state and the specific areas most likely to be affected by each of these hazards. In areas with high population concentration, major industrial activities, and history of major disaster events warrant special consideration.

Demographic information, population locations of people and animals, should be shared between the local jurisdictions and the state.

Keep in mind the following possibilities:

- Earthquakes
- Fires
- Floods
- Landslides
- Tornados/Hurricanes
- Volcanic Activity
- Severe weather, drought
- Foreign animal disease (FAD)
- Railroad accidents
- Oil/Chemical spills
- Nuclear accidents
- Electrical outage
- Dam levy failures
- Hazardous materials
- Transportation infrastructure
- Cyber

And of course, one must now add to the list terrorism. The U.S. Department of Homeland Security (DHS) has established objectives for a national effort to prevent terrorist attacks within the United States and reduce its vulnerability to terrorism, natural disasters, and other emergencies; and to minimize the damage, and recover from attacks, natural disasters, and other emergencies.

The following tables are taken from the Colorado State Emergency Operations Plan (March 2007) as samples of a Hazard Analysis. Colorado is divided into nine All-Hazard Emergency Management Regions. Table 2.4.1 provides a list of disaster event probabilities, based on historical data. The frequency time frame is from an average of recorded occurrences of a given event and should not be considered as an absolute indicator of when the next occurrence of an emergency or disaster event will happen. Because of the geological diversity within the state, it is difficult to establish a statewide probability of future occurrences.

There is a probability of the occurrence of major events striking simultaneously or within a close time frame. There is also the strong probability that the occurrence of one event will trigger one or more secondary events. Local and State emergency managers must plan for these secondary or cascading events. The correlation between the occurrence of a primary event and its secondary or cascading effect is shown graphically in Table 2.4.2.

6.   What is SEMS?

As a result of the 1991 Oakland Hills Firestorm, a law was passed by the CA legislature in 1993 to improve the coordination of state and local emergency response in California. The statute directed the governor's OES, in coordination with other state agencies and interested local emergency management agencies, to establish the *Standardized Emergency Management System (SEMS)*.

Table 2.4.1 Colorado Divided into Nine All-Hazard Emergency Management Regions—List of Disaster Event Probabilities, Based on Historical Data

	Avalanche	Drought	Earthquake	Flood	Landslide	Tornado	Wildfire	Winter Storm	Civil Disorder*	Dam Failure	HAZMAT	Subsidence	Transportation	Utility Disruption	Urban Fire (Major)*	Terrorism*
North central	1	1	2	3	3	3	3	3		3	3	1	3	3		
Northeast	1	2	1	3		3	3			3	2	2	2	2		
Northwest	3	3	1	2	3	2	2	2		2	1	1	1	2		
San Luis	2	3	1	2	1	2	2	2		2	1	1	1	2		
South central	2	2	2	2	2	3	3	2		2	3	3	3	3		
South	1	3	1	2	1	2	2	3		1	2	2	2	3		
Southeast	1	3	1	2	1	3	2	2		1	1	1	2	2		
Southwest	2	3	1	2	1	1	3	2		2	1	2	1	2		
West	3	2	1	2	3	2	3	2		2	2	3	2	2		

*Actual figures are unavailable.

Probabilities

High   3
Moderate   2
Low   1

(Based on State of Colorado, State Emergency Operations Plan, March 2007, Colorado Department of Local Affairs. Available at http://www.dola.state.co.us/dem/operations/seop2007/base_plan.pdf.)

Table 2.4.2 Occurrence of One Event Will Trigger One or More Secondary Events

	Avalanche	Drought	Earthquake	Flood	Landslide	Tornado	Wildfire	Winter Storm	Civil Disorder	Dam Failure	HAZMAT	Utility Disruption	Subsidence	Transportation	Urban Fire
Avalanche										►	►	►	►	►	
Drought							►								
Earthquake	►			►	►					►	►	►	►	►	►
Flood				►						►	►	►	►	►	
Landslide				►						►	►	►	►	►	
Tornado										►	►	►	►	►	
Wildfire				►	►					►	►	►	►	►	
Winter storm	►			►	►					►	►	►	►	►	
Civil disorder							►					►	►		►
Dam failure				►								►	►	►	
HAZMAT									►						
Utility disruption										►	►				
Subsidence														►	
Transportation							►				►			►	
Urban fire											►				
Terrorism	►									►	►	►	►	►	►

The ► indicates the types of secondary or cascading events that can be triggered by the primary event.
(Based on State of Colorado, State Emergency Operations Plan, March 2007, Colorado Department of Local Affairs. Available at http://www.dola.state.co.us/dem/operations/seop2007/base_plan.pdf.)

The SEMS is a statewide California system used in disaster events. The primary goal of SEMS is to aid in communication and response by providing a common management system and language, essential in the successful management of any incident. State agencies and local governments are required to use SEMS to participate in disasters.

The basic framework of SEMS incorporates the use of the Incident Command System (ICS), multiagency, or interagency coordination, the state's master mutual aid agreement, and mutual aid program.

SEMS is designed to be flexible and adaptable to the variety of emergencies that can occur in California and to meet the emergency management needs of all responders. By California law, state agencies must use SEMS when responding to emergencies involving multiple jurisdictions or multiple agencies. Local governments are strongly encouraged to use SEMS, and they must use SEMS in order to be eligible for state funding of certain response-related personnel costs.

SEMS is a management system. It provides an organizational framework and acts as the umbrella under which all response agencies may function in an integrated fashion. Training is essential to the effective use of SEMS at all levels.

Today the National Incident Management System (NIMS) is based on the same principles and structures that made SEMS so effective for the state of California.

7. What are the priorities of incident management?

The premise of the National Response Plan (NRP) and all state's plans is that all levels of government share the responsibility for working together in preventing, preparing for, responding to, and recovering from the effects of a disaster. Remember, all events begin and end locally. Each level of government will respond to an emergency or disaster to the extent of its available resources. Once these resources have been exhausted, mutual aid will be requested. If these are determined to be insufficient, then requests will go up the chain from local to state and state to federal government.

The priorities for incident management are to:

- Save lives and protect the health and safety of the public, responders, and recovery workers
- Ensure security of the homeland
- Protect and restore critical infrastructure
- Protect property and mitigate damages and impacts to individuals, communities, and the environment
- Facilitate recovery of individuals, families, businesses, governments, and the environment
- When appropriate, conduct law enforcement investigations to resolve the incident, apprehend the perpetrators, and collect and preserve evidence for prosecution. Note any indications of a terrorist act.
- Life-saving and life-protecting response activities have precedence over other emergency response activities, except when national security implications are determined to be of a higher priority.

One thing we need to remind ourselves in the veterinary community is that *people come before animals*. Like it or not, that's just the way it is.

8. What are the designated levels in the SEMS organization?

There are five designated levels in the SEMS organization; and the levels are activated as needed for an emergency. They are as follows:

- **Field Response Level** is where emergency response personnel and resources, under the command of an appropriate authority, carry out tactical decisions and activities in direct response to an incident or threat. Remember, all disasters start and end locally.
- **Local Government Level** includes cities, counties, and special districts. Local governments manage and coordinate the overall emergency response and recovery activities within their jurisdiction. Local governments are required to use SEMS when their Emergency Operations Center (EOC) is activated or a local emergency is declared or proclaimed in order to be eligible for state funding of response-related personnel costs.

- **Operational Area** encompasses the county and all political subdivisions located within the county including special districts.
  - ○ The operational area manages and/or coordinates information, resources, and priorities among local governments within the operational area.
  - ○ It also serves as the coordination and communication link between the local government level and regional level.
- **Region**—because of its size and geography, the state is usually divided into mutual aid regions. The regional level:
  - ○ Provides for the more effective application and coordination of mutual aid and other emergency related activities
  - ○ Manages and coordinates information and resources among operational areas within the region and also between the operational areas and the state level
- **The State Level**
  - ○ Manages state resources in response to the emergency needs of other levels
  - ○ Manages and coordinates mutual aid among mutual aid regions and between the regional level and state level
  - ○ Serves as the coordination and communication link between the state and the federal disaster response system
  - ○ Conducts operations from the State Operations Center (SOC) and is under the management of the Governor's Office of Emergency Services (OES)

9. What are the responsibilities of the State Operations Center (SOC)?

- Support the regions, state agencies, and other entities in establishing short-term recovery operations following disasters.
- Act as overall state coordinator in the event of simultaneous multiregional disasters such as earthquakes, fires, or floods. In this situation, provide interregional policy direction and coordination for emergencies involving more than one Regional Emergency Operations Centers (REOC) activation. Monitor and facilitate interregional communications and coordination issues.
- Compile and authenticate disaster status information obtained from all sources, in the form of Situation Reports ("SitReps"). These reports should be available to the governor's office, the legislature, state agencies, media, and others as appropriate.
- Provide on-going interagency coordination.
- Manage the state's Emergency Public Information program.
- Provide and maintain state headquarters linkage and inter-agency coordination with the Federal Response System.
- Assist in the planning for short-term recovery, and assist state agencies and REOCs in developing and coordinating recovery action plans.

10. What is mutual aid?

Incidents frequently require responses that exceed the resource capabilities of the affected response agencies and jurisdictions. When this occurs, mutual aid is provided by other jurisdictions and agencies. Mutual aid is voluntary aid and assistance by the provision of services and facilities including but not limited to fire, police, medical and health, communications, transportation, and utilities. Mutual aid is intended to provide adequate resources, facilities, and other support to jurisdictions whenever their own resources prove to be inadequate to cope with a given situation.

Nongovernment organizations (NGOs) (e.g., community-based organizations, collaboratives, private agencies, etc.) may participate in the mutual aid system along with governmental agencies. NGOs are an essential component of any disaster response, and their cooperation and level of participation should be established early in the planning process. Level of expectations, when and how they are to be deployed (and demobilized), responsibilities, limitations, liabilities, command and control, and other relevant factors should be clearly defined beforehand with a signed memorandum of understanding (MOU).

11. How does the state response fit with the local response?

During a disaster, if local resources are insufficient to meet existing needs, local government may request state assistance. When this assistance is requested; the Governor's OES will activate the State Disaster Plan. The ability to respond effectively at the state level largely depends upon planning accomplished between the state and local jurisdictions (REOC). Since the majority of volunteers, resources, and organization during a disaster originate in the local area, it is essential that counties and local agencies have animal response plans in place before disaster strikes.

The level of coordination required with the REOC will be determined by the type of emergency, the ability of the REOC to perform assigned functions, and the level of required interaction between the two state levels. While the REOC will have primary responsibility for state interaction with affected operational areas, the State SOC will perform the following activities, which require close interaction with the REOC:

- Prepare and release the State Situation Report—It will be the responsibility of the SOC to collect and authenticate material from all available sources, and to compile and release Situation Reports.
- Develop state-level public information announcements—In any major disaster that involves multiple state agencies, it is essential that there be coordination of the release of public information about the state response.
- Coordinate the involvement of all activated mutual aid systems to ensure they are functioning effectively and sharing information, and to ensure there is no resource ordering duplications taking place through the several mutual aid channels.
- Ensure REOC-SOC coordination takes place.

(See Chapter 2.3 on local response.)

12. How does the state response fit with the federal response?

The federal government has responsibilities to respond to national emergencies and to provide assistance to states when an emergency or disaster is beyond the states' capability to handle. The Department of Homeland Security has the overall responsibility for the coordination of federal emergency/disaster relief programs and supporting local and state government capabilities with resources.

The governor will review information collected to determine if a state emergency should be declared and if a presidential disaster declaration should be requested. If the governor finds that effective response to an event is beyond the combined response capabilities of the state and affected local governments, the governor may request the president declare a major disaster or emergency. The governor must submit a request for assistance to the president within 5 days of determining the need for emergency assistance and within 30 days of the event for a major declaration.

In the event of a catastrophic incident, where the magnitude and severity of damages are expected to be extreme and there is an immediate need for supplemental federal assistance, the governor may make an expedited request for a presidential disaster declaration. This request will not include specific estimates of damage and the amount of federal assistance necessary but will outline the anticipated impacts of the disaster.

The declaration triggers the implementation of federal disaster assistance programs, which are coordinated by the Federal Emergency Management Agency (FEMA), in cooperation with the state OES. Emergency Support Function (ESF) Annexes contain detailed information associated with a specific ESF. In a Presidential declaration, state ESFs will work directly with the corresponding national ESF. It is imperative that designated lead state departments understand the relationship between the state ESFs and the national ESFs.

Response and recovery operations in both state and federally declared disasters will be conducted in accordance with the standards set forth by the National Incident Management System (NIMS) and the National Response Framework (NRF). In the event of a Federal Disaster Declaration, ESF #11 (Agriculture and Natural Resources) will be activated by DHS/FEMA under the NRF (National Response Framework.)

The REOC(s) is the primary point of contact to provide status information and make resource requests to the state. State functional elements and counterpart federal personnel should work closely together at the same location when possible. ESF #11 includes the following functions:

- **Responding to animal and plant diseases and pests:** Includes implementing an integrated federal, state, tribal, and local response to an outbreak of a highly contagious or economically devastating animal/zoonotic disease, or an outbreak of a harmful or economically significant plant pest or disease. ESF #11 ensures, in coordination with ESF #8—Public Health and Medical Services, that animal/veterinary issues in natural disasters are supported. These efforts are coordinated by USDA's Animal and Plant Health Inspection Service (APHIS).
- **Ensuring the safety and security of the commercial food supply:** Includes the execution of routine food safety inspections and other services to ensure the safety of food products that enter commerce. This includes the inspection and verification of food safety aspects of slaughter and processing plants, products in distribution and retail sites, and import facilities at ports of entry; laboratory analysis of food samples; control of products suspected to be adulterated; plant closures; foodborne disease surveillance; and field investigations. These efforts are coordinated by USDA's Food Safety and Inspection Service (FSIS).
- **Providing for the safety and well-being of household pets:** Supports the Department of Homeland Security (DHS)/Federal Emergency Management Agency (FEMA) together with ESF #6—Mass Care, Emergency Assistance, Housing, and Human Services; ESF #8; ESF #9—Search and Rescue; and ESF #14—Long-Term Community Recovery to ensure an integrated response that provides for the safety and well-being of household pets. The ESF #11 effort is coordinated by USDA/APHIS.

13. Why plan for animal issues during a disaster?

In disasters, the first priority is the protection of life, property, and the environment. Unfortunately, in the past, this has not included a coordinated response for the evacuation, care, and sheltering of animals. Although the protection of human life is the highest priority in emergency response, recent disasters and follow-up research have shown that proper preparation and effective coordination of animal issues enhances the ability of emergency personnel to protect both human and animal health and safety. It is much more efficient, effective, and inexpensive to develop plans to address animal issues prior to an incident than during one. The following issues highlight why animal preparedness is necessary:

- **Refusal to evacuate and early return to unsafe areas.** Since human evacuation shelters do not allow pets in facilities, pet owners requiring sheltering must choose between deserting their animals, refusing to evacuate, or evacuating their animals to a predetermined site. Without advanced planning, this can be a difficult decision. Farmers and ranchers who depend on animals for their livelihood are often unwilling to leave their animals unsupervised in the event of a disaster. Some key facts to consider are:
  ○ Up to 25% of pet owners will fail to evacuate because of their animals; this represents 5% to 10% of the total population directed to evacuate.
  ○ From 30% to 50% of pet owners will leave pets behind, even with advance notice of evacuation.
  ○ Approximately 50% to 70% of people leaving animals behind will attempt to reenter a secure site to rescue their animals; this represents 5% to 15% of the total population directed to evacuate.
  ○ The 10% to 25% of individuals who refuse to evacuate or attempt to return to the evacuated areas because of their animals risk injury, exposure to hazardous materials, and their own lives, as well as those of emergency response personnel who must rescue them. The most effective and efficient way to minimize human and animal health and safety risks is for individuals and responding agencies to be properly prepared to address animal issues well in advance of a disaster.
- **Public health and safety risks caused by animals at large.** Animals that are not cared for by their owners during a disaster may become a public health and safety risk. Loose and displaced animals are possible carriers of disease (such as rabies and plague) and can become a nuisance or danger to people. Animals "at large" are the responsibility of local animal control officials.

- **Public relations considerations.** Society views animals as dependent upon human care and support. Many pets are considered integral parts of families. Animals and animal issues attract media attention. This is particularly true during a disaster. Public concern and support for animals during the disaster are higher now than ever. The failure to deal with animal issues in disasters not only results in utilizing more resources and placing additional human lives at risk, but can result in significant public outcry and negative media coverage.

14. Who is in charge of the state's animal plan?

In the CA SEMS organization, an animal services coordinator, who serves within the "Operations" section, is either a veterinarian, animal control officer, or other knowledgeable person trained in disaster response, animal care, and animal rescue.

In other states, it may be the state veterinarian, state Department of Food and Agriculture, or some other named entity.

15. Who are the players in the state's animal plan?

Two critical positions in the ICS are the Public Information Officer and the Liaison Officer.

- The *Public Information Officer (PIO)* develops and releases information about emergency operations to the news media, personnel involved in the response operations, and other appropriate agencies and organizations. The PIO is the only official spokesperson for the agency. Conflicting or inconsistent messages only lead to confusion and loss of the public's faith in the system.
- The *Liaison Officer* communicates with other agencies who may be intimately involved with the incident. An example would be the Cattlemen and Dairy Associations in the event of a foreign animal disease (FAD) outbreak.

It is important at the state level, just as it is in the local and federal levels, to develop a cadre of animal resources to aid in the event of a disaster. No single entity or organization can maintain enough resources on hand to adequately respond to a disaster.

Lead agencies must develop relationships with other groups, agencies, companies, etc., which can offer assistance during times of need. MOUs (memoranda of understanding) should be in place to clearly define roles and what is expected from each organization. The following is a list of possible stakeholders:

- *Voluntary Organizations*
  - State Veterinary Medical Association
  - American Veterinary Medical Association (AVMA)
  - Veterinary Medical Reserve Corps (VMRC)
  - Humane Societies/Society for the Prevention of Cruelty to Animals (SPCA)
  - State animal response team (SART)
  - Animal welfare groups
  - School groups (4-H, FFA, Animal Science Clubs, etc.)
  - Wildlife rehabilitation groups
  - Local food banks
  - Other disaster response agencies (Red Cross, Salvation Army, Code 3 Associates, etc.)
  - Animal clubs
- *Industry Groups*
  - Cattlemen, dairy, or equestrian associations
  - Farriers
  - Animal transporters
  - Pet food and supply businesses
  - Commercial animal industries (breeders, stables, kennels, beef, dairy, and poultry producers, etc.)
  - Horse track representatives
  - Fair organizations

16. How does the state manage volunteers during a disaster?

Experience has shown that when animals are impacted by disasters, a large number of self-responders will arrive to address the situation. These well-meaning, but untrained and emotionally driven, individuals can be very disruptive and create many law enforcement challenges. Additionally, these situations may encourage the arrival of "rescue groups." Some of these groups are well-trained and helpful, and some are not. Effective control of self-responding individuals and rescue groups is critical. This can occur only when a well-coordinated official response is in place. A county animal plan allows for appropriate identification and utilization of all available resources within the structure of the county animal response plan. This will minimize the intrusion of untrained and unsolicited volunteers in a crisis situation.

To facilitate this, local agencies need to develop relationships with bona fide volunteer organizations they know and trust. The volunteer organizations should be able to demonstrate levels of training (including ICS), accountability, and credentialing.

Level of expectations, when and how they are to be deployed (and demobilized), responsibilities, limitations, liabilities, command and control, and other relevant factors should be clearly defined beforehand with a signed MOU.

17. What is SART?

State animal response teams (SARTs) are interagency state organizations dedicated to preparing, planning, responding and recovering during animal emergencies in their respective states.

SART programs train participants to facilitate a safe, environmentally sound, and efficient response to animal emergencies on the local, county, state, and federal levels. The teams are organized under the auspices of state and local emergency management using the principles of the Incident Command System (ICS).

SARTs can be organized on the grassroots level with county animal response teams (CARTs). CARTs are under the jurisdiction of the county emergency management and include animal control officers, cooperative extension, sheriff's personnel, veterinarians, forestry officers, animal industry leaders and concerned citizens. (Figure 2.4.2). See Chapter 2.5 for more information on SART.

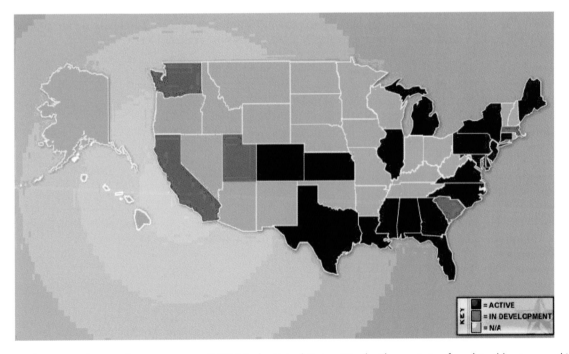

Figure 2.4.2 Statewide animal response teams (SARTs) in the United States. (Used with permission from http://sartusa.org/.)

18. We are now hearing about "medical and veterinary medical reserve corps." Describe what these organizations are and how they fit into the picture of disaster response.

The Medical Reserve Corps (MRC) is a national network of volunteer units that, under the sponsorship of the U.S. Surgeon General and local groups, supplement community resources for emergency response and public health. The MRC are looking for more veterinarians to join the ranks of physicians, nurses, pharmacists, dentists, and other health professionals who volunteer with community health teams. The 5-year-old corps has about 700 units, but 500 units do not have any veterinarians on their roster. Veterinarians and veterinary technicians can support the dual role of MRC units in responding locally to disasters and supporting the regular activities of health departments. Veterinarians could also serve as consultants on zoonoses, for example. The MRC structure allows health professionals to volunteer their full medical expertise during emergencies—because their unit will verify their credentials beforehand. The MRC is developing a mechanism to allow volunteers to help with a federal response outside their jurisdiction.

In several states, MRC units have formed specifically as a veterinary corps (VMRC) or animal response team. Now, the multidisciplinary MRC units are trying to incorporate more veterinarians. For example, the MRC unit in Las Vegas, under the sponsorship of the Southern Nevada Health District, counts a number of veterinarians among its members.

See Chapter 2.5 for more information on VMRC.

19. What is the role of the American Veterinary Medical Association (AVMA) in state animal responses during a disaster?

The AVMA created the Veterinary Medical Assistance Teams (VMAT) in 1993 as a private-federal partnership (with the Department of Health and Human Services) to provide veterinary emergency response at the national level. During deployment, VMAT members became temporary federal employees under the National Disaster Medical System (NDMS).

In late 2005–2006, the NDMS created their own National Veterinary Response Teams (NVRT) as a government program. Currently, the AVMA is exploring various directions for its VMAT program, such as assisting states during emergencies (see http://www.avma.org/onlnews/javma/may08/080515d.asp).

Suggested Reading
CA SEMS. http://www.oes.ca.gov/Operational/OESHome.nsf/Content/B49435352108954488256C2A0071E038?OpenDocument.
County Animal Disaster Preparedness and Response Planning Guide. http://www.cdfa.ca.gov/AHFSS/Animal_Health/Disaster_Preparedness.html.
DANR Guide to Disaster Preparedness, Division of Agriculture and Natural Resources, Veterinary Medicine Extension, University of California. www.vetmed.ucdavis.edu/vetext/INF-DI_DANRGuide.html.
Medical Reserve Corps. www.avma.org/onlnews/javma/nov07/071101n.asp.
SART. http://sartusa.org/.
STATE OF COLORADO, State Emergency Operations Plan, March 2007, Colorado Department of Local Affairs. http://www.dola.state.co.us/dem/operations/seop2007/base_plan.pdf.

CHAPTER 2.5
STATE ANIMAL AND AGRICULTURAL EMERGENCY PROGRAMS (INCLUDING STATE ANIMAL RESPONSE TEAM [SART] PROGRAMS AND STATE VETERINARY MEDICAL RESERVE CORPS [VMRC])

Kevin M. Dennison, DVM

1. What are state animal and agricultural emergency programs?

Each state has to develop mechanisms of addressing both animal and agricultural emergency management issues. Each state, however, has a unique statutory environment in which animal and agricultural issues are regulated. In addition, states have differing strengths and challenges, different risks, variable resources, and a unique political environment. For these reasons, we have 50 states that are addressing these issues through 50 variations and a wide variety of nomenclatures. Perhaps someday there will be more uniformity, but until that day, the state-to-state variations must be accepted in forging a national animal and agricultural emergency management system.

2. What are the two general mechanisms states have to address animal issues in disasters?

- State agencies, such as a department of agriculture, state veterinarian, or state emergency management agency can address these issues through exerting their statutory authorities and building direct partnerships with nongovernmental entities.
- States may develop programs that are designed to supplement state agencies through helping to coordinate multiple state-level stakeholders, building a partnership between the state and the private sector, supporting local animal or agricultural emergency response capacity, developing private sector funding resources, and facilitating the use of volunteers, including both animal professionals and citizen volunteers.

3. What are SART or similar programs?

The acronym SART can mean State Animal Response Team, State Agricultural Response Team, or State Animal Resource Team, depending on the state involved. In addition, there are several states using terminology close to SART, such as the State of Maine Animal Response Team (SMART), or Mississippi Animal Response Team (MART). A few other states use a very different nomenclature for programs that have some similar functions, such as the California Animal Response Emergency System (CARES), or Utah Emergency Animal Response Coalition (UEARC). For the purposes of this chapter, the term SART will be used broadly to include all state programs of this category.

4. Describe a brief history of the origin of SART?

Hurricane Floyd hit the Atlantic coast of the United States in 1999, creating havoc and major damage in North Carolina and several other states. Several key stakeholders in North Carolina, including the Department of Agriculture, North Carolina State University, and the veterinary medical community, developed a program to better prepare North Carolina to address animal issues in future disasters. The North Carolina State Animal Response Team (SART) was developed to facilitate all-hazards, all-species animal emergency response capacity and to build a partnership between the private sector and government. The program was managed through a newly formed charitable not-for-profit corporation in order to be able to supplement governmental funding with grants, sponsorships, and donations. In April 2003, the American Veterinary Medical Foundation funded a two-day session in Colorado whereby several North Carolina State Animal Response Team leaders facilitated a two-day strategic summit designed to explore exporting the SART concept to additional states. Colorado was selected based on a record wildfire year in 2002 and a willingness of the key stakeholders to participate in this event. The net result of the Colorado summit was to create the Colorado SART program within the Colorado Veterinary Medical Foundation, with Colorado SART beginning operations in July 2003.

Shortly thereafter, Florida and Georgia developed State Agricultural Response Team (SART) programs as governmentally administered programs to address critical needs in their states. Subsequently, North Carolina SART has continued to host additional summits in multiple states with the support of USDA (2004-2005) and later through grants from PetSmart Charities. Other states with SART-type programs include Pennsylvania, Massachusetts, Maine, Kansas, Virginia, Maryland, New York, Delaware, Lousiana, Mississippi, Texas, Oklahoma, and others. It should be noted that many other states developed a variety of programs without the SART nomenclature during this period. At the time of this publication, there are SART or similar programs in nearly three-fourths of the states.*

5. What are state Veterinary Medical Reserve Corps (VMRC) or similar programs?

Many states have developed VMRC programs under a variety of names, but we will use the acronym VMRC in this chapter to denote all similar state programs. Some states have VMRCs that fulfill some of the roles of a typical SART program (e.g., WY, OK); some states have VMRCs in addition to a SART program (e.g., CO, NC, FL). In some states, the VMRC is a unit of the Medical Reserve Corps program (e.g., CO, MN, OK) (see Question No. 6), and in some cases the VMRC is a program of the chief animal health official (e.g., ND, SD, MT, ID, NC, AZ). In some states the VMRC is focused on animal disease response, and in some states the program has a broader mission, including all-hazards emergency response. In all cases, VMRCs provide a mechanism to mobilize trained and credentialed veterinary professionals from the private sector to support the emergency needs of that state. At the writing of this chapter there are over 20 state VMRC programs in the United States.*

6. What is the Medical Reserve Corps (MRC)?

Medical Reserve Corps is a national program under the Office of the Surgeon General that provides a mechanism to involve voluntary medical professionals and support personnel in emergency preparedness, emergency response, and community public health efforts. MRC is affiliated with Citizen Corps, a federally coordinated set of community voluntary programs that also includes Community Emergency Response Teams (CERT), Volunteers in Police Service (VIPS), Neighborhood Watch, and Fire Corps. Medical Reserve Corps units are typically affiliated with local government, but MRC now includes an increasing number of statewide veterinary MRC units. This relationship has been productive in helping to bridge public health and animal health in emergency management. At the writing of this chapter, there are over 700 MRC units in our country with six state veterinary MRCs among them. These numbers continue to grow each year.

7. How do SART or VMRC programs contribute to state emergency management for animals and/or agriculture?

SART and VMRC programs provide several key services to their state, although the particular role of each program may vary with each respective state. In general, however, these programs provide the following:

- Support of planning and multiagency coordination efforts, helping to bring together the key stakeholders in order to build more functional animal and/or agricultural plans and work more effectively together in support of those plans
- Engage voluntary resources in support of the state plan through all phases (prevention/protection, preparation, response and recovery). SART programs are perhaps most importantly multiagency coordination entities even though their name often reflects response. In most incidents, local communities provide the vast majority of the response with augmentation from state and federal agencies when needed. In Texas, this issue was reflected when they named their SART program the Texas State Animal Resource Team.
- Cultivate and help manage the integration of nonprofit and private sector resources into emergency management. In some states, SART and/or VMRC programs provide a portal for public donations in support of state animal and agricultural emergency management efforts.
- Support local planning, training, and volunteer development efforts. Since all response starts locally, it is critical for state programs to invest substantial efforts in helping prepare local communities for that primary role.
- Most important, SART and VMRC programs do not replace or diminish the importance of the statutory authority and leadership of state agencies. These programs should work closely with these agencies, providing additional resources in support of those existing state authorities in order to create a more effective state animal and/or agricultural emergency management system.

8. How do SART programs contribute to local animal and agricultural preparedness?

Although exact mechanisms may vary from state to state, in general SART programs contribute to local animal and agricultural preparedness through the following:

- Attending local animal/agricultural planning meetings and helping to engage local voluntary and private sector entities in the planning process.
- Providing model support materials for local planning, such as a model plan, examples of other local plans, and sample operational guidelines that can be attached to local plans.
- Delivering training on animal and/or agricultural emergency management (including, but not limited to response) throughout the state.
- Promoting personal preparedness and business contingency planning throughout the state.
- VMRC programs may also provide some similar activities, particularly engaging veterinary professionals in supporting planning and response efforts within their home communities.

9. How do SART or VMRC programs contribute to personal and private sector preparedness?

Some examples of how SART or VMRC programs can contribute to personal and private sector preparedness include the following:

- Developing and/or distributing preparedness materials targeting preparedness for families with pets and/or livestock.
- Developing and/or distributing materials on biosecurity for both commercial livestock producers and "backyard" livestock operations.

- Maintaining an internet website that provides animal and/or agricultural emergency preparedness tools for families and businesses.
- Providing outreach at major events, such as a state fair or other public venue.
- Providing lecturers on the importance of animal and/or agricultural preparedness at conferences or other organizational meetings.
- Partnering with state agencies or nongovernment organizations, leveraging combined resources to create more effective outreach programs that include messages on animal and/or agricultural preparedness.
- Providing outreach to the animal service community (veterinarians, kennels, doggy daycare, grooming, pet retail, pet breeding, etc.) to encourage business contingency planning and participation in local preparedness efforts.
- Encouraging all animal response personnel, including volunteers to develop personal preparedness plans that include their pets and livestock.

10. How does a state develop SART, VMRC, or similar programs?

The key element in developing a state program such as a SART or VMRC program is gaining the support of the essential stakeholders (those state agencies, nongovernment organizations, and private sector businesses that have a major role in empowering animal emergency management). In many states, the key stakeholders would include the following:

- State Department of Agriculture or Board of Animal Health
- State animal health official (state veterinarian)
- State emergency management agency
- State public health agency
- State Medical Reserve Corps coordinator
- Academic institutions (veterinary medical colleges and/or land-grant universities
- Veterinary medical associations (veterinary and veterinary technician)
- State animal control association
- State animal welfare association
- Livestock associations
- Corporations or private foundations that support animal and agricultural issues in that state
- Other entities as appropriate for that state

In many states, the SART or VMRC program has been initiated after a formal meeting of all the critical stakeholders in a one- or two-day meeting or "summit." Such a meeting provides a chance to examine the risks, resources, and responsibilities within the group and achieve consensus on the needs and mechanisms of addressing building effective multiagency coordination, creating veterinary surge capacities, engaging volunteers, and supporting the development of local animal emergency plans and response capacities. Since no two states are identical with respect to these issues, every state will have a somewhat unique mechanism of addressing these important issues.

11. What agencies have statutory authority for animal and agricultural emergency response?

Authorities for animal emergency management are highly variable from state to state. Each state has a chief animal health official, most often called the "state veterinarian," but some states use other nomenclature. This person heads an agency that is responsible for livestock disease emergency response and in many cases animal health emergency response in companion animals as well. In a few states, however, the chief animal health official does not have any statutory authority beyond livestock. Companion animal authorities are highly variable from state to state. In some states, there is clear authority under the chief animal health official. In other states, the state public health agency may have significant responsibilities, but if not, another agency has authority to address companion animal issues or it may default to the state emergency management agency. Veterinary professionals need to consult with their state agencies to determine how these issues are addressed within their own state's statutory environment.

12. How can SART and VMRC programs engage private sector and voluntary resources?

SART and VMRC programs engage private sector and voluntary resources through the following:

- Developing a board, steering committee, or advisory committee that includes representatives of key state agencies and nongovernment entities. This process provides "ownership" of the issues to the members of this body and helps develop broadly accepted mechanisms for incorporating voluntary and private sector resources.
- Attending various state emergency management planning meetings (and there are a complex array of these), helping represent the perspective of animal, agricultural, voluntary and private sector entities at those meetings.
- Helping to establish volunteer training and credentialing standards.
- Providing volunteer training at the state and local level.
- Participating in general state and local table-top exercises, helping provide insight as to the use of voluntary and private sector entities in animal and/or agricultural emergency response and recovery.
- Organizing table-top and field exercises to provide voluntary and private sector resources with an opportunity to realize and evaluate their roles in animal and/or agricultural emergency management.
- Working with state agencies to develop animal and agricultural resource-typing programs that are consistent with FEMA guidelines and provide a mechanism to identify and mobilize voluntary and private sector teams and equipment.
- Providing capable personnel to train as part of the state emergency operations center to assist state agencies in managing animal and agricultural resources during emergency incidents, including the mobilization of voluntary and private sector resources.
- Working with the state chapter of Voluntary Organizations Active in Disaster (VOAD) to ensure coordination between state animal and agricultural voluntary resources and other voluntary sectors, including (for example) the American Red Cross, Salvation Army, Civil Air Patrol, Amateur Radio Emergency Services, United Way, Adventist Community Services, and other faith-based organizations.

13. Why do some states have SART or VMRC programs that are state run while others use a charitable organization to provide staff support?

Every state functions in a unique statutory and political environment. In some states, there is adequate capacity in state agencies to provide funding and staff support to the processes of multi-agency coordination, voluntary programs, and support of local planning and response capacities. In several states, however, a charitable organization was developed specifically to supplement these functions (e.g., NC, PA, MD), allowing for additional funding through foundations, corporate sponsorships, and private donations. In other states (e.g., CO and TX), the state veterinary medical foundation was asked to take on this role. In most cases where a charitable format is used, the state contributes significant funding as well, but the leverage of state funds with complementary private sector funding provides a better resource base. Each state needs to identify and develop such programs within the context of their own state statutory, political and financial environment. While it may seem like a simple decision, in actuality, it is a highly complex and sometimes contentious process that should be negotiated with due respect for the authorities, responsibilities, capabilities, and resources of all the stakeholders to this process.

14. Does a SART or VMRC program need paid staff support, or can it function primarily with voluntary management?

Some states have necessarily moved forward as much as they can without full-time program staff because of funding limitations. In these cases, management comes from time contributions from state agencies and from voluntary support from nongovernment organizations and dedicated individuals. Those states that have been able to provide resources to engage full-time program management have typically made substantially more progress than those without such support. Without full-time support, it is often difficult to attend the critical planning meetings and to build the broad networking connections that will more fully empower the SART or VMRC program. Even with full-time staff support, however, there is a constant need to keep the stakeholders engaged in the process. Several state SART directors have been challenged to accomplish this, since once a full-time director is engaged, there is a tendency to expect them to "take care of it." Keeping all the stakeholders adequately engaged and maintaining public interest in animal and/or agricultural emergency issues can be challenging, particularly in states where major disasters are less common.

15. What are the roles of SART or state VMRC programs in animal health emergencies?

Animal health emergencies, such as foreign animal disease outbreaks, are managed primarily under the statutory authority of the state chief animal health official and the U.S. Department of Agriculture. The roles of SART or state VMRC programs vary widely for these types of incidents, but the following assignments might be tasked to these programs:

- Helping to engage local and state stakeholders in raising awareness of animal health threats and helping promote local and state mitigation and preparedness efforts
- Including awareness of animal health emergencies within basic training for individual volunteers
- Including biosecurity information in outreach materials on animal and agricultural preparedness
- Identifying and training individuals and teams that can assist in various mission tasks related to an animal health emergency response. Some states have invested substantial efforts in training private sector veterinary medical professionals to respond under the chief animal health official during an animal disease emergency incident.
- Helping to identify and develop supporting mission capabilities that might include mental health support, logistical support for families isolated on their farms due to quarantine restrictions, public informational outreach, community surveillance, logistical support, and many more

16. How do state VMRC programs interact with various national or federal veterinary medical response programs?

State VMRC programs can effectively interact with multiple national veterinary medical emergency programs in the following ways:

- Individual state VMRC members should be encouraged to enroll in the National Animal Health Emergency Response Corps (NAHERC) in order to facilitate their deployment as paid USDA reserves in a major and/or extended emergency incident, such as a foreign animal disease outbreak. In 2008, discussions were just beginning between state VMRCs and NAHERC about the potential for collaborative training programs.
- State VMRC programs are beginning to collaborate on key issues through the National Alliance of State Animal and Agricultural Emergency Programs, and emerging organization designed to network and support SART, state VRMC, and similar programs.
- State VRMC members may also join federal programs that provide veterinary medical teams for disaster response, including the National Veterinary Response Teams (NVRTs), Disaster Medical Assistance Teams (DMAT), or National Medical Response Teams (NMRT) programs of the National Disaster Medical System (NDMS) in the Department of Health and Human Services. In addition, veterinarians may apply for enrollment in the U.S. Public Health Service (USPHS) Inactive Reserve programs. In both cases, veterinary professionals may be deployed as temporary paid Federal employees.
- The American Veterinary Medical Association (AVMA) has transformed the Veterinary Medical Assistance Team (VMAT) program from a partnership with the Federal government to an exclusively AVMA-operated program. This program, which in 2008 was just starting redevelopment, will provide teams of trained veterinarians

to states upon request. The new VMAT program will be designed to work closely with state VMRCs and will work to affiliate each regional team with a state in order to be able to deploy these teams via the Emergency Management Assistance Compact (EMAC) process (based on direct AVMA communication with the author in 2008).

• The American Veterinary Medical Foundation (AVMF) has provided tremendous support to state VMRCs, SART programs, and other state programs since 2003. AVMF provides start-up, challenge, and matching grants to state programs that involve the state's veterinary community.

17. What is the National Alliance of State Animal and Agricultural Emergency Programs (NASAAEP)?

The National Alliance of State Animal and Agricultural Emergency Programs (NASAAEP) is an emergency association of SART, state VRMC, and similar programs. Figure 2.5.1 shows the status of such state programs nationally as of May 2008. The voting membership will include SART, VRMC, or other programs acknowledged by the state's chief animal health official and the state's emergency management agency. Affiliate membership opportunities will be extended to national organizations, corporations, tribal nations, local communities, state and local organizations, and individuals. This organization will provide a networking and collaborative venue for state

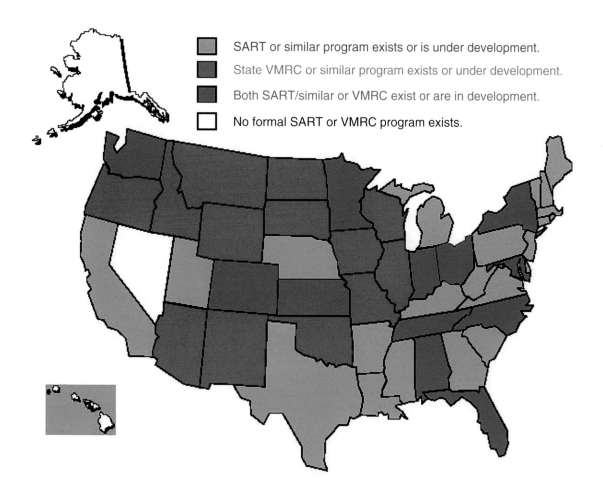

SART or similar program exists or is under development.

State VMRC or similar program exists or under development.

Both SART/similar or VMRC exist or are in development.

No formal SART or VMRC program exists.

Based on May 2008 data courtest of the
National Alliance of State Animal and Agricultural Emergency Programs

Figure 2.5.1 States with SART, VMRC, or no formal programs.

programs, federal agencies, and a broad array of affiliate members. While NASAAEP will not duplicate existing national organizational missions (e.g., U.S. Animal Health Association, National Assembly of State Animal Health Officials, and National Association of State Departments of Agriculture), this new organization will focus on the essential role of nongovernment partnerships, private sector contributions, local planning, and preparedness, and will serve to further the process of building state and local all-hazards, all-species animal and agricultural emergency management capabilities throughout our nation. NASAAEP is projected to be a charitable organization, allowing foundations, corporate sponsors, and the general public to contribute to this valuable effort.

18. How is NASAAEP projected to support local, state, and national animal and agricultural emergency management?

Since 2004, the network of state programs that has become NASAAEP has been working to connect state programs and mentor states as they develop new programs. The past and current activities include the following:

- Annual meetings of state programs and their national partners since 2004
- Monthly conference calls since January 2005
- Mentoring other states through state-to-state networking and information sharing, as well as SART Summit facilitation in many states through trainers from the NC SART program

19. What are some of the planned future activities of NASAAEP?

Future activities are projected to include:

- A dynamic web-based platform to facilitate communication and development of state and local animal and/or agricultural emergency management programs
- A broad-based annual conference on animal emergency management with appeal to multiple groups, from national stakeholders, to local programs and citizen volunteers
- A continued effort to work with all stakeholders, build partnerships at the national, state, and local level, and support efforts to develop and sustain effective credentialing, resource typing, and training standardization
- Work with states and national partners to create a broader base of financial support for state and local programs

Acknowledgments

*Statistics courtesy of the National Alliance of State Animal and Agricultural Emergency Programs (NASAAEP).

Suggested Reading

American Veterinary Medical Association. Disaster resources page including links to state resources. Available at http://www.avma.org/disaster/default.asp, 2008.

Extension Disaster Education Network site. Available at http://www.eden.lsu.edu/, 2008.

Medical Reserve Corps. Available at http://medicalreservecorps.gov, 2008.

National Alliance of State Animal and Agricultural Emergency Programs. Available at http://www.nasaaep.org (in development in 2008).

National Veterinary Response Team program (NDMS). Available at http://www.hhs.gov/aspr/opeo/ndms/teams/vmat.html, 2008.

USDA APHIS Veterinary Services, National Animal Health Emergency Response Corps. Available at http://www.aphis.usda.gov/vs/ep/naherc/, 2008.

Selected state program websites:
Alabama: http://www.alsart.org, 2008.
Arizona: http://ag.arizona.edu/ans/alirt/, 2008.

California: http://www.cdfa.ca.gov/AHFSS/Animal_Health/Disaster_Preparedness.html, 2008.
Colorado: http://www.cosart.org, 2008; http://www.cosart.org/COVMRC.htm, 2008.
Connecticut: http://www.ctsart.org, 2008.
Florida: http://www.flsart.org, 2008.
Idaho: http://www.agri.state.id.us/Categories/Animals/emergencyMgmt/indexemergencymgmt.php, 2008.
Iowa: http://www.iowaagriculture.gov/AgSec/IVRRT.asp, 2008.
Kansas: http://www.kssart.org, 2008.
Louisiana: http://lsart.org, 2008.
Maine: http://mainesmart.org, 2008.
Maryland: http://www.mdsart.org, 2008.
Massachusetts: http://www.smart-mass.org/, 2008.
Michigan: http://michigansart.org, 2008.
Minnesota: http://www.bah.state.mn.us/bah/emergency_planning/emergency_planning.html, 2008.
Nebraska: http://www.agr.state.ne.us/division/bai/ledrs.htm, 2008.
New Jersey: http://www.nj.gov/agriculture/divisions/ah/prog/emergency_preparedness.html, 2008.
New York: http://www.empiresart.org, 2008.
North Carolina: http://ncsart.org, 2008.
Oregon: http://www.oregonvma.org/resources/overt.asp, 2008.
Pennsylvania SART: http://pasart.org, 2008.
Texas: http://txsart.org, 2008.
Virginia: http://virginiasart.org, 2008.
Wyoming: http://wdh.state.wy.us/sho/prepare/wrvc.html, 2008.

CHAPTER 2.6
FEDERAL RESPONSE TO VETERINARY DISASTERS

Lorna L. Lanman, DVM

1. Describe a federally declared disaster and what determines the federal response?

The federal government maintains a wide array of capabilities and resources that can assist state governments in responding to incidents.

A federal law, The Stafford Act, establishes two incident levels—emergencies and major disasters:

- A *federally declared emergency* is defined as "any occasion or instance for which, in the determination of the President of the United States (President), Federal assistance is needed to supplement State, tribal, and local efforts and capabilities to save lives and to protect property and public health and safety, or to lessen or avert the threat of a catastrophe in any part of the United States."
- *Major disaster* means any natural catastrophe (including any hurricane, tornado, storm, high water, wind driven water, tidal wave, tsunami, earthquake, volcanic eruption, landslide, mudslide, snowstorm, or drought), or, regardless of cause, any fire, flood, *or* explosion, in any part of the United States, which in the determination of the president causes damage of sufficient severity and magnitude to warrant major disaster assistance under this Act to supplement the efforts and available resources of States, local governments, and disaster relief organizations in alleviating the damage, loss, hardship, or suffering caused thereby.

2. Describe progressive enhancement of the Stafford Act?

- The Stafford Act was named for Robert T. Stafford, (August 8, 1913—December 23, 2006), who was an American politician from Vermont. In his lengthy career, he served as the governor of Vermont, a U.S. representative, and a U.S. senator. A Republican, he is best remembered for his staunch environmentalism, his work on higher education, and for the Disaster Relief and Emergency Act for assistance in natural disasters.
- The Robert T. Stafford Disaster Relief and Emergency Assistance Act (Stafford Act) (Public Law 100-707) is a U.S. federal law designed to bring an orderly and systematic means of federal natural disaster assistance for state and local governments in carrying out their responsibilities to aid citizens.
- An amended version (1988) is the Disaster Relief Act (Public Law 93-288) creating the system in place today by which a presidential disaster declaration of an emergency triggers financial and physical assistance through the Federal Emergency Management Agency (FEMA). The Act gives FEMA the responsibility for coordinating government-wide relief efforts. It implements The Federal Response Plan, which includes the contributions from 28 federal agencies and nongovernment organizations, such as the American Red Cross.
- Congress again amended the Stafford Act by passing the Disaster Mitigation Act of 2000 (Public Law 106-390), and again in 2006 with the Pets Evacuation and Transportation Standards (PETS) Act (Public Law 109-308).

3. Describe what is meant by the "National Response Framework"?

The Stafford Act did not adequately recognize 21st-century threats. In recent years, our nation has faced an unprecedented series of emergencies and disasters. The Stafford Act needed to be further amended to establish a response level for catastrophic events (chemical, biological, radiological, nuclear attacks, or nuclear accidents). As a result, our national response structures have evolved and the response plan was improved to meet these threats.

The National Response Framework (NRF) is the next step in this evolution, and as such defines how we respond as a nation. Based on best practices and stakeholder input, the NRF presents the guiding principles that enable all response partners to prepare for and provide a unified national response to disasters and emergencies—from the smallest incident to the largest catastrophe.

4. Why change the name of the "National Response Plan" to the "National Response Framework"?

The NRF was adopted on March 22, 2008, and supersedes the 2006-updated National Response Plan. The update emerged from organizational changes within the Department of Homeland Security, as well as the experiences from responses to Hurricanes Katrina, Wilma, and Rita in 2005.

5. What are the intentions of the NRF?

- To define the principles, roles, and structures that organize how we respond as a nation to disasters and emergencies
- To establish a comprehensive, national, all-hazards approach to domestic incident response
- To ensure that communities, Native American tribes, states, federal government executives, private sector, nongovernment organization (NGO) leaders, and emergency management practitioners across the nation understand domestic incident response roles, responsibilities, and relationships in order to respond more effectively
- To describe specific authorities and best practices for managing incidents
- To build on the National Incident Management System (NIMS) that provides a consistent template for managing incidents

6. Describe why it is important that the NRF always be in effect?

It is not always obvious at the outset whether a seemingly minor event might be the initial phase of a larger, rapidly growing threat. The NRF allows for the rapid acceleration of response efforts without the need for a formal trigger mechanism. It also provides flexibility and scalability so **resources** can be implemented at any level, at any time.

7. Who coordinates the federal government's response to disasters?

- The president of the United States leads the federal government response effort and ensures that the necessary coordinating structures, leadership, and resources are applied quickly and efficiently to large scale and catastrophic incidents.
- The secretary of the Department of Homeland Security is the principal federal official responsible for coordination of all domestic incidents requiring multiagency federal response as outlined by law (Homeland Security Act of 2002) and by presidential directive. The secretary coordinates the federal government's resources available for use in response to or recovery from terrorist attacks, major disasters, or other emergencies.

8. List the six primary lanes of responsibility that guide the federal support at national, regional, and field levels.

Presidential directives outline the following six primary lanes of responsibility that guide federal support at national, regional, and field levels.

- A FEMA administrator serves as the principal advisor to the president, secretary of the Department of Homeland Security, and the Homeland Security Council on all matters regarding emergency management
- The U.S. Attorney General serves as the chief law enforcement officer, acting through the Federal Bureau of Investigation, and assumes lead responsibility for criminal investigations of terrorist acts or terrorist threats by individuals or groups inside the United States or directed at U.S. citizens or institutions abroad.
- Secretary of the Department of Defense (DOD). Many DOD components and agencies are authorized to respond to save lives, protect property and the environment, and mitigate human suffering under imminently serious conditions, as well as to provide support under their separate established authorities, as appropriate.
- Secretary of the Department of State is responsible for managing international preparedness, response, and recovery activities relating to domestic incidents and the protection of U.S. citizens and U.S. interests overseas.
- Director of National Intelligence Agency leads the Intelligence Community, serves as the president's principal intelligence advisor, and oversees and directs the implementation of the National Intelligence Program.
- Other department and agency heads. Under the NRF various federal departments or agencies may play primary, coordinating, and/or support roles based on their authorities and resources and the nature of the threat or incident.

9. What criteria are applied by the secretary of Homeland Security in deciding what type of response is warranted?

The type of response is dictated if and when any one of the following four conditions applies:

- A federal department or agency acting under its own authority has requested the assistance of the secretary.
- The resources of state and local authorities are overwhelmed and federal assistance has been requested by the appropriate state and local authorities.
- More than one federal department or agency has become substantially involved in responding to the incident.
- The secretary has been directed by the president to assume incident management responsibilities.

10. What are some of the duties of the FEMA administrator?

- Assists the secretary of Homeland Security to prepare for, protect against, respond to, and recover from all-hazards incidents
- Manages the operation of the National Response Coordination Center and provides for the effective support of all emergency support functions
- Makes recommendations to the president through the secretary of the Department of Homeland Security (DHS) on Stafford Act declaration requests
- Manages the core DHS grant programs supporting Homeland Security

11. Describe the Homeland Security Presidential Directive 5 (HSPD 5).

- This directive was established in February 2003 by President George Bush to enhance the ability of the United States to manage domestic incidents by establishing a single, comprehensive national incident management system (NIMS), in order to prevent, prepare for, respond to, and recover from terrorist attacks, major disasters, and other emergencies.

- The objective of the U.S. government is to ensure that all levels of government across the nation have the capability to work efficiently and effectively together, using a national approach to domestic incident management.
- With regard to domestic incidents, the U.S. government treats crisis management and consequence management as a single, integrated function.

12. What is the National Incident Management System (NIMS)?

- In 2004, the Department of Homeland Security released NIMS as required by Homeland Security Presidential Directive (HSPD 5)—Management of Domestic Incidents and HSPD-8 Preparedness. HSPD-5 established and designated the National Integration Center (NIC) Incident Management Systems Division as the lead federal entity to coordinate NIMS compliance. Its primary function is to ensure that NIMS remains an accurate and effective management tool through refining and adapting compliance requirements to address ongoing preparedness needs.
- NIMS provides a consistent nationwide template to enable all levels of government, the private sector, and NOGs to work together during an incident.
- NIMS provides a comprehensive framework to ensure that responders from across the country are organized, trained, and equipped in a manner that allows them to work together.
- Response actions are managed using the NIMS Command and Management, which includes the Incident Command System, Multiagency Coordination Systems, and Public Information.

13. List the benefits of NIMS in disaster response.

- Flexible framework that facilitates public and private entities at all levels working together to manage domestic incidents
- Standardized organizational structures, processes, procedures, and systems designed to improve interoperability
- Standards for planning, training, and exercising
- Personnel qualification standards are established.
- Equipment acquisition and certification standards
- Publication management processes and activities
- Interoperable communications processes, procedures, and systems
- Information management systems that use a commonly accepted architecture
- Supporting technologies, such as voice and data communications systems, information systems, data display systems, and specialized technologies

DHS/FEMA is conducting a final review of NIMS and will not conclude the process until August of 2008. The updated information may be accessed at http.//www.fema.gov/pdf/emergency/nrf/nrf-esf-all.pdf.

14. How does the federal government become involved in a disaster?

- Initial responsibility for managing domestic incidents generally falls on state and local authorities, and the federal government recognizes these roles and responsibilities in domestic incident management.
- When an incident occurs that exceeds or is anticipated to exceed state, tribal, or local resources, the federal government may provide resources and capabilities to support the state response.
- For incidents involving primary federal jurisdiction or authorities (e.g., on a military base or a federal facility or lands), federal departments or agencies may be the first responders and first line of defense, coordinating activities with state, territorial, tribal, and local partners.
- The federal government maintains a wide array of capabilities and resources that can assist state governments in responding to incidents.

The federal government also maintains working relationships with the private sector and NGOs.

15. Describe the progression of events leading to a response by federal resources.

The following actions demonstrate how federal agencies are likely to respond to assist state, tribal, and local governments that are affected by a major disaster or emergency (Fig. 2.6.1). Key operational components that may be activated include the National Response Coordination Center (NRCC), Regional Response Coordination Center (RRCC), Joint Field Office (JFO), and Disaster Recovery Centers (DRCs).

- The DHS National Operations Center continually monitors potential major disasters and emergencies. When advance warning is received, DHS may deploy—and may request that other federal agencies deploy—liaison officers and personnel to a state emergency operations center to assess the emerging situation. An RRCC may be fully or partially activated. Facilities, such as mobilization centers, may be established to accommodate federal personnel, equipment, and supplies.
- Immediately after a major incident, tribal and/or local emergency personnel respond and assess the situation. If necessary, those officials seek additional resources through mutual aid and assistance agreements and the state. State officials also review the situation, mobilize state resources, use interstate mutual aid and assistance processes such as the Emergency Management Assistance Compact to augment state resources, and provide situation assessments to the DHS/FEMA regional office. The governor activates the state emergency operations plan, declares a state of emergency, and may request a state/DHS joint Preliminary Damage Assessment (PDA). The state and federal officials conduct the PDA in coordination with tribal/local officials as required and determine whether the impact of the event warrants a request for a presidential declaration of a major disaster or emergency. Based on the results of the PDA, the governor may request a presidential declaration specifying the kind of federal assistance needed.
- After a major disaster or emergency declaration, an RRCC coordinates initial regional and field activities until a JFO is established. Regional teams assess the impact of the event, gauge immediate state needs, and make preliminary arrangements to set up field facilities (Fig. 2.6.2). If regional resources are or may be overwhelmed

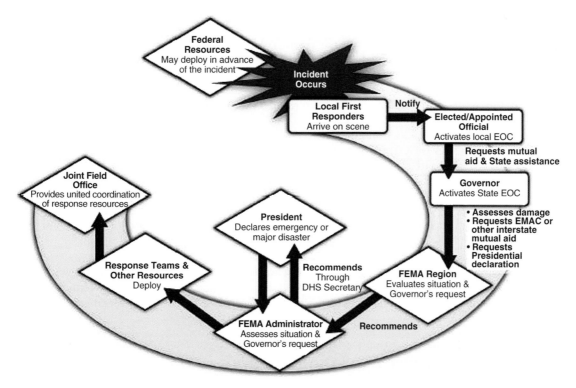

Figure 2.6.1 The progression of events leading to a response by federal resources. (Available from public domain: http://www.fema.gov/NRF.)

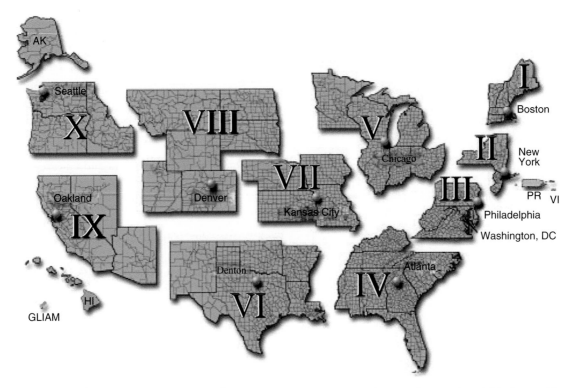

Figure 2.6.2 Federal Emergency Management Administration (FEMA) regions in the United States. (Available from public domain: http://www.fema.gov/pdf/emergency/nrf/nrf-core.pdf.)

or if it appears that the event may result in particularly significant consequences, DHS may deploy a national-level Incident Management Assistance Team (IMAT). IMATs will soon replace existing Emergency Response Teams (ERTs) at the national and regional level as well as the Federal Incident Response Support Teams (FIRST). The responsibilities of the IMATs are similar to the ERTs; however, the IMATs will be full-time employees concentrating on the response mission.
- Depending on the scope and impact of the event, the NRCC carries out initial activations and mission assignments and supports the RRCC.
- The governor appoints a State Coordinating Officer (SCO) to oversee state response and recovery efforts. A Federal Coordinating Officer (FCO), appointed by the president in a Stafford Act declaration, coordinates federal activities in support of the state.
- A JFO may be established locally to provide a central point for federal, state, tribal, and local executives to coordinate their support to the incident. The Unified Coordination Group leads the JFO. The Unified Coordination Group typically consists of the FCO, SCO, and senior officials from other entities with primary statutory or jurisdictional responsibility and significant operational responsibility for an aspect of an incident. This group may meet initially via conference calls to develop a common set of objectives and a coordinated initial JFO action plan.
- The Unified Coordination Group coordinates field operations from a JFO. In coordination with state, tribal, and/or local agencies, emergency support functions assess the situation and identify requirements. Federal agencies provide resources under DHS/FEMA mission assignments or their own authorities.

16. When do recovery operations begin?

- As immediate response priorities are met, recovery activities begin. Federal and state agencies assisting with recovery and mitigation activities convene to discuss needs.

- The Stafford Act Public Assistance program provides disaster assistance to states, tribes, local governments, and certain private nonprofit organizations. FEMA, in conjunction with the state, conducts briefings to inform potential applicants of the assistance that is available and how to apply.
- Throughout response and recovery operations, DHS/FEMA Hazard Mitigation Program staff at the JFO looks for opportunities to maximize mitigation efforts in accordance with state hazard mitigation plans.
- As the need for full-time interagency coordination at the JFO decreases, the Unified Coordination Group plans for selective release of federal resources, demobilization, and closeout. Federal agencies work directly with disaster assistance grantees (i.e., state or tribal governments) from their regional or headquarters offices to administer and monitor individual recovery programs, support, and technical services.

17. How is preparedness essential for effective response?

- The NRF contains an updated planning section that focuses on the critical importance of planning.
- Emergency planning is a national priority. To address this priority, the National Preparedness Guidelines have been developed. These guidelines are composed of four critical elements:
  - The first element is the National Preparedness Vision, which provides a concise statement of the core preparedness goal for the nation.
  - The next element is the National Planning Scenarios, which form a basis for coordinated planning, training, and exercising. These scenarios are planning tools that depict a full range from terrorist attacks to natural disasters.
  - The third element is the Universal Task List, which provides a menu of unique tasks linked to prevention, protection, response, and recovery strategies. This invaluable resource identifies the critical tasks for which response capabilities must be developed.
  - The final element is the Target Capabilities List, which defines specific response capabilities that all levels of government should possess.
- In addition to these elements, the National Preparedness Guidelines integrate key guidance documents such as the National Incident Management System, the National Infrastructure Protection Plan, and other national continuity policies and directives.
- Plans are continuous and evolving. They anticipate actions, maximize opportunities, and guide response operations. That is why plans are best described as "living" documents.
- Planning is the cornerstone of national preparedness. The NRF provides a foundation for unified planning for all response partners.

18. How do Emergency Support Functions (ESFs) respond in a disaster?

- NRF Organization is comprised of the core document, the 15 Emergency Support Function (ESF) Annexes, 8 Support Annexes, Incident Annexes, and the Partner Guides. The core document describes the doctrine that guides our national response, roles and responsibilities, response actions, response organizations, and planning requirements to achieve an effective national response to any incident that occurs.
- The following documents provide more detailed information to assist emergency managers in implementing the NRF:
  - Emergency Support Function Annexes serve as the primary operational level mechanism to provide assistance. ESFs group federal resources and capabilities into functional areas that are most frequently needed in a national response (e.g., Transportation, Firefighting, Search and rescue) (Table 2.6.1).
  - Support Annexes describe essential supporting aspects that are common to all incidents (e.g., Financial Management, Volunteer and Donations Management, Private-Sector Coordination).
  - Incident Annexes address the unique aspects of how we respond to seven broad incident categories (e.g., Foreign Animal Diseases, Agro-terrorism, Biological, Nuclear/Radiological, Cyber, and Mass Evacuation).
  - Partner Guides provide ready references describing key roles and actions for local, tribal, state, federal, and private-sector response partners.

These documents are available at the NRF Resource Center, http://www.fema.gov/NRF.

Table 2.6.1 Emergency Support Functions and ESF Coordinators

ESF #1—Transportation
ESF Coordinator: Department of Transportation
- Aviation/airspace management and control
- Transportation safety
- Restoration and recovery of transportation infrastructure
- Movement restrictions
- Damage and impact assessment

ESF #2—Communications
ESF Coordinator: DHS (National Communications System)
- Coordination with telecommunications and information technology industries
- Restoration and repair of telecommunications infrastructure
- Protection, restoration, and sustainment of national cyber and information technology resources
- Oversight of communications within the federal incident management and response structures

ESF #3—Public Works and Engineering
ESF Coordinator: Department of Defense (U.S. Army Corps of Engineers)
- Infrastructure protection and emergency repair
- Infrastructure restoration
- Engineering services and construction management
- Emergency contracting support for life-saving and life-sustaining services

ESF #4—Firefighting
ESF Coordinator: Department of Agriculture (U.S. Forest Service)
- Coordination of federal firefighting activities
- Support to wildland, rural, and urban firefighting operations

ESF #5—Emergency Management
ESF Coordinator: DHS (FEMA)
- Coordination of incident management and response efforts
- Issuance of mission assignments
- Resource and human capital
- Incident action planning
- Financial management

ESF #6—Mass Care, Emergency Assistance, Housing, and Human Services
ESF Coordinator: DHS (FEMA)
- Mass care
- Emergency assistance
- Disaster housing
- Human services

ESF #7—Logistics Management and Resource Support
ESF Coordinator: General Services Administration and DHS (FEMA)
- Comprehensive, national incident logistics planning, management, and sustainment capability
- Resource support (facility space, office equipment and supplies, contracting services, etc.)

ESF #8—Public Health and Medical Services
ESF Coordinator: Department of Health and Human Services
- Public health
- Medical
- Mental health services
- Mass fatality management

ESF #9—Search and Rescue
ESF Coordinator: DHS (FEMA)
- Life-saving assistance
- Search and rescue operations

Table 2.6.1 *Continued*

ESF #10—Oil and Hazardous Materials Response
ESF Coordinator: Environmental Protection Agency
- Oil and hazardous materials (chemical, biological, radiological, etc.) response
- Environmental short- and long-term cleanup

ESF #11—Agriculture and Natural Resources
ESF Coordinator: Department of Agriculture
- Nutrition assistance
- Animal and plant disease and pest response
- Food safety and security
- Natural and cultural resources and historic properties protection
- Safety and well-being of household pets

ESF #12—Energy
ESF Coordinator: Department of Energy
- Energy infrastructure assessment, repair, and restoration
- Energy industry utilities coordination
- Energy forecast

ESF #13—Public Safety and Security
ESF Coordinator: Department of Justice
- Facility and resource security
- Security planning and technical resource assistance
- Public safety and security support
- Support to access, traffic, and crowd control

ESF #14—Long-Term Community Recovery
ESF Coordinator: DHS (FEMA)
- Social and economic community impact assessment
- Long-term community recovery assistance to states, tribes, local governments, and the private sector
- Analysis and review of mitigation program implementation

ESF #15—External Affairs
ESF Coordinator: DHS
- Emergency public information and protective action guidance
- Media and community relations
- Congressional and international affairs
- Tribal and insular affairs

Available from public domain: http://www.fema.gov/pdf/emergency/nrf/nrf-core.pdf.

19. How have the federal government's responsibilities changed in a disaster involving animal victims?

The Pet Evacuation and Transportation Standards Act (PETS) was a bipartisan initiative in the U.S. House of Representatives to require a city or state seeking FEMA funding to accommodate pets and service animals in their plans for evacuating residents facing disasters. The bill passed the House of Representatives on May 22, 2006. Technically an amendment to the Stafford Act, it was signed into law by President George W. Bush on October 6, 2006. The bill is now Public Law 109-308.

The bill was initiated in the aftermath of Hurricane Katrina when the abandonment of many thousands of pets and other animals brought the matter of animal welfare to national attention. It is important to remember that the overarching objectives of response activities are life and safety, followed by protecting property and the environment. Many people do not evacuate because of their pets and livestock as many people do not think of their pets as property; thus numerous people stayed in harm's way when their pets were not allowed to be evacuated with them.

20. What are other major fundamental changes that are essential to the execution of the functions dealing with animals? (See Table 2.6.1.)

- ESF #6—Mass Care, Emergency Assistance, Housing and Human Services. ESF #6 is expanded in scope to include emergency assistance, the aid required by individuals, families, and their communities to ensure that immediate needs beyond the scope of the traditional "mass care" services. These services include: support to evacuations (including registration and tracking of evacuees); reunification of families; pet evacuation and sheltering; support to specialized shelters; support to medical shelters; nonconventional shelter management; coordination of donated goods and services; and coordination of voluntary agency assistance. DHS/FEMA executes the emergency assistance activity. In addition, the American Red Cross is no longer a primary agency for mass care; that responsibility has transferred to DHS/FEMA.
- ESF #11—Agriculture and Natural Resources. ESF #11 added a fifth primary function of Safety and Well-Being of Household Pets. Under USDA, ESF #11 will coordinate and support an integrated federal, state, tribal, and local response to ensure the safety and well-being of household pets. Supported activities include the evacuation, transportation, sheltering, husbandry, and veterinary care of affected animals as mandated in the Pets Evacuation and Transportation Standards Act of 2006.

21. Why does the NRF consider ESF #11 such a vital component of our nation's response network?

- Our nation's food and fiber system contributed at least $1.25 trillion to the U.S. Gross Domestic Product (GDP) in 2007.
- Nearly 16% of Americans work in the broad sector of food and fiber.
- U.S. agriculture exports grew by more than 15% in 2007 and with projected growth of nearly 11% more in 2008.
- Agricultural imports have risen from nearly $39 billion in 2000 to more than $65 billion in 2007.

22. What does the NRF challenge the USDA to do?

As part of Presidential Directives 7 and 9, USDA/APHIS, along with Homeland Security, other federal agencies, private industry, and state volunteers, is helping assess vulnerabilities in the food and agriculture sector and is directed to ensure the following:

- The U.S. food needs are met.
- The commercial food supply is safe and secure.
- Animal and plant diseases and pest situations are addressed.
- Household pets receive appropriate care.
- Important natural and cultural resources and historic properties are protected.

23. How is USDA/APHIS answering that challenge?

Since 1921, APHIS has offered an accreditation program for veterinarians. Accredited veterinarians have helped to eradicate brucellosis and tuberculosis among cattle. APHIS employs more than 8,500 people in all 50 states, several territories, and more than 30 foreign countries. It has designated 18 area emergency coordinators who are responsible for linking all local, state, and federal resources together to make the National Animal Health Emergency Management System work. These are the staff who would work with FEMA on animal health emergencies.

The USDA is developing a world-class animal disease biocontainment facility in conjunction with the DHS Science and Technology Directorate. This is the National Bio- and Agro-Defense Facility (NBAF). It will house the National Animal Disease Center, now located in an aging facility on Plum Island, off Long Island in New York. It establishes the National Animal Health Laboratory Network by partnering with the American Association of Veterinary Laboratory Diagnosticians to provide extra surveillance and capacity for testing and recovery in emergencies. This is a network of 54 medical and university laboratories and 4 federal laboratories located in 45 states.

The Veterinary Reserve Corps are veterinarians (often in private practices), who will supplement the permanent staff in outbreak situations. The USDA also maintains the cache of National Veterinary Stockpile. This stockpile includes personal protective equipment, vaccines, and other critical veterinary products available within 24 hours to supplement state and local resources to fight dangerous animal diseases.

24. What has become the nation's largest animal health emergency management and response organization?

The USDA National Animal Health Emergency Response Corps (NAHERC) is the largest national level animal emergency response corp. It is composed of veterinary medical officers (VMOs), animal health technicians (AHTs), veterinary medical students, and local animal response teams assimilated into an elite cadre within the emergency management response community. The NAHERC protects public health by providing a ready reserve of private and state veterinarians and veterinary technicians to combat threats to pets, livestock, and poultry in the event of a disaster or large outbreak of an exotic or foreign animal disease. NAHERC staff can be activated and supplement existing USDA-APHIS employees for periods of 3 weeks during domestic deployments or 30 days for international deployments. These positions are paid a salary on activation of the NAHERC. During a disaster, the size and scope of an incident can easily overwhelm conventional local animal health resources and could be devastating to the community as well as to the cattle, beef, and dairy industries. The NAHERC is an emergency response organization designed to provide large scale federal assistance during an animal event. Previously, NAHERC was activated and responded to the 2001 FMD outbreak in the United Kingdom (UK), the 2002 Low Pathogenicity Avian Influenza outbreak in Virginia, and the 2003 Newcastle disease outbreak in California/Arizona/Nevada. When an animal health emergency occurs, an immediate response is necessary to protect both animals and people in support of the NRF and Essential Support Function #11.

25. List some of the duties of the National Animal Health Emergency Response Corps (NAHERC)?

NAHERC staff duties during an outbreak or emergency event may include the following:

- Companion animal care
- Boarding and sheltering
- Conducting surveillance
- Examining herds or flocks for signs of disease
- Collecting specimens
- Vaccinating animals
- Conducting post-mortem examinations
- Euthanizing animals
- Supervising the disposal of animal carcasses
- Collecting epidemiologic information
- Inspecting livestock markets, trucks, and vehicles
- Other duties as assigned

26. Describe how Emergency Support Function (ESF) #8 now supports animal issues in disasters.

- The Secretary of HHS leads the ESF #8 response. ESF #8, when activated, is coordinated by the Assistant Secretary for Preparedness and Response. Once activated, ESF #8 functions are coordinated by the emergency management group (EMG) through the SOC.
- Health/medical/veterinary equipment and supplies. In addition to deploying assets from the Strategic National Stockpile (SNS), ESF #8 may request the Department of Defense (DOD) or the Veterans Administration (VA) to provide medical equipment, durable medical equipment, and supplies, including medical, diagnostic, and radiation-detecting devices, pharmaceuticals, and biologic products in support of immediate medical response operations and for restocking health care facilities in an area affected by a major disaster or emergency. When a veterinary response is required, assets may be requested from the National Veterinary Stockpile, which is managed by APHIS.
- Safety and security of drugs, biologics, and medical devices. ESF #8 may task the Department of Health and Human Services (DHHS) components to ensure the safety and efficacy of and advise industry on security measures for regulating human and veterinary drugs, biologics (including blood and vaccines), medical devices (including radiation emitting and screening devices), and other DHHS-regulated products.
- Agriculture safety and security. ESF #8, in coordination with ESF #11, may task DHHS components to ensure the health, safety, and security of food-producing animals, animal feed, and therapeutics. (Note: DHHS, through the Food and Drug Administration [FDA], has statutory authority for animal feed and for the approval of animal drugs intended for both therapeutic and nontherapeutic use in food animals as well as companion animals.)
- All-hazard public health and medical consultation, technical assistance, and support. ESF #8 may task DHHS components and regional offices and request assistance from other ESF #8 partner organizations in assessing public health, medical, and veterinary medical effects resulting from all hazards. Such tasks may include assessing exposures on the general population and on high-risk population groups; conducting field investigations, including collection and analysis of relevant samples; providing advice on protective actions related to direct human and animal exposures, and on indirect exposure through contaminated food, drugs, water supply, and other media; and providing technical assistance and consultation on medical treatment, screening, and decontamination of injured or contaminated individuals. While state, tribal, and local officials retain primary responsibility for victim screening and decontamination operations, ESF #8 can deploy any or all of the four National Medical Response Teams (NMRT) to assist with victim decontamination.
- Veterinary Medical Support, ESF #8 will provide veterinary assistance to ESF #11. Support will include the amelioration of zoonotic diseases and caring for research animals where ESF #11 does not have the requisite expertise to render appropriate assistance. ESF #8 will assist ESF #11 as required to protect the health of livestock and companion and service animals by ensuring the safety of the manufacture and distribution of foods and drugs given to animals used for human food production. ESF #8 supports DHS/FEMA together with ESF #6—Mass Care, Emergency Assistance, Housing, and Human Services, ESF #9—Search and Rescue, and ESF #11 to ensure an integrated response to provide for the safety and well-being of household pets and service and companion animals.

27. What is the National Disaster Medical System (NDMS)?

The NDMS is a federally coordinated system that augments the nation's medical response capability. The overall purpose of the NDMS is to establish a single integrated national medical response capability for assisting state and local authorities in dealing with the medical impacts of major peacetime disasters and to provide support to the military and the Department of Veterans Affairs medical systems in caring for casualties evacuated back to the United States from overseas armed conventional conflicts.

The NRF uses the NDMS, as part of the DHHS, Assistant Secretary for Preparedness Response, Office of Emergency Preparedness under Emergency Support Function #8 (ESF #8), Health and Medical Care, to support federal agencies in the management and coordination of the federal medical response to major emergencies and federally declared disasters including natural disasters, major transportations accidents, technological disasters, and acts of terrorism (including weapons of mass destruction events).

28. Describe what the acronyms DMAT, DMORT, NMRT, and NVRT stand for?

These acronyms describe various teams included in the National Disaster Medical System (NDMS).

- A *Disaster Medical Assistance Team (DMAT)* is a group of professional and paraprofessional medical personnel, physicians, physician assistants, nurses, pharmacists, respiratory therapists, paramedics, emergency medical technicians, and veterinarians organized to provide rapid-response medical care. DMATs are part of the NDMS and operate under the DHHS. Under the NRF, the 55 DMATs across the country are defined according to their level of capability and experience. Once a level of training and proficiency has been shown, the higher level of priority is given to the team. In addition to standard DMATs, there are DMATs that specialize in specific medical conditions such as crush injuries, burns, and mental health emergencies. DMATs are equipped with medical equipment and supplies, large tents, generators, and other support equipment (cache) necessary to establish a base of operations, are designed to be self-sufficient for up to 72 hours in a disaster area, and can treat up to 250 patients per day. The capability is similar to an urgent care-level health-care facility.
- A *Disaster Mortuary Operational Response Team (DMORT)* is made up of professionals (physicians, dentists, forensic scientists, police officers, medical examiners, funeral home directors, medical investigators, and other technical specialists) from all across the United States who volunteer to assist in the event of a mass fatality incident that overwhelms local and state resources. There are 10 DMORTs around the country and they are supported by 3 portable morgues. DMORT was deployed during the Oklahoma City Murrah Building bombing in 1995, the 9/11 attacks on the World Trade Center in New York City and the Pentagon, the 9/11 plane crash in Shanksville, Pennsylvania, the recovery of the remains of the astronauts of the Space Shuttle Columbia, and numerous other transportation accidents and natural disasters.
- The *National Medical Response Team (NMRT)* is a mass decontamination and medical care task force that is rapidly deployable anywhere in the United States or its territories. There are four NMRT within NDMS: East, DC, Central, and West. Only a handful of military assets respond faster than the NMRT. The Central team is the only response team in the system that has the ability to be loaded and ready to fly on commercial aircraft in 4 hours. The NMRT-Central uses SATCO Air Luggage Containers to store its equipment (over 25 tons), which allows the entire cache to be loaded onto any type of airframe with cargo capability; this includes FedEx, UPS, and commercial carriers. The NMRT-Central is now the only "all-hazard" team within NDMS and deploys with 60 medical and nonmedical specialists capable of decontaminating up to 1000 patients an hour or treating up to 200 patients a day in a medical setting.
- *National Veterinary Response Team (NVRT)*, formerly known as *Veterinary Medical Assistance Team (VMAT)*. The NVRT is a cadre of individuals within the NDMS system who have professional expertise in areas of veterinary medicine, public health, and research. In addition to supporting the mission requirements of NDMS under ESF #8, operational support may also be rendered by the NVRT to other federal partners such as the USDA under ESF #11, Agriculture, and FEMA under ESF #6, Mass Care, in the support of the Pets Evacuation and Transportation Standards Act. The NVRT provides assistance in identifying the need for veterinary services following major disasters, emergencies, public health, or other events requiring federal support, and in assessing the extent of disruption to animal and public health infrastructures. The NVRT is a fully supported federal program.

29. Describe some of the activities of the National Veterinary Response Team (NVRT).

- Assessing the veterinary medical needs of the community
- Medical treatment and stabilization of animals
- Animal disease surveillance
- Zoonotic disease surveillance and public health assessments

- Technical assistance to assure food safety and water quality
- Hazard mitigation
- Care and support of animals
- Certified as official federal responders to a disaster or emergency

30. Who are the National Veterinary Response Team members?

The NVRT members are private citizens who volunteer to be activated in the event of a disaster. The teams are comprised of individuals with diverse expertise and include veterinarians, animal health technicians, pharmacists, epidemiologists, safety officers, logisticians, communications specialists, and other support personnel. These individuals are assigned to designated teams that train in preparation for what might be experienced during a response. They are enabled by a regional cache of equipment, supplies, and pharmaceuticals. Team members are required to maintain the appropriate and current professional certifications and licensure of their discipline. NVRT personnel are intermittent federal employees when deployed. When members are activated during a deployment their licensure is recognized by the state(s) requesting assistance. Deployed team members are compensated for their duty time by the federal government. In an emergency or disaster response, the NVRTs provide assessments, technical assistance, public health, and veterinary services under the guidance of state and/or local authorities.

31. Describe the evolution of VMAT to NVRT.

Hurricane Andrew came ashore on the east coast of Florida in 1992, devastating south Florida. The NDMS responded by sending many DMAT teams to the area to provide emergent care for the residents of South Florida. There was no organized response for animal care until the U.S. Army Veterinary Command was deployed to provide organizational and veterinary medical assistance. Through the requests of many responders, including a DMAT commander who recognized this need, the American Veterinary Medical Association (AVMA) initiated a program to provide some financial support and sponsorship to Veterinary Medical Assistant Teams.

With the signing of a Memorandum of Understanding (MOU) in May 1993, veterinary services became incorporated into the Federal Response Plan for disaster relief as part of the National Disaster Medical System (NDMS). The AVMA's pioneering efforts in developing a world-class veterinary response team program (VMATs), resulted in this MOU between the AVMA and the U.S. Public Health Service. The agreement yielded 14 years of collaboration between the federal government and the AVMA. During this time the VMAT provided on-the-ground veterinary response during times of national emergencies, such as Hurricanes Floyd, Katrina, Rita, and other hurricanes; the World Trade Center; wildfires in Arizona; the avian influenza outbreak in Virginia; and a number of special events such as the Democratic National Convention, United Nations Meetings, and the Winter Olympics in Salt Lake City, Utah.

Our world has changed since 1993 and federal laws have changed to address new national security challenges. The AVMA developed the model of what is now the NDMS National Veterinary Response Teams (NVRTs). The AVMA also collaborates with other federal agencies, including the USDA. The completion, in August 1994, of an MOU between the AVMA and the USDA/Animal and Plant Health Inspection Service (USDA/APHIS) made it possible for VMAT to assist the USDA in the control, treatment, and eradication of animal disease outbreaks. Such a response would occur under the direction of the USDA. The MOU, originally signed in 1994, continues between the AVMA and the USDA. In addition, on January 26, 1998, the AVMA and American Veterinary Medical Foundation (AVMF) signed a statement of understanding (SOU) with The American Red Cross (ARC). In the SOU, during disasters, Red Cross volunteers refer all animal medical questions and needs to veterinarians affiliated with the national, state, county, or local veterinary medical associations.

32. What is the current status of VMAT?

What began as a privatized effort of the AVMA to assist with the care of animals, animal-related issues, and public health during a disaster, has become a federal program named the NVRTs as part of the National Disaster Medical

System (NDMS) under ESF #8 HHS/ASPR. The name "Veterinary Medical Assistance Team (VMAT)" was trademarked by AVMA and could no longer be used by the federal government as the name of the veterinary program within NDMS. The VMAT program was thus changed in 2007 to NVRT (the federal government's recently developed National Veterinary Response Team). Until the new national framework was adopted, VMATs were the only response teams recognized in the National Response Plan that provided veterinary medical treatment and addressed animal related issues resulting from natural and man-made disasters. Now, with the USDA being the lead agency for animal response and FEMA being charged with pet evacuation and sheltering, along with search and rescue personnel and dogs, NVRT will likely deploy in an assistance role to these ESFs.

The AVMA's Veterinary Medical Assistance Team program recently received the go-ahead from the executive board to move in a new direction, focusing on disaster preparedness and response activities at the state level. Now the AVMA-sponsored VMAT seeks to fill gaps at the state level. This program will offer services in the areas of early assessment, basic veterinary treatment, and training in disaster response.

A recent survey by the USDA found that only a small percentage of states have an animal response plan in place along with elements to support the plan. Many of the animal response teams at the state and county levels are still in the formative stages. The goal of this new state-focused AVMA-VMAT program is to work within the states' emergency response systems to assist in disaster preparedness and response. In some states, this may mean identifying which state resources are required following a disaster. In others, this may mean assisting the state in developing these critical resources.

The state-level AVMA-VMAT program will not supplant current state programs, such as animal response teams and veterinary corps, but attempt to enhance existing efforts and help establish programs where necessary.

Suggested Reading

http://emilms.fema.gov/IS800B/NRF0101summary.htm.
http://en.wikipedia.org/wiki/Stafford_Disaster_Relief_and_Emergency_Assistance_Act.
http://www.aphis.usda.gov/newsroom/speeches/content/2008/02/hs_defense_counci_final_2_12_08.shtml.
http://www.avma.org/disaster/vmat/.
http://www.avma.org/onlnews/javma/may08/080515d.asp.
http://www.fema.gov/about/stafact.shtm.
http://www.fema.gov/emergency/nims/nims_compliance.shtm.
http://www.hhs.gov/aspr/opeo/ndms/index.html.
http://www.hhs.gov/disasters/discussion/planners/playbook/hurricane/acronyms.html.
http://www.whitehouse.gov/news/releases/2003/02/20030228-9.htm.

CHAPTER 2.7
MILITARY ROLE IN VETERINARY DISASTER RESPONSE

Gary L. Stamp, DVM, MS

1. Provide some history for the role of the military in modern-day veterinary disaster response.

In late August 1992, Hurricane Andrew blew into South Florida and altered the entire landscape of the area and the lives of everyone in the region. Until Hurricane Katrina, this was considered to be the most devastating natural disaster ever encountered by the United States. The storm was disastrous for the animal population as well, causing numerous casualties and thousands of pets to be separated from their owners. Livestock and horses were equally impacted.

The local, regional, and federal response to this natural disaster was overwhelming and massive by all measurements, but also tremendously inefficient by consensus opinion of those involved. Why? An even more important question is "why does this underwhelming inefficiency still plague disaster response today," as evidenced by the Hurricane Katrina situation. What did we learn or *not learn* from previous experiences?

Following Hurricane Andrew, the American Veterinary Medical Association (AVMA) held a Disaster Medicine Symposium at their July 1993 annual convention. The papers from that symposium were published (*J Am Vet Med Assoc* 203:987–1010, 1993) as Hurricane Andrew "lessons learned" in hopes that the mistakes identified would be eliminated or at least minimized in future disaster responses. As we look forward it may be helpful to summarize the major failures and successes of that disaster response. Even though it has been 15 years, most are still reported in disaster relief after-action summaries since Hurricane Andrew:

- Failure to have or implement effectively a disaster response plan. At the time of Hurricane Andrew, there was little in the way of detailed planning to identify responsible organizations, designate area of responsibilities, etc.
- No clearly defined "chain of command" designating who is in charge. This caused fragmentation of effort, frustration, and conflict between organizations and the disaster relief team. The U.S. Army Veterinary Corps (VC) was asked for assistance to provide an equine specialist and small animal specialist to coordinate the respective relief efforts. The hope was that a "uniformed authority figure" would help coalesce and unify the groups toward a common purpose, as well as put in place a visible "chain of command."
- Failure of some volunteer animal welfare/humane organizations to work cohesively and reluctance to work "within the system." There was little control over the nongovernment organizations that insisted on establishing and conducting operations according to their own agenda.
- An ineffective communication and information management system severely hampered day-to-day operations in Hurricane Andrew. Cell phone networks were not well developed in 1993, and this resulted in clogging the communication channels that did exist and snarled the flow of information.
- Inadequate management of materials and supplies. Donations of medical and nonmedical supplies, including animal food, rapidly overwhelmed the response team's storage and handling capacity.
- No centralized system in place to process and account for the huge monetary donations. Several agencies set up their own collection points and little was ever known about the disbursement and use of the accumulated funds.
- Lack of animal identification. Microchipping had only just begun to be implemented in 1992 and was essentially not utilized at all. There was no real effective means to reunite lost and abandoned pets with their owners; this was perhaps the most significant animal-related disaster relief tragedy of Hurricane Andrew.

- Importance of reviving the operations of existing (predisaster) veterinary practices so that veterinary care in the local community can return to normal as soon as possible. Recognition that the most efficient system for delivering veterinary care was through the networks of existing clinics in the area, but several had been destroyed and others required major repair.
- Public health and zoonoses control are major issues in disaster response but are often overlooked and given a priority. This includes having a plan for carcass disposal, especially of large animals.
- Analysis of the Hurricane Andrew relief effort stimulated the development of many state disaster plans and the formation of the AVMA-VMAT program.

Hurricane Andrew was one of the first major involvements of the military, particularly the military veterinary services, in support of natural disaster relief efforts. Since that event, despite the documented participation of the VC, there has been a recurring question of what role, if any, the military can and should play in disaster relief.

2. Can the military services be used in disaster response? If so, under what circumstances? What determines if military resources can be used?

- Yes, the military can be used and is used to support and protect American lives and property.
- Disasters must be officially acknowledged, defined, and validated at the federal level to allow federal resources to flow. Specific definitions and criteria must be met to activate the Federal Response System to include support from the Department of Defense (DOD).
- Disaster Relief Act (Public Law 93-288) is the basis for the presidential disaster declaration of an emergency, which triggers financial and physical assistance through the Federal Emergency Management Agency (FEMA). The act gives FEMA the responsibility for coordinating government-wide relief efforts. (See details in Chapter 2.6.)
- The National Response Framework (NRF) adopted on March 22, 2008, outlines how we respond as a nation and presents the guiding principles that enable all response partners to prepare for and provide a unified national response to disasters and emergencies.

3. What and who authorizes the military to support relief efforts?

- The federal acts and laws mentioned above grant the authority for the military to provide support to civilian communities.
- Various memoranda of agreement (MOAs) or memoranda of understanding (MOUs) exist between federal departments to include Department of Homeland Security, FEMA, DOD, Department of Transportation, etc. Specifically, a memorandum entitled "DOD Support of Civil Authorities" from the chairman of the Joint Chiefs of Staff (DOD) dated 8 June 2007 details the roles, responsibilities, and limitations of DOD in providing assistance to civilian communities in a variety circumstances. This official document:
  - Outlines DOD support in scenarios ranging from natural disasters such as wildfires, floods, and hurricanes to terrorist actions and other "major national events"
  - Defines the coordination with other federal departments and agencies. Most relative for disaster support would be FEMA and the Department of Health and Human Services.
  - Specifies how and when military units or personnel will be deployed and how they can be used; also states how long they can remain
  - Identifies the military commands (i.e., unified major commands, subordinate commands, local commands, etc.) through which authority and resources flow to use military support
  - Designates the level of forces to be used, allowing for preapproved forces and the trigger points for activating and/or deploying
  - Emphasizes that deployment of DOD resources must not interfere with DOD mission priorities unless otherwise directed by the president or secretary of defense (SECDEF).
  - States that DOD support is on a reimbursable basis and outlines the documentation required for DOD to obtain reimbursement.

- Local and state authorities can request military support through a predetermined process between states and federal agencies, i.e., FEMA. It is important that state emergency management offices (EMO) are fully familiar with the process to request assistance and who their federal agency contacts are. If a written process is not in place, the EMO should develop and coordinate such procedures with the federal agencies, military commanders, etc.
- Requests for disaster support generally would be processed thru the Department of Homeland Security (DHS), FEMA, and DOD. Depending on the type and scope of the emergency, FEMA or DHS will determine what other federal agencies are needed to assist in the federal response. It is extremely important for disaster relief requests to be as specific as possible so the appropriate resources can be applied.
- Once it is determined that DOD support is required, official military orders would be issued directing the specific military units or personnel teams to respond. "Military orders" are official documents that can only be issued in accordance with military regulations and will specify who is responding for how long and for what purpose. The orders will also designate how funding will be handled for the military response.
- General support could also be requested through the state National Guard. This commonly is support for engineering service, security, evacuation, food/water distribution, etc. The National Guards do not have imbedded veterinary service capabilities, so this specific assistance would not be available from them.

4. What is the process to obtain military support for disaster relief?

- MOUs should be in place between state and federal agencies to streamline the process of obtaining military support and detailing specifically what agencies are officially authorized to make requests and through whom. Normally requests flow from the local office of emergency management through the state office of emergency operations to DHS or directly to FEMA.
- It is important to be as specific as possible regarding the type of military or federal support needed, i.e., engineering support for flood control, public health teams for food and water safety, mobile veterinary teams to assist livestock operations, field hospitals for urban small animal care, etc.
- When a military installation is located in the state or region where a disaster may occur (virtually every state), an MOU should be established and in place before the disaster. Local military commanders have authority to make agreements with civilian agencies to support them in time of emergencies to protect lives and property. This response can occur while a formal request goes forward to FEMA for broader support. This local commander-authorized response is time limited and services likely will be billed for later. For example, following Hurricane Andrew, Homestead Air Force Base provided shelters and logistical support as well as emergency medical service to the South Florida community. Likewise following the floods in South Dakota a few years ago, Grand Forks AFB provided key veterinary support as well as assistance in other areas.

5. Is there a cost to use military support for civil disaster response?

- Yes, military support is provided on a reimbursable basis. The Stafford Act and Economy Act are the legal directives that allow for and describe reimbursement procedures between agencies.
- Records will be kept to detail the personnel movement, payroll, supply, and equipment provided by the military and the costs passed on to the receiving state or local agencies receiving the military support.
- Strict funding and accounting directives are adhered to when military support is used. Unfortunately, transfer of funds from civilian agencies to military comptroller offices can be extremely complicated and may take months to complete.

6. Why and when should military support be considered?

- Military support should be considered when:
  - The disaster appears that it could or will exceed local response capabilities. Since Hurricane Andrew, it has been common for military installations and specific units in the region to be placed "on alert" during hurricane season.

- ○ Unique disaster requirements cannot be met in a timely manner by the civilian emergency management teams. This may include wildfires that require helicopter fire control, damage to a research laboratory that requires laboratory animal expertise, or disruption of food/water supply that requires mobile public health teams.
  - ○ Quick reaction response teams are needed before civilian teams can be available. Mobile veterinary units can normally be on site within 48 to 72 hours and specific individual personnel assets may be available in 24 hours or less. This rapid mobilization can fill the gap until large-scale civilian and federal support can be provided.
- Military support should also be requested when an authoritative presence would be beneficial to help calm and control the disaster scene (e.g., civil disobedience often accompanies a disaster). This certainly was the case in Hurricane Andrew when military units, including veterinary units, were deployed to not only provide specific technical and medical support but also to help organize and manage distribution of veterinary care which was very sporadic and uncontrolled.
- The military can be a quick response if the process to activate is in place prior to the disaster. Several military units have been established and are maintained with the purpose of being immediately deployable.

7. What unique capabilities and skill sets does the military offer?

- Regardless of the type of units responding, the most unique and valuable capabilities are deployability and self-sufficiency. Military units that respond to disasters would nearly always be fully deployable with their own transportation, communication, housing, and intrinsic support systems. Due to their self-sufficiency, the military team will be immediately functional upon arrival on site without placing further demands on the local systems which likely are already stressed. In contrast, a civilian disaster response team would normally require food/water, housing, communication support, and other services from the local disaster stricken infrastructure.
- The U.S. Army VC has six specialized (field) veterinary medicine teams of various size and configurations located in the United States that are fully deployable. Some portions of them have been sent to support Hurricanes Andrew, Hugo, Katrina, and Rita as well as to overseas locations.
- The VC possesses capabilities and trained specialists in nearly every area of veterinary medicine that is applicable to disaster relief. These include the following:
  - ○ **Clinical medicine:** The VC sends officers to advanced training to become board-certified specialists in internal medicine, emergency/critical care, radiology, surgery, and large animal medicine. Depending on the situation, these specialists may be deployed to the disaster site to augment general veterinary services and provide advanced clinical support for pets, military dogs, and search and rescue animals. Following Hurricane Andrew, equine and small animal medicine specialists were requested and sent to the region to coordinate the clinical medicine efforts.
  - ○ **Public health:** Food/water safety, zoonotic disease control, disease prevention and monitoring are major issues in nearly every large scale disaster. The Army has a large number of veterinarians board certified by the American College of Veterinary Preventive Medicine (ACVPM) who are quite knowledgeable in a wide range of public health issues. They are particularly adept working in a "field" environment where the basics of food and water safety and disease prevention must be addressed.
  - ○ **Lab animal (exotic) medicine:** These specialists can be invaluable if the disaster scene includes a research facility, zoo, or other exotic species facility. For example, a lab animal veterinarian was deployed to the Miami area after Hurricane Andrew to help with the loose primate problem after a research park was damaged. In another situation, an Army Lab Animal Medicine team was responsible for containing and cleaning up the Ebola virus ("Hot Zone") site in a Maryland civilian research facility several years ago, while Army veterinary pathologists were instrumental in identifying the viral agent.
  - ○ **Pathology:** Army VC pathologists are assigned all over the world and assist in disease surveillance, pathogen identification, infectious disease research, and other scientific activities. They are available to augment veterinary and public health teams as needed.
  - ○ **Scientists:** A number of veterinary scientists with doctorates in microbiology, virology, physiology, and pharmacology work in biomedical research, chem-bio defense, and related activities. These individuals can also be used to support disaster response if their expertise is needed.
  - ○ **Technician support:** The Army Veterinary service has several hundred animal medicine and food inspection enlisted personnel technicians who can be and are deployed as needed to support a disaster relief effort.
- **SMART-V Teams:** The Army VC possesses two Special Medical Augmentation Response Teams—Veterinary (SMART-V), one based on the East Coast and one on the West Coast. The mission of these teams is to assess initial destruction, degree of damage, determine the impending threat (risk), and convey recommendations for

immediate actions. The teams will have appropriate specialty personnel assigned depending on the disaster scenario, i.e., public health, clinical medicine, chem-bio experts, etc.

○ *East Coast SMART-V:* This unit is primarily focused on food and water safety issues relative to major public events of high significance. The team is activated and functions to ensure (as much as possible) that food and water at selected events pose no health risk.

○ *West Coast SMART-V:* The team currently focuses on avian influenza control but will modify the makeup of the team depending on the threat.

■ Air Force Biomedical Science Corps: The USAF does not have a veterinary service but does have veterinarians, nurses, and other biomedical officers who are specially trained in public health, food/water safety, and disease surveillance. They have mobile units that can be deployed to resolve public health challenges.

8. What general support functions can the military address?

• If needed, the military can provide the full spectrum of medical support to include mobile surgery teams, public health teams, field hospitals, decontamination units, epidemiology assessment teams, logistics support, evacuation, and more.

• Of course, nonmedical capabilities include, but are not limited to, transportation and evacuation, security, search/rescue, engineering support, logistics, information management, and communications. Because these assets are commonly found in state National Guard units, EMOs frequently use these them to have more control and flexibility and they would be less expensive than federal resources.

9. If military resources are incorporated into the response, who controls their activity?

• Generally, military units and personnel will have a military chain of command that flows from the SECDEF through the regional military command, USNORTHCOM, USSOUTHCOM, PACOM, etc. to local commanders.

• Normally a full colonel (06) or above will be a liaison between the military and the civilian authority. This office will coordinate across the military-civilian chain of command, will funnel requests for additional support through appropriate channels, and will ensure reports and documentation of the disaster relief are properly filed.

10. What are the advantages of having military support?

• **Total commitment:** It is well understood that that military brings many positive factors to the disaster relief effort. One of the most important advantages is that the military personnel and units are fully committed to the mission at hand. They will perform accordingly without a hidden or personal agenda that unfortunately deters the productivity of many other groups.

• **Disciplined execution:** Military units and individual personnel are disciplined in their approach, respect for authority and know the importance of working as a team. They will do as requested to the best of their ability.

• **Fully deployable and self-sustaining:** Being self-sufficient is extremely important when resources are scarce or unavailable. The military units involved in relief efforts can perform assistance activities without tasking or further burdening the disaster devastated community.

• **Display of authority:** Uniformed personnel convey a sense of authority which is very helpful and normally much appreciated by disaster victims and their community.

• **Versatile and flexible responders:** Military personnel are very flexible in their support role, usually taking a "do whatever necessary" attitude.

• **Full range of veterinary specialties and expertise:** Often overlooked or unknown is the level of veterinary expertise within the Army Veterinary Service. Several specialties exist and virtually every one that is needed is readily available to support disaster relief.

11. What are the limitations and disadvantages to using military resources?

- **Must be officially activated:** This can be difficult and seem bureaucratically impossible to achieve. At times the deployment is not timely due to administrative snarls that hold up mobilization and the request not being clear in defining the support needed.
- **Duration of support is specified:** Deployment to support disaster relief efforts is not open ended but set for a specified time which means that military orders must often be amended or reissued for the support to be extended.
- **Military chain of command:** Military units and individuals must follow the military chain of command and usually will not be subordinated to civilian leaders. This is not to say that the military members will not be totally committed to the objectives of the civilian emergency management team.
- **Limited availability:** The primary mission of the military is national security and many of the resources mentioned in this section are the very ones that also would deploy to support contingencies around the world. Additionally, in the mid and late 1990s there was dramatic decrease in active duty military units and total personnel; further, much of the active military was transferred into the reserve structure, thus making them not as readily available.

12. List some deployments where military support has been particularly effective in disaster response?

- Hurricane Andrew
- Hurricane Katrina
- 9/11
- Avian influenza outbreaks
- Other hurricanes
- Wildfires
- Floods
- Disasters outside United States

13. Summarize how the military will be an asset during a veterinary disaster response.

Military units/personnel can be a tremendous benefit in disaster relief efforts as they are well prepared to function self-sufficiently in a chaotic environment. They bring many valuable skills, as well as other positive attributes, but considering military mission priorities, should not be viewed as the cavalry coming to the rescue. A sound animal disaster response plan with the necessary agreements in place, coordinated up/down, and across all levels to include utilization of military resources, is the basis for successfully managing a veterinary disaster response.

Suggested Reading
Anderson R, Tennyson A. AVMA emergency preparedness planning. *J Am Vet Med Assoc* 1993;203:1008–1010.
Dee L. Lessons learned from Hurricane Andrew. *J Am Vet Med Assoc* 1993;203:986–988.
http://www.armymedicine.army.mil/tools/search/search.cfm.
http://www.fema.gov/about/stafact.shtm.
http://www.hhs.gov/disasters/discussion/planners/playbook/hurricane/acronyms.html.
http://www.veterinaryservice.army.mil/links.html.
Stamp G. Hurricane Andrew: Importance of coordinated response. *J Am Vet Med Assoc* 1993;203:989–991.

SECTION 3
PREPARATION

CHAPTER 3.1
FAMILY VERSUS BUSINESS DURING A DISASTER

Joan C. Casey

> Humanity is exalted not because we are so far above other living creatures, but because knowing them well elevates the very concept of life.
>
> Edward O. Wilson, *Biophilia*, 1984 Fl.R.

1. Why discuss the human-animal bond in disasters?

The human-animal bond is powerful. As families become more far-flung and people move frequently, sometimes great distances, pets become increasingly important members of the family unit. The American Veterinary Medical Association's 2007 *U.S. Pet Ownership and Demographic Sourcebook* has documented the following facts about animal ownership in America.

- There are more than 300 million companion animals in the United States, more than the total human population, and over 95% of pet owners view their pets as part of the family or as companions.
- Both 64.1% of households with children younger than age 6 and 74.8% of households with children older than 6 own at least one pet (Fig. 3.1.1). In fact, more American homes have pets than children.
- There are more dogs in the United States than there are people in any country in Europe, and there are more cats in the United States than there are dogs.
- A child in America today is more likely to grow up in a household with a pet than with a father in the home.
- More money is spent on pet food in the United States than on baby food.

2. Why are pets so important to families?

Pets assuage loneliness, encourage social interaction, and provide comfort (Fig. 3.1.2).

Animal-assisted therapies are becoming more common, everywhere from hospitals and nursing homes to rehabilitation centers for acute and chronic medical disorders. The University of Denver Graduate School of Social Work has an endowed chair for the Institute for Human-Animal Connection. Although animal-assisted therapy studies exist in other colleges, this is the first curriculum housed within a school of social work.

According to a *Small Business Trends* report on the pet industry, "Pet-related small businesses will be affected by a continuing increase in pet-related spending, higher awareness of pet health, greater uptake of pet insurance, and continued humanization of pets, integrating them into all aspects of our lives." Not only are pets traveling with their owners, included in hotel stays, and "writing" their own blogs, they are also recipients of large inheritances (i.e., Leona Helmsley) and beneficiaries of pet trusts.

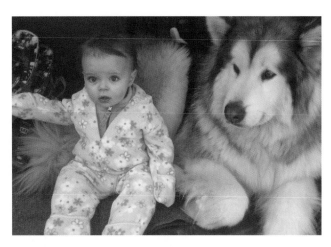

Figure 3.1.1   Pets are members of a family.

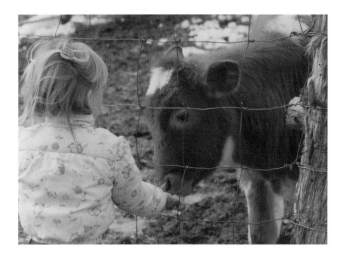

Figure 3.1.2   Animals assuage loneliness, encourage social interaction, and provide comfort.

3.   What is so important about animals in a disaster?

Most pertinent to this discussion is the fact that about 75% of pet owners will refuse to evacuate in a disaster if their pet(s) are not safe! And along with this fact is the expectation that services will be available for pets during a disaster. This will emotionally and psychologically affect a responder, veterinary hospital, and humane society.

4.   How can the veterinary hospital prepare their clients for a disaster?

Disasters do not always happen to "the other guy." A veterinary hospital could begin preparing their clients by viewing disaster preparation as they do routine vaccinations, etc. The annual exam is a great opportunity to communicate with clients to ensure that their expectations are the same as yours should a disaster or emergency occur. You need to know the need. Ensure that pets are identified with tags, licenses, and/or microchips and that the microchip registration is kept up to date. Create a packet for the client with the following information:

- A list of first-aid items
- Locations where the client can get medications including prescriptions
- Emergency information cards with alternate contacts for authorizing care of the pet, including a telephone number outside the immediate area
- Copies of vaccination records
- A checklist of items to include in an emergency kit such as leashes, food, carriers, etc.
- A list of telephone numbers to call to look for lost pets
- A photograph of the pet(s)
- A list of pet-friendly motels, if needed

Emergency responses will vary depending on the community. Rural communities have a tradition of working together to respond to emergencies. Urban communities are less closely knit. Identify pet owners that may be at more risk and, if possible, establish a way to check on these clients as soon as possible.

5. Does the veterinary clinic/hospital have an emergency plan?

Designate an OSHA officer or safety officer who will be responsible for turning off any utilities such as the gas and the anesthetic gas tanks. Ensure that there is emergency lighting available in the clinic. Keep a reserve supply of water on hand, and ensure that there are enough pharmaceuticals on hand to last several days.

The emergency plan is no good if it sits in the file cabinet. Discuss the plan regularly at staff meetings and hold practice scenarios. When possible, involve the local animal response team to help familiarize them with the clinic. Shape decisions based on shared values and goals. It is important that all staff understand their roles.

6. How will the animals be evacuated from the clinic?

Have the necessary plans and equipment in place should this be necessary and ensure that staff knows their location and proper use. Cat bags take up very little room and are handy for transporting cats or even snakes. Pillow cases can also be used in an emergency. Keep leashes and crates in the clinic to move and contain any dogs. Make similar provisions for other animals, such as reptiles, birds, small mammals, or exotics, that might be in the clinic.

Know which vehicles are available to move the critters. If possible, work with the local animal control, shelter, or animal response team. Ensure that everyone knows the location where the animals will be moved and how to get there safely.

7. Do humane societies have any obligation to assist a veterinary hospital in evacuating their patients?

Human safety is always paramount in any emergency. However, many animal control agencies and humane societies have emergency responders and rescue plans. But, once again, on the day of the disaster, it may be too late to ask for help. Develop an agreement with the local animal care and control organization to provide assistance should it be needed. Communicate what your needs may be, any hazards that they may expect to find at the hospital, and the location and the species of animals that may be at the clinic. It's all about mitigation and preparation.

8. What will happen if the hospital records are destroyed?

In addition to maintaining patient records at the clinic, it is important to keep a backup of all computerized records in an off-site location that can be accessed should the clinic suffer damage or destruction. Off-site backup of records is available through many of the internet security systems, or a manual backup can be done daily and copies kept off the premises.

9. How will veterinary prescriptions be refilled or replaced?

Most human pharmacies have the same or equivalent drugs. Make arrangements before a disaster occurs so that other pharmacists are familiar with you and your hospital. Disseminate this information to your clients so they will know who to call if you are not available.

10. If the veterinary hospital is full of animals, a disaster is impending, and the veterinarian is unable to contact all the owners to pick up their pets, what advice can be given?

Preparation, preparation, preparation! Pet owners will put their own lives at risk to ensure the safety of their animals. This is a matter of public safety, not just pet safety. Communicate with the incident command or public safety to alert them of the situation. Most communities have animal response teams already established. These responders are trained to handle animal emergencies and understand the incident command system and technical animal rescue. As part of the clinic's contingency plan, it is important to know who these teams are in the community.

11. A disaster has struck a community and all communication lines are down. What sort of notice should a veterinarian leave on his hospital door, and what information should be contained therein?

Be prepared for this possibility. The clinic may be unable to open due to the emergency, or the clinic veterinarians may be volunteering at an intake/triage center handling animals affected by the disaster. If possible, leave information on the hospital telephone message or website and post information on the hospital door about alternative clinics or about the animal triage/intake center. However, in disasters, access to telephone service or even transportation to the clinic may be unavailable. Include information about alternate clinics that have agreed to provide services as part of the emergency information provided to clients.

12. A disaster is impending, and the responder is trying to juggle priorities of his or her business and family. Where should those priorities lie?

Unless a responder is confident that his or her family and loved ones are safe, the responder is ineffective. The first priority for the responder will be to ensure the family's safety and then to respond as requested. A prearranged family emergency contact plan will provide that assurance more quickly. It is most important to be proactive. A veterinary clinic can develop memoranda of understandings (MOUs) with local animal control agencies and humane societies to provide assistance if needed and if they are able. For minor emergencies that do not threaten the entire community, prepare a list of staff who will respond and designate managers who will be responsible for requesting staff response. List managers in order of priority to ensure availability. If a designated person is not available, who is the backup? Be sure that everyone is "speaking the same language" and understands who will be responsible for which tasks.

13. A family has numerous pets and a small evacuation vehicle; what can be done with those pets when the family evacuates?

As the fire is coming over the hill, it's too late to plan. Before a disaster occurs, ensure that information about the importance of being prepared is made available through veterinary clinics, animal shelters, and animal publications. Pet owners and owners of livestock should have a plan about what they will do or who they will call for help. They should have supplies and medication for at least 3 days.

However, circumstances may mean that assistance is needed. In some recent fires, families were away for the day at work and school and the pets remained at their home. It was too dangerous for them to return for the animals. As part of an emergency plan, designated responders will be available to rescue these animals. Ensure that a contact telephone number for animal rescue is well-publicized throughout the community and at the incident command.

Along with the contact number, provide information about the location of emergency pet shelters and livestock holding grounds. Determine these locations prior to a disaster so that alternatives can be offered based on the location of the event and agreements kept in place for the use of the facilities.

An MOU with the Red Cross to establish a pet shelter next to their human shelter is very advantageous. Not only does it provide evacuees with a single destination location, it also helps them emotionally to have their pets where they can visit. Keep a roster of pretrained and prescreened volunteers to provide for intake, record keeping, triage, treatment, and care of the animals.

14. How will you identify your pet or livestock?

Keep a copy of your pet's licenses, vaccination records, and a photograph in the emergency kit. Ensure that your pet is microchipped in case a collar is lost and make sure that the microchip information in the database is up to date.

For livestock, ensure that brand inspection papers and other identification of the animals are parts of the animal emergency kit. Photographs are also good. In some disasters, livestock owners have painted their telephone numbers or other identifying marks on the sides of their horses or cattle.

15. A family goes to an evacuation shelter with their pets; the shelter refuses to allow the pets to enter. What recourse does the family have?

Create MOUs and agreements to establish pet shelters in coordination with human shelters prior to an event. Locations of these shelters must be well publicized, as previously mentioned. In addition, maintain a roster of previously accredited volunteers who are willing to foster animals displaced by the emergency and manage the volunteers from a central location. Ensure that this information is made available to human shelters. In some instances, MOUs with organizations such as United Way 2-1-1, Metro Volunteers, or Volunteers of America may be the most expedient way to work with volunteer foster homes. Before a disaster occurs, it is also beneficial to develop agreements with businesses willing to supply pet food and extra equipment such as animal airline crates, leashes, and other supplies (Fig. 3.1.3).

16. A family has a several horses, ostriches, and three boas. They have no way to evacuate these animals. Is there any advice you can offer?

Communities that have included animals in their emergency response plans will usually have an agreement with animal control or, in come cases, with the zoo to assist with the evacuation of exotic animals. Call the publicized telephone number for animal assistance, and they should be able to help. For the safety of the responders and the exotic pets, ask the family to ensure that the boas are caged!

Horses, ostriches, and other livestock also require specialized handling. Once again, those prior agreements with horse, livestock, and agriculture groups in the community are important. They will have access to trailers and the skills needed to manage livestock. Ensure that these resources are part of the community's emergency response plan. It is important for the owners of these animals and perhaps the clinic to make themselves aware of the resources that are available before the disaster occurs.

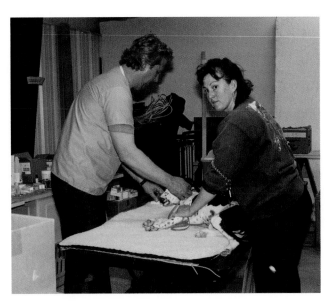

Figure 3.1.3 Volunteers are available to assist animal owners during a disaster.

Acknowledgment

The author is most appreciative of Dr. Ted Cohn, University Hills Animal Hospital, Denver, Colorado, and Philip Tedeschi, University of Denver, Graduate School of Social Work, for consulting on the information contained in this chapter.

Suggested Reading
U.S. Pet Ownership & Demographics Sourcebook. Schaumburg, IL, Center for Information Management; American Veterinary Medical Association, 2007.

CHAPTER 3.2
PREPARING YOUR PRACTICE FOR AN IMPENDING DISASTER

Gregory A. Rich, DVM

1. What type of disasters must I prepare myself and my veterinary clinic/hospital for?

The most common types of natural disasters are floods, tornadoes, hurricanes, and forest fires. Man-made fires or arson should also be considered in this group. Terrorist disasters have to be considered, but as of yet they have not damaged any veterinary clinic or hospital. Of these types of disasters, floods and hurricanes give the affected location the best opportunity for planning ahead, although if only for 24 to 48 hours. Disaster plans must be in place before the suspected disaster occurs. This makes deployment of the agenda flow smoother. Some types of fires give some warning, such as forest fires. As we have seen in California, though, wind changes may create a problem one day when there was none the day before. Arson and electrical fires often occur when the facility is closed. Tornadoes give only minutes of warning time, as do arson attacks, so there is little one can do to prepare the whole facility for these types of disasters.

2. What should I do to evacuate my facility?

Be prepared to have enough vehicles to evacuate the animals residing in the clinic. This seems like a daunting task, but careful preplanning can lead the disaster management team to find rental vans, animal shelter vehicles, school buses, or other transport available near your municipality.

For feline clinics, avian/exotic animal clinics, or outpatient facilities, a transport cage must be on hand for every cage in which there is an animal. Make sure when these animals leave the building that a copy of their records, medications, and enough food for each animal for 3 days go along with the pet(s). Boarding sheets and emergency contact numbers are critical for each pet to ensure early notification and reuniting the pet with the owner or relatives.

Watertight food containers are a must for transport of food to another location. All paperwork must be placed in watertight containers or resealable plastic bags.

3. How do I prepare the animals in my facility for evacuation?

As mentioned, all animals should have a copy of their records with them, or at least the client information and last medical page. All animals must be sent with a 3-day supply of food and fresh water. Any pet requiring medications, supplements, or treatments must have those items placed with their travel cage and in a watertight container. Pertinent medical supplies must be sent with the person evacuating the animals (i.e., heating pads, syringes, emergency medications, oxygen, etc.). It is the responsibility of the office manager and practice owner to make sure all boarding patients have current emergency contact numbers identified on the boarding check-in sheets. Data should include owner, emergency contact number, secondary in-town contact person, dietary instructions, medication(s) being administered, and length of time boarding. Out-of-town contact numbers should be listed if known. This information must be updated every time the pet is boarded at your facility.

4. What can I do to prepare the facility for a disaster?

A true disaster plan for the facility and the patients will set up a schedule of duties to be carried out by the staff. Someone needs to be in charge of securing the evacuation box. This item is for safe transport of vital legal documents, bank documents, architectural drawings, insurance papers and employee contracts/contact information. One or more persons should be dedicated to securing the cages for the pets and, if time permits, putting the animals in their transport cages if the time for evacuation is near.

Someone else should be in charge of moving the computers to higher ground and making backups of client data and other documents. All electrical cords should be unplugged, and if possible all equipment in the reception and waiting room areas should be put at counter height when facing flood or hurricane damage.

Pet foods and retail supplies should be moved to the highest shelves (minimum of 3 feet off the floor).

All moveable and vital medical equipment should be moved to an inside storage closet and off the floor. This includes, but is not limited to, microscopes, endoscopes, ultrasound machines, autoclaves, video equipment, and blood analyzers.

If time permits, the outside windows should be boarded in case of hurricanes and tornadoes.

5. How can I prepare my computers, my client files and my important documents for a disaster?

There are numerous ways to back up computer files. If you are just interested in client files, zip drives, disc backups or flash drives are sufficient to carry out this task. To back up the entire computer system, external hard drives are inexpensive, quick, and small enough to transport anywhere.

Off-site data storage is an idea that may be extremely valuable to large veterinary facilities. Many large medical businesses use this format for permanent data storage to protect their computer data in case of disasters as well as computer failure/viruses.

An extremely important fact is that two backups should be made and they should be sent with different team leaders to ensure that, in the case of an accident to one set of files, a second set is still viable.

With the advent of digital cameras, taking picture records of the facility and its contents has become an easy task to perform in-house. The entire clinic, including equipment, medications, retail items, and furniture, should be photographed and the files stored on CDs, thumb drives, or external hard drives.

6. What paperwork should I have backups/copies for?

It is critical to make copies of all financial, legal, real estate, and insurance documents NOW! Copies of these documents are best copied while there is time to commit to this task, not when a disaster is looming. I would highly recommend making paper copies and then having these most essential documents laminated. An evacuation box should be prepared. This box should be light enough to carry and water tight. Large "zip-lock" bags can be used to hold each category of paper files, bank records, computer backup materials, and valuable portable equipment. **Remember to make a box for your house, too.**

7. What materials should go into an "evacuation box"?

All bank documents, loan documents, real estate documents, employee contracts, leases, insurance papers, stocks/bonds, "money drawer," telephone lists, and computer backup materials and all clinic keys. It would be helpful to also have a copy of all state and federal drug licenses and permits, as well as association membership information.

EVACUATION BOX CHECKLIST

1) **Financial Papers**
   a. Loan documents   _____
   b. Checking/savings account   _____
   c. CD certificates   _____
   d. Stock certificates   _____
   e. Credit card statements   _____

2) **Insurance Papers**
   a. Health insurance   _____
   b. Disability insurance   _____
   c. Liability insurance   _____
   d. Auto insurance   _____
   e. Business umbrella policy   _____
   f. Business property insurance _____
   g. Business interruption insurance _____

3) **Business Documents**
   a. Leases   _____
   b. Employee contracts   _____
   c. Business contracts   _____
   d. Loans   _____
   e. Accounts receivable   _____
   f. DEA/state drug license   _____
   g. State veterinary license   _____
   h. Payroll data   _____
   i. Tax returns (3 years)   _____

4) **Telephone Lists**   _____
5) **Computer Backup**   _____
6) **Clinic/Storage/Drug Cabinet Keys** _____

8. How do I organize my staff to prepare for a natural disaster?

The office manager/practice owner will be in charge of delegating to other sections what tasks are needed to facilitate disaster preparations for your facility. He or she will be in charge of the master checklist and making sure the computers in the facility are safe and placed out of harm's way if possible.

Your head technician will be in charge of delegating to the technical staff how to secure the lab and all laboratory equipment (microscopes, hematology and blood chemistry analyzers), radiology equipment, and the entire surgery room. All electrical equipment should be unplugged and equipment light enough to be moved should be placed on countertops or placed in storage closets off the floor. Someone will be placed in charge of making sure copies of all paperwork and medications for hospitalized patients are placed in a central location and accessible to whomever is physically evacuating animals if necessary.

The kennel staff will be in charge of making sure all boarding data sheets are in a folder that will be placed in the evacuation box if an evacuation is planned. All food in the kennel, food storage closets, and the retail area should be placed off the floor in flood zones or placed in watertight containers in areas at risk of tornado, hurricane, and torrential wind/thunder storm damage. Placing food, supplements, and perishable goods in plastic bags or storage bins will be very helpful. All storage containers should be labeled for ease of locating items after the disaster has passed. A travel or transport cage must be readied for every cage holding an animal in your facility and placed by the animal's cage.

An extremely wise idea is to plan a run-through drill on a weekend or on a scheduled day off. This process will uncover gaps in the plan and allow for changes to be made before critical mistakes take place that may cause loss of data or patients or cause harm to a staff member.

9. How can I help my clients prepare for a natural disaster?

Advise all your clients to plan ahead. Offer pet carriers for sale year round. Make copies of this or other "disaster planning" guides to hand out. Have SBA Disaster Planning telephone numbers or local Office of Emergency Planning telephone numbers available to hand out to clients. The SBA, AVMA, and many local disaster agencies have free brochures that can be handed to the public.

10. What insurance should I maintain for disaster-related losses?

Update your contents insurance every 3 years. Most of us forget to update this information with our insurance agent at the time of new purchases. Business interruption insurance is invaluable if your insurance carrier is able to provide this type of policy. Business interruption insurance will pay you daily ongoing costs until the practice is open for business again. An umbrella package that covers overhead, liability, and building coverage in a critical need for all owners of veterinary practices. The liability policy hopefully will never be required, but in case animals get injured by the disaster or during the evacuation, this policy may save someone from financial ruin.

11. What telephone numbers are vital to me in case of a natural or man-made disaster?

This list may not be the exact list everyone prefers, but it is at least a beginning:

1. AVMA disaster assistance   _____
2. Insurance agent   _____
3. Insurance company   _____
4. Staff   _____
5. Personal physician   _____
6. Payroll specialist   _____
7. State veterinarian   _____
8. Local/state VMA   _____
9. Small Business Administration   _____
10. Small Business Disaster Centers _____
11. FEMA   _____
12. Accountant   _____
13. Employees (cell telephones)   _____

It is critical that telephone calls, faxes, or emails to any disaster agency, insurance company, or contractor be documented as to time/date/person spoken to. Documentation of correspondence will be essential in case communications are lost or mishandled. Keep a file for copies of all documents requested for quick reference in cases the information requested needs to be resent.

12. Which veterinary organizations should I contact regarding my situation?

Be involved in your local and state animal response plans. All counties/parishes are now required by law to have an animal plan. In helping, you will not only assist your clients and your practice, but you will be able to have answers for what is being done at the local and state level and what their plans are. All disasters are handled with the local response first, then the state, then the national level. Any requests that you need should be directed to the local office of emergency preparedness, but be prepared to use other sources. Document calls, expenses, and other costs that you have. Reimbursements can only be made if documentation is present. You may want to start with your local veterinary association. Your state VMA and the AVMA, as well as any national veterinary organizations you belong to, are all working on disaster plans that you can tap into when disaster occurs. They will be able to help and they will know your status. These organizations can quickly contact disaster relief organizations to come to your assistance and/or inform your colleagues of your situation in case help is needed to assist with veterinary care of the animals in your care.

Do your best to assist other veterinarians in the community if it is their clinic that is in trouble.

13. How should I keep in touch with my staff and clients after the disaster?

You should keep in touch with all your staff in the immediate period after the disaster. The various options are cell telephones (do not always work in national disasters), email, telephone number of an out-of-state relative your staff can contact, and/or the telephone number of the location you plan to evacuate to. You need to know if your staff members are safe. They need to know if you and your family are safe. You need to know when and where to tell them where to be to help with the clean up efforts and you need to let them know if they will be needed in an employee position in the postdisaster period. If you have business interruption insurance, you will need to calculate what staff you will maintain. If you plan to reopen soon after the disaster, you will need to redo work schedules and make plans on whether there will be any staff changes. If you plan to be out of business for an extended period of time, your staff needs to know so they can make plans to keep earning income.

Your clients are vital to the ability of your clinic/hospital to survive the postdisaster economic period. You must find a medium (newspaper, TV, radio, newsletters, and mail-outs) that will provide contact for the vast majority of your client base to let them know what the plans are for the clinic/hospital and where you will be seeing patients until the facility is rebuilt. Your telephone company is a vital player is this effort. Call your local telephone company and have them place a message on your main line informing callers of where you are, what your plans are, and how to obtain help for their pet. In the case of many major regional disasters, cell telephone towers may be rendered inoperable, so relying on cell telephones as a form of communication may not be possible. After Hurricane Katrina, residents in the directly affected areas could not be reached by cell telephone for up to 6 weeks in many cases.

14. Where should I plan to evacuate to?

Plan your evacuation destination by the location of a relative or colleague who will be able to house the animals you are evacuating with. Arrange ahead of time with a colleague the agreement to house animals from your facility in case you ever have to evacuate. In facilities located along the East Coast and the Gulf Coast, you may need to secure evacuation sites in several directions away from town, since hurricanes may force you to evacuate to the south one season and to the east the next. You should make arrangements to make this a reciprocal agreement.

15. Should I place my office manager/hospital manager in charge of anything?

The office manager/practice manager should be in charge of the checklist as well as overseeing the duties delegated to other sections of the facility. A basic checklist should at least include the following items:

1. Computer backup   _____
2. Client list   _____
3. Employee contact list   _____
4. Business insurance papers   _____
5. Contracts   _____
6. Lease/deed to property   _____
7. Payroll information   _____
8. Banking information   _____
9. Checking/savings books   _____
10. Emergency telephone list   _____
11. Health insurance papers   _____
12. Control drugs   _____
13. DEA registration   _____
14. State veterinary license   _____

16. Whom should I call as soon as the disaster has subsided, and how do I prioritize this list?

Priorities should rest on how much damage occurred and how many animals are in peril. If the animals are stable, I would call my insurance agent first, the state veterinarian second, and then the entire staff to update them on work needed to be attended to. If animals are in danger, call your state veterinarian or Office of Emergency Preparedness first, your insurance agent second, and other local veterinarians third, to seek help. There may be a local "animal response team" set up that your local or state Office of Emergency Preparedness is aware of.

17. Should I throw out everything that is damaged?

Definitely not! What you save you do not have to repurchase. Everything from microscope slides to surgical equipment may be completely unharmed, and if you let a salvage company clean out your facility, you have no idea what is still in usable condition. Every penny of insurance payments and disaster loans should go to replacing what is truly unsalvageable and essential for you to restart your practice. If you throw out good equipment, furniture, tables, or hard goods, you will find your insurance dollars will not completely replace every thing you lost or threw out. Your insurance proceeds are designed to replace the big ticket items that are damaged beyond repair. True, it would be nicer to have brand new everything, but this ideology will be very costly and insurance coverage is not designed to and, in reality, will not make you a profit.

18. How will disaster aid help me get back on my feet?

Insurance coverage will rarely cover 100% of the cost to replace equipment or property after a disaster. Government financial aid programs such FEMA, the Small Business Administration, and the Red Cross will be extremely helpful in bridging the gap between insurance coverage and replacement costs. There are numerous private aid programs in place to help in postdisaster aid to individuals and businesses. The AVMA, your state VMA, religious groups, and citywide recovery programs should be looked into in times of need in regard to disaster loans/grants.

19. Should I seek a disaster loan?

A resounding yes! Disaster loans can be the difference between restarting with nothing or restarting with a working capital and a new business loan. The main selling point is that the interest rate may be the most reasonable rate you have seen in decades.

20. What can I do about my monthly bank loan payments?

Consult your bank representative about grace periods. In cases of widespread national disasters, all banks may be offering grace periods for loan payments without you having to ask.

21. What can I do about my credit/debit card monthly payments?

Again, call the company for each and every card you hold; ask for a supervisor and explain the situation you are in, and ask if there is a grace period that may be applied to help defray finance charges while you are trying to rebuild your business and while you are recouping your business and financial losses.

22. Is the money I receive from my insurance and federal aid programs taxable?

Yes. Many people have been caught by this misunderstood fact. INCOME IS INCOME. Many of these items are taxable and if you spend all of your proceeds, you may be dearly surprised by the taxes due the following April. Consult with your financial advisor/accountant about any financial gains concerning insurance payments and disaster loans/grants.

23. How do I report donations from companies, clients, or rescue groups?

Consult with your financial advisor/accountant about any financial gains concerning insurance payments and disaster loans/grants.

24. Will veterinary supply companies help me get back on my feet?

Without a doubt! There will be many suppliers that will jump to assist you in the postdisaster period. There will be many forms of aid offered, from free pet food, to free supplies, to assistance with notifying the public and your client base of how to contact you or how to get help for their pets while your clinic is in the damage assessment/damage repair period.

25. How can I prepare better for future disasters?

Quarterly meetings with the entire staff are vital to the team's response effort. New hires can be caught up on their duties at these meetings. The entire staff should be handed updated telephone, email, and contact lists for the entire staff at these meetings. Make laminated wallet cards of the essential emergency telephone numbers for your staff to have in their possession. Supervisors should have input on any ways to make the plan run smoother since they are the ones carrying out many of the tasks.

26. How should I let my clientele know of my whereabouts if my clinic is too damaged to work out of or if I have evacuated and cannot return promptly?

The hospital or clinic's telephone company can set up a message for any caller to listen to that alerts the caller to any message you want to convey. Telephone calls may also be forwarded to a cell telephone or another location. It is recommended to place a sign at several locations inside the building in windows or glass doors (facing out) telling clients, rescue personnel and first responders of the whereabouts of the animals and the contact numbers of the hospital/clinic's management team. If you plan to have the clinic closed for an extended period of time, postcards and emails should be sent out letting everyone know the status of the clinic and the staff. Weekly or monthly updates are very reassuring to your loyal clients who need to know that you, your staff, and, in some instances, their pets are okay.

27. How should I prioritize my time between clinic and personal matters?

This is a very intricate matter that will vary depending on the management team at the office and the amount of support help available at home. No doubt both places (home and work) need to have game plans worked out well in advance of a disaster occurrence. Disaster planning will take the worry out of who should be delegated to perform what task and make sure all bases are covered. Lives may be at risk at either or both locations (flood, hurricane, and tornadoes), so details and job descriptions must be worked out in advance and documented on paper.

Suggested Reading
Cavanaugh D. Pensacola, FL, UWF Small Business Development Center. Available at www.sbdc.uwf.edu.
Littlefield, Martha. DVM, Assistant State Veterinarian, Louisiana; Malc@ldaf.state.la.us.

CHAPTER 3.3
PREPARING THE FARM AND ANIMALS FOR A DISASTER

Wayne E. Wingfield, MS, DVM

1. Describe the first step in preparing a farm for a disaster.

Before one can prepare for a disaster, a list of possible disasters and when they may occur should be obtained. Include all possible disasters such as firestorms, earthquakes, tornados, hurricanes, floods, blizzards, hazardous material spills, nuclear accidents, possible terrorist targets in the area, arson, and tsunamis. This part of the disaster plan is called "risk assessment."

2. Does the plan have to contain all the potential disasters?

No. It is unlikely your farm is going to be affected by a winter blizzard if you live in South Florida. Conversely, if you live in Colorado, it is highly unlikely you need to plan for hurricanes or tsunamis. An all hazards plan is desirable but most will customize their plan to their unique risks. Once the plan has been written each farm can decide which actions can be done in advance of the disaster and which actions will be required when the disaster strikes the farm.

3. When preparing a plan for each farm, is it necessary to write out the plan?

Absolutely! All disaster plans must be written to provide concise directions to family, employees, and responders. There is no guarantee you will survive the disaster and thus you need this plan to be available for review, practice, and implementation in the event of a disaster. Importantly, the plan needs to be created *before* the disaster strikes! Just like your other important documents, you need to keep your farm disaster plan in a safe, waterproof, fire resistant, and easily accessible location. Make sure all know where to locate the document.

4. List some other items to include in a farm's disaster plan.

- Names, addresses, and telephone numbers of important family contacts
- Names, addresses, and telephone numbers of neighbors and friends who might be available to lend assistance in the event of a disaster
- Names, addresses, and telephone numbers of trucking firms that might be available to move animals to temporary quarters
- Names, addresses, and telephone numbers of suppliers of feed for livestock

- Names, addresses, and telephone numbers of veterinarians who may be available to assist when animals are ill or injured following the disaster
- An inventory of animals on the farm with documentable evidence of animal identification.
- An inventory of farm equipment and machinery
- Ideally, an up-to-date inventory of all household and shop valuables

5. What steps can be taken to lessen the effects of a disaster on farm livestock?

- Avoid the disaster.
- Mitigate the effects of the disaster if it cannot be avoided.
- Shelter the animals when appropriate for the type of disaster.

6. Define "hazard mitigation."

Hazard mitigation is any action taken to eliminate or reduce the long-term risk to life and property from natural, man-caused, or technological hazards.

7. List some examples of hazard mitigation.

- Clearing brush and timber away from buildings
- Cloud seeding to reduce the intensity of a hurricane
- Storing farm equipment, implements, and fencing materials away from the likely approach of a disaster
- Anchoring homes or barns to the ground in order to withstand wind damage
- Digging water channels around buildings to redirect water
- Planting vegetation to absorb water
- Maintaining a safe distance from waterways for buildings and pens
- Constructing levees or permanent barriers to control flooding
- Maintaining roof structure soundness in all farm buildings
- Replacing glass windows and doors with solid materials or shutters

8. What should be done with pesticides, herbicides, and other potential animal toxins?

All toxins should be properly disposed of with the potential of a disaster in mind. You certainly do not want to bury used containers in an area likely to be flooded or near living quarters for the family, pets, or livestock. Containers of potential toxins must be secured to withstand flooding, high winds, fire, and pilfering.

9. How do good records for livestock help in the farm disaster plan?

By keeping accurate and up-to-date records on each animal on the farm, vaccinations, illnesses, injuries, and genealogy of the animals are available. These records need to include the product name, date of injection, and route of administration. It is not uncommon to see an outbreak of infectious diseases following floods. If your animals are vaccinated against the specific agent(s), they are more likely to be survivors.

10. List some of the items that should be available on each farm prior to a disaster.

- Battery-powered radios and/or televisions
- Flashlights, candles, portable generators
- Fuel and antifreeze for the generators
- Extra batteries
- Salt, gravel, and litter
- Ropes, halters, and animal restraint equipment
- Veterinary supplies (bandage materials, suture, antibiotics, antitoxins, and vaccines)

CONTROVERSY

11. Should you stockpile large amounts of hay and feed prior to a disaster?

Pro: Animal feed will be immediately available for the farm animals. You will not be forced to wait on feed from other locations.

Con: Damage to feed during a disaster is very likely. If hay or grain is wet, it will likely spoil before it can be fed. The one thing we can usually count on is the willingness of our neighbors, friends, and even local, state, and federal governmental agencies to help feed the animals. Experiences in numerous national disasters have shown that food supply for affected animals is usually more than adequate.

12. Who coordinates governmental disaster response?

A farm should be able to sustain itself for one to three days without expecting a government response. Disaster government response begins with local government. Depending on the size and scope of the disaster, local resources are frequently overwhelmed, thus necessitating state government response. Finally, if the state's emergency response is inadequate, it can request help from the federal government. In some disasters such as terrorism, the federal government will become involved almost immediately.

13. How does one decide to evacuate animals from the farm?

In the ideal world, it would be advantageous to move all animals from the path of a disaster. Obviously this will never happen! Instead, one must make decisions on sheltering in place, releasing the animals to pasture, or, as a last resort, transporting the animals from the disaster scene. Previously, some of the criteria used in deciding to evacuate included the following: sale value, breeding quality, stage of pregnancy, stage of production, or simply sentimental preference. If these criteria are to be used, the animals must be identified before the disaster strikes and are thus a part of the overall farm disaster response plan. Before evacuating there must be a plan in place that includes the route of evacuation; available help for moving the animals; transportation sources; the site where the animals will be relocated; the availability of restraint devices, halters, lead ropes, pens, feed, water, and veterinary attention; and, most important, that all animals must be identifiable by ear tag, tattoo, brand, registration papers, or microchip. Unfortunately, the best-made plans are usually disrupted by the same disaster one is evacuating from, and this will require altering plans after first checking to be sure routes, transportation, housing facilities, and personnel are available.

14.   What is the leading disaster for both horse and livestock owners?

Barn fires are likely the most common disaster affecting the farm.

15.   List some action items you can implement to reduce the likelihood of a barn fire.

- Prohibit all smoking in and around the barn.
- Do not store hay that has not been dried thoroughly prior to baling.
- Minimize the use of electrical appliances in the barn.
- Inspect and maintain all electrical systems on a regular basis.
- Avoid parking tractors, motorized farm equipment, and vehicles in or near the livestock barn.
- Discard any electrical appliance with a frayed electrical cord.
- Install a sprinkler system in livestock barns or, at the very least, install smoke detectors that will be audible from the farm house.

16.   What are some action items for managing poultry during a disaster?

- Fortunately, most commercial poultry facilities have been built on high ground and are less susceptible to flooding.
- With small poultry flocks, the birds need a high place to perch but also need access to food and clean water.

17.   What is meant by the phrase "sheltering in place"?

If evacuation is not possible, one must decide whether to confine livestock to an available shelter on the farm or leave the animals out to pasture. This decision must be based on the structural soundness of the shelter, the type and ferocity of the impending disaster, available barn space, number and species of animals, and disposition of these animal species. These tough decisions must be made and written into the farm disaster plan. Realistically, it is likely that most farm animals will be best turned out to pasture.

18.   What are some of the criteria you might use in deciding to release your livestock into your pasture?

- Power lines should not be strung through the pasture area.
- The presence of nonnative trees or shallow-rooted trees which are less likely to survive high winds should influence your decision.
- Woven wire appears to be the best fencing for hurricane-prone areas. It acts like a volleyball net; in many cases falling trees do not even take it down. It doesn't pull apart in high winds. Animals are less likely to get caught or tangled in it.
- Barbed wire fencing should not be loose around the pasture.
- Debris that could fly around during a disaster will be injurious to livestock.
- The pasture needs to provide ample space to move away from perceived threats. Releasing animals in small spaces (less than 1 acre) will not be adequate. These animals need to be evacuated.

19. If animals must be left unattended on the farm as the family is evacuated, how much food and water should be provided to the animals (Table 3.3.1)?

Table 3.3.1 Feed and Water Requirements for Animals

Animals	Water/day	Feed/day
Cattle		
In production	Summer: 9 gallons Winter: 7 gallons	20 pounds hay
Dry cows	Summer: 9 gallons Winter: 7 gallons	20 pounds hay
Weaning cows	Summer: 3 gallons Winter: 6 gallons	8–12 pounds hay
Pregnant cow	Summer: 7 gallons Winter: 6 gallons	10–15 pounds hay
Cow with calf	Summer: 9 gallons Winter: 8 gallons	12–18 pounds hay
Calf (400 pounds)	Summer: 6 gallons Winter: 4 gallons	8–12 pounds hay
Swine		
Brood sow and litter	3–7 gallons	8 pounds grain
Pregnant brood sow	3–6 gallons	2 pounds grain
!50 lb gilt or boar	3–5 gallons	3 pounds grain
Sheep		
Ewe with lamb	1 gallon	5 pounds hay
Ewe, dry	3 quarts	3 pounds hay
Weanling lamb	2 quarts	3 pounds hay
Poultry		
Layers	5 gallons/100 birds	17 lb/100 birds
Boilers	5 gallons/100 birds	10 lb/100 birds
Turkeys	12 gallons/100 birds	40 lb/100 birds
Horses		
All breeds	5 gallons/1000 lb	20 lb hay/1000 lb
Dogs and Cats		
All breeds	1 quart/animal	Free choice dry food

Based on Casper J, Heath SE, Linnabary RD. Preparing the farm and farm animals for a disaster. *Animal Welfare Information Center Newsletter* 1993;4:3–6.

20. What are the leading causes of death to large animals following a hurricane?

- **Collapsed barns:** Owners thought their animals were safer inside, but confinement takes away the animals' ability to protect themselves.
- **Kidney failure due to dehydration:** Wandering animals were deprived of food and water for days.
- **Electrocution:** Horses seek the lowest areas, in many cases this was a drainage ditch. Power lines are strung over drainage ditches and were blown down during the storm.
- **Fencing failure:** Wandering animals, although unharmed during the storm, were hit and killed on the roadways.

21. How does hurricane debris result in injury to farm animals?

Debris caused the most severe injuries. Many horses were euthanizatized due to entanglement in barbed wire and the resultant severe injuries. Debris injuries were found most often in the hindquarters, as horses turned their tails to the storm. Do not keep your animals in the barn to prevent debris injury. Debris injuries are severe, but in most cases treatable. If your barn collapses—*and there is no way to ensure that it won't*—farm animals have no chance to save themselves and are likely to panic if they cannot follow their instincts.

22. How can production records benefit the farmer following the disaster?

Production records are vital to the recovery phase of a disaster. With these records, there are numerous opportunities available for compensation of lost production costs. Your farm disaster response plan will include insurance and information regarding how to apply for these funds. The one caveat to recall is that you must insure the farm *before* the disaster occurs!

23. Any final thoughts on preparing the farm and farm animals for a disaster?

A farm disaster response plan will undoubtedly lessen the effects from the disaster. Economically, it is cheaper to prevent the problem or lessen the effects than to pay the costs of recovery.

Suggested Reading
Casper J, Heath SE, Linnabary RD. Preparing the farm and farm animals for a disaster. *Animal Welfare Information Center Newsletter* 1993;4:3–6.
http://doacs.state.fl.us/ai/.
http://www.fl-adpac.org.

CHAPTER 3.4
NOAH'S BURDEN: A PROLEGOMENON TO THE ETHICS OF VETERINARY DISASTER RESPONSE

Bernard E. Rollin, PhD

1. The most fundamental question pertaining to veterinarian involvement in disaster relief is a jarring, politically incorrect one— why spend (waste?) resources on animals when the same money could be spent to benefit humans?

An equally politically incorrect riposte is to point out that the person raising this question is very unlikely to take it seriously in his or her own life. Such a person very likely contributes to causes like Girl Scouts, Little League, sending the high school band on a European tour, or National Public Radio. If so, he or she is vulnerable to being hoisted on their own petard—why spend money on relative frivolities when people are starving? Why not forego dessert and give the money to Oxfam?

The answer, of course, is that few, if any, of us triage our moral concern in any rational way, scaled to need. We give charity based on our tastes and predilections and nonrational inclinations. Furthermore, as one of my cowboy students once responded to a similar challenge, "Morality is not a single shot shotgun." In essence, in a free society people may spend their money as they wish.

And there is no question that society has experienced a precipitous increase in concern for animals and their welfare since the early 1970s. This is evidenced in diverse ways by the passage of federal legislation in 1985 protecting the well-being of laboratory animals despite vigorous opposition from the research community: by Smithfield, the world's largest pork producer, abandoning sow stalls in virtue of consumer demand; by the most common topic on New York City cable television being animals; by fully 2,100 bills pertaining to animal well-being being floated in state legislatures in 2004; by people voting with their dollars for animal welfare–friendly products such as free-range eggs. Animal welfare concerns are ubiquitous across all areas of animal use. In such an environment, it is highly unlikely that society would countenance callous disregard of at least some animals in disaster situations, notably people's pets: this is evidenced by the public reaction to major failures to rescue companion animals after Hurricane Katrina.

2. In and of itself, of course, social fads are not moral justification, and appealing to them represents a classic ad populum fallacy. The key question, then, is whether there is a substantive moral substructure undergirding popular concerns.

The answer is yes. Historically, our actions toward animals were not the objects of examination by our full moral machinery. The only formalized societal ethic was represented by the anticruelty laws, proscribing deliberate, sadistic, purposeless, deviant, unnecessary, willful infliction of pain and suffering on animals, or outrageous neglect. This ethic, as Thomas Aquinas pointed out, existed more to ferret out and punish psychopathic individuals who might represent a danger to humans than to codify direct obligations to animals. (This insight is buttressed by recent research showing that animal cruelty is a major indicator of psychopathy.) Judicial history attests to the fact that "accepted" infliction of pain and suffering, i.e., that which, in the words of one judge, "ministers to the

501

necessity of man" broadly conceived, is invisible to the cruelty laws. Such pain-causing activities as steel-jawed trapping or hot-iron branding, for example, are exempt from cruelty prosecution. In short, if one considers the sum total of all suffering that animals experience at human hands, only a tiny fraction of that falls under the purview of the historically accepted social ethic for animals.

Work by philosophers over the last 30 years has challenged this limited ethic as inadequate. This challenge is based on the concept of what Peter Singer has aptly called "the expanding circle." Just as society has expanded the protection of our ethical umbrella and laws to cover disenfranchised humans—women, blacks, children, foreigners, non–property owners (the original citizens under the U.S. constitution were white, adult, native-born, male property owners), so we must judge the treatment of animals by more than just the blunt instrument of cruelty. This is true for two related reasons. First, one can identify no morally relevant reason for excluding animals from such protection and one can identify positive reasons for including them—to wit, that what we do *matters to them* (i.e., they are aware and can be harmed [or helped] by our actions). This insight provides a rational basis for the societal concern for animal treatment we mentioned earlier. In a nutshell, people wish to see animals protected from suffering in ways far beyond overt cruelty, hence the proliferation of laws and regulations in all areas of animal use.

Thus, extending moral concern to animals in disaster situations even as we do to humans would appear to be a rational ethical implication of changing societal ethics. But we as yet have no clear sense of what that means, or what sorts of animals are covered and in what way. If we looked at our obligations to humans affected by disasters, forms of aid vary considerably, from extensive to limited and from public money to private money along a spectrum.

3. What does rational ethical consideration suggest as answers to these questions? If we accept that all animals are to be included in the scope of moral concern, or are in the moral arena, how do we determine extents of obligations?

There are no firm rules of how this is done even in human ethics with regard to disaster aid—such questions as what we should be doing in Darfur, should we provide aid to civilians in enemy states, do we give priority to Europe or Asia—remain unresolved. Certainly some answers seem clear—for example, we help our own people before we help others, even as we feed our own children before feeding other people's children. This meager principle is of some value in determining our obligations to animals in disasters. Presumably all other things being equal, we should give priority to animals who mean a lot to people.

There is no doubt that pets have assumed an unprecedented role in human life, at least in American society, if not Western society in general. Repeated surveys indicate that as much as 95+% of the U.S. public view their companion animals as "members of the family." Divorce lawyers will attest to the fact that custody of pets in a divorce can be as great a source of tension as custody of the children.

4. It was not very long ago that grief over pet-loss subjected the grieving person to ridicule—today, such grief counseling is an academic discipline and an industry. What has occurred to effect such dramatic change?

The rise of a bond between humans and animals rooted not only in mutual symbiotic benefit, but also in something putatively more solid, did not occur until the twentieth century, with companion animals and the new sort of relationship we formed with them. While humans have enjoyed symbiotic relationships with dogs and, to a lesser extent, with cats for some 50,000 years, the bond was, as was the case with agricultural animals, one largely of mutual practical benefit. Dogs were useful as guardians of flocks, alarms warning of intruders, hunting partners, pest controllers, finders of lost people, haulers of carts, and finders and retrievers of game. In terms of mutual interdependence, dogs were very much analogous to livestock except that they were probably worth less.

In the past 50 or so years, however, dogs (and to a lesser extent, cats and other species) have become valued not only for the pragmatic, economically quantifiable purposes just detailed but for deep emotional reasons as well. These animals are viewed as members of the family, as friends, as "givers and receivers of love" as one judge put it—and the bond based in pragmatic symbiosis has turned into a bond based in love. This new basis for the bond imposes higher expectations on those party to such a bond on the analogy of how we feel we should relate to humans we are bound to by love and family. If a purely working dog is crippled and can no longer tend to the sheep, it violates no moral canon (except, perhaps, loyalty) to affirm that he needs to be replaced by another healthy animal and, like livestock, may be euthanized if the owner needs a functioning animal. (In practice, of course, people often kept the old animals around for supererogatory or "sentimental" reasons, but, conceptually, keeping them alive and cared for when they no longer could fulfill their function was not morally required any more than was keeping a cow alive that could no longer give milk.)

But insofar as an animal is truly perceived as an object of love or friendship, as companion animals have come to be perceived in the past 50 years, or as a member of the family, a different set of moral obligations are incurred. We do not euthanize or adopt out (let alone relinquish) a crippled child or sick spouse or aged parent—at most we may institutionalize them if we are unable to provide the requisite care. A love-based bond imposes a higher and more stringent set of moral obligations than does one based solely in mutual pragmatic benefit.

The rise of deep love-based relationships with animals as a regular and increasingly accepted social phenomenon came from a variety of converging and mutually reinforcing social conditions. In the first place, probably beginning with the widespread use of the automobile, extended nuclear families with multi-generations living in one location or under one roof began to vanish. At the beginning of the twentieth century, when roughly half of the public produced food for themselves and the other half of the public, significant numbers of large extended families lived together manning farms. The safety net for older people was their family, rather than society as a whole. The concept of easy mobility made preserving the nuclear family less of a necessity, as did the rise of the new idea that society as a whole rather than the family was responsible for assuring retirement, medical attention, and facilities for elderly people.

With the concentration of agriculture in fewer and fewer hands, the rise of industrialization, and as the post-Depression Dust Bowl and World War II introduced migration to cities, the nuclear family notion was further eroded. The tendency of urban life to erode community, to create what the Germans called *Gesellshaft* rather than *Gemeinschaft*, mixtures rather than compounds, as it were, further created solitude and loneliness as widespread modes of being. Correlatively, as selfishness and self-actualization were established as positive values beginning in highly individualistic 1960s, the divorce rate began to climb, and the traditional stigma attached to divorce was erased. As biomedicine prolonged our life spans, more and more people outlived their spouses, and were thrown into a loneliness mode of existence, with the loss of the extended family removing a possible remedy.

In effect, we have lonely old people, lonely divorced people, and, most tragically, lonely children whose single parent often works. With the best jobs being urban, or quasi-urban, many people live in cities or peripherally urban developments such as condos. In New York City, for example, one can be lonelier than in rural Wyoming. The cowboy craving camaraderie can find a neighbor from whom he is separated only by physical distance; the urban person may know no one, and have no one in striking distance who cares. Shorn of physical space, people create psychic distances between themselves and others. People may (and usually *do*) for years live 6 inches away from neighbors in apartment buildings and never exchange a sentence. Watch New Yorkers on an elevator; the rule is stand as far away from others as you can, and study the ceiling. Making eye contact on a street can be taken as a challenge, or a sexual invitation, so people do not. One minds one's own business, one steps over and around drunks on the street; "Don't get involved" is a mantra for survival.

Yet humans need love, companionship, and emotional support and need to be needed. In such a world, a companion animal can be one's psychic and spiritual salvation. An animal is someone to hug, and hug you back; someone to play with, to laugh with; to exercise with; to walk with; to share beautiful days; to cry with. For a child, the dog is a playmate, a friend; someone to talk to. The dog is a protector; one very unforgettable photograph shows a child of 6 in an apartment answering the door at night while clutching the collar of a 200-pound Great Dane, protected.

For many old people, the dog (or cat) is a reason to get up in the morning, to go out, to bundle up and go to the park ("Fluffy misses her friends, you know!"), to shop, to fuss, to feel responsible for a life, and to feel needed.

Thus, companion animals then, in today's world, provide us with love and someone to love, and do so unfailingly, with loyalty, grace, and boundless devotion. In a book that should be required reading for all who work with animals, author Jon Katz has chronicled what he calls the *New Work of Dogs*, all based on his personal experiences in a New Jersey suburban community. Here we read of the dog that a woman credits with shepherding her through a losing battle with cancer, as her emotional bed rock. Katz tells of the "Divorced Women's Dog Club," a group of divorced women united only by divorce and reliance on their dogs. He tells the tale of a dog who provides an outlet for a ghetto youth's insecurity and rage, and who is beaten daily. He relates the story of a successful executive with a family and friends, who in the end deals with stress in his life only by long walks with his Labrador, totaling many hours in a day. While raising the question of whether we are entitled to expect this of our animals, Katz explains that we do, and that they perform heroically.

Our pets have become sources of friendship and company for the old and the lonely, vehicles for penetrating the frightful shell surrounding a disturbed child, beings that provide the comfort of touch even to the most asocial person, and inexhaustible sources of pure, unqualified love.

The above considerations indicate why we must reasonably give more weight to an animal with which a person is emotionally bonded than to one who is not so bonded in a situation demanding triage decisions. In effect, this means that we should save companion animals as we save the humans to whom they are bonded, a point that was all too intuitively evident during Hurricane Katrina, when people risked their lives and refused rescue when their animals could not leave with them. This has been evident intuitively for many years, when firemen, for example, risk their lives to rescue a family pet. We can be morally certain that they do so for some combination of the reasons discussed above, both the recognition that what happens to animals matters to them, and the recognition of the profound importance of the animals to their humans.

5. Describe the variety of problems that arise in disaster relief, even if we give pride of phase to people's companion animals.

One such issue devolves around postdisaster medical care. Who should bear the cost of such treatment? While one may reasonably affirm that the costs should accrue to the animals' owners, what if the owners are rendered financially destitute? Furthermore, in the case of the poor, they may have never been in a financial position to pay for catastrophic illness or injury even before a disaster. Yet an animal may mean as much to such a person as to an affluent person, or quite possibly mean more, as "all the person has left." In this case, disaster simply magnifies a problem already inherent in society.

Another issue is provided by the example of Hurricane Katrina. Suppose an animal is separated from its owner, but rescued and placed in a foster home or adoptive home. Assuming the original owner is located after some time, should the animal be returned to the original owner?

In my view, the answer is "yes." Precedent exists in human situations during the Holocaust, when children, often infants, were placed with non-Jewish families to protect them, and then grew up as members of that family. The Holocaust ended, and the birth parent or parents, who may not have seen the child for many years, and have not had any part in their lives, now demand the return of the child. Heart-wrenching though such scenarios may be, the children were usually returned to the birth parent. The strong claim of a natural parent who did not relinquish the child willingly to getting the child back is generally seen to trump the adoptive parent's claim. In the end, someone must suffer. It seems intuitively clear that the birth parent, who has suffered greatly, should be given every chance to rebuild his or her life. Certainly the harm to the adoptive parent is significant, but in the end their primary role was to *save* the child for as long as necessary, not necessarily to have it forever!

6. We can reasonably move on to asking about our obligations to other animals, notably livestock and "wild" animals. Since neither set of animals stand in the same relationship to humans as companion animals (except for some horses), we must explore which group gets triage priority. We will argue that "it depends."

To begin with livestock: such animals, while rarely (though sometimes) members of the family, do stand in a special relationship to humans. In particular I am referring to animals raised under animal husbandry, rather than "animal science," defined as the application of industrial methods to production of animals. It is noteworthy that, if we look at the approximately 11,000 years of animal domestication, industrialized agriculture has been extant for approximately .006% of that time—the rest of the time animal agriculture was husbandry.

The traditional account of the growth of human civilization out of a hunter-gatherer society invariably invokes the rise of agriculture (i.e., the domestication of animals and the cultivation of crops). This, of course, allowed for as predictable a food supply as humans could create in the vagaries of the natural world—floods, droughts, hurricanes, typhoons, extremes of heat and cold, fires, etc. Indeed, the use of animals enabled the development of successful crop agriculture, with the animals providing labor and locomotion, as well as food and fiber.

This eventuated in what has been called the "ancient contract" with animals, a highly symbiotic relationship that endured essentially unchanged for thousands of years. Humans selected among animals congenial to human management, and further shaped them in terms of temperament and production traits by breeding and artificial selection. These animals included cattle—dubbed by Calvin Schwabe the "mother of the human race"—sheep, goats, horses, dogs, poultry and other birds, swine, ungulates, and other animals capable of domestication. The animals provided food and fiber—meat, milk, wool, leather; power to haul and plow; transportation; and sometimes served as weaponry, as in the case of horses and elephants. As people grew more effective at breeding and managing the animals, productivity was increased.

As humans benefited, so simultaneously did the animals. They were provided with the necessities of life in a predictable way. And thus was born the concept of husbandry, the remarkable practice and articulation of the symbiotic contract.

"Husbandry" is derived from the Old Norse words *hus* and *bond*; the animals were bonded to one's household. The essence of husbandry was care. Humans put animals into the most ideal environment possible for the animals to survive and thrive, the environment for which they had evolved and been selected. In addition, humans provided them with sustenance, water, shelter, protection from predation, such medical attention as was available, help in birthing, food during famine, water during drought, safe surroundings, and comfortable appointments.

Eventually, what was borne of necessity and common sense became articulated in terms of a moral obligation inextricably bound up with self-interest. In the Noah story, we learn that even as God preserves humans, humans preserve animals, exemplifying the ethics of our obligations to animals in disasters. The ethic of husbandry is in fact taught throughout the Bible; the animals must rest on the Sabbath even as we do, one is not to seethe a calf in its mother's milk (so we do not grow insensitive to animals needs and natures); we can violate the Sabbath to save an animal. Proverbs tells us that "the wise man cares for his animals." The Old Testament is replete with injunctions against inflicting unnecessary pain and suffering on animals, as exemplified in the strange story of Balaam who beats his ass, and is reprimanded by the animal's speaking through the grace of God.

The true power of the husbandry ethic is best expressed in the 23rd Psalm. There, in searching for an apt metaphor for God's ideal relationship to humans, the Psalmist invokes the good shepherd:

> The Lord is My shepherd; I shall not want.
> He leadeth me to green pastures,
> He maketh me to lie down beside still waters,
> He restoreth my soul.

We want no more from God than what the good shepherd provides to his animals. Indeed, consider a lamb in ancient Judaea. Without a shepherd, the animal would not easily find forage or water, would not survive the multitude of predators the Bible tells us prowled the land—lions, jackals, hyenas, birds of prey, and wild dogs. Under the aegis of the shepherd, the lamb lives well and safely. In return, the animals provide their products and sometimes their lives, but while they live, they live well. And even slaughter, the taking of the animal's life, must be as painless as possible, performed with a sharp knife by a trained person to avoid unnecessary pain. Ritual slaughter was, in antiquity, a far kinder death than bludgeoning; most important, it was the most humane modality available at the time.

The metaphor of the good shepherd is emblazoned in the Western mind. Jesus is depicted as both shepherd and lamb from the origin of Christianity until the present in paintings, literature, song, statuary, and poetry, as well as in sermons. To this day, ministers are called shepherds of their congregation, and "pastor" derives from "pastoral." And when Plato discusses the ideal political ruler in the *Republic*, he deploys the shepherd–sheep metaphor: The ruler is to his people as the shepherd is to his flock. Qua shepherd, the shepherd exists to protect, preserve and improve the sheep; any payment tendered to him is in his capacity as wage earner. So, too, the ruler, again illustrating the power of the concept of husbandry on our psyches.

The singular beauty of husbandry is that it was at once an ethical and prudential doctrine. It was prudential in that failure to observe husbandry inexorably led to ruination of the person keeping animals. Not feeding, not watering, not protecting from predators, not respecting the animals' physical, biological physiological needs and natures, what Aristotle called their *telos*—the "cowness of the cow," the "sheepness of the sheep"—meant your animals did not survive and thrive, and thus neither did you. Failure to know and respect the animal's needs and natures had the same effect. Indeed, even Aristotle, whose world view was fully hierarchical with humans at the top, implicitly recognized the contractual nature of husbandry when he off-handedly affirmed that though the natural role of animals is to serve man, domestic animals are "preserved" through so doing. The ultimate sanction of failing at husbandry—erosion of self-interest—obviated the need for any detailed ethical exposition of moral rules for husbandry: Anyone unmoved by self-interest is unlikely to be moved by moral or legal injunctions! And thus one finds little written about animal ethics and little codification of that ethic in law before the twentieth century, with the bulk of what is articulated aimed at identifying overt, deliberate, sadistic cruelty, hurting an animal for no purpose or for perverse pleasure, or not providing food or water.

Under husbandry, the need to help animals in disaster is self-evident. Not only is such help directly related to the philosophical underpinnings of husbandry, it has been internalized by husbandry-based producers. The largest group of such people is Western ranchers. And, of the 15,000 whom I have addressed, one can barely find any who fail to feel a moral obligation to the animals in their charge.

7. That attitude is beautifully encapsulated in the following anecdote: About 3 years ago, I was visiting a rancher friend in Wyoming and having dinner at his home along with a dozen other ranch people. I asked the dinner guests how many of them had ever spent more money on medical treatment for their cattle than the animal was worth in economic terms?

All replied in the affirmative. One woman, a fifth-generation rancher, asked with something of an edge, "What's wrong with that, Buster?" I replied, "Nothing from my perspective. But if I were an agricultural economist, I would tell you that one does not spend $25 to produce a widget that one sells for $20." She fairly spat her reply: "Well, that's your mistake, Buster. We're not producing widgets, were taking care of living beings for whom we are responsible!"

Virtually every rancher I have encountered across the United States and Canadian West would respond in a similar vein. Even if they do not spend cash, ranch people often sit up all night for days with a marginal calf, warming the animal by the stove in the kitchen, and implicitly valuing their sleep at pennies per hour! Children of ranch families often report that the only time their father ever blew up at them was when they went to a dance or a sporting event without taking care of the animals. These ranchers represent the last large group of agriculturalists in the United States still practicing animal husbandry.

Thus, giving aid to farm animals raised under husbandry conceptually parallels our discussion of aid to companion animals. In both cases, direct obligation to the animals is potentiated by the obligation to the animal's owners. When the British killed their cattle herd in order to control foot and mouth disease, the effect on farmers was devastating. The grief of British cattle farmers, leading sometimes to a refusal to witness the killing, and to psychological trauma to many farmers and even to suicide, has been well documented. That trauma is so devastating that it led Nussbaum et al. to argue that veterinarians trained in disaster relief need to be prepared to address the psychological issues, since "in disaster-stricken areas, up to 80% of the casualties can be psychologic." Here, then, is an ethical issue associated with disaster relief that needs to be stressed, since few veterinarians see themselves as rendering psychological first aid.

In the case of industrialized agriculture, the psychological burden on producers will, in most cases, be far less because industrialized producers, particularly very large entities, tend to see themselves as more like manufacturers than shepherds. Once again, an anecdote can point out this difference dramatically.

Consider the story told to me by one of my colleagues in Animal Science at Colorado State University. This man told of his son-in-law who had grown up on a ranch but could not return to it after college because it could not support him and all of his siblings. (Notably, the average net income of a front range rancher in Colorado, Wyoming, or Montana is about $35,000!) He reluctantly took a job managing a feeder pig barn at a large swine factory farm.

One day he reported a disease that had struck his piglets to his boss. "I have bad news and good news," he reported. "The bad news is that the piglets are sick. The good news is that they can be treated economically." "No," said the boss. "We don't treat! We euthanize (by dashing the baby pigs' heads on the side of the concrete pen)." The young man could not accept this. He proceeded to buy the medicine with his own money and clock in on his day off, and treated the animals. They recovered, and he told the boss. The boss's response was, "You're fired!" The young man pointed out that he had treated them with his own time and money, and was thus not subject to firing. He did, however, receive a reprimand in his file. Six months later he quit and became an electrician. He wrote to his father-in-law, "I know you are disappointed that I left agriculture, Dad. But this ain't agriculture!"

Thus, though the ancient contract with domestic animals was inherently sustainable, it was not in fact sustained with the coming of industrialization. Husbandry was born of necessity, and as soon as necessity vanished, the contract was broken. The Industrial Revolution portended the end of husbandry, for humans no longer needed to respect their animals to assure productivity. In symbolic advertisement of the breaking of our sustainable contract with animals, in the mid-twentieth century academic departments of animal husbandry in the United States became departments of animal science, with industry replacing husbandry. The values of productivity and efficiency replaced the values of husbandry, to the detriment of animals, sustainability, the environment, agriculture as a way of life, rural communities, stewardship, and a respectful, moral stance toward the living things we built our civilization on.

Animal husbandry may be characterized as putting square pegs in square holes, round pegs in round holes, and creating as little friction as possible in doing so. Failure at husbandry meant that one's animals did not produce; failure to respect animal needs and natures hurt oneself as well as the animals. This was suddenly overridden by technological tools, as it were "technological sanders," that allowed us to force square pegs into round holes, and round pegs into square holes, and where, at least in the short run, productivity flourished at the expense of respect for animal needs and natures.

I do not, of course, intend to suggest that, as a matter of logical necessity, *every person* using industrial methods does not care about his or her animals. But there is unquestionably such a strong tendency inherent in the nature of such systems. One of the managers of the largest swine production operation in Colorado some years ago was an accountant who was honestly puzzled when I asked him about his knowledge of swine. "What does that have to do with managing this facility?" he asked.

So clearly the obligation based on a concern for animals as anything other than economic units to people does not loom as large in industrial agriculture. As far as the animals themselves are concerned, however, we are equally obliged to help, particularly since these animals are often put into danger by the systems we keep them in (e.g., the floods in North Carolina that killed many pigs in confinement). In addition, we have truncated their natural abilities to survive, and they are totally dependent on us in the event of disaster, unable even to escape.

8. What of "wild animals" caught in a disaster?

Few people have discussed our obligation to such animals. My own tendency is to affirm that we should leave them alone. For example, I have argued that we have no obligation to save the rabbit from the fox or to try and impose a vegetarian diet on predatory carnivores, although some philosophers feel otherwise. Thus, in my view, if a tornado strikes the Galapagos, I don't think we have any duty to help beyond what we owe animals as moral objects.

The moral dimension changes significantly, however, if the harm experienced by "wild animals" is as a result of human interference or effect on their environment. And very often we have had deleterious effects on their ability to fend for themselves. Some years ago, Rocky Mountain sheep in Wyoming suffered a chlamydial eye infection, blinding them so that they were falling off cliffs and dying of hunger and thirst. The authorities refused to treat this infection, on the grounds that it was a "natural disaster." This is disingenuous, since the infection was acquired from human livestock. In my view, we here have a paradigmatic duty to treat, since the infection would not be there were it not for us. Similarly, in many cases, we simply do not know the causes of animal problems. I recall seeing an impala with a stick buried in its side in South Africa. This sort of thing—wounding— happens all the time, without our knowledge or, as in my case, without an ability to intervene. On the other hand, as even hunting ethics decrees, when an animal is suffering due to something humans have done (e.g., a badly aimed shot), we have a duty to alleviate the animal's suffering.

As a general principle, I would articulate as a maxim, "If humans are directly or indirectly responsible for a disaster befalling animals, humans have a duty to ameliorate the problem well beyond their simple obligation to the animals as moral objects." The *Chlamydia* case described here is a good example, as is fire started by humans, floods caused by dams bursting, disease spread from livestock, or disease created by ground, air, or water pollution, as has famously occurred with massive fish kills. A similar example can be found in damage to animals occasioned by global warming, if indeed humans are responsible for this phenomenon.

On the other hand, if a disaster is natural, such as volcanic activity, hurricane, or tsunami, the amelioration of animal suffering is more a matter of charity than of duty, since humans bear no responsibility.

Laboratory animals and zoo animals are similar to animals in industrial agriculture. We have deprived them of their natural abilities to cope or escape and made them totally dependent on us. Many such animals could not survive outside of the highly artificial environments we have adapted them to. Thus, we have a responsibility to ensure that they not suffer in the event of a disaster, even if that obligation is met by humane euthanasia as an alternative to starvation or drowning. In the case of zoo animals, some may enjoy quasi-pet status, as did the polar bears Klondike and Snow, born and reared at the Denver Zoo, whose survival and maturation became something with which the public identified.

Veterinarians often receive harsh criticisms from the public for euthanizing animals during disasters. The public must be educated to understand that euthanasia may be the only modality for ending animal suffering for physical or medical reasons or because of lack of resources for treating animals. If the public is not so educated, veterinarians may experience what I called "moral stress" 25 years ago. Moral stress occurs paradigmatically when humane society workers or veterinarians kill healthy animals for owner or societal convenience and grows out of the conflict between such killing and one's fundamental motive for working in the field. If such stress is engendered by societal lack of understanding of euthanasia during disaster, the veterinarians' physical and mental health may suffer great damage.

9. How would I summarize some of the ethical dilemmas noted here?

There are a vast number of individual ethical issues that arise in massive endeavors like disaster response, many of them unprecedented. In such cases we must, as we so often do, "muddle through." Our discussion has been designed to show that incurring the burden of dealing with such situations is morally justifiable and indeed obligatory, although it entails engaging a wide range of moral problems about animals that society has hardly begun to address.

Suggested Reading

Katz J. *The New Work of Dogs: Tending to Life, Love and Family*. New York, Villand, 2003.

Nussbaum KE, et al. 2007. Psychologic first and veterinarians in rural communities undergoing livestock depopulation. *J Am Vet Med Assoc* 2007;231:692.

Rollin BE. *Animal Rights and Human Morality*. 3rd ed. Buffalo, NY, Prometheus Books, 2006.

SECTION 4
RECOVERY

CHAPTER 4.1
CARE FOR THE CAREGIVER: PSYCHOLOGICAL AND EMOTIONAL FACTORS IN VETERINARY DISASTER RESPONSE

Dennis Michael Baker, MA, LPC, and P. J. Havice-Cover, MA, LPC, CAC III

Taking care of the psychological needs of those who provide medical and protection services for animals and, by default, their owners during a catastrophic event is a critical function that has been traditionally overlooked. Casualty factors in disaster response for these professionals include burnout, stress-related illnesses and somatic complaints, interpersonal conflicts (Lawrence, 2006), depression, high rates of suicide (Bartram and Baldwin, 2008), and vicarious trauma.

1. What is stress, and how can it affect me during a disaster?

Stress is the feeling of overload of internal and/or external pressure we experience when we are faced with changes. When events happen that are outside of the normal range of what we have come to expect, we are out of our comfort zone of predictability. If your car always starts and then it does not start, it causes stress. Too much stress, however, such as stress experienced in a disaster, can cause reactions that are less than helpful. Extreme stress can cause the brain to send out distress signals that tell us to fight, flight, freeze, or faint to escape the stressor. These are the most common extreme distress reactions. While these distress signals can be useful in certain life or death situations, they can interfere with optimal functioning when one of these signals is activated during a high stress event. In an evacuation where time is of the essence and stress levels are high, reactions may take the form of one of the four stress reactions. Those whose automatic reaction is to freeze or fight may be a liability and interfere with their own rescue.

2. Can stress also be a positive force?

While stress is often seen as a negative factor, it can also be a positive force that can motivate us to take action. Without *any* stress, we see no reason to do things differently. When stress levels are low, we maintain the status quo and carry on business as usual. Figure 4.1.1 illustrates the concept of how a healthy amount of stress increases performance, but when stress becomes excessive, it causes ill effects and decreases performance.

3. Are there types of catastrophic events that cause more stress for veterinarians than others?

While all catastrophic events cause stress, some events have been shown to be more disturbing than others (Norris et al., 2005). Current theory on extreme psychological effects shows that human-caused events such as arson and terrorism create more dissonance because of the intentional destruction versus an act of nature or an accident, which is easier to justify. In a natural disaster or accidental occurrence, we assume that it is unintentional. It is explainable and therefore it may be excused. Intentional destruction, on the other hand, prompts anger because the act was done to someone or something with the purpose of hurting, scaring, or disabling.

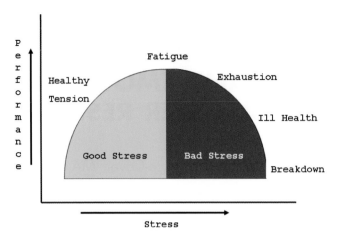

Figure 4.1.1   A healthy amount of stress increases performance, but when stress becomes excessive it causes ill effects and decreases performance.

Intentional harm is unpardonable. Animal cruelty or events that have cascading effects that cause injury are difficult, if not impossible, to overlook. It seems the world is not a safe place. Omissions, on the other hand, lead us to conclude incompetence for things such as failing to protect or relocate pets or livestock when there is impending devastation of a credible threat. The threat may be weather related as in extreme heat or cold, flood, hurricane, or fire, or it may be a preventable disease. Omission offenses are more common than willful harm, and therefore, while still not acceptable, are more psychologically pardonable. Finally, accidents or acts of nature are unpredictable and are usually justifiable because of the perception that the wrongdoer had little or no warning and was a victim of the circumstances.

4.   What are some constructive ways to deal with the stress veterinarians face during a disaster?

You want to help. You want to be able to stay focused on the most critical needs. One of the most promising evidence-informed strategies for dealing with disaster stress is psychological first aid (PFA) (National Child Traumatic Stress Network, 2006). Like the medical form of first aid, PFA is intended to restore function, stabilize, and determine if a call for an advanced level of help is necessary. The difference between medical first aid and PFA is that PFA is focused on psychological stabilization. An adverse stress reaction can be dangerous to the person's well-being or to those around the person affected by a challenging situation. PFA is flexible and can be used by behavior health professionals or by a layperson who understands the purpose and goals.

5.   How is psychological first aid administered?

PFA is composed of eight steps to help a distressed person regain their emotional equilibrium. These steps are as follows:

1. **Contact** and **Engagement**—Make a connection with the distressed person.
2. Ensure their **Safety** and **Comfort**
3. **Stabilization** through calming techniques
4. **Information Gathering**—What are their concerns?
5. **Practical Assistance**—Do they have the basics?
6. **Connection with Social Supports**—Who can they connect to, besides you?
7. **Information on Coping**—Normalizing their reaction to stress
8. **Linkage with Collaborative Services**—What agencies can assist them?

A way to help refocus and stabilize is to help a person focus on his or her breathing. One stress management breathing technique uses a 12-count system where you ask the person to breath in through the nose to the count of 4 (e.g., 1, 2, 3, 4) and hold it for the count of 4, then blow it out through the mouth to the count of 4. Have the person continue until he or she reports feeling better or, if this does not provide relief, have him or her cease this exercise and consult with a medical and/or behavioral health specialist.

6. What are some other considerations for coping with disaster-related stress?

Other ways to cope with stress are to maintain optimism and hope. Looking forward to better days and reminding yourself that things will not always look as glum as they do right now can be resilience building. Hope allows us to see past the current stressful event. By managing your stress, you can maximize your effectiveness.

7. I feel helpless when I'm unable to give the best care possible to each case because there are so many veterinary needs during a disaster. How can I deal with this?

It feels uncomfortable when we are forced to make difficult decisions based on unfortunate circumstances. Keep in mind that you *are* making a difference if you are trying to help. You want to give each case your best efforts, and it seems like all you have time to do is a second-rate, quick fix at best. We all want to save the town from destruction and make it all better—after all we are helpers. However, more often than not the unsung heroes are the ones taking care of the details like bandaging and relocating pets and livestock. It helps maintain perspective.

8. How can I maintain perspective when things look so bleak?

Reframing is a technique for looking at a situation from a different perspective. In a disaster, it may involve reevaluating the reasons for using an altered standard of care. During stressful situations, most people try to do the best they can under the circumstances. We operate under certain assumptions most of the time and have standard operating procedures. We feel comfortable knowing protocol and procedures, and it may be uncomfortable when we are faced with the challenge of treating more cases with fewer resources at an inferior level than you usually do.

For example, we can look at it from the "glass is half-empty" perspective in having to turn away pet owners with animals with minor injuries as a painful reality and curse the blighted, poorly managed, systems that did not plan well enough so this did not happen. Or we could see it as a "glass-is-half-full" perception and see the value of providing *lifesaving* care to as many pets as we are able that have *serious* injuries when services must be rationed due to an overwhelming need. When triage is necessary, the focus is on doing the greatest good for the most cases. *Triage* simply stated means sorting the treatable cases with the best chance for survival.

9. Animal owners sometimes get angry when we cannot save their pet or livestock from an injury or illness. During a disaster, those concerns escalate. What suggestions can you offer for dealing with unhappy clients?

Anger and grief are common reactions when unpleasant things happen. In a disaster, the world as we knew it has changed for the worse. When bad things happen, we want an explanation and answers to why this happened.

Sometimes blames gets assigned in an attempt to say, "If they would have done _____, this wouldn't have happened." This may or may not be a true statement but the point is—what can we do now? It is uncomfortable to be around angry people. In everyday situations, we usually try to avoid confrontation, hoping for the storm to blow over, or we defend ourselves. In the case of hostile pet or livestock owners, it may be helpful to listen to concerns they have and find something in their statement you both agree on. For example, if they are talking about how their beloved pet should never have died and you could have done more, you may agree on the part about how unfair it feels to lose a valued family member.

10. Sometimes during crisis things seem to escalate. Are there ways to avoid this?

Defending your actions about not doing enough gives the angry person fuel to continue their attack. No matter how you say you did all you could, they may still be angry and it could escalate. A sincere "I am very sorry" seems inadequate. However, it can provide the bridge to understanding that you tried and you are sorry you could not save their loved one. A word of caution, saying "I'm sorry" and following it with the word "but" or "however" means, "I am not taking any responsibility." It can intensify the anger they already feel.

Anger management does not mean you do not get angry, it means you have effective coping mechanisms for dealing with the annoyances that can build up to anger. Anger management means dealing with the minor issues that are irritating by reframing, selectively ignoring some things, discussing it with someone whom it also affects, or fixing the problem. Managing stress and anger at the minor irritation level allows you to have more energy to devote to the issues you choose to address.

11. How can a veterinarian help with issues of grieving over animal loss?

Despite the best-laid plans, the loss of companion animals and livestock may be unavoidable. While most practicing veterinarians are likely to be familiar with specific aspects of animal loss and bereavement, not everyone on the emergency response team will be—neighbors and other community members supporting individual and family losses may also be relatively unaware of these issues.

The intensity of grief over the death of a beloved animal may take the owner by surprise, but this can be attributed to the special nature of the bond and to the role that the animal played in the person's life. Grieving over an animal has long been a disenfranchised process. Even with the recent focus of animal losses, our society has not fully acknowledged or sanctioned such mourning. The likelihood of disenfranchised grieving increases considerably in the event of livestock loss on farms in a disaster. In cases where the decision to euthanize an animal has been involved in the loss, the event may aggravate a sense of guilt, regret, or even failure. The need to cull healthy herds to contain an epidemic may be particularly devastating. It is supportive and therapeutic for the veterinarian to tell clients that grieving an animal loss is normal and that it is unnecessary and even unhealthy to minimize these feelings (Podrazik et al., 2000; Stutts, 1996).

12. What are the psychological impacts for epidemic livestock loss?

Recent livestock epidemics that required extensive depopulation or culling offer many lessons in the emotional toll that can be anticipated as well as what interventions may be helpful. An outbreak of ovine Johne's disease in Australian sheep in 1995 required that the government quarantine farms and depopulate flocks. The program was suspended in 1999 because of mounting reports of severe emotional and social distress in farmers, nonfarming rural families, and government employees who had to implement the destocking program. Destocking caused multiple losses beyond the actual loss of the herds of healthy sheep, leading to financial downturn and stigma. Destocking was described by farmers as traumatic and emotionally shattering: "We could hear the lambs bleating even after leaving the sheep yards, and we were no longer able to watch." Farmers who were forced to kill their own flocks early in the program were the most profoundly affected. The government staff witnessing or conducting the slaughter were traumatized as well and were subject to open hostility, exhaustion, and burnout. Rural businesses blamed farmers, and both blamed the government (Department of Natural Resources and the Environment Investigatory Committee to the Parliament of Victoria Australia, 2000).

The most recent outbreak of foot-and-mouth disease in Great Britain required the government to destroy nearly 4 million animals to stop the epidemic. Estimated losses to the food, agriculture, and tourist industries exceeded $10 billion (U.S. General Accounting Office, July 2000). Many farmers and families were profoundly affected psychologically, and the social infrastructure of many rural communities was severely stressed.

13. What role can veterinarians play in the psychological impact of epidemic livestock loss?

Concerning the Great Britain foot-and-mouth outbreak, veterinarians who were interviewed thought that farmers found it easier to talk to veterinary surgeons, who were perceived as being able to relate to the loss of the animals, than to community caseworkers or government staff. Agencies offering practical information, such as the unions, rural farm bureaus, and veterinary surgeons, received the most calls and frequently found themselves offering emotional support (Deaville & Jones, 2001). Many of these frontline contacts found their inability to help distressed farmers so debilitating and emotionally taxing that a government-sponsored program of on-site counseling and debriefings was developed for these employees. The report noted that, initially, the workload literally doubled in veterinary practices but that there was an early increase in the use of mental health services.

14. When dealing with the psychological impact of epidemic livestock loss, what should I be looking for?

Women are often the first to seek emotional help for themselves or their families. Seven of ten callers to rural information lines were women worried about their husbands' mental health. Although the husband farmers were frequently identified as the cause of concern, the report identified two high-risk groups that were likely to be overlooked: farmer's wives, who tended to neglect their own welfare to care for their families, and children who were moved into village communities to continue schooling. Children were separated from farming parents on infected farms in the midst of great uncertainty and turmoil, with the added anxiety of seeing parents and relatives in distress. Some children lost livestock that had become pets. "Playground feuding" sometimes occurs between farming children over the perceived blame for bringing the disease to an area.

15. How can I help the people who are involved with epidemic livestock loss?

The reports from both the ovine Johne's disease epidemic in Australia and the foot-and-mouth epidemic in the United Kingdom provide examples of interventions that were thought to be helpful. Livestock officers in Australia set up network groups of farmers to discuss economic recovery and how to develop new business skills. These groups were facilitated by the livestock officer but run by the farmers. As the group focused on educational issues, psychological and emotional themes were also aired, while the livestock officer served the role of an **understanding listener**. This facilitator would then move the discussion to issues over which farmers felt they had control. Examining individual circumstances in a group in which the agenda was ultimately set by the farmers offered participants a means of renewing and establishing networks as well as restoring a sense of control. It is noted that, for the most part, farmers did not use government-established counseling centers that would have required the farmer to initiate the call (Department of Natural Resources and the Environment Investigatory Committee to the Parliament of Victoria Australia, 2000). The importance of active outreach was repeatedly emphasized.

Another highly successful approach was begun late in the Australian sheep epidemic. After an infected animal was identified on a farm, the local veterinarian known to the farmer would visit the family with an offer of help and ongoing support through the process of culling the herd. The offer was not pressed but a second visit was made several days later, giving the farmer a chance to absorb the acute shock of the diagnosis without being left unsupported for too long. Outside veterinarians were available to meet other practice obligations, freeing the local professional to tend to his or her own clients who had been acutely affected by the epidemic.

16. What kinds of things can we do to prepare a client for the psychological impact of an epidemic livestock loss?

Anticipating the psychological impact of epidemic livestock loss on different constituencies in rural communities ensures that plans can be developed before a disaster strikes. Preparing local communities through public education programs will mitigate the inevitable distress experienced by individuals and institutions. Drawing attention to such high-risk groups as farm women and children facilitates outreach and encourages help-seeking. Schools and faith-based and civic organizations can play important roles in prevention, support, and recovery. Educating the veterinary community about psychological stresses after disasters is also a critical part of emergency preparedness.

The more the community understands about resources that will be activated or deployed if such a disaster occurs, the more quickly they can avail themselves of these services. In rural communities, rapid availability of veterinary medical care to the animal community will be equally important. Veterinarians who are attuned to their farm families' strengths and vulnerabilities are valuable assets in outreach planning and emotional recovery.

17. What are some of the risks to veterinarians when they are first responders?

As first responders, veterinarians are vulnerable to the impacts of traumatic stress in natural and terrorist disasters and may themselves become a high-risk group. Like their physician counterparts, they are likely to minimize the emotional impact of the disaster they are involved in, overdedicate themselves to work, sacrifice rest and respite, and risk exhaustion and burnout. In the culling of herds in the United Kingdom, veterinarians expressed a profound sense of sorrow and anger at having to slaughter the lives they had dedicated themselves to protect and heal. When Veterinary Medical Assistance Team teams were deployed to care for the search and rescue dogs at the World Trade Center, they confronted an unimaginable devastation that traumatized the entire nation (Nolen, 2001).

18. Why do people stay in harm's way regarding their pets during disasters?

The importance of understanding the power of the relationship between people and their pets is apparent during disaster evacuations. According to several studies, animal owners will risk danger to themselves and may not evacuate disaster areas unless they are assured of their animals' well-being (Lockwood, 1997). Moreover, the most common reason people return to an evacuation site is to rescue their pets. Today over 60% of households have pets, an increase from 56% of households in 1988, and close to 100% of today's pet owners identify their pets as members of the family (American Veterinary Medical Association, 2003). Many pet owners view their pets as enhancing the quality of family life by minimizing tension between family members. Human attachment to animals may really be a unique bond, similar to but different from human attachment to humans.

19. Have the laws changed concerning the evacuation and housing of pets during disasters?

Health safety regulations in the recent past did not allow pets in public emergency shelters. Further, very few emergency planners took into account the rescue or evacuation of pets and livestock. However, in the wake of Hurricane Katrina, when thousands of pet owners were forced to leave their pets outside the Superdome in New Orleans and be evacuated, a public outcry started a push of new federal legislation to address this issue. In October 2006, Congress passed the Pets Evacuation and Transportation Standards Act (PETS Act), which required local and state emergency preparedness authorities to include in their evacuation plans how they will accommodate household pets and service animals in the event of a major disaster. Since 2006 and based on this law, most local and state planners have been addressing this issue.

20. During a disaster response, I have heard and seen a lot of disturbing things. Sometimes I wonder if what I do matters and if I should stay in this line of work. Are these common reactions?

Not only are these common reactions during disaster response and recovery, these are job-related hazards for those in the health care fields under normal circumstances. Some of the contributing factors to these feelings are burnout, compassion fatigue, and vicarious trauma. *Burnout* involves being emotionally exhausted, having a negative or hostile outlook toward patrons and less productive work activity. *Compassion fatigue* comes from caring too much and being unable to turn off work thoughts. *Vicarious*, or secondary, *trauma* is a stress reaction that may occur when you hear or see too many terrible things. It causes a change in your outlook—the world looks like a dark, negative, hostile planet. One of the most important factors in recovery from these is having support from others. Being able to share the thoughts helps to make sense of it and discover that what you are doing really does make a difference.

Suggested Reading

Bartram DJ, Baldwin DS. Veterinary surgeons and suicide: Influences, opportunities and research directions. *Vet Rec* 2008;162:36–40.

Department of Natural Resources and the Environment Investigatory Committee to the Parliament of Victoria Australia. *Inquiry Into Control of Ovine Johne's Disease (OJD) in Victoria. Chapter 11: Social impacts.* October 31, 2000.

GovTrack.US. H.R. 3858–109th Congress (2005): Pets Evacuation and Transportation Standards Act of 2006. Available at www.govtrack.us/congress/bill.xpd?bill=h109-3858.

Lawrence C. Shock central: Veterinarian suicides. Available at corralonline.com.

Lockwood R. *Through Hell and High Water: Disasters and the Human-Animal Bond.* Washington, DC, The Humane Society of the United States, March 1997. Available at www.fema.gov/library/equine.shtm.

National Child Traumatic Stress Network and Center for PTSD, *Psychological First Aid: Field Operations Guide.* 2nd ed. July 2006. Available at www.nctsn.org and www.ncptsd.va.gov.

Nolen SR. VMATs aid rescue efforts in New York City. *J Am Vet Med Assoc* November 1, 2001 Available at www.avma.org/onlnews/javma/nov01/s110101a.asp.

Norris FH, Bryne CM, Diaz E, Kaniasty K. *The range, Magnitude, and Duration of Effects of Natural and Human Caused Disasters: A Review of the Empirical Literature.* Washington, DC, U.S. Department of Veterans Affairs, National Center for Posttraumatic Stress Disorder, 2005.

Podrazik D, Shackford S, Becker L, et al. The death of a pet: Implications for loss and bereavement across the lifespan. *J Person Interperson Loss* 2000;5:361–396.

Public Health Emergency Preparedness: Terrorism and mental Health. 2008 New York City Department of Health and Mental Hygiene. Available at http://www.nyc.gov/html/doh/html/browse/browse-emergency.shtml.

Stutts JC. Bereavement and the human-animal bond. *Vet Tech* 1996;17:429–433.

The health impact of the foot and mouth situation on people in Wales: The service providers' perspective. A summary report to the National Assembly for Wales by the Institute of Rural Health. May 2001. Available at www.irh.ac.uk/publications/respub.php.

U.S. Department of Health and Human Services. *A Guide to Managing Stress in Crisis Response Professions.* DHHS Publication No. SMA 4113. Rockville, MD, Center for Mental Health Services, Substance Abuse and Mental Health Services Administration, 2005.

U.S. General Accounting Office. *Foot and Mouth Disease: To Protect U.S. Livestock, USDA Must Remain Vigilant and Resolve Outstanding Issues.* Washington, DC, GAO, 02-808, July 2002.

CHAPTER 4.2
DISASTER ASSISTANCE FOR HOMEOWNERS, RENTERS, AND BUSINESS OWNERS

Eugene A. Adkins, DVM

1. Does the homeowner and renter need to prepare and practice a disaster plan?

Yes! Before a disaster strikes, each household should develop a plan that will include all of their pets. To ensure the plan is functional, it must be practiced *before* a disaster occurs. Every 3 months, the plan should be reexamined and updated and changes made known to the entire family.

2. What should be included in a disaster plan for households with pets?

- Write out a disaster plan for all of your animals and practice the plan to identify flaws.
- Prepare an evacuation plan and practice this plan.
- Make sure you have an up-to-date inventory of all your pets so all may be accounted for in the event of a major disaster.
- Train your four-legged pets to go up and down stairs to facilitate rescue.
- Keep written directions on how to reach your house close to the telephone in the event you must relate directions to responders.
- Assemble an animal evacuation kit (discussed in detail later).
- Be sure vehicles to be used in evacuation are well maintained and full of fuel.
- Have some emergency cash available. In a disaster, electricity may be out and ATMs may be unusable.
- If your house/apartment has an emergency generator, make sure it is in good working order and you have fuel for the machine.

3. If you are not at home, how can you identify the fact you have pets that may be inside?

Preplace stickers on or near the front and rear doors, pasture entrances, and barn and tack room doors. These stickers should identify the types of animals and locations of evacuation kits.

4. What additional information should be immediately available to rescuers should you not be at home?

- Provide an inventory of all pets, their names, behavioral quirks, whether they have an identification collar, whether they have a microchip for identification, and specific animal information such as breed, color, identifying marks, gender, and a photograph of each animal.

- Provide a list of evacuation kits you have prepared and where to find them.
- To facilitate a successful rescue, provide muzzles, leashes, halters, lead ropes, handling gloves, catch nets, and other animal restraints as required.
- Whenever you leave your home/apartment, inform a neighbor that you will be out of town and that your animals are either leaving with you or are within the house/apartment. Provide the neighbor an inventory of animals that can be shared with rescue personnel should a disaster strike in your absence.
- In your disaster plan, you should provide a presigned letter that releases your neighbor from responsibility if one of your animals becomes injured or escapes during evacuation.
- Your disaster plan should also include a presigned veterinary medical treatment authorization. This letter should be shared with your veterinarian and neighbor.

5. List means of identification of animals prior to a disaster (Table 4.2.1).

Table 4.2.1   Means of Identification of Animals before a Disaster

Small Animals	Horses	Livestock
Collar tag	Microchip	Neck chain
Microchip	Tattoo	Ear notches
Tattoo	Halter tag	Leg band
Temporary neck band	Neck collar	Ear tag or triage tag
Waterproof pouch attached to collar with identification information inside	Leg band or triage tag	Brand
Mark reptiles with a waterproof permanent felt-tipped marker	Mane clip	Livestock marking crayon
Clear, complete information on cage/housing for confined animals	Luggage tag braided into the tail or mane	Non-toxic, non-water soluble spray paint
Triage tag	Clipper-shaved information in the horse's hair	Wattle notching
	Permanent marker on horse's hooves	Ear tattoo
		Back or tail tag

6. List the items you should have immediately available in all households prior to a disaster.

- Flashlight and plenty of extra batteries or emergency crank-rechargeable battery lights
- Portable, battery-operated (and extra batteries) or an emergency radio with crank-rechargeable batteries
- First-aid kit and manual
- Supply of nonperishable food and water for 72 hours
- Manual can/bottle opener and spoon
- Essential medications
- Cash and credit cards
- Important family documents and veterinary records
- Include at least one complete change of clothing and footwear for each family member. Included in this change are the following suggestions: sturdy shoes or work boots, hats and gloves, rain gear, thermal underwear, blankets, sleeping bags, underwear, warm jacket/wool sweater, and several pairs of warm socks (not cotton).
- Animal evacuation kit

7. What is included in a small animal evacuation kit?

- Provide a list of animals, how they can be identified (breed, age, gender, collar, microchip, etc.) AND include a comment regarding the behavioral quirks of each ("easily frightened," "possible biter," "likely to hide in the laundry room during a storm," "afraid of lightning," etc.).
- Provide an emergency contact list that includes your personal information and contact information of the neighbor(s) and your veterinarian.
- A map of the area with possible evacuation routes or alternative sheltering with names, contact information, and location
- Two-week supply of food (dry and/or canned)
- Manual can opener
- Spill-proof food and water dishes
- Two-week supply of water in large plastic jugs with secure lids
- Feeding instructions for each animal. Include foods to avoid in the event of individual animal allergies.
- Provide copies of veterinary records and proof of ownership (registration papers, rabies tag certificates, digital or color photographs, etc.)
- Pet first-aid kit (See Chapter 1.18.)
- Pet medications. List each animal separately and include the name of the drug, dosage, and frequency of administration. For drugs requiring special handling (i.e., refrigeration), indicate where the drug is located so the rescuer may easily access the medication.
- Cage/carrier for each animal. Each should be labeled with the pet's information as well as your contact information.
- Familiar items to make the pets feel more comfortable
- Newspaper for bedding
- Paper towels
- Heavy duty trash bags
- Heavy (welder) gloves for handling cats
- Leash and collar or harness for each animal
- Litter, litter pan, litter scoop
- Muzzles (canine and feline)
- Stakes or tie-outs

8. What suggestions can you offer in maintaining your evacuation kit?

- Store the evacuation kit in a convenient place known to all family members and at least one neighbor.
- Items are best stored in air-tight plastic containers or bags.
- Every 6 months, replace all water and food to keep both fresh.
- Revisit your disaster plan every year and update or change the plan as required to keep it current.
- Check with your veterinarian or pharmacist regarding medications and how often they should be replaced.
- Keep your animal census current.

9. Where can I find information regarding evacuation of horses and livestock?

See Chapters 1.20 and 3.3.

10. Why is it important to include an emergency communication plan?

- Unfortunately, family members are often separated during a disaster. An emergency communication plan that is known to all family members will define a plan for reuniting after the disaster.
- Use an out-of-state relative as a "family contact". Following a disaster, local telephone lines are often jammed or destroyed. Interestingly, one can often make long distance calls even during the disaster as long as the lines are functional.
- It is very important that each family member knows who the emergency contact person will be and has the name, address, telephone number (land line and cell phone), and perhaps even a facsimile number. You can easily place this information in a side pocket of a child's school backpack for easy access. Keep this information updated at least twice each year.

11. Why is it important to alert rescuers to behavioral quirks of your pets?

Behavior of animals often changes drastically during a disaster. Normally quiet and friendly animals may become fractious and scared. All animals need to be closely observed and provided a safe and secure enclosure.

12. If you are evacuated to a local shelter, can your pet come with you?

Yes, dogs and cats can be evacuated to a temporary animal shelter adjoining shelters for people. It is unlikely your pet will be joining you in your shelter as your fellow victims sometimes have aversions or allergies to animals and there is often limited space. Knowing your pet is close by provides you some assurance of the animal's well-being and you can likely visit frequently to help assure the pet of your availability and also to help shelter personnel care for your animal. If your pet is a boa constrictor or iguana, you will likely not be allowed to bring it along. Be sure to check this out before a disaster so you can make alternative plans.

13. Describe how you might arrange for sheltering your animals in the event of a disaster.

Temporary animal shelters are included in local disaster management plans. You can obtain information from your local disaster management office and identify where these shelters are scheduled to be located. Obviously things often change during a disaster so listen to newscasts or contact your veterinarian prior to the disaster so you have an idea of where to relocate your pet. All animals to be housed in a shelter will be required to have an identification tag and/or microchip, current licensure, and vaccinations.

14. What are you going to do if your pet is a bird and there is an impending disaster?

- Identification and proof of ownership are important as noted earlier for pets, horses, and livestock.
- Transportation and housing of birds become more critical as they are so susceptible to stress-induced illness and death.
- Try to keep your bird separated from other birds to decrease the likelihood of disease transmission.
- Keep your bird out of drafty areas.
- Use small, secure, covered carriers to transport your bird.

- Environmental temperature control is very important for birds. With a blizzard or cold weather, you must warm your vehicle before moving your bird.
- Be extra careful and vigilant when transferring your bird to a different cage at the sheltering location.
- Birds should be kept in quiet, clean environments.
- Provide clean food and water daily.
- Should your bird appear ill, lower the perch, food, and water bowl within the cage and seek veterinary attention as soon as possible.
- In addition to many of the items listed in the small animal evacuation kit, include the following items:
  - Avian dietary supplements
  - Plant misters to cool the bird during excessively hot weather
  - Hot water bottles to keep the bird warm during excessively cold weather

15. What are you going to do if your pet is a reptile or amphibian?

- Reptiles and amphibians cannot be released prior to the disaster and must be confined in a manner to protect the animal and prevent its escape.
- Use pillow cases, cloth sacks, or small transport cages to move animals to a shelter.
- At the shelter carefully transfer your "pet" to a secure cage or enclosure.
- Since reptiles do not usually require daily feeding, determine beforehand whether the animal needs to be fed. Often the stress of feeding and the stress of a disaster make it even more hazardous for the animal.
- The shelter should ideally be in a quiet, environmentally controlled area away from heavy human traffic, loud noises, and vibrations.
- Plan for an escape of your pet.
- In addition to items listed in the pet evacuation kit above consider inclusion of the following items:
  - Dietary supplements
  - Water bowl that will allow soaking of the animal
  - Spray bottle for misting
  - Heating pad (ideally battery operated) and towels to cover it to protect the animal from thermal injury. Include extra batteries.
  - Supplies for handling animal

16. What sort of disasters should you prepare for?

Practically any disaster can strike at any time. You need to be aware of the types of disasters seen in your locale. Obviously, you will not experience a hurricane in Wyoming and it is highly unlikely you will experience a blizzard in Florida. Disasters such as fires, wildfires, flooding, severe thunderstorms and lightning, extreme heat, high winds, tornados, hazardous materials spills, and terrorist attacks are usually unpredictable. Knowing if you are located near an earthquake fault or volcano provides you information to allow the family to prepare for such a disaster. Your local disaster response agency will have a list of likely disasters in your area and will surely share this information with you.

17. Weather forecasters often use the words "watch" or "warning" to alert a community to an impending disaster. What is the difference?

A "watch" (i.e., flood watch, tornado watch, blizzard watch, etc.) indicates there is a strong possibility for one of these disasters to occur in a specific locale within a specific time frame. A "warning" means the weather event is either occurring or expected to occur and a specific area is designated with immediate danger being imminent.

18. Who else might provide you with good information regarding the disasters that may or have occurred in your locale?

Your insurance agent is an excellent source of information. Insurance companies keep vital records of past events in order to predict future disasters. It makes good sense to visit with your agent yearly to assess needed changes in your insurance coverage for your property and possessions.

19. There is an impending disaster in your area. Now what are you going to do?

If an evacuation order has been issued, evacuate your family and animals as early as possible. By evacuating early you will decrease the chance of becoming a victim of the disaster.

20. List some check-off items you can use in the event you must evacuate your animals quickly.

- Account for all your animals.
- Make sure all animals have some sort of identification securely attached.
- Place animals in their individual transportable cages.
- Secure leases on larger animals.
- Load your larger animal cages/carriers into your vehicle. This will serve as temporary housing until the animals can be relocated.
- Load your animal evacuation kit(s) and supplies.
- Call your prearranged animal evacuation site to confirm availability of housing.
- Implement your equine/livestock evacuation plan (if applicable).
- Take recommended evacuation routes to the pre-arranged animal shelter facility.

21. The disaster has passed and now it's time to pick up the pieces. How do you prepare to reenter the area with your animals?

- Pick up your animals from the shelter if you are certain it will be safe to return them to your home following the disaster.
- Survey the home and property inside and out of the house to identify and remove dangerous materials and wildlife (i.e., snakes, skunks, etc.), sharp objects, and contaminated water.
- Closely examine your animals. If you have any questions, call your veterinarian.
- Be aware that familiar landmarks and scents have likely changed and this may be stressful to your animals.
- If you have horses and livestock, check for debris that may injure them and check that all fences are intact before releasing them to a pasture. Never release the animals after dark. You need to watch them move into the pasture to be assured they will adapt to their surroundings.
- Do NOT release dogs and cats outside following a disaster. There will be many objects that might injure them, they will be confused and may run away, or may encounter wildlife or other stray animals.
- Release birds, amphibians, and reptiles only after you are sure they are calm and in an enclosed space.
- Feeding animals should start with small servings, free-choice water, and observe for any gastrointestinal signs (vomiting, diarrhea, retching, abdominal discomfort, etc.).
- Provide as quiet an area as possible for your pets to sleep all they want. They will be as exhausted as you and sleep/rest will help them recover from the stresses of being away from home, being housed in a strange place, and having strangers feeding and caring for them.
- Begin the arduous task of cleaning up and trying to return your family and animals to a life that was once "normal."

22. The disaster has passed but prior to evacuation you were unable to locate your pet(s). You evacuated without them and now you have returned home. Your pet is nowhere to be found. List some items we have learned from previous disasters regarding the return of lost pets following a disaster.

- The longer the pet is lost, the less likely he or she is to be found.
- Animals lost over 4 weeks are rarely returned.
- Animals that had some sort of identification are 10 times more likely to be reunited with their owners.
- Cats are frequently left behind in a disaster.

23. Provide some guidance on what to do if you have lost a pet in a disaster.

- Physically go to Animal Control and animal shelters and look for your pet. Do not depend upon a telephone description to a receptionist to result in the correct identification of your pet.
- You must physically return to facilities sheltering animals on a daily basis for at least 2 weeks after a major disaster if you hope to find your pet.
- Your disaster plan included pictures of your pet. Take those photographs, create a poster, place the poster in a waterproof casement, and distribute them to your neighborhood and leave them with animal control, local law enforcement, veterinarians, and sheltering facilities as well. Be sure to include the animal's name, your name and contact information, and behavioral quirks that might help recognize your pet.
- Online resources are also available following a disaster. Your local news channels, radio stations, and papers will usually list the websites you should check. Some websites you might try include the following:
  - Go to Google.com and enter a search for websites specializing in lost and found pets.
  - www.1888pets911.org
  - www.dogsonly.org/Lost_and_found.html
  - www.fidofinder.com/
  - www.findthatpet.com/
  - www.globalpetfinder.com
  - www.hsus.org/pets/pet_care/finding_a_lost_pet.html
  - www.missingpet.net
  - www.petfinder.com/
  - www.petrescue.com
  - www.pets911.com

Suggested Reading

Animals in disasters. Available at http://www.training.fema.gov/EMIWeb/downloads/b-1.pdf.

Disaster preparedness. Available at http://www.avma.org/disaster/default.asp.

Disaster response guide. Available at http://www.avma.org/disaster/responseguide/E_owners.pdf.

Farm Service Administration. Available at http://www.fsa.usda.gov/pas/disaster/default.htm.

FEMA. Available at http://www.fema.gov.

Heath SE, et al. Observations from the Oakland fire storms. *J Am Vet Med Assoc* 1998;212:504.

Heath SE, Beck AM, Kass PH, et al. Risk factors for pet evacuation failure after a slow-onset disaster. *J Am Vet Med Assoc* 2001;218:1905–1910.

Heath SE, Voeks SK, Glickman LT. Epidemiologic features of pet evacuation failure in a rapid-onset disaster. *J Am Vet Med Assoc* 2001;218:1898–1904.

Red Cross. Available at http://www.redcross.org.

Saving the family. Available at http://www.avma.org/disaster/saving_family_brochure.pdf.

APPENDIX 4.2.1
DISASTER ASSISTANCE FOR HOMEOWNERS AND RENTERS

Homeowners, renters, and business owners who suffered damages or losses as a result of the disaster may be eligible for assistance from a variety of state, federal, and voluntary agencies. Types of assistance include the following:

Program/Agency	Assistance	Eligibility	Specific Criteria
Emergency Assistance Coordinated by the American Red Cross and Voluntary agencies active in disaster. www.redcross.org www.fema.gov/news/ newsrelease.fema?id=34772	Emergency food, clothing, shelter, and medical assistance.	Available to individuals and families with disaster related emergency needs.	Also makes referrals to church groups and other voluntary agencies
Home/Personal Property Disaster Loans Small Business Administration (SBA). http://www.sba. gov/disaster	Low-interest loans for restoring or replacing uninsured or underinsured disaster-damaged real and personal property.	For individuals located in counties included in the presidential-declared disaster.	Loans limited to amount of uninsured, SBA-verified losses. Maximum loans: $200,000 real property $40,000 personal property
Disaster Housing Assistance Administered and funded by FEMA. http://www.fema. gov	Provides grants for temporary housing or for emergency repairs needed to make a residence livable until more permanent repairs can be made.	Available to homeowners and renters whose permanent homes are uninhabitable because of the disaster. Homeowners	Housing assistance grants are coordinated with any insurance coverage an individual might have. Grants made to homeowners who can return to their homes with minimal repairs. Homeowners with more substantial property damage may qualify for temporary housing grants for rent. Mobile homes provided if no rental resources available.
		Renters	Renters may qualify for rental assistance. Mobile homes provided if no rental resources available.
Individual and Family Grant Program Administered by state. Funded by FEMA. http://www. fema.gov	Grants to meet serious disaster related needs and necessary expenses not covered by insurance or other federal, state, or voluntary agencies.	Persons with serious unmet needs who do not qualify for a SBA disaster loan.	Maximum grant of $13,900 depending upon family composition and needs. Average grant = $2000 –$4000.

Business Disaster Loans

Small Business Administration www.sba.gov/services/ disasterassistance/index. html

Loans for the repair or replacement of destroyed or damaged business facilities, inventory, machinery or equipment. Economic Injury Disaster Loans also may be available for working capital to assist small businesses during the disaster recovery period.

Businesses located in counties included in the presidential-disaster declaration. Small businesses located in the disaster area.

$1,500,000 loan limit to repair or replace damaged real and personal property.

Tax Assistance

Internal Revenue Service. http:// www.irs.ustreas.gov/prod/hot/ fema.html

Expedited federal tax deductions for casualty losses to home, personal property, or household goods. Assistance and information on state income tax returns can also be obtained from the State Dept. of Revenue.

Individuals and families with disaster-related losses that exceed 10% of the adjusted gross income for the tax year by at least $100.

Under certain circumstances the IRS allows certain casualty losses to be deducted on Federal income tax returns for the year of the loss or through an immediate amendment to the previous year's return.

Disaster Unemployment Assistance

May be available through the state unemployment office and supported by the U.S. Department of Labor. www.state.ar.us/esd/ WorkersUnempBenefits/A_uidua. htm

Benefits available to individuals out of work because of the disaster.

Available to individuals out of work because of the disaster, including self-employed persons, farm owners, and others not covered under regular unemployment insurance.

Maximum 26 weeks benefits. Proof of income required. Must register with state's employment services office.

Farm Assistance

Farm Service Agency. http://www. fsa.usda.gov/pas/disaster/ default.htm

Emergency loans for physical or production losses.

Available to farmers who were operating and managing a farm at the time of the disaster.

Loans limited to the amount necessary to compensate for actual losses to essential property and/or production capacity.

Insurance Information

State Insurance Commissioner, American Insurance Association, FEMA, and National Flood Insurance Program. www.fema. gov/business/nfip/

Assistance and/or counseling regarding ways to obtain copies of lost policies, file claims, expedite settlements, etc.

Individuals and families with disaster-related losses.

Legal Assistance

Coordinated by FEMA, Young Lawyers Division of the American Bar Association. www.femainfo.us/ Disaster_Assistance_Overview-Legal_Aid.shtml

Free legal advice, counseling, and representation for low-income disaster victims.

Individuals and families with disaster-related legal issues.

Applicable to such matters as replacing legal documents, transferring titles, contracting problems, will probates, insurance problems, and certain landlord-related problems.

Social Security Benefits

Social Security Administration http://www.ssa.gov

Assistance expediting delivery of checks delayed by the disaster Assistance in applying for Social Security disability and survivor benefits.

Individuals eligible for Social Security.

Veterans Benefits

Department of Veterans Affairs http://www.va.gov

Assistance with information about benefits, pensions, insurance settlements, and VA mortgages.

Help in applying for VA death benefits, pensions, and adjustments to VA-insured home mortgages.

Consumer Services
www.governmentguide.com/
consumer_services.
adp?id=16101558

Counseling on consumer problems such as product shortages, price gouging, and disreputable business practices.

Aging Services
www.aoa.gov/; www.aahsa.org/

Services to the elderly such as meals, home care, and transportation.

Individuals covered by the Older Americans Act.

Crisis Counseling
www.fema.gov/assistance/
process/additional.shtm;
www.emsc.nysed.gov/crisis/
counsel.htm

Referrals and short-term counseling for mental health problems caused by the disaster.

Reducing Future Losses
Project Impact Administered by FEMA; http://www.fema.gov

Guidelines for mitigating the effects of future disasters such as roof repairs, hurricane shutters, care for damaged vegetation, working with construction contractors, the building permit process, etc.

Aid to Persons Facing Mortgage Foreclosure
Administered and funded by FEMA; www.fema.gov/news/ newsrelease.fema?id=5492

Amount of actual rental or mortgage payments

Individuals who have lost their jobs or businesses because of a major disaster.

Affected individuals who:
– Are unable to make mortgage or rental payments as a result of disaster-related financial hardship.
– Have received written notice of foreclosure or eviction from mortgage lender or landlord

Based on http://www.avma.org/disaster/responseguide/E_owners.pdf

CHAPTER 4.3
AMERICAN VETERINARY MEDICAL FOUNDATION: DISASTER ASSISTANCE

Wayne E. Wingfield, MS, DVM

1. What is the American Veterinary Medical Foundation (AVMF)?

Founded in 1963, the American Veterinary Medical Foundation (AVMF) is a 501c3 organization that raises and disburses funds for initiatives supporting its mission statement: "Advancing the care of animals with an emphasis on disaster preparedness and response, and animal health studies."

2. What does the AVMF recommend for all veterinary practices prior to a disaster?

It is essential that a veterinary practice have a written disaster plan that includes the following:

- Emergency relocation of animals
- Medical record backup
- Continuity of operations
- Security
- Insurance and legal issues

3. What information should be included in your emergency relocation of boarded or hospitalized animals?

- Leashes, carriers, and other species-specific supplies
- Appropriate, prearranged animal transportation
- Temporary animal holding location
- 24-hour client contact list (off-site access)
- Secure and weather-resistant patient identification
- In conjunction with appropriate legal council, involving your staff, clients, and their pets in disaster planning and disaster drills can help ensure community buy-in and dedication to the plan.

4. What should be included in your plan for backing up records?

- Off-site computer backup (fireproof safes will not prevent melting)
- Off-site copies of important documents
- Itemized inventory (on-site and off-site)
- Digital storage

5. List some items important in developing a plan for continuity of operations.

- Communications (do not rely on land lines, cell phones, or pagers)
- Alternate power source (i.e., generators with regular maintenance) and training for staff; ideally, professionally installed and able to provide long-term power to the entire facility)
- Generator fuel source
- Continued refrigeration
- List of suppliers with current 24-hour contact information
- Alternate human and animal food and water sources in case of contamination
- Five to seven days' worth of food and water for on-site staff and patients
- Five to seven days of personal medications for on-site staff
- Alternate practice location (within your vicinity)
  - Contact your local and state Veterinary Medical Association for potential resources.
  - Yours may be the only practice affected in area (i.e., hospital fire).
- Minimize inconvenience to your clients.
  - Eliminate a need for your clients to obtain services elsewhere.
  - Adopt a sister practice (outside your vicinity).
    - Pay the sister practice a percentage of your income for the use of their facility.
    - Set up a reciprocal arrangement.
  - Contact your local and state Veterinary Medical Association for potential resources.
  - Avoid a gap in client services.
- Practice disaster drills together, uniting two communities that may not have otherwise communicated.

6. List some things useful in providing security to your practice in case of emergency.

- Local fire department: free inspection and evacuation drills
- Water system independent from electrical system
- Oxygen tanks isolated for safety
- Secure practice from theft and looting
- Unobstructed escape routes
- Emergency lighting
- Multiple exits
- Regular disaster/evacuation drills (local fire department, local police, clients)
- Office phone-tree (24-hour numbers)
- Prearranged off-site meeting location for staff
- Prearranged conference call capability to keep all staff informed
- Encourage and help to develop each employee's personal family disaster plan (if they are prepared at home, they will be better able to assist the practice).
- Hazardous materials inventory with Material Safety Data Sheets (accessible off-site)
- Employee identification cards (access to disaster-stricken area)

7. What are some of the legal and liability issues to consider before a disaster?

- Current and comprehensive insurance policy
- Discuss the details of disaster drills with your legal counsel to make sure you are covered for any injuries that might occur during the drill.
- Safely store all receipts for all purchases.
- Videotape and photograph inventory.
- In the event the practice is damaged, it is important to take measures to avoid further damage (e.g., if a practice's roof is damaged in a disaster but the contents in the building are ruined because of subsequent rains, your

possessions may not be covered by your insurance policy if the rain is deemed "after the initial disaster" and you did not take steps to secure a tarp over the top of your building, preventing further damage).
- Familiarize yourself with tax laws and deductible disaster expenses.
- Business Owners Policy, AVMA PLIT, 800-228-PLIT, www.avmaplit.com

8. What are some of the items you should check to be sure your insurance addresses?

- Business interruption (continuing expenses); find out exactly when it ends and what triggers the end.
- Extra expense (payment of overtime pay and relocation expenses)
- Professional extension (injury/loss/death of animals)
- Loss of income
- Personal property (replacement value)
- Automatic inflation
- Fire damage
- Water damage
- Debris removal/cleanup
- Comprehensive building and structure replacement
- Coverage of rented and leased equipment
- Interruption of power, heating/air, water, and sewage
- Coverage of worker's compensation
- General and professional liability

9. How does the AVMF assist during and following a disaster?

The AVMF Animal Disaster Relief and Response Fund provides support for emergency veterinary aid for the health, safety, and welfare of animals affected by disasters at the local level, emergency preparedness at the state level, and the Veterinary Medical Assistance Teams (VMATs) at the national level.

10. Describe how a veterinarian may apply for assistance from the AVMF following a disaster.

- One purpose of the AVMF is to ensure the medical care of animal victims of disaster, and this is accomplished by providing veterinarians an opportunity to apply for financial assistance.
- Currently, awards are for disasters that occur only after February 3, 2008.
  - Up to $5,000 can be issued per grantee for out-of-pocket expenses, which are defined as the actual cost of medical supplies purchased as directly from a vendor.
  - Modest boarding costs may be covered.
  - Professional/staff time, overhead costs, equipment usage fees, and taxes are not reimbursable.
  - Travel associated with disasters of significant magnitude to affect a significant number of animal victims, veterinarians, and/or veterinary clinics affecting several states may be reimbursed, such as gas, lodging, airfare, and car rental.
- All awards are based on merit and availability of funds.

11. Describe the eligibility criteria used by AVMF for these reimbursement expenses.

- Must apply in writing
- Must be a licensed veterinarian or staff member, such as a licensed veterinary technician
- Must have provided for the medical care of animal victims of the disaster listed on the application (Table 4.3.1)

Table 4.3.1   Criteria for Awarding Reimbursement Expenses to Qualified Applicants Are as Follows

Item	Cat/small pet like ferret <10 lb	Dog <40 lb	Dog >40 lb
Per Animal:			
Boarding/housing	$5/day	$10/day	$10/day
Spay	$25	$40	$50
Neuter/minor surgery	$10	$25	$35
Major surgery	$20	$35	$45
Heartworm treatment	$200	$200	$250
Other:			
Physical exam	$5/animal		
Any injection	$6/animal		
CBC	$8/animal	In-house lab work	
Urinalysis	$4/animal	In-house lab work	
Profile	$15/animal	In-house lab work	
Heartworm check	$5/animal	In-house lab work	
Cytology (ear swab, etc.)	$5/animal	In-house lab work	
Fecal exam	$3/animal	In-house lab work	
Misc. lab work	Actual cost	As charged by outside lab	
Radiographs (x-rays)	$10/animal plus $5/sheet of film		
Ultrasound	$15/animal		
Fluids	$7/day ($5 +$2/liter of fluid)		
Oral medication	1–$3/day	Provided by facility	
Dispensed drugs or supplies	Actual cost	As charged by vendor	

Based on http://www.avmf.org/clientuploads/documents/AnimalHealthCareReimbursement020308.pdf.

12.   Describe the application procedure for reimbursement expenses from the AVMF.

Forms are available at www.avmf.org. Print a form and write clearly or type. Fill in all the boxes. Incomplete forms will be returned. If you cannot print the form, call the AVMF Grants Coordinator at 1-800-248-2862, ext. 6691, and a form will be mailed to you.

Request up to $5,000 in box 6a. If the amount requested in box 6a is insufficient to cover your needs, please note the final amount that would meet your needs in box 6b and anticipate that the initial award will be no more than $5,000. Checks will be payable to the person/entity named in box 7g.

13.   What is the deadline for application?

Applications must be received no later than 9 months following the disaster.

14. How does one receive more information regarding these grants?

American Veterinary Medical Foundation
Grants Coordinator
1931 N. Meacham Road Suite 100
Schaumburg, IL 60173

Suggested Reading and Sources

http://www.avma.org/disaster/vet_practices_brochure.pdf.
http://www.avmf.org/clientuploads/documents/AnimalHealthCareReimbursement020308.pdf.

EMERGENCY RESPONSE CONTACTS DIRECTORY

KEY FEDERAL GOVERNMENT AGENCY WEB SITES

Centers for Disease Control and Prevention (CDC)
  http://www.cdc.gov/
Department of Agriculture (USDA)
  http://www.usda.gov/
Department of Defense (DOD)
  http://www.defenselink.mil/
Department of Energy (DOE)
  http://www.energy.gov/
Department of Health and Human Services (DHHS)
  http://www.hhs.gov/emergency/
Department of Homeland Security (DHS)
  http://www.dhs.gov/
Department of the Interior
  http://www.doi.gov/
Department of Transportation (DOT)
  http://www.dot.gov/
Disaster Medical Assistance Teams (DMAT)
  http://www.dmat.org/
Disaster Mortuary Operational Response Teams (DMORT)
  http://www.dmort.org/
Environmental Protection Agency (EPA)
  http://www.epa.gov/
Federal Aviation Administration (FAA)
  http://www.faa.gov/
Federal Bureau of Investigation (FBI)
  http://www.fbi.gov/
Federal Emergency Management Agency (FEMA)
  http://www.fema.gov/
Food and Drug Administration (FDA)
  http://www.fda.gov/
International Medical Surgical Response Team (IMSURT)
  http://www.imsurtwest.com/
National Animal Health Emergency Management System (NAHEMS)
  http://emrs.aphis.usda.gov/nahems.html
National Disaster Medical System (NDMS)
  http://www.hhs.gov/aspr/opeo/ndms/index.html
National Institutes of Health (NIH)
  http://www.nih.gov/
National Interagency Fire Center
  http://www.nifc.gov/

National Medical Response Team (NMRT)
  http://www.nmrtcentral.com/
National Response Center
  http://www.nrc.uscg.mil/nrchp.html
National Veterinary Response Teams (NVRT or VMAT)
  http://www.vmat.org/
Naval Maritime Forecast Center/Joint Typhoon Warning Center
  http://metocph.nmci.navy.mil/
Nuclear Regulatory Commission (NRC)
  http://www.nrc.gov/
Office of Preparedness and Emergency Operations
  http://www.hhs.gov/aspr/opeo/index.html
Ready.Gov (from the U.S. Department of Homeland Security)
  http://www.ready.gov/
Substance Abuse and Mental Health Services Administration (SAMHSA)
  http://www.samhsa.gov/
U.S. Army Corps of Engineers
  http://www.usace.army.mil/
U.S. Army Veterinary Command
  http://vets.amedd.army.mil/vetcom/
U.S. Coast Guard Command Center
  http://www.uscg.mil/hq/commandcenter/
U.S. Geological Survey Earthquake Hazards Program
  http://earthquake.usgs.gov/
U.S. Geological Society Volcano Center
  http://volcanoes.usgs.gov/

IMPORTANT TOPICAL WEB SITES

Agency for Toxic Substances and Disease Registry (ATSDR)
  http://www.atsdr.cdc.gov/
American Association of Equine Practitioners
  http://www.aaep.org/
American Cat Fanciers Association
  http://www.acfacats.com/
American Humane
  http://www.americanhumane.org/site/PageServer
American Kennel Club
  http://www.akc.org/
American Quarter Horse Association
  http://www.aqha.com/
American Red Cross
  http://www.redcross.org/
American Society for the Prevention of Cruelty to Animals (ASPCA)
  http://www.aspca.org/site/PageServer
American Veterinary Identification Devices (AVID)
  http://www.avidid.com/
American Veterinary Medical Association
  http://www.avma.org
Animal and Plant Health Inspection Service (APHIS)
  http://www.aphis.usda.gov/
Animal Blood Bank
  http://www.animalbloodbank.com/
Animal Blood Bank and Restore Health Center
  http://www.hemopet.org/

Animal Poison Control Center
   http://www.aspca.org/
Animal Rescue
   http://www.code3associates.org/
Biological Agents
   http://www.bt.cdc.gov/agent/agentlist.asp
BioSense
   http://www.syndromic.org/pdf/work3-JL-BioSense.pdf
Bureau of Explosives
   http://boe.aar.com/
Chem/Bio Terrorism Links
   http://www.chem-bio.com/links/misc.html
Chemical Agents
   http://www.bt.cdc.gov/chemical/
Chemical Spills
   http://www.chemicalspill.org/EPCRA-facilities/ehs.html
CHEMical TRansportation Emergency Center (ChemTrec)
   http://www.chemtrec.org/Chemtrec/
Colorado Veterinary Medical Reserve Corps
   http://cosart.org/COVMRC.htm
Control of Communicable Diseases Manual (James Chin)
   http://www.amazon.com/Control-Communicable-Diseases-Manual-James/dp/087553242X
County Animal Response Teams
   http://cosart.org/county_animal.htm
Days End Farm Horse Rescue
   http://www.defhr.org/
Delta Society
   http://www.deltasociety.org/
Emergency Response Guidebook 2008
   http://www.labelmaster.com/ERG/
Epidemic Information Exchange (Epi-X)
   http://www.cdc.gov/epix/
Epidemic Intelligence Service (EIS)
   http://www.cdc.gov/eis/
Euthanasia Guidelines (AVMA)
   http://www.avma.org/onlnews/javma/sep07/070915b.asp
First Responder's Field Guide to Hazmat and Terrorism Response (Jill Meryl Levy, 2006 Edition)
   http://www.amazon.com/Responders-Hazmat-Terrorism-Emergency-Response/dp/0965151697
Foodborne Diseases Active Surveillance Network (FoodNet)
   http://www.cdc.gov/foodnet/
Health Alert Network (HAN)
   http://www.phppo.cdc.gov/han/
HomeAgain Microchip
   http://www.homeagainid.com/
Houston SPCA
   http://hspca.convio.net/site/PageNavigator/homepage_new
Humane Euthanasia of Sick, Injured, and/or Debilitated Livestock
   http://lacs.vetmed.ufl.edu/HumaneEuthanasia/
Humane Society of the United States (HSUS)
   http://www.hsus.org/
InfoPet Microchip
   http://www.infopet.biz/
International Pet Travel Microchip Information
   http://www.pettravel.com/passports_pet_microchip.cfm
International Wildlife Rehabilitation Council
   http://www.iwrc-online.org/

Jane's Mass Casualty Handbook: Pre-hospital
   http://catalog.janes.com/catalog/public/index.cfm?fuseaction=home.ProductInfoBrief&product_id=84857
Laboratory Response Network (LRN)
   http://www.bt.cdc.gov/lrn/
National Animal Control Association
   http://www.nacanet.org/
National Association for Search and Rescue (NASAR)
   http://www.nasar.org/nasar/
National Association of Wildlife Rehabilitators
   http://www.nwrawildlife.org/home.asp
National Disaster Medical System (NDMS)
   http://ndms.dhhs.gov/
National Hurricane Center
   http://www.nhc.noaa.gov/
National Response Plan (NRP)
   http://www.dhs.gov/nrp/
National Response Team (NRT)
   http://www.nrt.org/
National Weather Service (NOAA)
   http://www.nws.noaa.gov/
NIOSH Pocket Guide to Chemical Hazards
   http://www.cdc.gov/niosh/npg/
Pandemic Influenza
   http://www.pandemicflu.gov/
Pesticide Hotline
   http://chppm-www.apgea.army.mil/ento/hotken.htm
Radiological Agents
   http://www.bt.cdc.gov/radiation/
Rocky Mountain Poison and Drug Center
   http://www.rmpdc.org/
Safe Drinking Water Hotline
   http://www.epa.gov/ogwdw/drinklink.html
Severe Acute Respiratory Syndrome (SARS)
   http://www.cdc.gov/ncidod/sars
State Animal Response Teams (SART)
   http://nc.sartusa.org/
   http://cosart.org/
Strategic National Stockpile (SNS)
   http://www.bt.cdc.gov/stockpile/index.asp
United Animal Nations
   http://www.uan.org/
Veterinary Emergency and Critical Care Society (VECCS)
   http://www.veccs.org/
West Nile Virus (WNV)
   http://www.cdc.gov/ncidod/dvbid/westnile/index.htm

ANIMAL CONTROL EQUIPMENT AND SUPPLIES

Aazel Corporation (animal control equipment)
   http://www.aazelcorp.com
Animal Care Equipment and Services, Inc. (animal control equipment and supplies)
   http://www.animal-care.com
Ark Shelter Software (shelter software)
   http://www.arksoftware.com

Business Computing (shelter software)
 http://www.youramerica.net
Crawford Industrial Group, LLC (animal cremation and incineration systems)
 http://www.crawfordequipment.com
 http://www.animal-cremation.com
Critter Control (animal facts/wildlife trivia)
 http://www.crittercontrol.com/?doc=resources
C Specialties, Inc. (small animal products, animal control equipment)
 http://www.cspecialties.com
Deerskin Manufacturing, Inc. (animal transport units)
 http://deerskinmfg.com
Harford Systems (animal transport units)
 http://www.harfordsystems.com
HDL Software (Licensing Software)
 http://www.hdlcompanies.com
Jones Trailer Company (animal transport units)
 http://www.jonestrailers.com
Ketch-All Company—The Original Animal Control Pole
 http://www.Ketch-All.com
Matthews Cremation Division (animal cremation and incineration systems)
 http://www.matthewscremation.com
Mavron, Inc. (animal transport units)
 http://www.mavron.com
PetData (animal licensing)
 http://www.petdata.com
Petfinder.com (free online service for shelters)
 http://www.Petfinder.com
RoseRush Services, LLC (animal control and shelter software)
 http://www.ShelterPro.com/
Swab Wagon Company (animal transport bodies)
 http://www.swabwagon.com
T-Kennel (animal housing, cages)
 http://www.T-Kennel.com
Tomahawk Live Trap Company (traps, animal control equipment)
 http://www.livetrap.com
Wildlife Control Supplies (wildlife control and animal handling)
 http://www.wildlifecontrolsupplies.com/
Wolfe Pack Press, Inc. (publications)
 http://www.wolfepackpress.com
Wolverine Coach (animal transport units)
 http://www.wolverinecoach.com

INDEX